Priorities for Health Promotion and Public Health

Priorities for Health Promotion and Public Health brings together the evidence behind the UK's public health priorities into one comprehensible textbook.

Taking one theme per chapter, the book examines the social and environmental influences that shape people's health; health inequalities; poverty and health; mental, emotional and spiritual health; sexual health; physical inactivity; diet; tobacco; alcohol; drugs; weight; cardiovascular disease; cancer; diabetes and dementia. The book takes a holistic approach, combining scientific and epidemiological evidence with the subjective experiences of those who undergo these health journeys. Each chapter explains the causes of poor health and the evidence behind the recommendations for good health and ends by demonstrating the health benefits of positive action. This is a core text for those studying health promotion or public health, and a supplementary text for students of healthcare and social care. The book focusses on adults' health in the UK, with examples from the four nations, and provides some contextual international information where relevant.

Priorities for Health Promotion and Public Health is an ideal companion for busy practitioners who work across the wider sectors that support people's health and wellbeing. It is also an essential textbook for students new to health promotion and public health.

Dr Sally Robinson led the public health team at Canterbury Christ Church University from 2003 to 2018. For over 30 years, she has developed, led and taught a wide range of courses for undergraduates, postgraduates and professionals working in public health, healthcare and education.

Priorities for Health Promotion and Public Health

Explaining the Evidence for Disease Prevention and Health Promotion

Edited by Sally Robinson

Routledge
Taylor & Francis Group
LONDON AND NEW YORK

First published 2021
by Routledge
2 Park Square, Milton Park, Abingdon, Oxon OX14 4RN

and by Routledge
52 Vanderbilt Avenue, New York, NY 10017

Routledge is an imprint of the Taylor & Francis Group, an informa business

British Library Cataloguing-in-Publication Data
A catalogue record for this book is available from the British Library

Library of Congress Cataloging-in-Publication Data
Names: Robinson, Sally, editor.
Title: Priorities for health promotion and public health : explaining the evidence for disease prevention and health promotion / edited by Sally Robinson.
Description: Milton Park, Abingdon, Oxon ; New York, NY : Routledge, 2021. |
Series: Canterbury public health series |
Includes bibliographical references and index. |
Summary: "Priorities for Health Promotion and Public Health brings together the evidence behind the UK's public health priorities into one comprehensible textbook. Taking one theme per chapter, the book examines the social and environmental influences that shape people's health; health inequalities; poverty and health; mental, emotional and spiritual health; sexual health; physical inactivity; diet; tobacco; alcohol; drugs; weight; cardiovascular disease; cancer; diabetes and dementia. The book takes a holistic approach, combining scientific and epidemiological evidence with the subjective experiences of those who undergo these health journeys.
Each chapter explains the causes of poor health, the evidence behind the recommendations for good health and ends by demonstrating the health benefits of positive action. This is a core text for those studying health promotion or public health, and a supplementary text for students of healthcare and social care. The book focusses on adults' health in the UK, with examples from the four nations, and provides some contextual international information where relevant. Priorities for Health Promotion and Public Health is an ideal companion for busy practitioners who work across the wider sectors that support people's health and wellbeing. It is also a core textbook for students new to health promotion and public health"– Provided by publisher.
Identifiers: LCCN 2020044003 (print) | LCCN 2020044004 (ebook) |
ISBN 9780367820282 (hardback) | ISBN 9780367423414 (paperback) |
ISBN 9780367823689 (ebook)
Subjects: LCSH: Health promotion–United Kingdom. |
Public health–United Kingdom. | Medicine, Preventive–United Kingdom.
Classification: LCC RA427.8 .P7534 2021 (print) |
LCC RA427.8 (ebook) | DDC 362.10941–dc23
LC record available at https://lccn.loc.gov/2020044003
LC ebook record available at https://lccn.loc.gov/2020044004

ISBN: 978-0-367-82028-2 (hbk)
ISBN: 978-0-367-42341-4 (pbk)
ISBN: 978-0-367-82368-9 (ebk)

Typeset in Sabon
by Newgen Publishing UK

This book is dedicated to Peter Main, senior lecturer at Canterbury Christ Church University until 2003. This is the book his work inspired.

Contents

Figures

Tables

Boxes

Contributors

Tristi Brownett leads the BSc (Hons) Public Health and Health Promotion course at Canterbury Christ Church University. Prior to joining the university, Tristi worked as an occupational health nurse in both public and privately owned workplaces. Her teaching includes environment and health, health protection, work and health, and community development. Her scholarship has included measuring flourishing and wellbeing in a variety of workplace and community settings. Currently, she is researching how festivals promote wellbeing.

Joanne Cairns is undertaking a research fellowship, funded by Yorkshire Cancer Research at Hull York Medical School (HYMS), on inequalities and cancer screening uptake. Before moving to HYMS, Jo was a lecturer in health promotion and public health at Canterbury Christ Church University (2017–2019). Previously, Jo worked for Alcohol Research UK as a senior research and policy officer (2016–2017). She also worked as a post-doctoral research associate and teaching fellow at Durham University (2012–2016) upon successful completion of her PhD in health geography. Jo's research and teaching experience are interdisciplinary spanning across social sciences, public health and medicine.

Pat Chung is a senior lecturer in occupational therapy at Canterbury Christ Church University. She supervises MSc and PhD students' research projects. Previously, she worked as a senior occupational therapist in clinical settings including mental health for older people, hospices and geriatric rehabilitation. Her research interests include dementia, activity engagement and a person-centred approach, caregiving, falls prevention and ageing and mental health. She has been involved in dementia-related post-doctoral research funded by NIHR and the UK Occupational Therapy Research Foundation.

Elisabetta Corvo earned a degree in Jurisprudence before moving into public health and health promotion at Canterbury Christ Church University. Her PhD explored the effectiveness and transferability of an English model of health promotion, based on participation in singing groups for older adults, to Italy. She was research fellow for the Department of Public Health and Infectious Disease in Sapienza University of Rome. Her current research concerns health literacy, social capital and new social networks, and arts and health. Her teaching includes research methods and social aspects of health.

Athene Lane-Martin led training for the local public health workforce training team within the NHS before joining Canterbury Christ Church University. Athene has extensive experience working in health promotion services. She worked as a community alcohol and drugs worker for young people, and then became a mental health promotion specialist. Her qualifications span postgraduate arts and psychology. Athene's teaching includes communicating health, health psychology, health promotion and mental health promotion.

Sally Robinson led the public health team at Canterbury Christ Church University from 2003 to 2018 and is now a Visiting Reader. She has developed, led and taught a wide range of courses for undergraduates, postgraduates and professionals working in public health, healthcare and education. She is an experienced supervisor of PhDs and external examiner to other universities. Her research and scholarship have centred on public health nutrition, health promotion and children's health and wellbeing.

Rajeeb Kumar Sah was a medical doctor who worked with disadvantaged communities before moving into university education at Canterbury Christ Church University. His PhD examined social and cultural factors affecting sexual lifestyles and relationships of young people. He is particularly interested in international aspects of health, and his research concerns young people, sexual health, social inclusion, heath inequalities, migrant health and ethnography. He leads the MSc Global Public Health and his teaching includes global health, major health and lifestyles, epidemiology and public health.

Gail Sheppard worked as an exercise physiologist in NHS cardiac rehabilitation prior to entering university education at Canterbury Christ Church University. From 2018, Gail has led the public health team at Canterbury Christ Church University. Her current PhD research focuses on sedentary behaviour in the workplace. Gail has been a member of the British Association of Cardiovascular Prevention and Rehabilitation (BACPR) since 2009, acting as scientific officer from 2011 to 2015. She was co-editor of BACPR's second edition of *Cardiovascular Prevention and Rehabilitation in Practice* guidelines (2020).

Trish (Patricia) Vella-Burrows is a principal research fellow at the Sidney De Haan Research Centre for Arts and Health and a visiting lecturer in arts and health at Canterbury Christ Church University. As director of the International Network for Research and Applied Practice, she is currently researching the impact of music on people with degenerative neurological conditions. She is interested in developing models of care for people with dementia which integrate the holistic needs of family carers, care staff and those for whom they care.

Preface

Priorities for Health Promotion and Public Health brings together the evidence behind the UK's public health priorities into one textbook. Today's public health workforce comprises people from all sectors. They enter from backgrounds in education, law, business, social sciences, local government and so forth. Only some have backgrounds in biomedicine, healthcare or a scientific health-related discipline. Similarly, students enter undergraduate studies with very varied backgrounds, often with only sketchy memories of any human biology. This text seeks to step into the gap between the detailed biomedical texts written for students of biomedicine/healthcare, which take the reader through the systems of the body in minute detail, and the short descriptions of diseases and risky behaviours written for the general public. It also aims to put the scientific and epidemiological evidence into a holistic context. Students and practitioners of health promotion/public health need to understand disease prevention at a deep enough level to comprehend the reasons behind public health advice, to question it, and to be confident when communicating with others. This book is written for them.

Acknowledgement

With thanks to Noah Silver for graphic design.

Part I

Social and environmental determinants of health

1 Social context of health and illness

Sally Robinson

Key points

- Introduction
- Traditional model
- Medical model
- Social model
- Models of health and illness today
- Why understanding models of health and illness matters
- Summary

Introduction

How a society deals with preventing ill health and promoting good health will depend on what people believe about the factors that influence their health. Different approaches are called models of health, or models of health and illness. Duncan (2007) explains how these models often reflect the discipline or profession of the author. Sociologists often describe the medical model and the social model (Gillespie and Gerhard, 1995; Yuill *et al.*, 2010). Meredith Turshen (1989), who specialises in public health policy, suggests that there are five models: germ theory, genetics, lifestyles, multiple causes, and social. The sociologist Peter Aggleton (1990) presents four: traditional, positivist (biomedical and social), interactionist and structuralist. Here we present three models: traditional, medical and social.

Traditional model

The traditional model is the oldest approach to preventing illness, treating illness and promoting good health. It was the dominant model of health and illness practised across Europe before 1800 by the ancient Greeks, Romans and Christians, and today it underpins what Europeans sometimes call folk beliefs or alternative medicine such as traditional Chinese medicine, Ayurvedic medicine, homeopathy and herbalism. Central to this model are concepts of holism and balance (Aggleton, 1990). Holism means that the body and mind are one. People are whole humans within a whole universe, as if they are permeable to their environment. Health means that opposing forces, elements or qualities within themselves or between themselves and other people, or the environment, are in balance and harmony. As illness is the result of imbalance, the prevention and treatment of illness aims to restore the person back to balance. Traditional beliefs are defined as personalistic or naturalistic.

Personalistic beliefs

Personalistic beliefs refer to supernatural forces, often personified as a witch, spirit or god who casts illness in the form of a spell, a punishment, or a mystical force which enters and possesses a person. Balance, and therefore health, is maintained by constant vigilance, such as wearing amulets, fasting, lighting candles; ill health is treated by extinction of the cause. In Christianity, the New Testament cites demons, sin and acts of God as the three causes of illness (Unschuld, 1991). God may prevent or cure illness in response to prayer, repentance and pilgrimage. In 1487 English clerics published the Malleus Maleficarum, the authoritative guide to identifying and dealing with witches, the personification of evil, who were blamed for spreading destruction and disease (Ussher, 1989). Personalistic beliefs remain prevalent across the world today (Murdock, 1980). In the Gambia people believe in the buwaa, a witch who sucks the life force from their victims until they become sick and die, and the Jinne, an invisible creature that enters and possesses a person, causing illness. Marabouts are well respected religious figures who use prayer, healing, clairvoyance and other rituals (O'Neill *et al.*, 2015).

Naturalistic beliefs

Naturalistic beliefs are based on the concept that the nature around us influences our inner nature and therefore our health. Four important concepts are humours, theory of the 'airs', contagion and miasma.

Humours

Ayurvedic medicine was first recorded in India in 600 BC (Aggleton, 1990). It is based on the belief that a person comprises three humours: wind (vayu), gall (pitta) and mucus (Kapha). In the West, humoural theory began in ancient Greece. Jouanna (2012) explains how Hippocrates (460–375 BC) and others believed a person comprised four humours: black bile, yellow bile, blood and phlegm. Each humour corresponded to the properties hot, dry, wet and cold and to the four seasons:

> Blood, hot and wet, predominates in spring; yellow bile, hot and dry, in summer; black bile, cold and dry, in autumm; and phlegm, cold and wet, in winter.
>
> (Jouanna, 2012 p.335)

Galen, a Roman physician writing in the second century AD, focused on the importance of mixing and balancing four qualities: hot, cold, wet and dry. One was the opposite of the other. If these were in balance, the person was healthy; if separated or out of balance, the person was ill. Galen attributed moral and physical characteristics to the qualities. For example, the combination of cold and dry was associated with a white, hairless body, cold to the touch and a cowardly, retiring character. This was not humoural theory, but Jouanna (2012) says Galen read the work of Hippocrates and others, and in correspondence suggested a relationship between the four humours yellow bile, black bile, blood and phlegm and the four elements fire, water, air and earth; and also a relationship between the four humours and people's character. After Galen, the theory of the four temperaments, phlegmatic, sanguine, bilious and melancholic, was incorporated between the fourth and sixth centuries AD.

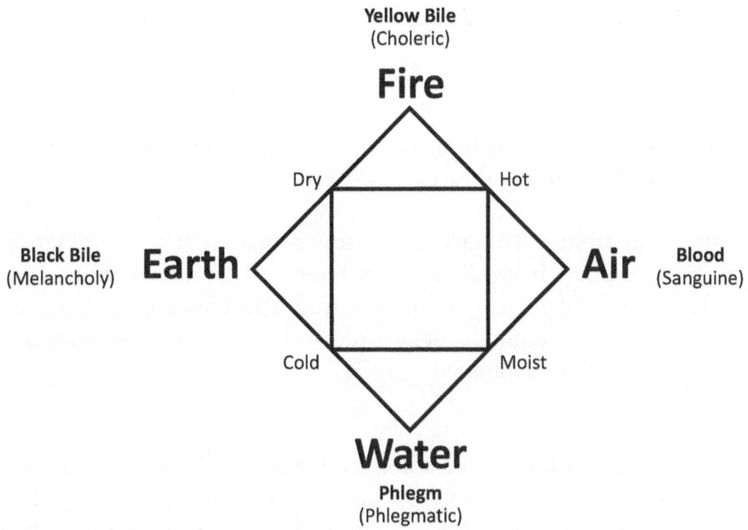

Figure 1.1 Integrated theory of humours, qualities, elements and temperaments

Two broad approaches emerged for returning the humours back into balance (Dubos, 1984; Moon, 1995). The first was named after the Greek goddess of health, Hygeia, who emphasised cleanliness, harmony, care, a sensible lifestyle, attention to the conditions in which people lived and illness prevention. The second was named after Asclepius, the heroic Greek god of healing, who advocated direct bodily intervention using surgery and herbal remedies to bring about cure. Common tools used by a practitioner of the naturalistic tradition include bloodletting using cutting or leeches; applying a heated glass vessel to the skin (cupping); purging using laxatives, emetics or diuretics; and the provision of herbs and other forms of nourishment such as meditation, exercise or yoga (Weintraub *et al.*, 2008; Ling *et al.*, 2012).

Theory of the 'airs'

The integrated theory incorporates the idea that people are part of the wider cosmos, the sun, moon, seasons and climate. Astrology can play a significant part. Herzlich and Pierret (1991) describe these ideas as the theory of the 'airs'. Traditional Chinese medicine describes a constant exchange of energy between each person and the universe (Aggleton, 1990). Helman (1984) reported Londoners' descriptions of the cold, wet weather entering the skin, perhaps through having wet hair, and causing the runny nose and watery eyes of a cold. The antidote to the cold, wet symptoms was to keep warm and dry.

Contagion

The plagues of the fourteenth, fifteenth and sixteenth century encouraged the belief that disease could be contagious, passed from one person to another through touch, through the sharing of objects or from a distance (Herzlich and Pierret, 1991). Beliefs about contagion led to quarantine, the practice of isolating sick people from the healthy by locking them in their homes or in isolation hospitals (Champion, 1995; Porter, 1995). They also led to the promotion of cleanliness and hygiene.

Miasma

Miasma, the stench of putrid, foul-smelling air, was thought to be absorbed through the skin and cause illness. Herzlich and Pierret (1991) write:

> The corrupt air ... attributed to various causes: a 'malignant' combination of heat and humidity, miasmas from the ground, the marshes in the country, putrid effluvia from the corpses of men and animals, and also emanations from living bodies and soiled clothing, stagnant air in excessively narrow town streets – all these ideas converged and intermingled.
>
> (p.77)

In the 1700s, the industrial revolution prompted overcrowded living around the new factories across England. With greater squalor and coal-burning came air pollution and high death rates from infectious diseases. In 1837, the registration of births, marriages and deaths began. The 1842 annual report recorded, per million people living in England, 616 died of smallpox, 704 died of scarlet fever, 902 of whooping cough, 668 of typhus, 2004 of pneumonia and 3922 of consumption (respiratory tuberculosis) (General Register Office, 1842). The prime suspect was miasma in the air. Figure 1.2 shows a meteorology report submitted as part of the 1849 annual report.

Cholera epidemics began in 1832 and killed thousands through sickness, diarrhoea and dehydration (Underwood, 1947). Edwin Chadwick, a lawyer and social activist, led an inquiry into sanitation and wrote *The Sanitary Conditions of the Labouring Population* in 1842. It linked people's poor living conditions to their poor life expectancy and led to the Public Health Act 1848. The Act set out to provide sewers and improve drainage, provide clean drinking water and remove refuse from streets. It introduced the inspectors of nuisances and sanitary inspectors, the forerunners of today's environmental health officers. Their numbers were increased after the Sanitary Act of 1866 (Stewart *et al.*, 2005). Chadwick's argument was economic, improving the public's health would reduce money needed for the poor, but underpinning the action was the imperative to reduce the miasma that was causing disease.

Florence Nightingale (1820–1910) was the founder of modern, professional nursing, but also a highly influential scholar, theorist, social reformer, statistician and pioneer of public health (McDonald, 2004). Her belief in miasma underpinned her vigorous promotion of cleanliness and fresh air to prevent the spread of infection in home and hospital. Above all, she believed in the Spirit of God on whom, she wrote, health and recovery depended. Her work drew upon naturalistic and personalistic beliefs, and reflected the feminine Hygeian tradition of cleanliness, environment, prevention and care, at a time when male doctors were advancing the Asclepian tradition, using medical science to understand and treat the human body.

> *In the traditional model, we protect and promote health by being in harmony with our physical and metaphysical environment.*

Meteorology. 349

On the Meteorology of the Years 1841 to 1847, compiled from the published Greenwich Magnetical and Meteorological Volumes, and from the Weekly Tables furnished by the Astronomer Royal to the Registrar-General, by James Glaisher, Esq., of the Royal Observatory at Greenwich.

YEARLY METEOROLOGICAL TABLE.

YEAR.	Mean Reading of the Barometer from 12 Observations taken daily reduced to 32° Fahrenheit.	THERMOMETER. Highest Reading during the Year.	THERMOMETER. Lowest Reading during the Year.	THERMOMETER. Mean. Of the Highest Readings from one Observation daily.	THERMOMETER. Mean. Of the Lowest Readings from one Observation daily.	THERMOMETER. Mean. Differnce in Degrees.	THERMOMETER. Mean Reading from 12 Observations daily.	THERMOMETER. Dew Point. Mean of 12 Results daily.	THERMOMETER. Self-Registering. Highest in the Sun. During the Year.	THERMOMETER. Self-Registering. Highest in the Sun. Mean.	THERMOMETER. Self-Registering. Lowest on the Grass. During the Year.	THERMOMETER. Self-Registering. Lowest on the Grass. Mean.	In the Water of the Thames at Greenwich, by Self-Registering Thermometers read once a-day. Mean. Of the Highest.	In the Water of the Thames at Greenwich, by Self-Registering Thermometers read once a-day. Mean. Of the Lowest.	Difference between the Dew Point Temperature and Air Temperature. Mean.	Difference between the Dew Point Temperature and Air Temperature. Mean of the greatest in each Month.	Difference between the Dew Point Temperature and Air Temperature. Mean of the least in each Month.	Difference between the Mean Temperature and the Average Temperature of 25 Years.	WIND. General Direction.	WIND. Pressure in lbs. on the Square Foot. Greatest Pressure during the Year.	WIND. Pressure in lbs. on the Square Foot. Mean Pressure.	The Mean Amount of Horizontal Movement of the Air in each Week.	Mean Amount of Cloud 0—10.	Rain in Inches.
	Inches.	°	°	°	°	°	°	°	°	°	°	°	°	°	°	°	°	°		lbs.	lbs.	Miles		Inches.
1841	29·687	82·8	4·0	58·5	43·7	14·8	48·7	43·7	107·0	74·1	12·0	37·2	- -	- -	5·0	- -	- -	—0·6	S. W.	24·0	- -	- -	6·7	33·3
1842	29·832	90·5	23·2	57·9	43·0	14·9	49·6	45·0	121·2	72·2	12·5	35·4	- -	- -	4·6	- -	- -	+0·3	W. S. W.	21·0	- -	- -	6·3	22·6
1843	29·765	89·8	20·3	57·7	43·5	14·2	49·4	45·7	110·8	70·9	7·0	35·0	- -	- -	3·7	- -	- -	+0·1	W. S. W.	25·0	- -	- -	6·9	24·5
1844	29·776	87·6	18·8	57·3	42·4	14·9	48·6	43·7	115·0	70·7	7·9	34·6	- -	- -	4·9	- -	- -	—0·7	W. S. W.	17·0	- -	800	6·7	25·0
1845	29·742	86·0	7·7	56·2	41·5	14·7	47·6	43·2	111·6	67·4	-6·0	34·5	- -	- -	4·4	- -	- -	—1·7	W. S. W.	13·0	- -	900	6·7	22·3
1846	29·733	93·3	18·8	61·1	44·8	16·3	51·3	46·2	116·5	75·4	9·0	38·1	55·2	53·4	5·1	10·9	1·0	+2·0	S. W.	12·0	0·3	860	7·0	25·3
1847	29·811	86·0	12·0	56·7	42·7	14·0	49·5	43·8	114·8	73·0	9·0	35·1	52·2	50·6	6·0	12·0	1·5	+0·2	S. W.	16·5	0·3	870	7·0	17·6

Figure 1.2 Meteorology in England, 1841 to 1847

Source: Registrar-General, 1849 p.349 Wellcome Collection made available under a CC BY 4.0 licence https://creativecommons.org/licenses/by/4.0/

Medical model

The medical model of health and illness is one where an individual becomes ill either because of a physiological malfunction or because a harmful external agent has entered the body (Aggleton, 1990). It is based on science and is strongly associated with medicine.

The rise of medical science

The origins of the scientific approach to health and illness are debated, but Mosley (2010) identifies the Italian Renaissance as a pivotal moment when people began to trust their own eyes and believe what they could see, rather than trusting what they had been told they could see. For example, physicians believed for centuries that the human liver had three lobes because Galen had said so, despite being able to see and count four, such was the power of belief. Mosley identifies Leonardo da Vinci (1452–1519) as a pioneer of the new thinking and cites the artist's observational, detailed drawings of the human body as his evidence. Later, Vesalius (1514–1564) published his work on anatomy in 1543. René Descartes (1590–1650) challenged the concept of holism by arguing that the physical body could be considered as separate to the mind, dualism. This facilitated the Church to focus on the mind, and physicians to focus on the body using scientific method (Moon, 1995).

Scientific method comprises careful, objective, observation; gathering and documenting empirical (real) measurable evidence; and testing a hypothesis through controlled experiments. The method reveals whether a cause produces an observed effect. This approach can lead to the discovery of eternal and immutable universal laws of science. The scientific study of the body, biomedicine, seeks to find universal causes of disease and treatments. Reductionism means breaking the body down into parts, systems and organs and studying them in increasing detail. William Harvey was an early practitioner of the scientific, reductionist, experimental study of the body which led to his discovery of blood circulation in 1628 (Lubnitz, 2004).

We can illustrate the transfer of society's allegiance away from the traditional model and towards the scientific medical model through accounts of smallpox and cholera. Germ theory established the model as the most influential of the twentieth century.

Smallpox

Smallpox, a deadly infectious disease, was prevalent in the 1700s. Many knew that catching cowpox from cows protected people from smallpox. Pead (2003) writes that the Turkish idea of introducing live smallpox into the skin through an incision (inoculation) was introduced to England in 1722 by Lady Mary Montague, but it had a high risk of infection or death. In 1774 Benjamin Jesty, a farmer, was the first to insert pus from an infected cow's udder into the arms of his wife and sons. The local community was horrified, but the family were protected from later smallpox epidemics.

Twenty-two years later, in 1796, the physician Edward Jenner carried out the same procedure as Jesty. He documented and disseminated his use of scientific method, observation, investigation and deduction, and published his findings in 1798. The UK

Vaccination Act 1853 made vaccination with cowpox compulsory. In an era when the theory of the airs, contagion and miasma dominated public understandings of health and illness, people resisted the law, they wanted freedom of choice and the medical profession took much convincing (Reidel, 2005). History recorded Jenner as a celebrated scientist and the first vaccinator. Jenner prevailed where Jesty the farmer did not, because he had influential friends and scientific and professional credentials (Pead, 2003).

Cholera

In 1854, six years after the Public Health Act aimed to tackle the causes of miasma, the physician John Snow plotted cases of cholera onto a map of Soho in London. On removing the handle from the water pump in Broad Street, the cases of cholera in the vicinity reduced. Halliday (2001) describes how Snow presented the evidence that unclean water was the cause of cholera to a Parliamentary committee, but the committee continued to believe that the poisonous air was the problem, not the water. It would be after Snow's death that the British Government realised Snow had been right.

John Snow is widely credited as the founder of epidemiology, the application of scientific method to analysing the spread and pattern of disease among populations. Snow believed that cholera was spread by 'morbid matter' passing from the excrement of a sufferer into food or water, and then being ingested by another. He believed that the 'germ of the disease' multiplied internally (Singer, 2009). As medical science continued its reductionist path, it was sub-dividing itself beyond merely physicians and surgeons into further specialities: epidemiology, microbiology and then bacteriology. It was the bacteriologist Robert Koch who provided the detailed, observable evidence of the cholera bacillus in 1883 (Blevins and Bronze, 2010).

Germ theory

Berche (2012) explains how Louis Pasteur, a research scientist in France, discovered that microorganisms were the cause of decay, rotting and fermentation of living things. In 1861, he proposed that this theory of germs could explain all infectious diseases. He named his treatment vaccination after 'vacca', the Latin for cow, in tribute to Jenner. Building on Pasteur's work, Joseph Lister developed antiseptics which could treat wounds and prevent gangrene, which led to the introduction of sterile conditions for surgery. At the same time, according to Blevins and Bronze (2010), Robert Koch, a doctor in Germany, identified which specific microorganisms, bacteria, caused specific diseases and founded the discipline of bacteriology. He identified tubercle bacillus as the cause of tuberculosis, and its predominance in sputum. This led to the sterilisation of clothes and bed linen, and to the restriction of spitting in public places. His work also confirmed that access to clean water was necessary to prevent cholera. Pasteur's work focused on protecting individuals through immunisation, while Koch's work aimed to protect communities though better hygiene and public health.

In 1848, medical officers for health were introduced in England (Hardy, 2001). Their epidemiological work became the branch of medicine called public health medicine. By 1900, the records showed a dramatic fall in infectious diseases such

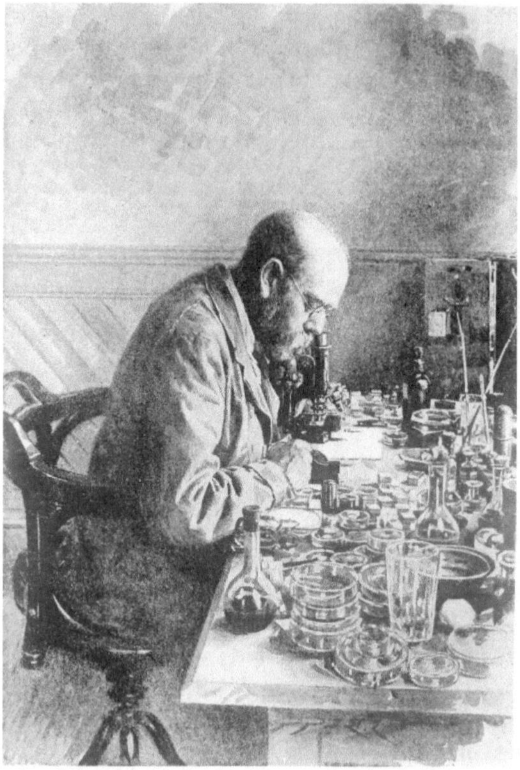

Figure 1.3 Robert Koch (1843–1910) working in South Africa
Source: Wellcome collection made available under a CC BY 4.0 licence http://creativecommons.org/licenses/by/4.0

as smallpox, respiratory tuberculosis and scarlet fever in England and Wales, and it was widely believed to be due to the advancement of medical science (McKeown, 1976). During the twentieth century money and support went into the development of vaccines and antibiotics. Doctors became associated with miraculous cures and respect for the profession soared. Infectious diseases continued to fall, and by the middle of the century international vaccination programmes were developed for the eradication of infectious diseases (Hajj *et al.*, 2015).

Wider scientific developments

The rise of science had not only helped to develop medical science, but understandings of biomechanics and physiology had informed the rise of exercise science and sports medicine (Berryman and Park, 1992). The 'Chemical revolution' in France in 1785 advanced chemistry, and informed nutritional science and the profession of nutritionists (Carpenter, 2003). Psychology, which emerged from philosophy, adopted the scientific method in 1879 and developed into a number of branches, including health psychology (Hothersall, 2003). These disciplines and professions could also trace their roots from the traditional model of the Greeks and Romans. All used experimental science and some also used epidemiology to inform their work.

Medical influence on healthcare

Separate, was the medically dominated field of healthcare. During the twentieth century the process of reductionism led to specialisations such as gastroenterology, cardiology, psychiatry and obstetrics. Surgeons with dental skills successfully lobbied to become the profession of dentistry in 1921 (Nettleton, 1988). Others became the professions 'allied to medicine' such as physiotherapists, occupational therapists, radiographers and dietitians. A range of healthcare specialist scientists to support the medical professionals emerged, such as haematologists, pathologists, histopathologists, and electron microscopy, nuclear medicine and radiotherapy physics. Medicine influenced the course of nursing, bringing it closer to medicine than Florence Nightingale would have wanted (McDonald, 2004). Each profession practised the medical model focusing on fixing the body, organs, systems or cells through diagnosis, treatment, cure, care and rehabilitation back to the normative view of health as the absence of disease. In this climate, the UK National Health Service began in 1948.

Disease prevention

Disease prevention can be traced back the goddess Hygeia. In England, the Public Health Acts 1848 and 1875, and the introduction of the Central Council for Health Education in 1927, were important landmarks, but in the context of science, Bown (2003) takes us to 1747 when James Lind, a surgeon, began dietary experiments on HMS Salisbury. Lind's work led the English Admiralty to issue a daily ration of lemon juice to all Royal Navy sailors to prevent scurvy (Figure 1.4). Scurvy caused blackened gums, loose teeth, ulcers in the mouth and legs, general malaise and sometimes death. Between 1795 and 1815, the Royal Navy bought 1.6 gallons of lemon juice, a factor that helped the healthy sailors stop Napoleon from invading England.

During the early twentieth century the non-infectious, non-communicable, diseases such as cardiovascular disease and cancer became the main causes of early death. From 1910 to 1950 nutritional scientists had identified most of the major vitamins and minerals, and understood how deficiencies led to disease (Mozaffarian *et al.*, 2018). Vitamin C was named as the preventative for scurvy. Elsie Widdowson and Robert McCance published the first edition of the Composition of Foods in 1940, based on a body of work into the chemistry of food. During the 1950s, the physiologist Ancel Keys demonstrated that saturated fat was significantly associated with high blood cholesterol and coronary heart disease (Keys *et al.*, 1956; Pett *et al.*, 2017). Epidemiologists confirmed that smoking caused lung cancer (Doll and Hill, 1954) and that a physically active job was protective against coronary heart disease (Morris and Crawford, 1958). These breakthroughs helped to develop measurements of the probability of a population acquiring disease, relative to the amount of risky behaviour they undertook. Avoiding the risks of smoking, saturated fat and inactivity became a key strategy for disease prevention (Nettleton, 2013). Exercise physiologists, nutritionists, psychologists, dentists, doctors, dietitians and other professions, all adopted an approach to disease prevention based on a model of health and illness underpinned by science.

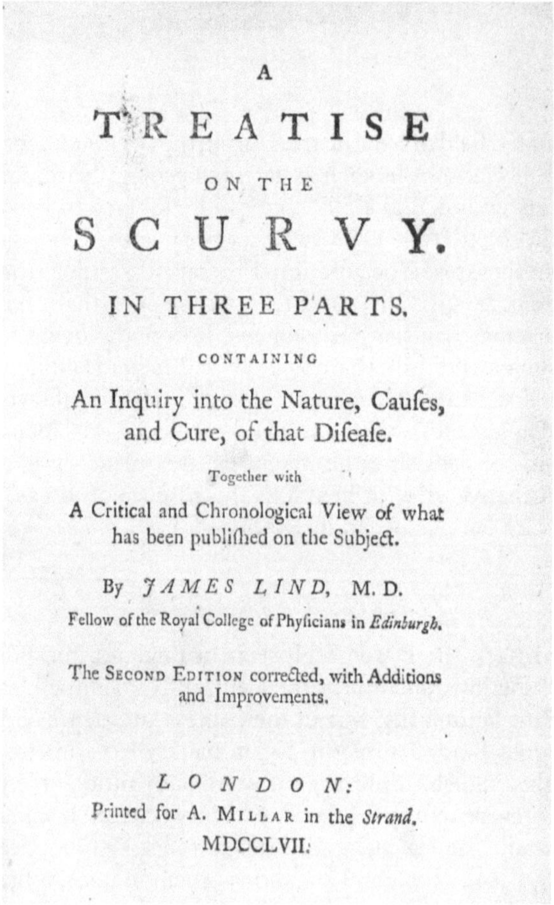
A

TREATISE

ON THE

SCURVY.

IN THREE PARTS,

CONTAINING

An Inquiry into the Nature, Cauſes, and Cure, of that Diſeaſe.

Together with

A Critical and Chronological View of what has been publiſhed on the Subject.

By *JAMES LIND*, M. D.

Fellow of the Royal College of Phyſicians in *Edinburgh.*

The SECOND EDITION corrected, with Additions and Improvements.

LONDON:

Printed for A. MILLAR in the *Strand.*

MDCCLVII.

Figure 1.4 A treatise on the scurvy by James Lind, 1757

The medical model

The medical model sees a person as the sum of their body parts, right down to their cells, and this concept led to the creation of hospitals, laboratories and specialisms to fix, treat, cure and repair the body machine using technology, drugs, nutrients and surgery. Jewson (1976) describes how medicine defines disease by its internal, hidden causes, which requires expert, objective diagnosis based on physical examination and chemical tests of body substances. It is disease-centred. Jewson describes how the patient, an object of the clinical gaze, waits for the consensus of opinion imposed and controlled by the scientific, most often medical, community. This consensus creates normative universal standards, such as defining a body temperature of 36.4°C to 37.6°C as healthy, and a degree either side as unhealthy. Normally, the individual is not held responsible for becoming ill. Experts aim to restore the machine to good working order.

Epidemiologists study populations and analyse patterns of disease and their causes. A lack of vitamins and minerals, too much saturated fat, physical inactivity and smoking are key causes of bodily malfunction and disease. They are risk factors for disease and they need to be avoided or removed. The population, now an object of surveillance, waits for the consensus of opinion imposed and controlled by the scientific, most often medical, community. This consensus creates normative universal standards for healthy living such as no smoking, daily nutritional recommendations for calories and nutrients, and guidelines about how much and at what level we need to exercise. The model treats lifestyle like any other medical condition, there is a cause and an effect. The population is often held responsible for their health-related behaviour. Experts persuade people to change their behaviour, to comply, to avoid the 'dangerous' risks that could damage the mechanics of their bodies.

During the late twentieth and into twenty-first century, the medical model, and its reductionist approach, led to the discovery of the human genome and genetic engineering. Current evidence continues to demonstrate that our diet, smoking, alcohol, physical inactivity and obesity are important risk factors for disease and early death (ONS, 2017). The creation and dissemination of evidence-based standards for treatment and disease prevention receives both private and public funding and is led by bodies such as the World Health Organization, National Institute for Health and Care Excellence (NICE) and Cochrane Library.

Challenges to the medical model

The limitations of the medical model are predominantly that those who work with it ignore the wider social, psychological, cultural, political and economic factors that influence health. In seeking 'one size fits all' universality, it ignores individual differences and wider perceptions. It is based on a belief that someone is healthy if an expert can find no disease, and keeping healthy means minimising risk factors.

The medical model, as practised by doctors, has been much criticised and this is due to the extraordinary power that the medical establishment wields. The social revolution of the 1960s swept away unquestioning deference to those in authority, and by the 1970s there were challenges to medicine. Foucault (1973) argued that the medical establishment replaced the Church in claiming power over health and illness, and its self-belief disallowed any criticism from outsiders. Medicine's pretence of having a neutral, objective stance was a mirage. This was leading to poor, sometimes deadly, medical practice based on supporting colleagues and precedents rather than scientific evidence (Cochrane, 1972; Tew, 1998). The anti-psychiatry movement argued against medical control of mental health and illness (Crossley, 1998) and Oakley (1993) argued against the medical control of childbirth. Thomas McKeown (1976) presented epidemiological evidence and argued that the dramatic reduction in many infectious diseases in the nineteenth century owed more to environmental public health measures, nutrition and improved standards of living introduced in Victorian times than to medical science such as vaccinations.

McKeown's graph, shown in Figure 1.5, shows how respiratory tuberculosis was falling before the bacillus was first identified by Robert Koch, and decades before the administration of medicine to treat the disease or vaccination to prevent it.

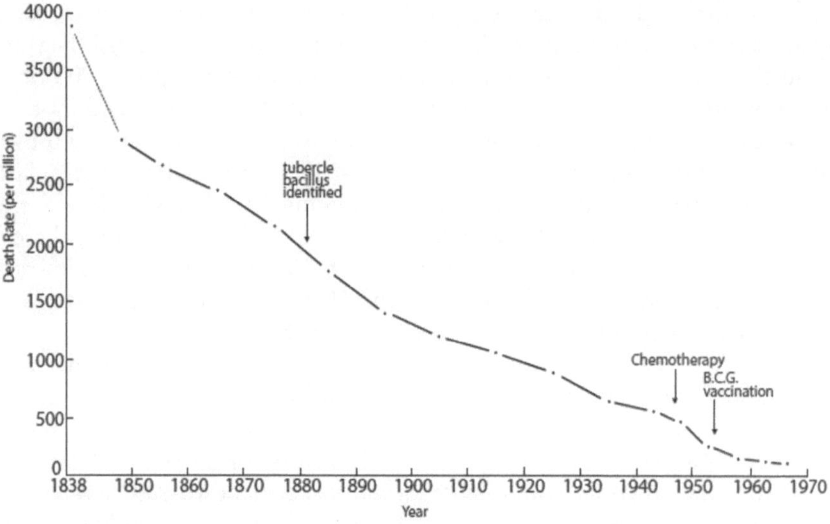

Figure 1.5 McKeown's analysis of death rates from respiratory tuberculosis in England and Wales 1838 to 1967

Source: McKeown, 1976 p.81. Reproduced with permission from the Nuffield Trust

McKeown wrote:

> The appraisal of influences on health in the past suggests that we owe the improvement, not to what happens when we are ill, but to the fact that we do not so often become ill; and we remain well, not because of specific measures such as vaccination and immunization, but because we enjoy a higher standard of nutrition and live in a healthier environment ... However it by no means follows that these influences have the same relative importance today as in the past.
>
> (McKeown, 1976 p.94. Reproduced with permission of Nuffield Trust.)

Table 6.1 from McKeown's report shows that medicine had little effect between 1848 and 1971, but more during 1948 to 1971 (Figure 1.6). He argued that in the context of improved standards of living, such as a healthy environment and good nutrition, medicine helped to speed up the decrease in disease.

Ivan Illich (1976), a theologian, philosopher and critic of medicine, used the term iatrogenesis to describe how the medical system was harmful to human health because of the negative side-effects of clinical treatments, such as medicines and surgery. He argued that it reinforced dependence on doctors, creating a sick society of consumers who wanted technical solutions for managing every aspect of their health and well-being, indeed much of their life including their death.

Thinking point:

> Consider the handling of COVID-19 coronavirus when it spread to the UK in early 2020. With reference to the views of Hygeia, Asclepius and Illich, think

TABLE 6.1. *Estimated number of deaths from respiratory tuberculosis prevented by use of chemotherapy: England and Wales.*

	1948-1971	1848-1971
Estimated by extrapolation*	273,727	4,337,265
Actual	133,891	4,237,429
Deaths prevented	139,836	139,836
Proportion of deaths prevented	51%	3.2%

*Of 1921-46 rates

Figure 1.6 McKeown's analysis of the effectiveness of medical intervention in the reduction of respiratory tuberculosis 1948 to 1971

Source: McKeown, 1976 p.83. Reproduced with permission from the Nuffield Trust.

about the slogan 'Protect the NHS. Save Lives', the building of COVID hospitals and the acquisition of ventilators alongside rising death rates in care homes which amounted to a sixth of all COVID-related deaths by April 2020.

Today, the power of medicine in the Western world is evident in our common language. A question about a person's health often elicits a reply about illness and disease, and quickly turns to healthcare services whose main focus is treatment, cure, rehabilitation and sometimes disease prevention. Professions are described as 'alternative' or 'complementary' or 'allied' to medicine. Despite acknowledgement that most doctors know very little about nutrition, physical activity or understanding the psychosocial dimensions of health behaviour (Adams *et al.*, 2010; Adamski *et al.*, 2018), they nevertheless encroach into these fields (Mosely, 2014; Chatterjee, 2017). The addition of the word 'medical', 'prescription' or the endorsement of a doctor opens doors to which other professions can only dream. This is partly because of the relationship between medicine and the media. Karpf (1988) explains the phenomenon:

> Television and radio stations, as cultural institutions, naturally breathe in and exhale the prevailing ideas about medical authority and expertise ... the media not only share dominant beliefs about medicine, they also help to strengthen them ... as evidenced by the number of times that doctors are brought into TV programmes to comment on an area of life which most of us would never in practice consult them about, even on ('lifestyle') issues they feel they can do nothing about ... Medicine has provided the vocabulary and framework through which to think about problems, and subjects are increasingly recast in pathological or therapeutic terms ... By using phrases such as 'research shows', 'doctors agree', and 'scientists say' – valuable shorthand when time is short – broadcasters also imply that research is incontestable, and the medical profession unanimous ... broadcasting has an unlimited need for the authoritative commentator ... Medicine's privileged social status makes it perfectly suited to the task.
>
> (p.131–133)

Table 1.1 Models of health and illness

	Traditional	*Medical*	*Social*
Concept of a human being	Holistic, mind and body are one, whole person is integrated with whole universe.	Body as machine, mind and body are separate, the body is the sum of its parts.	Holistic, mind and body are one and influenced by the social context in which we live.
Health is	Balance within person and between the person and the wider physical and metaphysical environment.	Absence of disease or illness.	Absence of disease and physical, mental and social wellbeing.
Causes of poor health and illness	Internal imbalance, imbalance with the environment/universe or a supernatural force.	Malfunction of the body caused by a gene, a microorganism, a blockage or break. These are sometimes caused by risky health-related behaviours.	Social, economic and physical environment and its influence on people's psychology, health-related behaviours and biology. These are shaped by culture and inequalities in power.
Process of defining health or ill health	Subjective. Listen to people's descriptions of their symptoms and feelings, observe their appearance and temperament, consider natural environment, astrology, religious guidance	Objective. Reductionist, observation of signs and symptoms, process of diagnosis by physical examination and chemical tests of body substances, measurement against normative medical standards.	Objective and subjective. Observation of the relationship between population health and social, economic and environmental factors. Listening to people's perceptions and experiences of health and illness.
Aims of prevention and health promotion	Maintain harmony with nature and supernatural forces.	Protect body machine from causes of infection and malfunctions.	A healthy social, economic and physical environment for all.
Aims of treatment	Restore balance. Person-centred.	Fix the machine, restore homeostasis. Disease-centred.	Equal health chances for all people regardless of where they live. Culturally sensitive.
Source of expert knowledge	Religious leaders, naturopaths, complementary/alternative medical practitioners.	Medical scientists and practitioners.	All people, cross-disciplinary and multi-professional.

In the medical model, we protect and promote health by avoiding germs and having healthy behaviours that will keep our body in good working order.

Social model

The social model suggests that the underlying causes of ill health and the determinants of good health are not biological, but social. The World Health Organization (2008) sums this up by asking:

> Why treat people ... then send them back to the conditions that made them sick?

People create cultures and environments which affect our bodies, beliefs and behaviours and these determine our health, and our perceptions of our health.

A new era for health

In the 1970s, a new language emerged to 'reclaim' the word health from the medical model. The governments of Canada (Lalonde, 1974) and the UK (DHSS, 1976) agreed that health was a matter beyond healthcare. They acknowledged McKeown's work on the importance of the physical and social environment whilst continuing to blame individuals for their, "... grisly litany of destructive lifestyle habits and their consequences" (Lalonde, 1974 p.16). At the start of the 1980s, 'blaming the individual' was challenged by the World Health Organization's Global Strategy for Health For All by the Year 2000 (WHO, 1981). It declared that "health problems and socioeconomic problems are interlinked" (p.19), health was a "fundamental human right and a worldwide social goal" (p.34) and it was not merely the absence of illness. Health For All was a vision, a movement and a strategy for all governments of the world to achieve health for everyone across the world. In this way, attention was drawn to a better understanding of the social, economic and physical environment; and to psychosocial, cultural and structural influences on our health.

Box 1.1 Global Strategy for Health for All by the year 2000

> "... in 1977 in resolution WHA30.43 that by the year 2000, *all* people in *all* countries should have a level of health that will permit them to lead a socially and economically productive life. This implies that the level of health of all people should be at least such that they are capable of working productively and of participating actively in the social life of the community in which they live. Health for all does not mean that in the year 2000 doctors and nurses will provide medical care for everybody in the world for all their existing ailments; nor does it mean that in the year 2000 nobody will be sick or disabled. It does mean that health begins at home, in school and in factories. It is there, where people live

and work, that health is made or broken. It does mean that people will use better approaches than they do now for preventing disease and alleviating unavoidable disease and disability, and have better ways of growing up, growing old and dying gracefully. It does mean that there will be an even distribution among the population of whatever resources for health are available. It does mean that essential health care will be accessible to *all* individuals and families in an acceptable and affordable way, and with their full involvement. And it does mean that people will realize that they themselves have the power to shape their lives and the lives of their families, free from the avoidable burden of disease, and aware that ill-health is not inevitable."

(Source: WHO, 1981 p.31, 32. Reproduced with permission from the World Health Organization)

Social, economic and physical environment

In 1980, the Black Report demonstrated that British people, across all ages, experienced health differently. Men working in professional and managerial occupations, and women married to these men, experienced better health and longer lives than those in semi-skilled or unskilled jobs (Black *et al.*, 1982). This inequality was due to social, economic and environmental factors. Better-off people were not only richer, but they tended to live in healthier environments. A healthy environment included clean water and good sanitation, but also minimal traffic, no pollution, green spaces, and a good education, diet, housing and working conditions. It prompted the question of whether it was fair that someone born into relatively deprived circumstances should be condemned to a shorter life and more ill health than someone born into relatively better circumstances.

Psychosocial factors

Michael Marmot, a social epidemiologist, studied how the social determinants of health affect our psychology and then our biology. The Whitehall Studies were a collection of research studies into the health, illness and death of members of the British Civil Service who worked for the government within the Whitehall area of London. The studies showed how a social gradient existed within one geographical area. Men in the lowest grades of employment died younger from coronary heart disease than the men in higher grades (Marmot *et al.*, 1984). The lower the grade of employment, the less control the civil servants had over their work. Jobs with high demand and low control were associated with greater coronary heart disease (Bosma *et al.*, 1997). Wilkinson and Marmot (2003) brought together a body of research to show how low control, continuous anxiety, low self-esteem, relative poverty, social isolation and social exclusion due to stigmatisation or discrimination all cause long-term stress which increases the probability of having high blood pressure, heart attacks, stroke, depression, aggression, infections and diabetes.

Structural factors

The World Health Organization revitalised its commitment to 'Health for All', social justice and equity by setting up the Commission on Social Determinants of Health in 2004 (WHO, 2010). Today, it is widely recognised that health and illness do not strike individuals randomly, but some groups of people experience better health and longer life due to the way society is organised (Lieberman *et al.*, 2013; Yang *et al.*, 2018). We might define the powerful and weak as: capitalist employers versus workers, men versus women, industry (e.g. food, tobacco, alcohol) versus consumers, white versus black, or doctors versus patients. The powerful dismiss, label and control the weak, and their knowledge, to keep their power (Aggleton, 1990). Lack of power reduces access to education, healthcare, income, employment, influence and other factors which support good health.

Nettleton (2013) explains how industry and the media encourage people to be consumers of health, fitness and certain types of food to achieve their brand of lifestyle, beauty, body and wellbeing. The culture of health aspirations meets the culture of risks to our health, such as messages about disease prevention, safety and harm minimisation. People's perceptions and attitudes towards health and illness reflect how they negotiate their day-to-day experience of their relationships, social norms and material circumstances. For example,

> ... I've smoked and as soon as I found out I was pregnant I stopped, and now I wouldn't dream of it. But I suppose if you live where everybody is smoking around you, it's just what you do, isn't it?
>
> (Adult living in North East England quoted in Garthwaite and Bambra, 2017 p.271)

In 2010, Marmot concluded that inequalities in health could not simply be attributed to genetics, biology or 'bad behaviour', they were caused by structural differences in society and putting them right had to include action by those who had the power to do so, it was about justice for all.

Social determinants of health

The social determinants of health are

> ... the conditions in which people are born, grow, live, work and age. These circumstances are shaped by the distribution of money, power and resources at global, national and local levels. The social determinants of health are mostly responsible for heath inequities – the unfair and avoidable differences in health status within and between countries.
>
> (Reprinted from World Health Organization, 2019)

The social determinants of health can have a dual meaning in that the phrase is used to describe the determinants of health and also the determinants of inequalities in health (WHO, 2010).

Figure 1.7 shows Dahlgren and Whitehead's (1991) conception of factors that threaten health, promote health and protect health. The outer layer, the structural

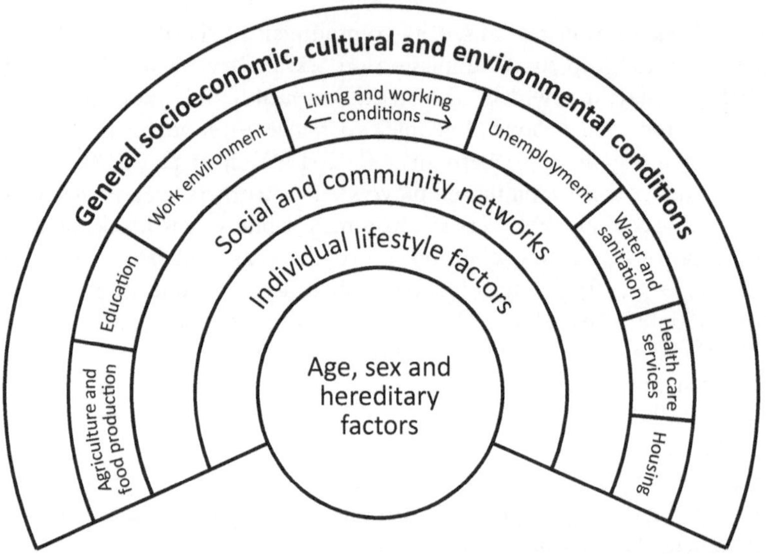

Figure 1.7 The main determinants of health

Source: Dahlgren and Whitehead, 1991 p.11. Reproduced with permission from the Institute for Futures Studies.

environment, influences material and social conditions such as housing, education and agriculture. These influence social support from family, friends and the local community. These layers influence individual lifestyles. At the centre are the biological factors over which we have little control. Dahlgren and Whitehead used the framework to show how policies designed to improve health needed to act across the levels.

Social-ecological models

Social ecology considers human beings and their habitat as an ecosystem of interdependent elements. An ecosystem is an area where living things, such as animals and plants, exist alongside the environment of water, earth, sun, soil and so forth. Each element of the eco-system has a role to play in keeping the whole area healthy. Barton and Grant (2006) put people at the centre of their health map, which focuses on health and sustainable development. They write:

> The [human] settlement is set within its bioregion and the global ecosystem on which it ultimately depends. Broader cultural, economic and political forces which impact on well-being are represented. Thus all the elements of ... health are included, spread out to reflect the ecosystem of the local human habitat.
>
> (Barton and Grant, 2006 p.253)

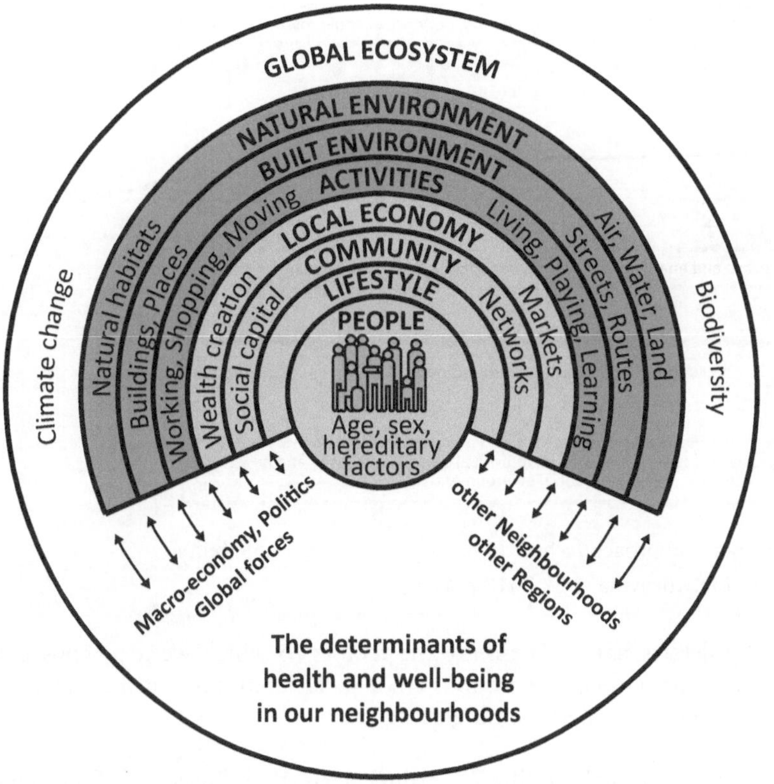

Figure 1.8 A health map
Source: Barton and Grant, 2006 p.252. Reproduced with permission from Sage Publications.

Life course approach

Some social ecological models focus on how the environment interacts with our biology across the life course. The World Health Organization (2000) explains how epidemiologists who take a life course approach study patterns of health and disease across people's lives and generations. They aim to understand how physical and social factors affect people's health from gestation through childhood to older age, and to the next generation. There are critical periods such as during childhood where exposures can do long-term damage. The cumulative effect of positive and negative influences determine our lifetime experience of health and illness.

The Commission on Social Determinants of Health (WHO, 2010) describe the interrelationships between

- socio-economic and political context, e.g. government policies and culture
- structural and socio-economic position. This concerns hierarchy, power, prestige and discrimination, e.g. income, education, occupation, social class, gender, race/ethnicity

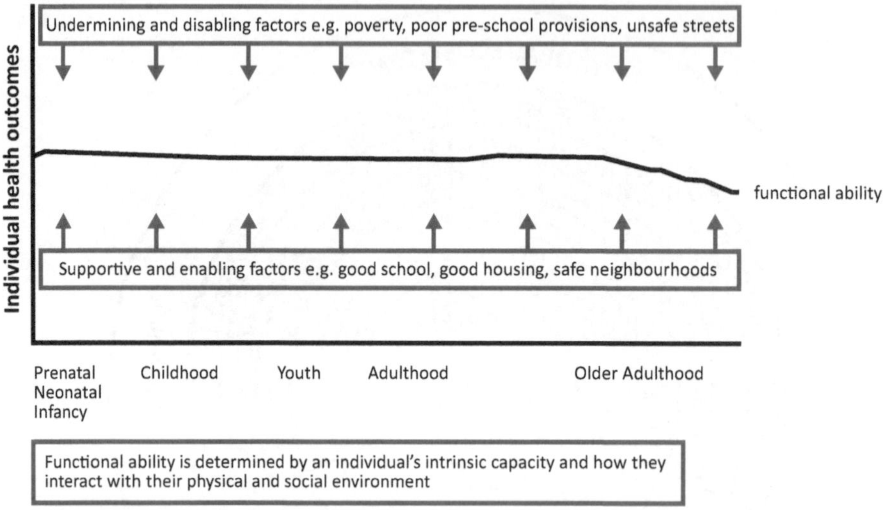

Figure 1.9 Life course approach to health, measured as functional ability
Source: adapted from Kuruvilla *et al*, 2018 p.41

- intermediary determinants. These are the factors to which we are exposed and how vulnerable or resilient we are to them, e.g. social and physical environment, psychosocial, behavioural and biological factors

These interact with individuals at different points across their life course. Some people suffer more ill health and die early, while others, at the top of the social gradient, have relatively longer healthier lives. This is discussed in more detail in Chapter 3.

Lay perceptions

So far, this chapter has described ways of thinking about health and illness which have been shaped by 'experts/professionals' including those from the religious, scientific and social scientific communities. During the upheaval of the 1970s, the idea emerged that lay people, the 'non- professionals or experts', have not only the 'right to health' (WHO, 1981), but the right to interpret what health and illness means to them based on their own experiences. Perceptions often reflect the traditional, medical or social models. Views that reflect a traditional model include:

> "Health is the most important blessing that the Lord has granted us," and, "Because illness is in the hands of God the Great and Almighty."
>
> (Muslim adults living in the United Arab Emirates, quoted in Elbarazi *et al.*, 2017 p.4)

> When I feel weak and tired, I know I have too much yin or cold in my body ... After I drink the herbal juice, I feel my body is balanced in yin and yang, which produces strength and energy for me.
>
> (Chinese elder living in the USA, quoted in Torsch and Ma, 2000 p.475)

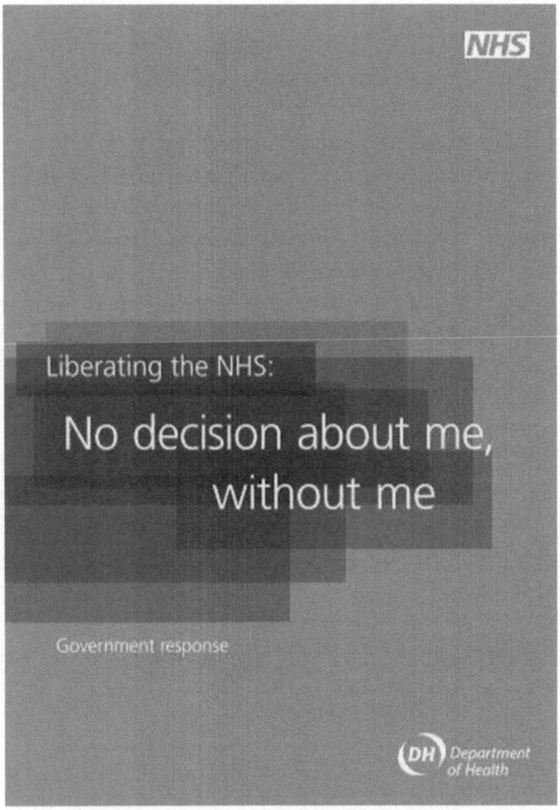

Figure 1.10 No decision about me without me
Source: DH, 2012. Reproduced under the terms of the Open Government Licence v3.0

Views that reflect a medical model include:

> Health is [pause] not what I am. To not be so tired, to not have as many shakes.
> (Canadian person with chronic illness quoted in McKague and Verhoef, 2003 p.708)

> If you move around, you won't kick the bucket. If you keep your body active, your body stays healthy ...
> (Chinese elder living in the USA, quoted in Torsch and Ma, 2000 p.482)

> I don't think that because I had that lump ... I think the percentage of risk is always there for everybody.
> (Woman in outer London quoted in Calnan and Johnson, 1985 p.66)

Views that reflect a social model include:

> Pollution, kinds of additives in our food, hormones that are used in food. I think those kind of things affect your health.
> (Canadian woman quoted in McKague and Verhoef, 2003 p.710)

> I think [the longer life expectancy] is cos them in [affluent area] have jobs and they have loads of money. They've got good work and they've got good living.
>
> (Adult living in North East England quoted in Garthwaite and Bambra, 2017 p.271)

People's perceptions of health and illness often include factors such as habits, self-care, the environment, relationships, money and their own constitution (Macintyre *et al.*, 2006). People may describe themselves as healthy when they have a disease, and use words such as having 'energy', physical ability and/or psychosocial vitality (Blaxter, 2010). Doctors may enter a patient's frame of reference by using phrases associated with the traditional model, 'caught a chill', rather than the medical model, 'infected by bacteria' (Helman, 1984). A person's perception can change according to context, whether they are a consumer or producer. Professionals are also lay people in another context. Perceptions can be individual and social, personal and public, lay and professional (Duncan, 2007; Nettleton, 2013).

Many organisations acknowledge the importance of lay perceptions by inviting customers, clients, patients, victims of crime and so forth to input into strategies to protect and improve their health. For example, the UK Department of Health committed to listen to people's views of their healthcare in No Decision About Me, Without Me (DH, 2012) (Figure 1.10).

> *In the social model, we protect and promote health by attending to the social conditions in which people live and promoting equality.*

Models of health and illness today

By the early twenty-first century, we had learnt that germs and health-related behaviours were influenced by the social, economic and physical environment in which people live and work. Today we see the reductionism of the medical model advance further in the quest to find '*the* underlying biological root cause of the causes of disease(s)', whilst recognising the vital role of the environment and how it cumulatively shapes people's health at both the micro level of the gene to the macro level of the society in which we journey through our whole life course. As we travel this bumpy road, we continue to turn to traditional ways of finding the balance within and without ourselves. The three models still exist, but we are beginning to see them more as an integrated whole, as the examples of low-grade inflammation, epigenetics and adverse childhood experiences show.

Low-grade inflammation: medical model

When we are injured or invaded by harmful bacteria or viruses, the body responds by local or systemic inflammation. As the immune system acts to repair the damage, it produces heat and sometimes swelling. Normally, once we are well, the inflammation reduces and disappears. In recent years, researchers have discovered that the inflammation does not always 'switch off', it remains at a chronic low level throughout the body. This is called low-grade inflammation or systemic chronic inflammation

Table 1.2 Contributors to chronic low-grade inflammation and long-term consequences

Factors which promote low-grade inflammation	*Long-term consequences associated with low-grade inflammation*
Environmental/industrial pollution	Cardiovascular disease
Chronic stress	Cancer
Physical inactivity	Type 2 diabetes
Poor diet	Chronic kidney disease
Imbalance of the microbiome	Depression
Tobacco/tobacco smoke	Non-alcoholic fatty liver disease
Alcohol	Autoimmune disorders e.g. rheumatoid arthritis
Drugs	Neurodegenerative disorders
Excess body fat/overweight/obesity	Osteoporosis
Loneliness/isolation	Sarcopenia (loss of muscle)
Chronic infections	
	Metabolic syndrome
	Hypertension (high blood pressure)
	Hyperglycaemia (high blood glucose)
	High blood cholesterol

Source: Furman *et al.* (2019).

and it damages the body's cells. It accumulates with age. The level of inflammation can be measured by a blood test. There is a significant body of research that suggests many of the major non-communicable diseases are caused by low-grade inflammation (Table 1.2). Rather than unhealthy behaviours and poor mental and emotional health causing disease, it seems they encourage low-grade inflammation which is, at least in part, the direct culprit. Current research seeks to understand how we may prevent, screen, diagnose and treat low-grade inflammation.

Epigenetics: social-ecological model/life course approach

We inherit genes which are made up of DNA. Genes can be turned on (expressed) or turned off (repressed) so that we can develop liver cells, skin cells, brain cells or whatever cells we need. The process of gene expression/repression is called epigenetics and it is influenced by the cells' environment. The environment can refer to inside the uterus or the environment inside the body. The body is influenced by factors such as diet, inactivity, weight, alcohol, the air, pollution, stress, calm and the whole experience of life. As we age, more genes associated with low-grade inflammation are expressed. Some conditions such as some cancers, Parkinson's disease, muscular dystrophy, Alzheimer's disease and multiple sclerosis are associated with epigenetic errors. Understanding genes is advancing possibilities for genetic screening for an increasing number of debilitating conditions and gene therapy which seeks to correct genetic 'defects' to prevent diseases. Recent studies suggest that maternal low-grade inflammation influences the genes of the foetus, who is more likely to grow up to have low-grade inflammation and then the health conditions that it promotes, such as cancer and cardiovascular disease (Furman *et al.*, 2019).

Adverse childhood experiences: social-ecological model/life course approach

In the mid-1990s, the Centres for Disease Control and Prevention in the United States of America carried out a study into the effect of child abuse and neglect, which they collectively called adverse childhood experiences (ACEs), on later life (Felitti *et al.*, 1998). Researchers asked adults to complete questionnaires about their childhoods and their current health. They found the more the respondent had been exposed to abuse or household dysfunction as a child, the more likely they were to report current cardiovascular disease, cancer, respiratory disease, bone fractures, liver disease and poor self-rated health. The links between the adverse childhood experiences and later disease were smoking, drug misuse, alcohol misuse, overeating or sexual behaviours, as these were also frequently reported. The researchers suggested that these health-risk behaviours were conscious or unconscious ways of achieving a psychological or physical benefit, they were coping strategies in the face of the stress of abuse, violence and other forms of family dysfunction. Further research has led the Centres for Disease Control and Prevention to declare:

> Simply put, our childhood experiences have a tremendous, lifelong impact on our health and the quality of our lives. The ACE Study showed dramatic links between adverse childhood experiences and risky behaviour, psychological issues, serious illness and the leading causes of death.
>
> (CDC, 2020)

Box 1.2 The health risks of cumulative adverse childhood experiences

Compared to people with no ACEs, those with four or more are:

4 times more likely to be a high-risk drinker
6 times more likely to smoke tobacco or e-cigarettes
6 times more likely to have had sex under 16 years old
6 times more likely to have had or caused unintended teenage pregnancy
11 times more likely to have smoked cannabis
14 times more likely to have been a victim of violence in the previous year
15 times more likely to have committed violence against another person in the previous year
16 times more likely to have used crack cocaine or heroin
20 times more likely to have been imprisoned at some point

(Source: adapted from Bellis *et al.*, 2015 p.5)

ACEs cannot be divorced from the society in which children live. Chen and Lacey (2018) followed 7,464 people who were born in 1958 in Britain and found more ACEs were associated with greater low-grade inflammation in adulthood. The authors write:

Table 1.3 Adverse childhood experiences and health problems in adulthood, 2020

Adverse childhood experiences (ACEs)	*Adult health problems with which ACEs are associated*
Emotional abuse	Autoimmune disease
Physical abuse	Cancer
Sexual abuse	Chronic obstructive pulmonary disease
Emotional neglect	Disability
Physical neglect	Frequent headaches
Mother treated violently	Poor health-related quality of life
Substance abuse in household	Cardiovascular disease
Mental disorders in household	Liver disease
Separation/divorce	Type 2 diabetes
Imprisonment of a household member	
	Alcohol misuse
	Drug misuse
	Obesity
	Sexual risk behaviour
	Smoking
	Depression
	Hallucinations
	Stress disorder, post-traumatic stress disorder
	Borderline personality disorder
	Suicidal behaviours
	Limits to life opportunities e.g. adult education, employment, potential income

Source: CDC (2020).

> Our findings suggest that the occurrence of ACEs appears to set children down a path of life course disadvantage, particularly with regards to educational attainment, socioeconomic position and the uptake of risky behaviours ... health-threatening behaviours exacerbate inflammatory tendencies via impaired interpersonal relationships and poor self-management capacities.
>
> (p.588)

Mindfulness: traditional model

Mindfulness is the process of individuals paying quiet attention to their emerging thoughts and feelings in the present moment. They are observing and experiencing the senses offered by the world around them. It is

> ... knowing directly what is going on inside and outside ourselves, moment by moment ... This means waking up to the sights sounds, smells and tastes of the present moment.
>
> (NHS, 2018)

The origins of mindfulness are thought to come from Buddhism, and there is a growing body of evidence which suggests it can help with anxiety, depression and stress (Hofmann *et al.*, 2010; Parmentier *et al.*, 2019; Janssen *et al.*, 2018). These are causes and consequences of low-grade inflammation. There is some research to suggest mindfulness may reduce chronic low-grade inflammation, at least in middle-aged/older adults and those who are overweight, raising the possibility it may become an important disease-prevention intervention (Villalba *et al.*, 2019).

Why understanding models of health and illness matters

Understanding models of health and illness provide frameworks with which to understand differing perspectives and enable us to question and to better design interventions for protecting and promoting people's health. They encourage us to question

- who defines what health and illness mean for an individual, and for a whole community
- the balance between personal health choices versus the community's health
- where lies the cause or blame for ill health
- what factors protect and promote good health
- who is responsible for preventing ill health and promoting good health

Thinking point:

> Imagine having frequent headaches and visiting three practitioners, one who works with a traditional model, one with a medical model and one with a social model. What might each say about the causes of your headaches? What advice might they give you to prevent these headaches?
>
> Imagine that 90% of a town is suffering from frequent headaches, and three practitioners, who work with a traditional model, a medical model and a social model, write a piece for a local newspaper. What might each write about the causes of the headaches? What might they say about how to prevent these headaches?

Summary

This chapter has

- described traditional, medical and social models of health and illness
- placed the evolution of models of health and illness within historical and social change
- outlined how a scientific approach towards health and illness became more dominant during the twentieth century
- described the challenges to the medical model and the rise of the social model of health
- provided examples of social ecological models that represent contemporary understandings of health and illness
- described the life course approach to health and illness
- explained the contribution of lay perceptions about health and illness
- demonstrated how the three models exist today, but within an increasingly integrated view of health and illness

Further reading

Moon, G., and Gillespie, R. (1995) *Society and health*. London: Routledge
Napier, A.D. (2017) *Culture matters: using a cultural contexts of health approach to enhance policy making*. Copenhagen: World Health Organization (Europe)
Nettleton, S. (2020) *The sociology of health and illness*. 4th edn. Cambridge: Polity Press

Useful websites

World Health Organization *Social determinants of health*. Available at: www.who.int/social_determinants/en

References

Adams, K.M., Kohlmeier, M., Powell, M., and Zeisel, S.H. (2010) 'Nutrition in medicine: nutrition education for medical students and residents', *Nutrition in Clinical Practice*, 25(5), pp.471–480

Adamski, M., Gibson, S., Leech, M., and Truby, H. (2018) 'Are doctors nutritionists? What is the role of doctors in providing nutrition advice?', *Nutrition Bulletin*, 43, pp.147–152

Aggleton, P. (1990) *Health*. London: Routledge

Barton, H., and Grant, M. (2006) 'A health map for the local human habitat', *The Journal for the Royal Society for the Promotion of Health*, 126(6), pp.252–253

Bellis, M., Ashton, K., Hughes, K., Ford, K., Bishop, J., and Paranjothy, S. (2015) *Adverse childhood experiences and their impact on health-harming behaviours in the Welsh adult population*. Cardiff: Public Health Wales

Berche, P. (2012) 'Louis Pasteur, from crystals of life to vaccination', *Clinical Microbiology and Infection*, 18(Suppl.5), pp.1–6

Berryman, J.W., and Park, R.J. (eds) (1992) *Sport and exercise science. Essays in the history of sports medicine*. Illinois: University of Illinois

Black, D., Morris, J.N., Smith, C., and Townsend, P. (1982) '*The black report*', in Townsend, P., Davidson, N., and Whitehead, M. (eds) *Inequalities in health*. London: Penguin, pp.29–213

Blaxter, M. (2010) *Health*. 2nd edn. Cambridge: Polity Press

Blevins, S.M., and Bronze, M.S. (2010) 'Robert Koch and the "golden age" of bacteriology', *International Journal of Infectious Diseases*, 14(9) e744–e751. doi: 10.1016/j.ijid.2009.12.003

Bosma, H., Marmot, M.G., Hemingway, H., Nicholson, A.C., Brunner, E., and Stansfield, S.A. (1997) 'Low job control and risk of coronary heart disease in Whitehall II (prospective cohort) study', *BMJ*, 314(7080), pp.558–565

Bown, S.R. (2003) *Scurvy: how a surgeon, a mariner, and a gentleman, solved the greatest medical mystery of the age of sail*. New York: Thomas Dunne Books

Calnan, M., and Johnson, B. (1985) 'Health, health risks and inequalities: an exploratory study of women's perceptions', *Sociology of Health and Illness*, 7(1), pp.55–75

Carpenter, K.J. (2003) 'A short history of nutritional science: part 1 (1985-1885)', *The Journal of Nutrition*, 133 (3), pp.636–645

Centres for Disease Control and Prevention (2020) *Adverse childhood experiences (ACEs)*. Available at: www.cdc.gov/violenceprevention/acestudy/index.html (Accessed 5th September 2020)

Champion, J. (1995) *London's dreaded visitation: the social geography of the great plague in 1665. Historical Geography Research Series No. 31*. Edinburgh: University of Edinburgh

Chatterjee, R. (2017) *The 4 pillar plan: how to relax, eat, move and sleep your way to a longer healthier life*. London: Penguin Life

Chen, M., and Lacey, R.E. (2018) 'Adverse childhood experiences and adult inflammation: findings from the 1958 British birth cohort', *Brain, Behavior, and Immunity*, 69(2018), pp.582–590

Cochrane, A.L. (1972) *Effectiveness and efficiency: random reflections on health services*. London: Nuffield Provincial Hospitals Trust

Crossley, N. (1998) 'R.D. Laing and the British anti-psychiatry movement: a socio-historical analysis', *Social Science Medicine*, 47(7), pp.877–889

Dahlgren, G., and Whitehead, M. (1991). *Policies and strategies to promote social equity in health*. Stockholm, Sweden: Institute for Futures Studies

Department of Health (2012) *Liberating the NHS. No decision about me, without me*. London: Department of Health

Department of Health and Social Security (1976) *Prevention and health. Everybody's business*. London: Her Majesty's Stationery Office

Doll, R., and Hill, A.B. (1954) 'The mortality of doctors in relation to their smoking habits', *British Medical Journal*, 4877, pp.1451–4877

Dubos, R. (1984) 'Mirage of health', in Black, N., Boswell, D., Gray, A., Murphy, S. and Popay, J. (eds) *Health and disease*. Milton Keynes: Open University Press, pp.4–9

Duncan, P. (2007) *Critical perspectives on health*. Basingstoke: Palgrave Macmillan

Elbarazi, I., Devlin, N.J., Katsaiti, M., Papadimitropoulos, E.A., Shah, K.K., and Blair, I. (2017) 'The effect of religion on the perception of health states among adults in the United Arab Emirates: a qualitative study', *BMJ Open*, 7 doi:10.1136/bmjopen-2017–016969

Felitti, V.J., Anda, R.F., Nordenberg, D., Williamson, D.F., Spitz, A.M., Edwards, V., Koss, M.P., and Marks, J.S. (1998) 'Relationship of childhood abuse and household dysfunction to many leading causes of death in adults. The Adverse Childhood Experiences (ACE) Study', *American Journal of Preventive Medicine*, 14(4) pp.245–258

Foucault, M. (1973) *The birth of the clinic*. London: Routledge

Furman, D., Campisi, J., Verdin, E., Carrera-Bastos, P., Targ, S., Franceschi, C., Ferrucci, L., Gilroy, D.W., Fasano, A., Miller, G.W., Miller, A.H., Mantovani, A, Weyand, C.M., Barzilae, N., Goronzy, J.J., Rando, T.A., Effros, R.B., Lucia, A., Kleinstreuer, N., and Slavich, G.M. (2019) 'Chronic inflammation in the etiology of disease across the life span', *Nature Medicine*, 25(12), pp.1822–1832

Garthwaite, K., and Bambra, C. (2017) '"How the other half live": lay perspectives on health inequalities in an age of austerity', *Social Science and Medicine*, 187, pp.268–275

General Register Office (1842) *Fourth annual report of the registrar general of births, deaths, and marriages, in England*. London: Her Majesty's Stationery Office

Gillespie, R., and Gerhardt, C. (1995) 'Social dimensions of sickness and disability', in Moon, G., and Gillespie, R. (eds) *Society and health. An introduction to social science for health professionals*. London: Routledge, pp.79–94

Hajj, I.H., Chams, N., Chams, S., El Sayegh, S., Badran, R., Raad, M., Gerges-Geagea, A., Leone, A., and Jurjus, A. (2015) 'Vaccines through centuries: major cornerstones in global health', *Frontiers in Public Health*, 3 (269), pp.1–16. doi: 10.3389/fpubh.2015.00269

Hardy, A. (2001) *Health and medicine in Britain since 1860*. Basingstoke: Palgrave

Halliday, S. (2001) 'Death and miasma in Victorian London: an obstinate belief', *BMJ*, 323(7327), pp.1469–1471

Helman, C. (1984) 'Feed a cold, starve a fever', in Black, N., Boswell, D., Gray, A., Murphy, S., and Popay, J. (eds) *Health and disease*. Milton Keynes: Open University Press, pp.10–24

Herzlich, C., and Pierret, J. (1991) 'Illness: from causes to meaning', in Currer, C., and Stacey, M. (eds) *Concepts of health, illness and disease. A comparative perspective*. Oxford: Berg, pp.73–96

Hoffmann, S.G., Sawyer, A., Ashley, W., and Oh, D. (2010) 'The effects of mindfulness-based stress reduction on anxiety and depression: A meta-analytic review', *Journal of Consulting and Clinical Psychology*, 78(2) pp.169–183

Hothersall, D. (2003) *History of psychology*. 4th edn. Maidenhead: McGraw-Hill Education

Illich, I. (1976) *Limits to medicine: medical nemesis: the exploration of health*. London: Marion Boyars

Janssen, M., Heerkens, Y., Kuijer, W., van der Heijden, B., and Engels, J. (2018) 'Effects of mindfulness-based stress reduction on employees' mental health: a systematic review', *PLoS ONE*, 13(1) doi:10.1371/journal.pone.0191332

Jewson, N.D. (1976) 'The disappearance of the sick man from medical cosmology, 1770–1870', *Sociology*, 10, pp.225–44

Jouanna, J. (2012) *Greek medicine from Hippocrates to Galen: selected papers*. (Translated by Neil Allies). Edited with preface by Philip van der Eijk. Leiden, The Netherlands: Brill

Keys, A., Anderson, J.T., Aresu, M., Biörck, Brock, J.F., Bronte-Stewart, B., Fidanza, Fl, Keys, M., Malmros, H., Poppi, A., Posteli, T., Swahn, B., and del Vecchio, A. (1956) 'Physical activity and the diet in populations differing in serum cholesterol', *The Journal of Clinical Investigation*, 35(10), pp.1173–1181

Karpf, A. (1988) *Doctoring the media*. London: Routledge

Kuruvilla, S., Sadana, R., Montesinos, E.V., *et al.* (2018) 'A life-course approach to health: synergy with sustainable development goals', *Bulletin of the World Health Organization*, 96(1) pp.42–50

Lalonde, M. (1974) *A new perspective on the health of Canadians. A working document*. Ottawa: Government of Canada

Lieberman, L., Golden, S.D., and Golden, S.D. (2013) 'Structural approaches to health promotion: what do we need to know about policy and environmental change?' *Health Education and Behaviour*, 40(5), pp.520–525

Ling, Y., Yang, D., and Shao, W. (2012) 'Understanding vomiting from the perspective of traditional Chinese medicine', *Annals of Palliative Medicine*, 1(2), pp.143–160

Lubnitz, S.A. (2004) 'Early reactions to Harvey's circulation theory: the impact on medicine', *Mount Sinai Journal of Medicine*, 71(4), pp.274–280

Macintyre, S., McKay, L., and Ellaway, A. (2006) 'Lay concepts of the relative importance of different influences on health; are there major socio-demographic variations?' *Health Education Research*, 21(5), pp.731–739

Marmot, M.G., Shipley, M.J., and Rose, G. (1984) 'Inequalities in death-specific explanations of a general pattern?' *The Lancet*, 323(8384), pp.1003–1006

Marmot, M. (2010) *Fair society, healthy lives. The Marmot review*. H.M. Government: London

McDonald, L. (ed) (2004) *Florence Nightingale on public health care: volume 6 of the collected works of Florence Nightingale*. Ontario: Wilfrid Laurier University Press

McKague, M., and Verhoef, M. (2003) 'Understandings of health and its determinants among clients and providers at an urban community health center', *Qualitative Health Research*, 13(5), pp.703–717

McKeown, T. (1976) *The role of medicine. Dream, mirage or nemesis?* London: Nuffield Provincial Hospitals Trust. Available at: www.nuffieldtrust.org.uk/files/2017-01/1485273106_the-role-of-medicine-web-final.pdf (Accessed 29th October 2018)

Moon, G. (1995) 'Health care and society', in Moon, G., and Gillespie, R. (eds) *Society and health. An introduction to social science for health professionals*. London: Routledge, pp.49–64

Mosley, M. (2010) *The story of science. Power, proof and passion*. London: Mitchell Beazley/Octopus

Mosley, M. (2014) *The fast diet: lose weight, stay healthy, live longer*. London: Short Books

Morris, J.N., and Crawford, M.D. (1958) 'Coronary heart disease and physical activity of work', *British Medical Journal*, 2, pp.1485–1496

Mozaffarian, D., Rosenberg, I., and Uauy, R. (2018) 'History of modern nutrition science – implications for current research, dietary guidelines and food policy', *BMJ*, 361 doi: 10.1136/bmj.k2392

Murdock, G.P. (1980) *Theories of illness: a world survey*. Pittsburgh: University of Pittsburgh

National Health Service (2018) *Mindfulness*. Available at: www.nhs.uk/conditions/stress-anxiety-depression/mindfulness/ (Accessed 5th September 2020)

Nettleton, S. (1988) 'Protecting the vulnerable margin: towards an analysis of how the mouth came to be separate from the body', *Sociology of Health and Illness*, 10(2), pp.156–169

Nettleton, S. (2013) *The sociology of health and illness*. 3rd edn. Cambridge: Polity Press

Oakley, A. (1993) *Essays on women and health*. Edinburgh: Edinburgh University Press

Office of National Statistics (2017) *An overview of lifestyles and wider characteristics linked to healthy life expectancy in England*. Available at: https://bit.ly/2Vv3Swa (Accessed 21st October 2018)

O'Neill, S., Gryseels, C., Dierickx, S., Mwesigwa, J., Okebe, J., d'Alessandro, U., and Peeters Grietens, K. (2015) 'Foul wind, spirits and witchcraft: illness conceptions and health-seeking behaviour for malaria in the Gambia', *Malaria Journal*, 14(167) doi 10.1186/s12936-015-0687-2

Parmentier, F.B.R., Garcia-Toro, M., Barcia-Campayo, J., Yañez, A.M., Andrés, P., and Gili, M. (2019) 'Mindfulness and symptoms of depression and anxiety in the general population: the mediating roles of worry, rumination, reappraisal and suppression', *Frontiers in Psychology*, 10(505) doi:10.3389/fpsyg.2019.00506

Pead, P.J. (2003) 'Benjamin Jesty: new light in the dawn of vaccination', *The Lancet*, 362(9401), pp.2104–2109

Pett, K.D., Kahn, J., Willett, W.C., and Katz, D.L. (2017) *Ancel Keys and the seven countries study: an evidence-based response to revisionist histories. White paper. The True Health Initiative*. Available at: www.truehealthinitiative.org/wordpress/wp-content/uploads/2017/07/SCS-White-Paper.THI_.8-1-17.pdf (Accessed 19th October 2018)

Porter, R. (1995) *Disease, medicine and society in England, 1550–1860*. 2nd edn. Cambridge: Cambridge University Press

Reidel, S. (2005) 'Edward Jenner and the history of smallpox and vaccination', *Baylor University Medical Center Proceedings (BUMC Proceedings)*, 18(1), pp.21–25

Registrar-General (1849) *Eighth annual report of the registrar-general of births, deaths and marriages, in England*. London: Her Majesty's Stationery Office

Singer, M. (2009) *Introduction to syndemics. A critical systems approach to public and community health*. San Francisco: Jossey-Bass

Stewart, J., Bushell, F., and Habgood, V. (2005) *Environmental health and public health*. London: Chadwick House

Tew, M. (1998) *Safer childbirth? A critical history of maternity care*. 3rd edn. London: Free Association Books

Torsch, V., and Ma, G.X. (2000) 'Cross-cultural comparison of health perceptions, concerns, and coping strategies among Asian and Pacific islander American elders', *Qualitative Health Research*, 10(4), pp.471–489

Turshen, M (1989) *The politics of public health*. London: Zed Books

Underwood, E.A. (1947) 'The history of cholera in Great Britain', *Proceedings of the Royal Society of Medicine*, 41(3), pp.165–173

Unschuld, P. (1991) 'The conceptual determination (űberformung) of individual and collective experiences of illness', in Currer, C., and Stacey, M. (eds) *Concepts of health, illness and disease. A comparative perspective*. New York: Berg, pp.51–70

Ussher, P. (1989) *The psychology of the female body*. London: Routledge

Villalba, D.K., Lindsay, E.K., Marsland, A.L., Greco, C.M., Young, S., Brown, K.W., Smyth, J.M., Walsh, C.P., Gray, K., Chin, B., and Creswell, J.D (2019) 'Mindfulness training and systematic low-grade inflammation in stressed community adults: evidence two randomized controlled trials', *PLoS ONE*, 14(7) doi: 10.1371/journal.pone.0219120

Weintraub, M.I., Mamtani, R., and Micozzie, M.S. (eds) (2008) *Complementary and integrative medicine in pain management.* New York: Springer

Wilkinson, R., and Marmot, M. (eds) (2003) *Social determinants of health: the solid facts.* 2nd edn. Copenhagen: World Health Organization (Europe)

World Health Organization (1981) *Global strategy for health for all by the year 2000.* Geneva: World Health Organization

World Health Organization (2000) *The implications for training of embracing a life course approach to health.* Geneva: World Health Organization

World Health Organization (2008) *Closing the gap in a generation: health equity through action on the social determinants of health.* Available at: www.who.int/social_determinants/final_report/media/csdh_report_wrs_en.pdf (Accessed 9th October 2019)

World Health Organization (2010) *A conceptual framework for action on the social determinants of health.* Geneva: World Health Organization

World Health Organization (2019) *Social determinants of health.* Available at: www.who.int/social_determinants/sdh_definition/en/ (Accessed 9th October 2019)

Yang, J.S., Mamudu, H.M., and John, R. (2018) 'Incorporating a structural approach to reducing the burden of non-communicable diseases', *Globalization and Health*, 14(1) doi.org/10.1186/s12992-018-0380-7

Yuill, C., Crinson, I., and Duncan, E. (2010) *Key concepts in health studies.* London: Sage

2 Environment and health

Tristi Brownett and Joanne Cairns

Key points

- Introduction
- Climate change
- Air pollution
- Built environment
- Housing
- A healthy environment
- Summary

Introduction

Abraham Maslow (1943) argued that all human beings need food, air, water and shelter in order to survive and maximise health and wellbeing. This chapter discusses the physical environment and focuses on climate change, air pollution, the built environment, housing and sustainability.

Climate change

Climate refers to the long-term average weather pattern that one can expect in a given location at a given time of year (Royal Meteorological Society, 2018). Climate change means that there is a systemic change affecting the weather pattern. The collection of climate statistics helps us to know what weather to expect, to plan and then adapt as needed. As a result of global warming, the interacting weather systems behave differently and affect the climate in each region.

Until recently, changes to climate and weather patterns were considered a normal part of the planet's life cycle, and scientists have demonstrated that over two million years the planet has undergone significant climate change (Le Treut *et al.*, 2007). It is now generally agreed that human activity, since the industrial revolution, has accelerated this natural process. Climate change is widely acknowledged to be one of the biggest public health challenges of our times, and the Lancet Commission on Health and Climate states that it is undermining 50 years of global public health progress (Watts *et al.*, 2015).

Global warming

Planet Earth is surrounded by an atmosphere of five gaseous layers. These layers help to protect the planet and give it properties such as the air we breathe and an ability to maintain moisture. Within the atmosphere is the stratosphere, which contains ozone gas. Ozone absorbs heat and protects humans from the sun's ultraviolet (UV) radiation. As there is limited air movement in the stratosphere, chemicals and particles can become trapped for long periods. This is problematic as some of these chemicals such as chlorofluorocarbons (CFCs) found in coolants and aerosol propellants are known to deplete the ozone layer, thus allowing more heat from UV radiation to penetrate the earth. The ozone layer has become thinnest at the north and south poles, and the intensification of UV radiation and heat reaching the earth is contributing to the melting of polar ice caps. As the ice melts, it is inevitable that oceans will rise, and low-lying countries will experience flooding. It is encouraging that scientists have found the ozone layer can recover if humans limit their use of CFCs, causing the heat from the UV radiation to reduce and the earth to cool (Knight, 2011).

Ozone depletion is not entirely responsible for climate change because as the earth orbits around the sun there is also a natural global warming of the planet. This natural warming is exacerbated by solar events such as solar flares or the trapping of particles and gases from volcanic eruptions, sea salt and Saharan dust (Highwood, 2018). The recent escalation in global warming is due to an increase in these trapped gases and particles which affect the usual functioning of the stratosphere and its neighbouring troposphere. These gases, which are sometimes called greenhouse gases, include carbon dioxide, methane, nitrous oxide, CFCs and hydrofluorocarbons (HFCs). When released into the stratosphere, they accumulate and essentially act as a planetary quilt allowing heat from the sun to enter the earth's stratosphere, but not to escape so easily. This is the enhanced 'greenhouse effect' (IPCC, 1988).

Table 2.1 Anthropogenic and non-anthropogenic contributions to global warming

Anthropogenic/human-made factors	*Non-anthropogenic/external factors over which humans have no control*
Burning fossil fuels, e.g. power plants, factories, oil for homes and transport	Changes in the Earth's orbit
Landfill releases methane	Solar radiation
Petroleum and natural gas industries release methane	Volcanic activity
Agriculture, e.g. grazing animals release methane	
Aerosols may release CFCs	
Fertilizers, used in industry and for refrigeration, release nitrous oxide	
Deforestation (cutting down trees and plants which absorb carbon dioxide)	
Urbanisation (increased air pollution and waste disposal issues)	

Sources: Environmental Protection Agency (2017); National Research Council (2010); National Geographic Society (2019).

The release of greenhouse gases into the earth's atmosphere is caused by the burning of the carbon-based, finite/non-renewable, fossil fuels, coal, gas and oil, for energy. As these activities have increased over the last century, so has the amount of carbon dioxide released into the environment. In the natural environment trees absorb carbon dioxide and helpfully release oxygen, rebalancing the atmosphere. Unfortunately, we have seen the destruction of many forests to clear the land for large-scale agricultural businesses, negatively influencing the natural repair process. Additionally, modern farming and manufacturing practices also release greenhouse gases such as methane, nitrous oxide, CFCs and HFCs and, without intervention, it is becoming unlikely that the planet can heal itself.

The Intergovernmental Panel on Climate Change (2018) states that in the last 120 to 170 years the planet has warmed by 0.87°C compared to pre-industrial times. During the last 30 years there has been unprecedented warming at around 0.2°C per decade. The Panel predict that if people continue to produce greenhouse gases at the present rate of anthropogenic activities, the average global surface air temperature could rise to 1.5°C above previous levels by 2030. It might go even higher. Future rising temperatures will depend on the rate of greenhouse gas emissions produced.

Consequences of climate change for people's health

The increased rate of global warming is a major concern because changes in weather patterns have negative impacts on human health. This burden affects the most vulnerable people of the world and substantially exacerbates inequalities in health, discussed in Chapter 3. Our health is affected by environmental warming and heatwaves, air quality and emissions, ultraviolet radiation, heavy rainfall and flash floods, drought, freezing weather, allergens and vector-borne diseases and conflict and displacement.

Environmental warming and heatwaves

As temperatures rise, we experience more heat waves. The body's normal reaction to heat is to cool down by increasing surface blood flow and sweating. Smith and colleagues (2015) explain that children and older people are particularly vulnerable as their bodies are less able to regulate their core body temperatures than others. With ageing, older people become less aerobically fit, meaning their bodies do not transport and use oxygen as well. Heat may exacerbate existing health conditions, and dehydration can lead to the loss of important mineral salts, leading to a strain on muscles, including the heart. Prolonged heat can disrupt sleep, leading to poor concentration, mental distress and fatigue. An increase in hospital admissions and deaths, linked to heat waves, was observed in the UK in 2003, and again in the summer of 2018 (HCEAC, 2018). In response, public health teams developed surveillance, early warning systems and heatwave plans (PHE, 2019).

Air quality and emissions

Rising temperatures and emissions of greenhouse gases affect the quality of the air. As populations grow, more energy is consumed. This results in higher levels of greenhouse gas emissions. In the residential sector, the amount of fuel used is heavily influenced by external temperatures. For example, in 2010 when temperatures were

Table 2.2 Health impacts of climate change

Health problem	*Caused by*	*Climate change factor*					
		Environmental warming and heatwaves	*Air quality and emissions*	*Heavy rainfall/ flash floods*	*Freezing weather*	*Drought*	*UV (sun) exposure*
Breathing difficulty	Air pollution	✓	✓				✓
	Fungal spores	✓					
	Fluctuating seasonal temperatures	✓			✓		
	Damp exposure			✓			
	Increased pollen	✓					
Cardiac and renal difficulty	Dehydration	✓				✓	
	Age vulnerability	✓	✓	✓	✓	✓	✓
Skin cancer and cataracts	Increased UV exposure						✓
Mental distress	Adaptation to extreme weather events	✓	✓	✓	✓	✓	✓
	Loss of/damage to home			✓			
	Financial hardship (cost of adapting)	✓		✓	✓		
	Human loss	✓	✓	✓	✓	✓	✓
Vector-borne disease	Human and animal migration	✓	✓	✓	✓	✓	✓
	Biological contamination of buildings by exotic species/ pathogens/household pests	✓		✓		✓	
Food poisoning	Contamination by spores	✓					
	Microbiological hazards	✓		✓			
	Environment no longer appropriate for food storage	✓		✓		✓	✓

the coldest in Britain since 1987, people increased their heating, causing a significant rise in domestic gas emissions (DECC, 2012). The UK Government introduced the Climate Change Act in 2008, which aims to reduce greenhouse emissions by 80% in 2050 compared to 1990. This Act was followed by the Clean Growth Strategy in 2017 (H.M. Government, 2017).

Ultraviolet radiation

Ultraviolet radiation (UV) is part of the electromagnetic spectrum emitted by the sun. It contains UVA and UVB rays. UVA penetrates deep into people's skin, causing premature ageing. UVB triggers a chemical reaction that provides people with vitamin D, but it also causes sunburn. Both UVA and UVB rays can cause skin cancer, and this can occur from sun beds as well as the natural sun. In the UK about 85% of skin melanomas are caused by too much ultraviolet radiation, and the advice is for people to use a combination of shade, clothing and sunscreen (Cancer Research UK, 2020).

Heavy rainfall/flash floods

Increased rainfall and severe weather are consequences of climate change. The worst, immediate impact of storms and flash flooding is loss of life through drowning, but more pervasive is the damage to homes and businesses that can take months to dry out and repair. Sewage can wash into rivers and buildings, creating the potential for microbiological health hazards such as those which cause gastrointestinal illness. The

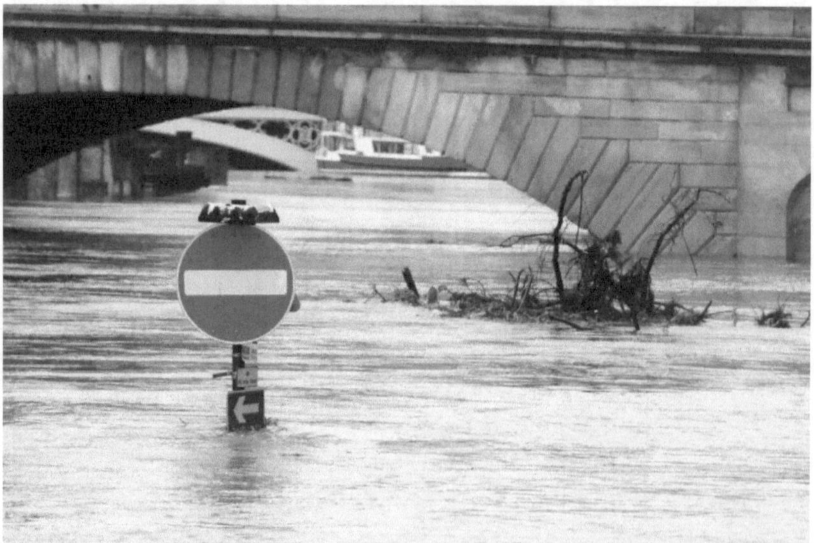

Figure 2.1 Flooding of the River Ouse, York, 2013
Source: JaneHYork/Shutterstock.com

loss of people's income, possessions and personal security is devastating and where livestock is drowned and crops destroyed, the potential for starvation and famine is high. Families and communities may not recover for years. Without help, especially international support for poorer countries, disease and death rates will rise primarily due to a lack of shelter, a lack of reliable, affordable and accessible energy which we call 'energy security' and the transmission of diseases (IPCC, 2014).

Drought

Drought, storms and floods affect the quality of soil. The soil determines the type of crops that can be grown to provide food for humans and animals. The weather and seasons are essential to the quantity and quality of the world's food production. To have food security, food needs to be reliable, available and affordable to people.

Freezing weather

Many epidemiological studies have demonstrated an increased risk of death as temperatures drop below a threshold (Bunker *et al.*, 2016; Gasparrini *et al.*, 2015; Yu *et al.*, 2012). There may be a link between arctic warming and the extreme weather incidents seen in the UK over the last decade, but more research is needed (Hanna *et al.*, 2017). In February/March 2018, the UK experienced icy blizzards caused by Storm Emma meeting easterly winds, called the 'Beast from the East', and

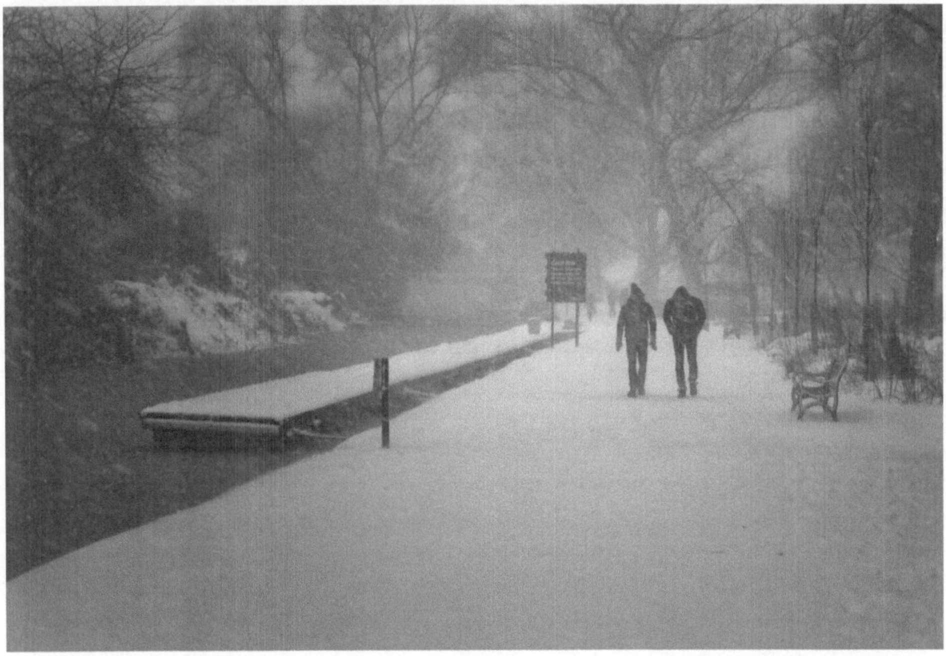

Figure 2.2 Beast from the East, Edinburgh 2018
Source: Ludovic Farine/Shutterstock.com

- 10 people died
- more than 18,000 people were without power
- the Environment Agency issued 15 flood warnings and 36 flood alerts across the country
- military personnel assisted emergency services in responding to the freezing conditions
- widespread disruption to railways, roads and airports throughout the day made it difficult for commuters to go to work
- hospitals struggled as staff were unable to get to work
- thousands of schools were closed

(Jones, 2018)

Allergens and vector-borne diseases

Climate change affects the seasons which influence the distribution of pollen and the growth of fungal spores. These are linked to allergies, such as hay fever and asthma. With an increasing number of allergens, we see more people being affected, more severe allergies and breathing (respiratory) conditions.

Climate change also affects the local ecology. It affects the delicate balance of ecosystems, where the local habitat supports living plants and animals, including the smallest organisms. Vectors are organisms that carry pathogens which cause disease in humans and/or animals (e.g. mosquitoes, ticks, flies and lice). Vector-borne diseases include zika, malaria, dengue, haemorrhagic fever and plague. Climate change is altering habitats in ways that better support vectors and therefore the spread of diseases (Campbell-Lendrum *et al.*, 2015). About 17% of infectious diseases across the world are attributable to vector-borne diseases causing 700,000 annual deaths (WHO, 2017).

Some vector-borne diseases are emerging in new places. In southern Europe we are seeing malaria and tick-borne encephalitis, and in eastern Europe, West Nile virus has recently emerged (ECDPC, 2019). Within the UK, Lyme disease, spread by ticks, is sufficiently common to be endemic, requiring routine surveillance (PHE, 2018a). Furthermore, statistical models predict that anophelines, mosquitoes which are capable of carrying the parasite that causes malaria, and mosquitoes that spread other infectious diseases such as dengue fever and West Nile virus, are likely to be able to survive and breed in parts of Europe, including the UK, in the near future. This is because changes to the climate are expected to make it more suitable for these vectors over the next 10 to 15 years (Medlock and Leach, 2015). In response, the UK has

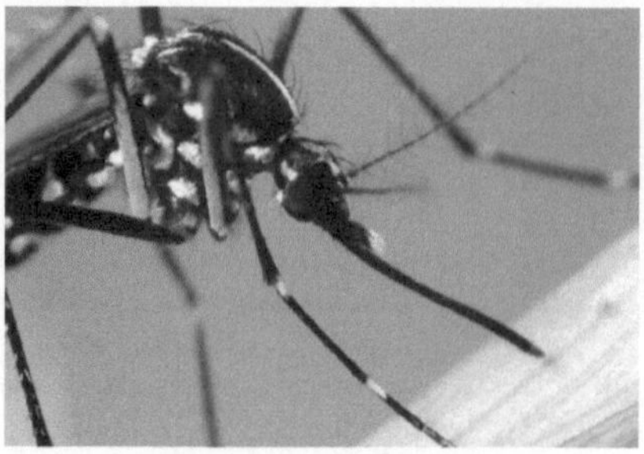

Figure 2.3 Asian tiger mosquito (*Aedes albopictus*)
Source: InsectWorld/Shutterstock.com

introduced a mosquito surveillance programme that seeks to identify any non-native mosquitoes, including those brought into the country via imported goods. Since 2016, the programme, at the time of writing, has identified two separate episodes of *Aedes albopictus* eggs in Kent. These are laid by Asian Tiger mosquitoes, which carry tropical diseases such as dengue fever and zika. The eggs were subsequently destroyed.

Conflict and displacement

Increasingly the world's population is seeing the displacement of people due to extreme climate change disasters, such as the 2004 Asian tsunami, in which emergency shelters were set up for 100,000 people (UN Refugee Agency, 2004). The term 'climate refugee' describes those who have been forcibly displaced as a direct consequence of climate change disasters.

International response to climate change

Whether or not climate change can be stopped is highly contested. Some scientists suggest it may be too late (e.g. Steffen *et al.*, 2018). A series of international climate negotiations aim to slow down the rate through the implementation of the Paris Agreement (UN, 2015a). This aims to keep the increase in global temperature to below 2% and reduce carbon dioxide emissions. In Europe, countries agreed to reduce emissions by 40% by 2030 compared to 1990. They hope to achieve this by developing renewable, 'green', energy sources, such as wind, solar and hydro energy to replace non-renewable fossil fuels and reduce the total amount of energy used. In December 2018, global delegates at Katowice in Poland agreed international strategies to make the Paris Agreement and its subsequent standards workable and measurable (UN Climate Change, 2018).

> *Climate change is causing changes to the weather which lead to significant threats to the public's health.*

Air pollution

The air we breathe is made up of nitrogen, carbon dioxide and oxygen along with other trace elements. Today, most parts of the globe experience air pollution which affects the delicate balance of these gases. Air pollution is associated with abnormal foetal development and chronic diseases throughout the life course, such as type 2 diabetes, heart disease and asthma (PHE, 2018b). In the UK, the Royal College of Physicians (2016) estimates that outdoor air pollution contributes to about 40,000 deaths a year.

Air pollutants

Air pollutants comprise particulates, ground-level ozone, petrol and diesel.

Particulates

The air contains small particles of solids or liquids, called particulates. These particulates may be natural, such as soil and pollen, or from anthropogenic sources such as dust from construction, vehicle brakes or road surfaces. Fossil fuels release

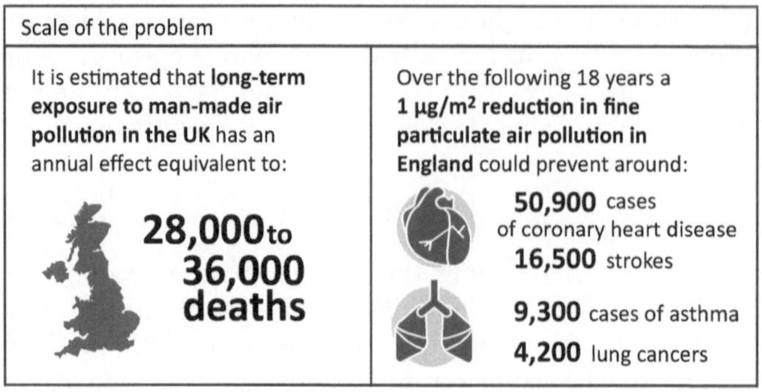

Figure 2.4 Air pollution, the scale of the problem
Source: PHE, 2018b. Reproduced under the terms of the Open Government Licence v.3.0

airborne particulates such as carbon. Particulates may be visible as smoke, haze or smog. Particulates irritate and inflame people's eyes and airways, and long-term exposure can be permanently damaging, causing respiratory conditions, heart and lung diseases and premature death (PHE, 2018b).

Ground-level ozone

Petrol, solvents, perfumes, air fresheners, furniture, laminate flooring and other products release non-methane volatile organic compounds (NMVOCs) into the air. These react with other air pollutants in the presence of sunlight to produce ground-level ozone. Sunny hot weather, urban heat islands and anthropogenic activities such as industrial production and traffic escalate this process, as does the burning of fossil fuels to keep warm in cold weather. Ground-level ozone causes inflammation of the throat, lungs, nose, mouth and eyes, as well as damaging local ecosystems (DEFRA, 2019).

Petrol and diesel

Many fuels used for transport are significant producers of greenhouse gas emissions and air pollution. For example, petrol contained tetraethyl lead from the beginning of the motor industry, because it enhanced the performance of the internal combustion engine. When it became known that lead is a poison, the UK introduced non-leaded petrol in 1972. By the 1980s, leaded petrol was no longer used across most countries in the world, and vehicles using alternative fuels to petrol are now being developed (Yeh, 2007). Lead particulates can still be found in the air around metal smelting plants and the manufacturers of batteries, but cleaner recycling practices of lead-acid batteries are being introduced (Li *et al.*, 2019).

In a bid to reduce both lead pollution and carbon dioxide emissions, the UK Government initially encouraged people to trade in cars with petrol engines for those which run on diesel. However, in 2013, a series of motor industry scandals revealed diesel exhaust fumes contain both harmful gases (in terms of being respiratory irritants and excessive production of greenhouse gases) and particulates such as benzene, 1,3-butadiene, formaldehyde and polycyclic aromatic hydrocarbons, all of which are volatile organic compounds and major pollutants. In Paris, diesel cars are banned and in Madrid all vehicles are banned in the heart of the city. The UK government will ban sales of petrol and diesel cars by 2030. Currently, road tax is used to discourage UK drivers from owning higher-polluting cars. London motorists pay a 'congestion charge', which is more expensive for higher-polluting vehicles, and a vehicle ban is being considered in some areas of the country.

Tackling air pollution

The Daily Air Quality Index (DAQI) is an instrument used in the UK to measure air pollution levels (low, moderate, high or very high). When meteorological factors cause high levels of air pollution, the public may be advised to avoid being outside at certain peak times, to take less polluted routes to work and schools, and to keep doors and windows closed. Some may be advised to take medicines such as asthma inhalers as a preventative measure.

Managing air pollution requires political leadership, such as legislation like the UK's Clean Air Acts of 1956 and 2019, and new engineering solutions. Individuals can contribute by

- changing their travel behaviour
- planting more trees in urban areas
- avoiding the use of diesel-fuelled vehicles
- encouraging business and personal use of renewable energy
- increasing active travel (walking/cycling)

Built environment

The built environment consists of the buildings, roads, infrastructures that supply energy and those that remove waste. It may include elements of the natural environment such as fields and rivers. Over the last two centuries, towns and cities across the world have become environments densely populated with people. Today, more than half of the world's population reside in urban areas (UN, 2014). The planning and management of the built environment is an important influence on people's health and wellbeing.

Many modern towns and cities are built from materials such as tarmac, asphalt and concrete. These retain and reflect UV radiation and prevent water evaporating from the soil below. When buildings are built close together, the circulation of air is lowered. Anthropogenic heat, that is heat produced by human activities, adds to the collection of factors that create an urban heat island, an area that is significantly warmer than the surrounding natural environment. Today a built environment, an urban heat island, can be up to 10 degrees warmer than the neighbouring rural environment (Heaviside *et al.*, 2017). During heatwaves, the relentless heat and humidity can be lethal for older adults and children. Some people may use air conditioning, but air conditioning systems contribute to global warming because they release heat into the environment, and the energy required to run the system may depend on carbon-based fossil fuels.

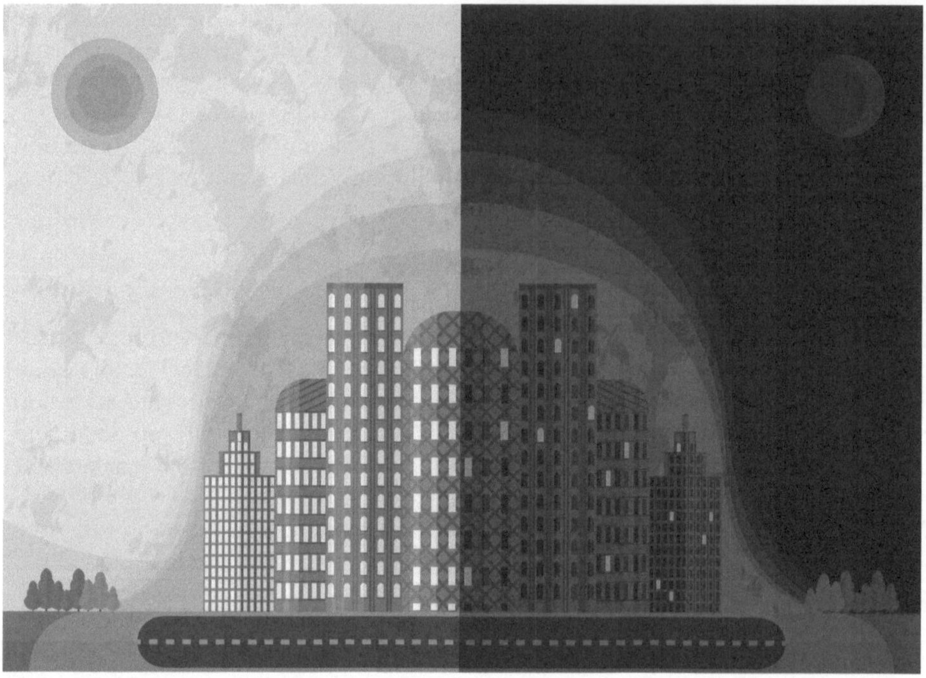

Figure 2.5 Urban heat island
Source: ValentinaKru/Shutterstock.com

Obesogenic environments

Obesogenic environments describe places that promote weight gain by encouraging the intake of calories and discouraging physical activity (Government Office for Science, 2007). These may be built environments where there is a wide choice of accessible, calorie-rich, convenience foods available through shops, markets, home deliveries, fast-food outlets and restaurants. They may also be the 'food deserts' that are found in socio-economically deprived areas, both urban and rural, where there are fewer options and a reliance on cheaper, high fat/sugar/calorie foods (Cummins and Macintyre, 2002). An obesogenic environment is also one that creates both real and perceived barriers to physical activity. Foster and Giles-Corti (2008) show how the interconnection of the physical/built environment, the social environment and individual factors can deter activity. For example, poor street lighting may deter people from going jogging due to their fears about personal safety. Weight gain is a key risk factor for diseases such as cardiovascular disease, cancer and type 2 diabetes.

Environments and health

Poor-quality housing is associated with poor health outcomes. In a study of UK data from 1996 to 2002, the housing factors which were significantly associated with worse mental and physical health, especially for women, included

- shortage of space
- noise from neighbours
- street noise
- too dark, not enough light
- lack of adequate heating facilities
- condensation
- damp walls, floors and foundation
- rot in window frames or floors
- pollution, grime or other environmental problems
- vandalism or crime in the area

(Pevalin *et al.*, 2008)

Green space is an important determinant of health (Pearce, 2017). Between 2007 and 2011, McEachan and colleagues (2016) found that pregnant women living in areas of little greenspace were significantly more likely to report depressive symptoms compared to those living in greener areas. Green and blue spaces, such as parks and lakes, are also important for stress relief (de Vries *et al.*, 2016).

A healthy built environment

A healthy built environment is one which recognises the multiple factors that impact on human health. For example, the UK's Healthy New Towns programme seeks to design environments which connect communities and promote health (NHS, 2018a): for example, by providing cycling lanes and a range of sports facilities, limiting takeaway hot food outlets, installing water fountains within parades of shops and initiatives to grow and cook local food.

Housing

Housing refers to the buildings or structures in which people live, providing a physical shelter and a psychosocial environment in which to feel safe and thrive. In the UK, poor housing has been linked to poor health outcomes that cost the National Health Service about £2.5 billion per year (Nicol *et al.*, 2015).

Physical structure of housing

Lead

The design, materials and construction of buildings can influence health. For example, lead has been linked to neurological and cardiovascular conditions (Sanders *et al.*, 2009; Navas-Acien *et al.*, 2007). Lead in paint dust can be inhaled and lead in pipes can be absorbed into the drinking water. In the southeast of England, naturally occurring calcium deposits tend to coat the inside of lead pipes, reducing the risks, but in the north, and especially the old industrial cities such as Manchester, the risks may be higher (Drinking Water Inspectorate, 2011). In the UK, it has been illegal to use lead pipes for drinking water since 1989, and where older houses are appropriately renovated and managed the risks for occupiers reduce.

Humidity and damp

Poor ventilation, badly fitting doors and windows, or a leaking roof are some of the structural problems that contribute to excess damp, condensation and poor air quality. Humid and damp environments support the growth of fungal spores which irritate people's airways and can be deadly for those with pre-existing health conditions, such as cystic fibrosis and asthma (NHS, 2018b). *Aspergillus*, a fungus normally found in compost heaps, can grow in heating and air conditioning systems. Inhaled *Aspergillus* spores can lead to aspergillosis, a debilitating condition that impedes breathing and causes a high body temperature, weight loss and the coughing of blood.

Carbon monoxide

Carbon monoxide is a colourless, odourless and tasteless gas that we can inhale with ease. It is a product of the incomplete burning of wood and the carbon-based fossil fuels: gas, oil, and coal. Poorly maintained boilers, coal fires and wood burners can produce carbon monoxide, and poor ventilation can enable it to accumulate (Green *et al.*, 1999). Once inhaled, it replaces the oxygen in red blood cells, causing dizziness, shortness of breath, tissue damage and potentially death (NHS, 2019).

Radon gas

Radon gas is a naturally occurring radioactive gas that emanates from rocks and soil. In the UK, most homes are exposed to low levels, but higher levels are found in areas rich in granite. Prolonged radon exposure is particularly harmful to lungs, kidneys and bone marrow (Keith *et al.*, 2012). It is responsible for 9% of lung cancer deaths in European countries and around 1,400 cases annually in the UK (Milner *et al.*, 2014), though not all cases emanate from radon in the home. We can prevent risks to health by good under-floor ventilation or the fitting of a radon sump which acts like an exhaust pipe, removing harmful gasses out of the ground and away from the house. Public Health England (2020) produces maps of radon levels for the UK and encourages the population to get their property tested if they live in a high-risk area.

Cold homes

Poorly insulated homes are expensive to heat and lose heat. They cause a range of health problems for their occupants. Marmot and colleagues (2011) found that cold homes in England were associated with a five-fold increase in mental health problems, in addition to increased numbers of winter deaths and exacerbations of ailments such as arthritis and asthma in the elderly and very young. The loss of heat from a house in a built environment will add to the urban heat island. Houses may not be adequately heated if the occupants experience fuel poverty. In England, this means that their fuel costs are above average, and it would leave them with a residual income below the poverty line (DEBIS, 2019). In 2017, 2.532 million (10.9%) households (10.9%) were classed as fuel poor, a slight decrease (0.2%) from the previous year (DEBIS, 2019).

The psychosocial environment of housing

The psychosocial environment relates to whether a house provides a sense of safety and security. It is about whether a house feels like a home. A house that is located within a well-lit neighbourhood, with low crime and neighbours who are perceived as trustworthy feels very different to one that is located within an area of high crime. For example, Mason and colleagues (2013) explored perceptions of safety and the impact on walkability in deprived neighbourhoods in Glasgow: people who felt safe tended to walk more.

Thinking point:

> If people feel they are living in an unsafe neighbourhood, consider how this may affect their behaviour and their health.

Homelessness, rough sleeping and changing accommodation

Homelessness is a situation where there is shelter but the place is not emotionally supportive, affordable, decent or secure, and human rights might not be met (Fitzpatrick and Watts, 2010). Homelessness can also include sofa surfing. According to Shelter (2006), being homeless is subtly different to rough sleeping, which refers to sleeping outdoors or in buildings that are not intended for habitation. The root causes of homelessness are both individual, such as anti-social behaviour, relationship breakdown, domestic violence, ill-health, substance misuse, debt and eviction, and structural, such as welfare reforms, poverty, job loss and a lack of affordable housing (MHCLG/DWP, 2019). Both homelessness and rough sleeping have catastrophic impacts on people's personal security, physical and mental health and their sense of autonomy.

Some people may avoid homelessness or rough sleeping, but they find themselves unwillingly moving accommodation because it is too expensive or being placed in emergency accommodation. Moving frequently is stressful. It often necessitates changing jobs, schools and registering with a new local general practice or health centre. Warfa and colleagues (2006) held discussion groups with 34 Somali refugees who had escaped from war and were living in London. Single people moved residence more frequently than families, but it took up to five years before most had permanent accommodation. Some moved from one deprived area to another deprived area with no improvement in their socio-economic environment. The experience of these forced moves felt chaotic, and they spoke of a sense of powerlessness, stress and significant disruption to family life. For example, one person said:

> ... someone who never wanted to come here but had to come here ... never registered with a G.P., having ... poor health ... he is moved again, there's no stability.... It might not create a physical health problem, but that is a major mental problem.
>
> (male, professional, Warfa 2006 p.510)

Housing stock

Housing stock refers to the total number of dwellings, including houses, flats, bungalows and maisonettes, in an area (Wilcox *et al.*, 2017). Recent reports from

Table 2.3 Advantages and disadvantages of building on brownfield and greenfield sites

Advantages	
Brownfield	*Greenfield*
Better for the environment as space and buildings are recycled. Cleaned of any industrial hazards left by previous industry and operations on that site (remediation). Addresses housing demands. Located in urban locations providing access to essential infrastructure: • water, energy and sewerage services • road and transport networks • amenities such as hospitals, schools and shops Can improve the look and feel of the existing urban environment. Easier to get planning permission as the land has been built on previously.	Sites may be cheaper to purchase. No cost for remediation. New builds do not need to take account of any old buildings that must be kept due to their heritage and architectural importance, addressing the needs of the future at an affordable rate. New builds and their location may have higher desirability.
Disadvantages	
Brownfield	*Greenfield*
Remediation is expensive. Contaminants from industrial processes may affect soil quality, affecting the growth of plants, and domestic pets/animals will not be able to graze within the garden. Demolishing and rebuilding former industrial buildings will need to be carefully managed to avoid contaminants harmful to health being released into the environment, potentially polluting air, land and water. The remaining district may continue to be industrialised, resulting in less desirability of the location. Conversely, development of the district may lead to desirability, affecting the affordability of house prices.	Potential to contribute to urban sprawl as towns and cities grow beyond their historic boundaries, making green sites less available and accessible within the locality. Costs to develop local infrastructure may be excessive and may not fall upon the builder but instead the regional authorities. Pre-existing communities may complain that they are being pushed out or resist change as they do not wish to see green spaces developed. Planning permission may be more difficult to achieve.

the UK Housing Review describe an overall shortage of housing stock, and there are parts of the country where the supply/demand varies significantly. In parts of England the quantity of housing stock is close to what is needed but the quality needs much improvement. Too often, the types of houses being built are unaffordable for the majority. Successive governments have recognised the need for a wide range of housing stock and there is much debate about whether it should be built on brownfield or greenfield sites. Brownfield land is typically former industrial sites which are now redundant and intended for redevelopment. Greenfield land is that which has been used as a public amenity or for agricultural purposes. There are advantages and disadvantages to building on both.

Location

The location of housing is vital to residents' health. If poorly planned, it can result in residents being hard to reach, isolated or unable to access healthy foods and employment. They could be living near roads that expose them to noise and air pollution.

Box 2.1 Billy Connelly living in Drumchapel

Billy Connelly, the Scottish comedian, was moved from a cramped Glasgow tenement when he was 14 years old.

> "Drumchapel seemed like a promised land at first ... but then the scales began to fall from our eyes. We started to feel very cheated. Because there were houses there but there was [nothing] else. There were no amenities whatsoever: no shops, cafés, pubs, cinemas, not even any churches. Nothing ... It was weird. There was nowhere to buy groceries. If we needed bread, or tea, we had to wait for the little green vans that operated as mobile shops to call around once a day. We'd avidly listen out for them in the same way that kids listen for ice-cream vans ... It was a crime ... We had nowhere to go or to let go of our emotions. We boys would gather in little gangs and just wander around the streets. We weren't looking for mischief – we were looking for something, anything, to do, before we gave up and all went off to bed. Even as a boy, it was obvious to me that things like cafés, cinemas and theatres are essential to a sane and normal life. If you live in a town with none of those things, a dullness descends on the place and an anger develops among the people. It felt like the council had played a dirty trick on us. It was as if they thought that all we people were good for was to go to work, come back home to our houses and quietly watch TV until we died. To me, it was a nasty way of thinking and it showed a real contempt for us. I think it would be a very good idea to make town planners live in the places that they plan."
>
> (Source: Connelly, 2018, p.31, 32)

Healthy housing

Housing Europe, the European Federation for Public, Cooperative and Social Housing, have a vision that all Europeans should have

> ... access to decent and affordable housing for all communities which are socially, economically and environmentally sustainable and where everyone is enabled to reach their full potential.
>
> (Pittini *et al.*, 2017 p.5)

Taylor (2018) argues there are four housing-related pathways that need to be addressed to improve people's health.

- Stability – no disruptions to employment, education, social networks and healthcare

- Quality and safety – no exposure to substandard housing such as damp, pests, cold, accident hazards or overcrowding
- Affordability – no stress related to finding the rent/mortgage, more income for fuel and other health essentials
- Neighbourhood – away from high-volume roads, near to public transport, pedestrian crossings, nutritious food outlets, social cohesion and support

Unhealthy environments, including the air and buildings, significantly contribute to poor health and major diseases.

A healthy environment

Barton's (2005) health map, shown in Chapter 1, shows a conceptual anthropocentric model of a healthy ecosystem, with people's health and wellbeing at the centre of seven spheres:

- global ecosystem – climate change, biodiversity
- natural environment – natural habitats, air, water, land
- built environment – buildings, places, streets, routes
- activities – working, shopping, moving, living, playing, learning
- local economy – wealth creation, finance markets
- community – social capital, social networks
- lifestyle – activity, diet, substance use

These are interacting spheres and all seven need to be considered when designing a healthy environment.

Thinking point:

Considering each of the seven spheres, what are the challenges to creating a healthy environment?

Environmental stewardship

Environmental stewardship means conserving, protecting and restoring natural ecosystems and their biodiversity. In England, the Department for Environment, Food and Rural Affairs (DEFRA) works closely with the administrations of Wales, Scotland and Northern Ireland, and acts on behalf of the UK on international matters. It is responsible for food, air and water along with safeguarding the natural environment. It works with agencies and statutory bodies to care for forestry, nature and water supplies to protect the environment and ensure its sustainability. This includes developing land that can cope with excessive flood waters, forestry management or enabling access for education.

Sustainability

The concept of sustainability recognises that the natural systems on earth, the ecosystems, are interconnected and resources are finite. There is concern that the way people are using the earth's resources is leading to a deterioration of the natural environment. This is fast reaching an ecological 'tipping point' which will make it harder for all living things to survive (Koons, 2012). Biodiversity, a variety of plants and animals, is vital for maintaining healthy ecosystems. For biodiversity to thrive, it requires clean air, soil and water and, in turn, these supply the nourishment needed by all living things. As these become disrupted or depleted, the ecosystems become imbalanced, and eventually clean air, soil, water, and then food, land security and energy become scarce. Human conflicts are likely to erupt over highly prized commodities and inequalities in health will widen.

Perhaps the most well recognised definition of sustainability is from the Report of the World Commission on Environment and Development: Our Common Future:

> Sustainable development is development that meets the needs of the present without compromising the ability of future generations to meet their own needs.
> (Bruntland 1987 p.41)

This report recognises that as the planet becomes more populated we place increased burdens upon it. Its ability to support the essential needs and living standards of people, especially those in developing economies, is at risk. Human economic activities, and activities which relate to how we live, often impact directly and negatively upon the environment. Therefore, sustainable development is about how humans can interact with the environment in new ways which maintain healthy ecosystems and life on earth is both equitable and peaceful.

Three pillars of sustainability

Sustainability is a global challenge for everyone. Since the 1980s there has been international consensus that any intended planned action needs to take into consideration its impact on society, the economy and the environment. These 'three pillars of sustainability' are visually presented as circles or pillars (Purvis *et al.*, 2018).

The 'three pillars' concept was embedded into the 2030 Agenda for Sustainable Development, which makes clear that sustainable initiatives must balance the need to foster social equity among and between communities, with the need to provide economic opportunities such as employment, and the need to protect the natural environment (UN, 2015b). This requires people to make complex decisions. Examples of sustainable initiatives include active travel, 'think global act local' and environmental stewardship.

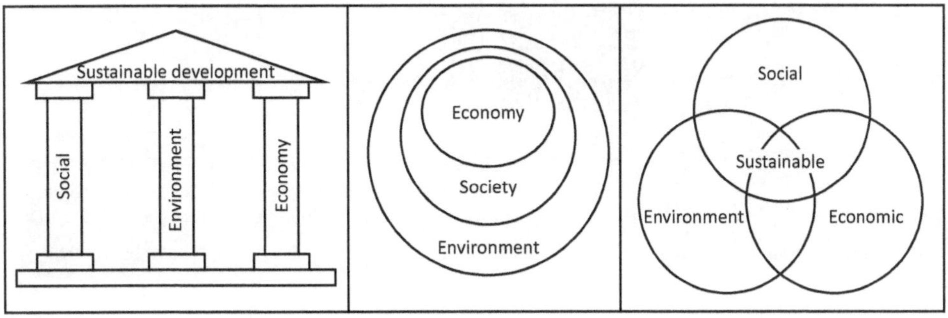

Figure 2.6 Three pillars of sustainability

Active travel

Active travel means replacing motorised transport with human activated travel, such as walking, cycling or scooting, which produce fewer air pollutants, less traffic congestion and fewer road traffic accidents (PHE, 2016). Active travel reduces sedentary behaviour, which is linked to a range of physical health conditions including obesity, and it has also been found to increase social contact and improve mental health (PHE, 2016).

'Think global act local'

'Think global act local' is a sustainability mantra, adopted from the environmental movements of the late 1960s, that encourages individuals and corporations to consider the global impact of their actions. For individuals, it means to recycle, reuse, repair, share, or restore objects to cut down on the number of items produced and subsequently discarded, because this helps sustainable growth. For businesses, it means taking 'corporate social responsibility' for the impact of their activities on the community and environment. This includes reducing the amount of greenhouse gases that their activities produce, otherwise known as their 'carbon footprint'; introducing an ethical supply chain which means ensuring fair wages, having responsible employment practices; and ensuring that raw materials are 'responsibly sourced', meaning that they are not being grown, produced or made, in a way that has a negative impact on the planet.

Sustainable development goals

The United Nations (2015b) set out the 17 sustainable development goals in their 2030 Agenda for Sustainable Development. These aim to tackle climate change,

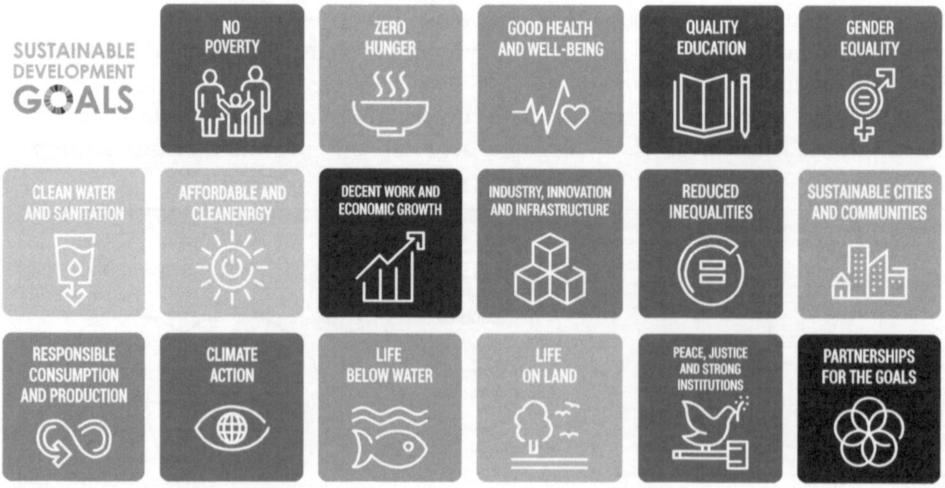

Figure 2.7 Sustainable development goals
Source: ALX1618/Shutterstock.com

Table 2.4 Sustainable development goals

1	No poverty	End poverty in all its forms everywhere
2	Zero hunger	End hunger, achieve food security and improved nutrition and promote sustainable agriculture
3	Good health and wellbeing	Ensure healthy lives and promote wellbeing for all at all ages
4	Quality education	Ensure inclusive and equitable quality education and promote life-long learning opportunities for all
5	Gender equality	Achieve gender equality and empower all women and girls
6	Clean water and sanitation	Ensure availability and sustainable management of water and sanitation for all
7	Affordable and clean energy	Ensure access to affordable, reliable, sustainable and modern energy for all
8	Decent work and economic growth	Promote sustained inclusive and sustainable economic growth, full and productive employment and decent work for all
9	Industry, innovation and infrastructure	Build resilient infrastructure, promote inclusive and sustainable industrialisation and foster innovation
10	Reduced inequalities	Reduce inequality within and among countries
11	Sustainable cities	Make cities and human settlements inclusive, safe, resilient and sustainable
12	Responsible consumption and production	Ensure sustainable consumption and production patterns
13	Climate action	Take urgent action to combat climate change and its impacts
14	Life below water	Conserve and sustainably use the oceans, seas and marine resources for sustainable development
15	Life on land	Protect, restore and promote sustainable use of terrestrial ecosystems, sustainably manage forests, combat desertification, and halt and reverse land degradation and halt biodiversity loss
16	Peace, justice and strong institutions	Promote peaceful and inclusive societies for sustainable development, provide access to justice for all and build effective, accountable and inclusive institutions at all levels
17	Partnerships for the goals	Strengthen the means of implementation and revitalise the global partnership for sustainable development

Source: Adapted from UN (2015b p.14).

reduce poverty and deprivation, improve health, education, and economic growth, and reduce inequalities.

Summary

This chapter has

- defined climate change and explained why it is a global public health priority
- described the factors that create and reduce air pollution
- examined how the built environment impacts people's health
- discussed how housing affects people's health through its physical structures, its role as a psychosocial environment and location
- illustrated the characteristics of a healthy environment, including sustainability

Further reading

Friis, R.H. (2012) *Essentials of environmental health*. 2nd edn. London: Jones and Bartlett

Pruss-Ustun, A., Wolf, J., Corvalan, C., Bos, R., and Neira, M. (2016) *Preventing disease through healthy environments: a global assessment of the burden of disease from environmental risks*. Geneva: World Health Organization

Useful websites

Bristol Health Partners *Supporting healthy inclusive neighbourhood environments (SHINE)*. Available at: www.bristolhealthpartners.org.uk/health-integration-teams/supporting-healthy-inclusive-neighbourhood-environments-hit

World Health Organization *Climate change*. Available at: www.who.int/health-topics/climate-change

References

Barton, H. (2005) 'A health map for urban planners. Towards a conceptual model for healthy, sustainable settlements', *Built Environment*, 31(4), pp.339–355

Brundtland, G.H. (1987) Report of the World Commission on Environment and Development: Our Common Future, The World Commission on Environment and Development. Available at: www.un-documents.net/our-common-future.pdf (Accessed 12th April 2018)

Bunker, A., Wildenhain, J., Vandenbergh, A., Henschke, N., Rocklöv, J., Hajat, S., and Sauerborn. R. (2016) 'Effects of air temperature on climate-sensitive mortality and morbidity outcomes in the elderly; a systematic review and meta-analysis of epidemiological evidence', *EBioMedicine*, 6, pp.258–268

Campbell-Lendrum, D., Manga, L., Bagayoko, M., and Sommerfeld, J. (2015) 'Climate change and vector-borne diseases: what are the implications for public health research and policy?' *Philosophical Transactions of The Royal Society B Biological Sciences*, 370(1665) doi.org:10.1098/rstb.2013.0552

Cancer Research UK (2020) *Sun, UV and cancer*. Available at: www.cancerresearchuk.org/about-cancer/causes-of-cancer/sun-uv-and-cancer (Accessed 9th April 2020)

Connelly, B. (2018) *My grand adventures in a wee country*. London: Penguin/Random House

Cummins, S., and Macintyre, S. (2002) ' "Food deserts" evidence and assumption in health policy making', *BMJ*, 325(7361), pp.436–438

Department of Energy and Climate Change (2012) UK Energy in Brief 2012. Available at: www.decc.gov.uk/en/content/cms/statistics/publications/brief/brief.aspx (Accessed 9th April 2020)

Department of Energy, Business and Industrial Strategy (2019) Annual fuel poverty statistics in England, 2019 (2017 data). *Office of National Statistics*. Available at: https://assets.publishing.service.gov.uk/government/uploads/system/uploads/attachment_data/file/829006/Annual_Fuel_Poverty_Statistics_Report_2019__2017_data_.pdf (Accessed 5th September 2019)

Department for Environment and Rural Affairs (2019) *Clean air strategy 2019*. London: Department for Environment and Rural Affairs, Department for Business, Energy and Industrial Strategy, Department for Transport, Department of Health and Social Care, HM Treasury, Ministry of Housing, Communities and Local Government

de Vries, S., ten Have, M., van Dorsselaer, S., van Wezep, M., Hermans, T., and de Graaf, R. (2016) 'Local availability of green and blue space and prevalence of common mental disorders in the Netherlands', *British Journal of Psychiatry Open*, 2(6), pp.366–372

Drinking Water Inspectorate (2011) Drinking water 2010: public water supplies in the Northern region of England. DEFRA July 2011. Available at: http://dwi.defra.gov.uk/about/annual-report/2010/northern.pdf (Accessed 13th November 2019)

Environmental Protection Agency (2017) *Causes of climate change*. Available at: https://19january2017snapshot.epa.gov/climate-change-science/causes-climate-change_.html (Accessed 5th April 2020)

European Centre for Disease Prevention and Control (2019) *West Nile virus in Europe in 2019 – human cases, updated 30 August*. Available at: https://ecdc.europa.eu/en/publications-data/west-nile-virus-europe-2019-human-cases-updated-30-august (Accessed 6th September 2019)

Fitzpatrick, S., and Watts, B. (2010) 'The "right to housing" for homeless people', in O'Sullivan, E., Busch-Geertsema, D., Quilgars, D., and Pleace, N. (eds) *Homelessness research in Europe*. Brussels: FEANTSA, pp.105–122

Foster, S., and Giles-Corti, B. (2008) 'The built environment, neighbourhood crime and constrained physical activity: an exploration of inconsistent findings', *Preventive Medicine*, 47(3), pp.241–251

Gasparrini, A., Guo, Y., Hashizume, M., Lavigne, E., Zanobetti, A., Schwartz, J., Tobias, A., Tong, S., Rocklöv, J., and Forsberg, B. (2015) 'Mortality risk attributable to high and low ambient temperature: a multicountry observational study', *Lancet*, 386 (9991), pp.369–375

Government Office for Science (2007) *Foresight. Tackling obesities: future choices – project report*. London: Department for Innovation, Universities and Skills

Green, E., Short, S., Shuker, L.K., and Harrison, P.T.C. (1999) 'Carbon monoxide exposure in the home environment and the evaluation of risks to health – a UK perspective', *Indoor Built Environment*, 8(3), pp.168–175

Hanna, E., Hall, R.J., and Overland, J.E. (2017) 'Can artic warming influence UK extreme weather?' *Royal Meteorological Society*, 72(11), pp.346–352

Heaviside, C., Macintyre, H., and Vardoulakis, S. (2017) 'The urban heat island: implications for health in a changing environment', *Current Environmental Health Reports*, 4(3), pp.296–305

Highwood, E. (2018) Aerosols and climate, Royal Meteorological Society. Available at: www.rmets.org/resource/aerosols-and-climate (Accessed 12th April 2020)

H.M. Government (2017) The clean growth strategy. Available at: https://assets.publishing.service.gov.uk/government/uploads/system/uploads/attachment_data/file/700496/clean-growth-strategy-correction-april-2018.pdf (Accessed 9th April 2020)

House of Commons Environmental Audit Committee (2018) Heat waves: adapting to climate change. Ninth report of session 2017–19. Available at: https://publications.parliament.uk/pa/cm201719/cmselect/cmenvaud/826/826.pdf (Accessed 12th April 2020)

Intergovernmental Panel on Climate Change (1988) *Climate Change: the IPCC scientific assessment*. Cambridge: Cambridge University Press

Intergovernmental Panel on Climate Change (2014) Climate change 2014: impacts, adaptation and vulnerability. Available at: www.ipcc.ch/report/ar5/wg2/ (Accessed 6th April 2020)

Intergovernmental Panel on Climate Change (2018) Global warming of 1.5. Available at: www.ipcc.ch/sr15/ (Accessed 12th April 2020)

Jones, H. (2018) 'Snow disruption continues with roads, railways, hospitals and airports hit – as happened. Summary', *The Guardian*, 3rd March 2018. Available at: www.theguardian.com/uk-news/live/2018/mar/02/uk-weather-snow-disruption-storm-emma-beast-from-the-east-live (Accessed 7th April 2020)

Keith, S., Doyle, J.R., Harper, C., Mumtaz, M., Tarrago, O., Wohlers, D.W., Diamond, G.L., Citra, M., and Barbar, L.E. (2012) *Toxicological profile for Radon*. Atlanta: Agency for Toxic Substances and Disease Registry

Knight, S. (2011) Climatic systems. *Royal Geographic Society*. Available at: www.rgs.org/schools/teaching-resources/dr-sylvia-knight-answers-questions-on-climatic-sys/ (Accessed 1st May 2019)

Koons, J.E. (2012) 'At the tipping point: defining an Earth Jurisprudence for social and ecological justice', *Loyola Law Review*, 58(2), pp.349–390

Le Treut, H., Somerville, R., Cubasch, U., Ding, Y., Mokssit, A., Peterson, T., Prather, M., Qin, D., Manning, M., Chen, A., Marquis, M., Averyt, K., Tignor, M., Miller, H.L., and Solomon S. (2007) 'Historical overview of climate change science' in *Contribution of Working Group I to the Fourth Assessment Report of the Intergovernmental Panel on Climate Change*. Available at: www.ipcc.ch/report/ar4/wg1/ (Accessed 9th April 2020)

Li, M., Yang, J., Liang, S., Houa, H., Hua, H., Liua, B., and Kumard, R.V. (2019) 'Review on clean recovery of discarded/spent lead-acid battery and trends of recycled products', *Journal of Power Sources*, 436(1) doi:10.1016/j.jpowsour.2019.226853

Marmot, M., Geddes, I., Bloomer, E., Allen, J., and Goldblatt, P. (2011) The health impacts of cold homes and fuel poverty. Available at: https://friendsoftheearth.uk/sites/default/files/downloads/cold_homes_health.pdf (Accessed 7th September 2018)

Maslow, A. (1943) 'A theory of human motivation', *Psychological Review*, 50(4), pp.370–396

Mason, P., Kearns, A., and Livingston, M. (2013) '"Safe going": the influence of crime rates and peceived crime and safety on walking in deprived neighbourhoods', *Social Science and Medicine*, 91C:15–24 doi:10.1016/j.socscimed.2013.04.011

McEachan, R.R.C., Prady, S.L., Smith, G., Fairley, L., Cabieses, B., Gidlow, C., Wright, J., Dadvand, P., van Gent, D., and Nieuwenhuijsen, M.J. (2016) 'The association between green space and depressive symptoms in pregnant women: moderating roles of socioeconomic status and physical activity', *Journal of Epidemiology and Community Health*, 70(3), pp.253–259

Medlock, J.M., and Leach, S.A (2015) 'Effect of climate change on vector-borne disease risk in the UK', *Lancet Infectious Disease*, 15(6), pp.721–730

Milner, J., Shrubsole, C., Das, P., Jones, B., Ridley, I., Zaid, C., Hamilton, I., Armstrong, B., Davies, M., and Wilkinson, P. (2014) 'Home energy efficiency and radon related risk of lung cancer: modelling study', *BMJ*, 348 doi:10.1136/bmj.f7493

Ministy of Housing, Communities and Local Government and Department for Work and Pensions (2019) Cause of homelessness and rough sleeping: rapid evidence assessment. Available at: www.gov.uk/government/publications/causes-of-homelessness-and-rough-sleeping-feasibility-study (Accessed 13th November 2019)

National Research Council (2010) *Advancing the science of climate change*. Washington DC: The National Academies Press

Navas-Acien, A., Guallar, E., Silbergeld, E.K., and Rothenberg, S.J. (2007) 'Lead exposure and cardiovascular disease – systematic review', *Environmental Health Perspectives*, 115(3), pp.472–482

National Geographic Society (2019) Causes and effects of climate change. Available at: www.nationalgeographic.com/environment/global-warming/global-warming-causes/n (Accessed 20th April 2020)

National Health Service (2018a) Healthy by design? The healthy new towns network prospectus. Available at: www.england.nhs.uk/wp-content/uploads/2018/01/healthy-by-design-healthy-new-towns-network-prospectus.pdf (Accessed 13th November 2019)

National Health Service (2018b) Available at: www.nhs.uk/conditions/aspergillosis/ (Accessed 11th November 2019)

National Health Service (2019) Carbon monoxide poisoning. Available at: www.nhs.uk/conditions/carbon-monoxide-poisoning/ (Accessed 13th November 2019)

Nicol, S., Roys, M., and Garrett, H. (2015) The cost of poor housing to the NHS. BRE Trust. Available at: www.bre.co.uk/filelibrary/pdf/87741-Cost-of-Poor-Housing-Briefing-Paper-v3.pdf (Accessed 9th April 2020)

Pearce, J. (2017) The great outdoors: why green space is a determinant for health throughout life. Available at: https://vhscotland.org.uk/wp-content/uploads/2017/11/Jamie-Pearce-University-of-Edinburgh.pdf (Accessed 13th May 2020)

Pevalin, D.J., Taylor, M.P., and Todd, J. (2008) 'The dynamics of unhealthy housing in the UK: a panel data analysis', *Housing Studies*, 23(5), pp.679–695

Pittini, A., Koessl, G., Dijol, J., Lakatos, E., and Ghekiere, L. (2017) The state of housing in the EU 2017. Housing Europe. Available at: www.housingeurope.eu/resource-1000/the-state-of-housing-in-the-eu-2017 (Accessed 9th April 2020)

Public Health England (2016) Working together to promote active travel: a briefing for local authorities. Available at: https://assets.publishing.service.gov.uk/government/uploads/system/uploads/attachment_data/file/523460/Working_Together_to_Promote_Active_Travel_A_briefing_for_local_authorities.pdf (Accessed 13th November 2019)

Public Health England (2018a) Lyme disease epidemiology and surveillance. Available at: www.gov.uk/government/publications/lyme-borreliosis-epidemiology/lyme-borreliosis-epidemiology-and-surveillance (Accessed 10th July 2019)

Public Health England (2018b) Health matters: air pollution. Available at: www.gov.uk/government/publications/health-matters-air-pollution/health-matters-air-pollution (Accessed 6th September 2019)

Public Health England (2019) Heatwave plan for England. Available at: https://assets.publishing.service.gov.uk/government/uploads/system/uploads/attachment_data/file/801539/Heatwave_plan_for_England_2019.pdf (Accessed 9th April 2020)

Public Health England (2020) UK maps of radon. Available at: www.ukradon.org/information/ukmaps (Accessed 8th April 2020)

Purvis, B., Mao, Y., and Robinson, D. (2018) 'Three pillars of sustainability: in search of conceptual origins', *Sustainability Science*, 14(101), pp.681–695

Royal College of Physicians (2016) Every *breath* we take: the lifelong impact of air pollution. Available at: www.rcplondon.ac.uk/projects/outputs/every-breath-we-take-lifelong-impact-air-pollution (Accessed 18th February 2019)

Royal Meteorological Society (2018) *Climate: what is climate change?* Available at: www.rmets.org/resource/what-climate-change (Accessed 1st May 2019)

Sanders, T., Liu, Y., Buchner, V., and Tchounwou, P.B. (2009) 'Neurotoxic effects and biomarkers of lead exposure: a review'. *Reviews on Environmental Health*, 24(1), pp.15–45

Shelter (2006) Street homelessness. Available at: https://england.shelter.org.uk/__data/assets/pdf_file/0011/48458/Factsheet_Street_Homelessness_Aug_2006.pdf (Accessed 9th April 2020)

Smith, S., Elliot, A.J., Hajat, S., Bone, A., Smith, G.E., and Kovats, S. (2015) 'Estimating the burden of heat illness in England during the 2013 summer heatwave using syndromic surveillance', *Journal of Epidemiology and Community Health*, 70(5), pp.459–465

Steffen, W., Rockström, J., Richardson, K., Lenton, T.M., Folke, C., Liverman, D., Summerhayes, C.P., Barnosky, A.D., Cornell, S.E., Crucifix, M., Donges, J.F., Fetzer, I., Lade, S.J., Scheffer, M., Winkelmann, R., and Schellnhuber, H.J. (2018) 'Trajectories of the earth system in the anthropocene', *Proceedings of the National Academy of Sciences*, 115(33), pp.8252–8259

Taylor, L.A. (2018) 'Housing and health: an overview of the literature', *Health Affairs Health Policy Brief*, June 7th doi:10.1377/hpb20180313.396577

United Nations (2014) World's population increasingly urban with more than half living in urban areas. Available at www.un.org/en/development/desa/news/population/world-urbanization-prospects-2014.html (Accessed 6th September 2019)

United Nations (2015a) Paris Agreement. Available at: https://unfccc.int/files/essential_background/convention/application/pdf/english_paris_agreement.pdf (Accessed 9th April 2020)

United Nations (2015b) Transforming our world: the 2030 agenda for sustainable development. Available at: www.un.org/ga/search/view_doc.asp?symbol=A/RES/70/1&Lang=E (Accessed 23rd November 2019)

United Nations Climate Change (2018) Katowice Climate Change Conference – December 2018. Available at: https://unfccc.int/process-and-meetings/conferences/katowice-climate-change-conference-december-2018/katowice-climate-change-conference-december-2018 (Accessed 6th September 2019)

United Nations Refugee Agency (2004) UNHCR steps up response to Asian tsunami catastrophe. Available at: www.unhcr.org/news/press/2004/12/41d2c9374/unhcr-steps-response-asian-tsunami-catastrophe.html (Accessed 5th September 2019)

Warfa, N., Bhui, K., Craig, T., Curtis, S., Mohamud, S., Stansfeld, S., McCrone, P., and Thornicroft, G. (2006) 'Post-migration geographical mobility, mental health and health service utilisation among Somali refugees in the UK: a qualitative study', *Health & Place*, 12(4), pp.503–515

Watts, N., Adger, W., Agnolucci, P., *et al.* (2015) 'Health and climate change: policy responses to protect public health', *Lancet*, 386 (10006), pp.1861–1914

Wilcox, S., Perry, J., Stephens, M., and Williams, P. (2017) 2017 UK housing review. Briefing paper. Chartered Institute of Housing. Available at: www.cih.org/resources/PDF/1UKHR%20briefing%202017.pdf (Accessed 13th November 2019)

Yeh, S. (2007) 'An empirical analysis on the adoption of alternative fuel vehicles: the case of natural gas vehicles', *Energy Policy*, 35(11), pp.5865–5875

Yu, W., Mengersen, K., Wang, X., Ye, X., Guo, Y., Pan, X., and Tong., S. (2012) 'Daily average temperature and mortality among the elderly: a meta-analysis and systematic review of epidemiological evidence', *International Journal of Biometeorology*, 56(4), pp.569–581

3 Inequalities in health

Sally Robinson, Athene Lane-Martin and Elisabetta Corvo

Key points

- Introduction
- Health inequalities and health inequities
- Examples of inequalities in health
- Causes of inequalities in health
- Why health equality matters
- Summary

Introduction

When we are born, we do not share equal chances of good health and a long life. This chapter will show how some parts of the population suffer poorer health from all conditions, and a greater number of early deaths, than other parts of the population. It will discuss the social causes of these inequalities. Many believe that inequalities in people's health experiences are unfair and reducing them has become a major focus for how we protect and promote the population's health today.

Health inequalities and health inequities

Health inequalities

Health inequalities are differences in health status between individuals, groups or populations. Inequalities in health occur because of the unequal distribution of the social determinants of health, summarised as money, power and resources (World Health Organization, 2018).

Social gradient of health

People's social position tends to reflect their money, power and/or resources. When we plot people's social position against people's health, we see a social gradient. The higher the social position, the better experience of health they will have. Those who have a lower social position experience poorer health and earlier deaths. We call the difference between the top and the bottom of the social gradient of health the 'health gap'.

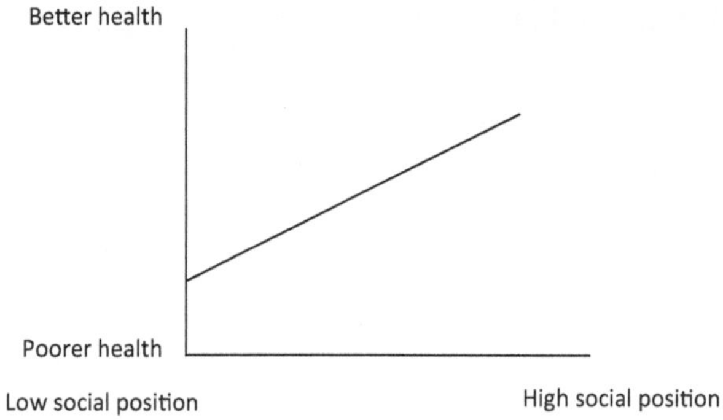

Figure 3.1 The social gradient of health

Health inequities

Inequalities in people's health are important because they are associated with people's whole life chances. Some people are doomed to a shorter life and greater ill health due to social factors that are beyond their control. These are not merely differences, but the differences are unfair, unjust, and politically, socially and economically unacceptable (WHO, 2008; 2010; Marmot, 2010). The World Health Organization makes clear,

> Health inequities are *avoidable* inequalities in health between groups of people … [that] arise from inequalities within and between societies.
>
> (WHO, 2018)

To achieve health equity for all, the World Health Organization (2008; 2010) believes that the world needs to work towards becoming a more equal society in order that all people can have equal chances of experiencing a long and healthy life.

> *A social gradient in health can be seen when we plot people's social position against their health experiences. To many, these health inequalities are unfair, health inequities.*

Examples of inequalities in health

We measure people's health in many ways such as by age at death, number of years of healthy life, amount of diseases, quality of life or by indicators of wellbeing. To demonstrate some inequalities in health, we have used the measures of life expectancy, early death rates, limitations to day-to-day activities due to a health problem or disability, and self-reporting of poor health or disability. Health inequalities are found between places and between people.

Inequalities in health between places

People who live in different places have different experiences of health.

International inequalities

Table 3.1 shows current forecasts for life expectancy, meaning the average number of years that people in different countries are expected to live. People's greater wealth seems to be associated with longer life expectancy. However, Sweden has a higher life expectancy than the wealthier United States of America, which suggests that other factors might be involved.

Regional inequalities

Estimates of people's life expectancy, at time of birth, vary according to where someone is born. Recent data shows those born in the south east are expected to live longer than the England average, and those born in the north east are expected to have shorter lives (Figure 3.2).

Life expectancy also varies according to whether someone lives in a more, or less, deprived area. Deprivation includes lower incomes, higher unemployment, lower skills and educational attainment, higher rates of premature deaths and lower quality of life, more crime, poor access to housing and services and a poor-quality indoor and outdoor environment (Ministry of HCLG, 2019). The Office of National Statistics (2018a) divided both England and Wales, separately, into 10 divisions, deciles, based on greater and lesser deprivation. Each decile represents 10% of the population. They compared the least deprived areas with the most deprived areas.

- In England, males born in the least deprived areas could expect to live 9.3 years longer, and females 7.4 years longer, than those born in the most deprived areas.

Table 3.1 World comparisons of wealth per person versus life expectancy

Country	*World ranking according to wealth per person* (GDP per capita in international dollars)*	*Life expectancy***
Qatar	1 (134,623)	78.1 years
United States of America	12 (64,767)	78.5 years
Sweden	18 (54,071)	82.4 years
United Kingdom	29 (46,782)	81.4 years
Bangladesh	142 (4,993)	72.7 years
Liberia	185 (1,423)	62.9 years
Central African Republic	190 (746)	53 years

Sources: Adapted from *Ventura (2019); **World life expectancy (2018).

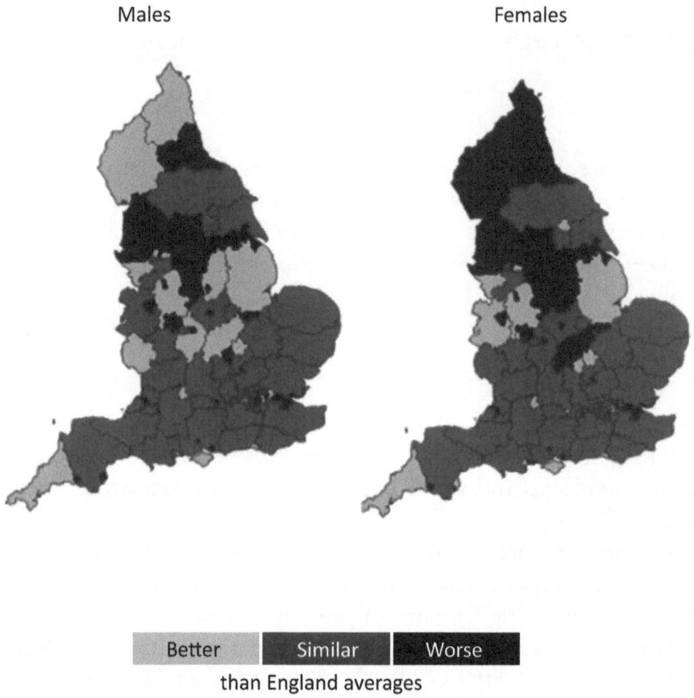

Figure 3.2 Health inequalities in England based on life expectancy at birth 2015 to 2017
Source: PHE, 2019a. Reproduced under the terms of the Open Government Licence v.3.0

- In Wales, males born in the least deprived areas could expect to live 8.9 years longer, and females 7.3 years longer, than those born in the most deprived areas.
- When the Office of National Statistics estimated healthy life expectancy, that is years lived in very good or good health, they found a gap between the least and most deprived areas of more than 18 years for people in England and more than 17 years for those in Wales.

Men born in the relatively deprived area of Tower Hamlets in London are expected to live to an average age of 79.3 years (PHE, 2019b) and men born in Kensington and Chelsea, a very wealthy area only nine miles (14.4 kilometres) away, can expect to live to about 83.3 years (PHE, 2019c). Table 3.2 shows that more people die at a relatively young age in Tower Hamlets than in Kensington and Chelsea, from a range of conditions. In thinking about the reasons for these inequalities, we might consider social determinants of health such as deprivation, income and employment.

Table 3.2 Inequalities in health between Tower Hamlets and Kensington and Chelsea, 2019

	Tower Hamlets	*Kensington and Chelsea*
Death rates		
(age-standardised rate per 100,000 population under 75 years of age)		
Deaths under 75 years from all causes	361.1	245.7
Deaths from cardiovascular disease under 75 years	94.3	43.5
Deaths from cancer under 75 years	123.7	102.6
Socio-economic determinants of health		
Deprivation score	35.7	23.4
Children (under 16) in low-income families	30.3% of population	20.5% of population
Employment rate (16–64)	73% of population	61.7% of population
Health-related behaviour		
Hospital admission rate for alcohol-related conditions*	492.6	476.1
Smoking prevalence in adults (18 years and over)	20.3% of population	14.9% of population
Physically active adults (19 years and over)	67.2% of population	72.8% of population
Excess weight in adults (18 years and over)	49.1% of population	50% of population

Note: *age-standardised rate per 100,000 population

Sources: Public Health England (2019b; 2019c).

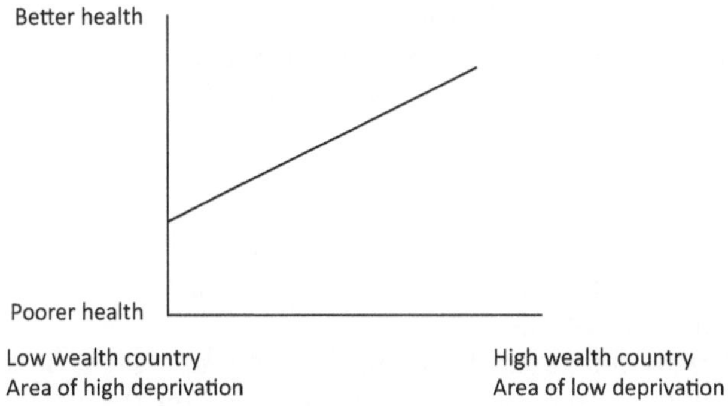

Figure 3.3 Examples of the social gradient of health between places

Health-related behaviours in places

People living in Tower Hamlets have worse health-related behaviours in terms of excess alcohol, smoking and low levels of physical activity, compared to Kensington and Chelsea. They also have a higher proportion of overweight people, a risk factor for poor health. This pattern is mirrored across England, where we see a relationship

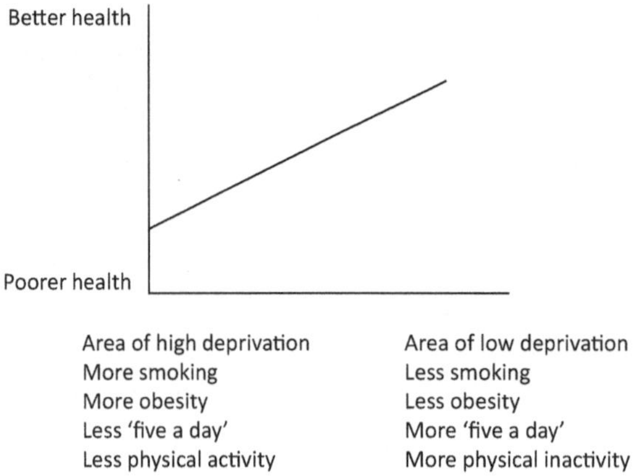

Figure 3.4 Examples of the social gradient of health between places and health-related behaviours

between geographical areas of deprivation, shorter lives lived in good health, and higher levels of smoking, obesity, poorer consumption of fruit and vegetables ('five a day') and physical inactivity (ONS, 2017a).

> *We find inequalities in health when we compare people who live in different places.*

Inequalities in health between people

We also find inequalities when comparing one group of people with another group of people, even when they live in the same geographical area. Here we consider ethnicity, sex, gender, education, income, occupation and socio-economic position.

Ethnicity

People's race normally refers to biological or physical differences between groups of people, whereas ethnicity is a broader concept relating to nationality, citizenship, colour, race, language, religion and customs.

Bhopal and colleagues (2018) compared deaths in Scotland across 13 different ethnic groups of people. They found that death rates were lower, for the same age, among the 12 ethnic minority groups compared to the majority White Scottish population. The Chinese had the lowest death rates of all. The authors concluded that place of birth, inside or outside of the UK or the Republic of Ireland, and people's health-related behaviours seem to explain some of the differences between ethnic groups in Scotland.

The Scottish Government (2015) looked at how different ethnic groups in Scotland answered a question on the Census, "Are your day-to-day activities limited because

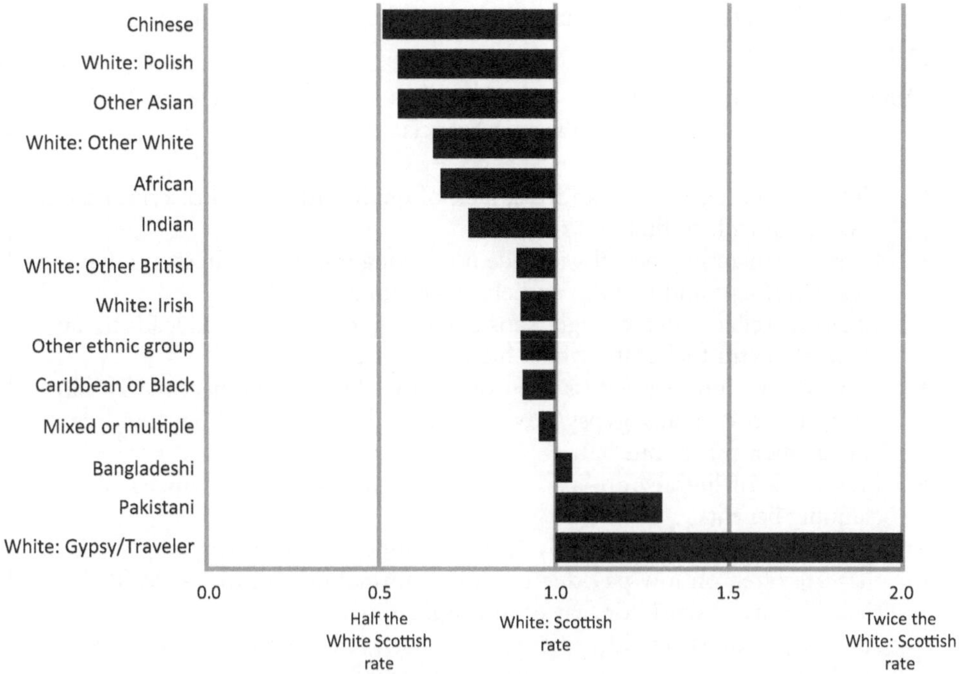

Figure 3.5 Ethnic inequalities in health for women, 2011 – age-standardised ratios of long-term limiting health problem or disability for ethnic groups compared to the 'White Scottish' group

Source: Scottish Government, 2015 p.5. Reproduced under the terms of the Open Government Licence v3.0

of a health problem or disability which has lasted, or is expected to last, at least 12 months?" Women from the Bangladeshi, Pakistani and gypsy/traveller groups reported experiencing limitations to their daily activities due to poor health more than the White Scottish population (Figure 3.5). The remaining 10 ethnic groups reported limitations less frequently than the White Scottish population. Among men, only the Pakistani and gypsy/traveller populations reported higher rates of poor health or disability than the male White Scottish group.

The gypsy/travellers in Scotland appeared to experience the worst health. They reported poor health three and a half times more than the White Scottish group. Gypsy/travellers also compared poorly to the rest of the population in terms of accommodation (housing/sites), literacy, school education outcomes, poverty, discrimination and a lack of trust in services (Scottish Government, 2013; The Social Marketing Gateway, 2013). The Scottish Government set up a Ministerial Working Group and invited gypsy/travellers to contribute. Box 3.1 presents a summary what two gypsy/travellers told the committee about their lives.

Box 3.1 Gypsy/travellers' presentation to the Scottish Ministerial Working Group

Ministerial Working Group on Gypsy/Travellers Minutes: 4th October 2018
"Mary Jean Williamson and Virginia Francis told the group:

- Not having a permanent address, lack of qualifications and discrimination make it difficult to find work
- Barriers to claiming benefits include not having proof of address, not having a bank account and moving on before a claim is completed
- Gypsy/travellers can face higher costs of living: moving around leads to days off work, extra fuel costs, which increases poverty
- Reliance on internet access is problematic. Sites don't necessarily have internet access, many gypsy/travellers don't have smart phones and can't afford credit for mobile data
- Low levels of literacy are also a barrier to accessing employment, and to claiming benefits
- Where gypsy/travellers (mainly women) work in mainstream employment, they are often on low pay due to lack of formal qualifications. Many hide their identity at work for fear of discrimination
- An address sometimes identifies as a gypsy/traveller site which can also lead to discrimination, especially in relation to employment
- Barriers to traditional forms of employment are getting worse, and it is becoming impossible to make a living, e.g. requirements for a registered address for trading standards, requirement for formal qualifications, cold-calling laws
- Information that is used in relation to gypsy/travellers may not be up to date, for example information quoted about number of sites is out of date as some have closed recently
- Also need to look more at housing need for gypsy/travellers – overcrowding on current sites is a big issue. The biggest problem in relation to poverty is adequate provision of permanent accommodation to meet gypsy/travellers' needs
- Gypsy/travellers don't know where to go for help. Trust in services or individuals providing support is critical and takes time to build."

(Source: Scottish Government, 2018. Reproduced with permission from the Chair of the Working Group)

Thinking point:

> What social determinants of health might explain why the gypsy/traveller population suffered poorer health and deaths at a younger age, compared to the other 12 ethnic groups?

Sex and gender

According to the UK Government (ONS, 2019a),

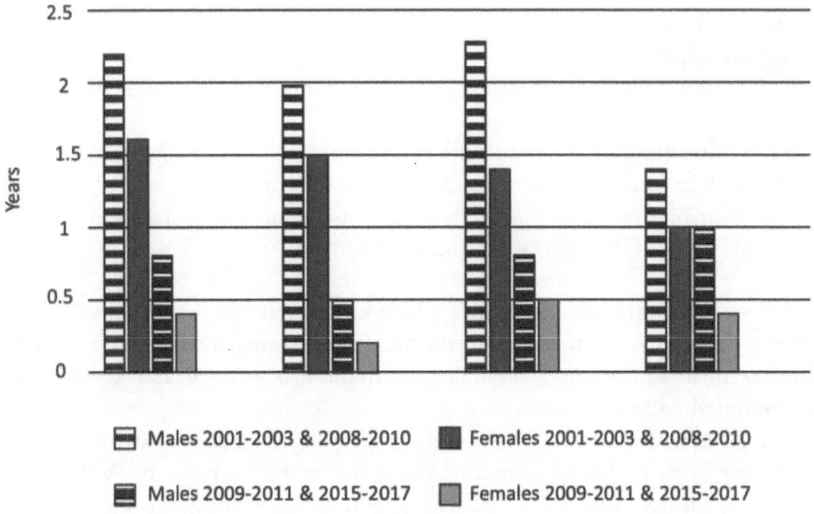

Figure 3.6 The gain in life expectancy at birth for UK males and females 2001 to 2003 and 2008 to 2010 compared to 2009 to 2011 and 2015 to 2017

Source: adapted from ONS, 2018b p. 4, 5

Table 3.3 Sex differences in life expectancy, healthy life expectancy and disability-free life expectancy in the UK

	Males	*Females*	*Difference*
Mean age of death/life expectancy at birth (years)			
1980–1982	71	77	6
1985–1987	71.9	77.7	5.8
1990–1992	73.1	78.7	5.6
1995–1997	74.2	79.1	4.9
2000–2002	75.6	80.3	4.7
2005–2007	77.1	81.4	4.3
2010–2012	78.7	82.6	3.9
2015–2017	79.2	82.9	3.7
Proportion of life expectancy in 'good or very good health' (%)			
2000–2002	80.2%	77.6%	2.6%
2009–2011	79.9%	77.4%	2.5%
2015–2017	79.7%	76.7%	3%
Proportion of life expectancy spent being disability-free (%)			
2014–2016	78.9%	74.9%	4%
2015–2017	79.2%	74.7%	4.5%

Sources: ONS(2014a; 2014b; 2017b; 2018b).

SEX

- refers to the biological aspects of an individual; their anatomy and physiology
- is male, female or intersex
- is assigned at birth

GENDER

- is a social construction
- is an internal sense of self
- is a set of behaviours and attributes which are labelled feminine, masculine or transgender
- identity may not match the sex to which someone was assigned at birth
- is where an individual may see themselves as a woman, a man, as having no gender, or non-binary gender which means someone identifies as being somewhere on a spectrum between man and woman

The UK Office for National Statistics (2019b) is working to collect accurate gender-identity data so we can examine the health of transgender people and make comparisons to those who identify as male or female. For now, we can see differences in male and female health outcomes.

Life expectancy in the UK has been rising, but Figure 3.6 shows how the rate has decreased for both males and females in recent years. Females in Wales had the smallest increase, followed by males in Wales. Females live longer, on average, than males in the UK (Table 3.3). Although life expectancy has been rising over the last few decades, the gap between males and females is narrowing. A higher proportion of male lives are spent in 'good health' and 'disability-free' compared to females, and recently this gap has widened. A male, born with no disabilities, can expect to live an average 16.5 years with a disability, and a female 20.9 years (ONS, 2018b). Common mental disorders are more prevalent in females than males (Table 3.4) but, in the UK, three-quarters of suicides have been among males, since the mid-1990s (ONS, 2019c).

We have noted that when we compare where people live, their health-related behaviour, their ethnicity and sex we find inequalities in health. Here we focus on gender because

> Gender affects most of the known factors related to health, including education, income, occupation, social networks, physical and social environments and health services. Accordingly, gender has a significant influence on health and well-being throughout life.
>
> (Hassanzadeh *et al.*, 2014 p.1)

Heise and colleagues (2019) created a model to explain how gender affects health and contributes to health inequity. Figure 3.7 shows we are born with a biology that determines our sex. We immediately enter the gender system, that is social pressure for

Table 3.4 Percentage of men and women in England who experienced a common mental disorder 'in the past week', 2014

	Male	*Female*
Asian/Asian British	12.9%	23.6%
Black/Black British	13.5%	29.3%
Mixed/multiple/other	10.5%	28.7%
White British	13.5%	20.9%
White other	13.1%	15.6%

Source: McManus *et al.* (2016).

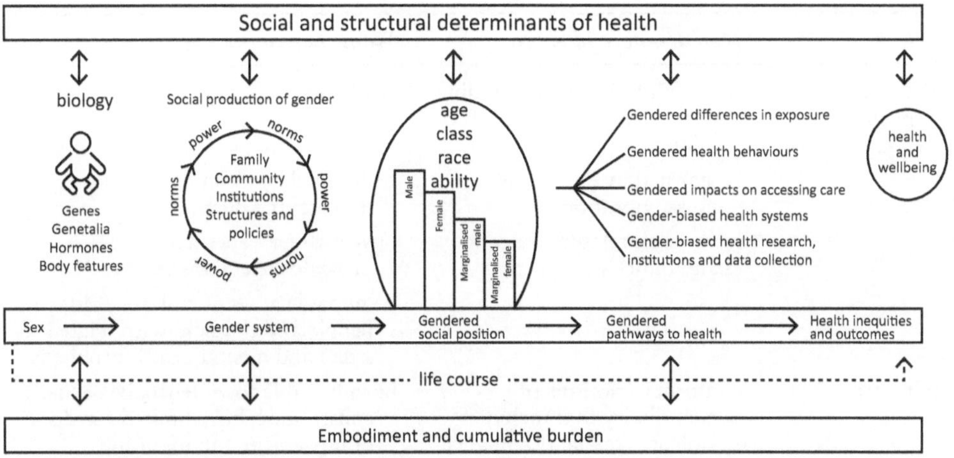

Figure 3.7 Conceptual framework of the gender system and health
Source: adapted from Heise *et al*, 2019 p.2443

children to conform to feminine and masculine cultural expectations. Usually gender systems are patriarchal: they give greater value, resources, power and status to that which is considered masculine. Gendered socialisation, where society encourages feminine attributes such as vulnerability and emotionality, and masculine attributes of strength and independence, leads to females limiting their horizons and males embracing theirs. There is social pressure to conform and to deviate from these binary gender expectations may lead to social exclusion. This process results in the person's gendered social position, which is heightened or diminished by the place they live, ethnicity, social class, ability versus disability, and other forms of power and causes of inequality.

Health inequalities can have a biological basis, such as diseases of sex-specific organs. Health inequity, unfair differences, can be encouraged by gendered social and structural factors, such as market forces, laws and policies which influence men and women's working conditions and wages. In recognition of this, the United Nations included gender equality in their action plan for the planet, Sustainable Development Goal 5: To achieve gender equality and empower all women and girls (UN General Assembly, 2015). Heise and colleagues (2019) use international evidence to explain how the person's gendered social position affects their health through five interacting pathways, which lead to health inequity (Table 3.5).

Education

There is clear evidence that having more education is associated with better health and longer life (Clark and Royer, 2013). European research shows how low education is associated with more

- binge drinking of alcohol
- smoking

Table 3.5 Gendered pathways to health with examples

Pathways	*Men are more likely to*	*Women are more likely to*
Differences in exposure	work in physically demanding jobs such as construction or mining	work in service or care
	be harmed by chemicals, noise, vibrations	be harmed by cleaning chemicals, hair dyes, textile dust
	have work-related accidents and injuries	have asthma, repetitive musculoskeletal disorders
		be unpaid carers of children, older people and the sick, with related stress and mental health problems
Health behaviours	conform to notions of masculinity that include violence, sexual dominance, sexual freedom and risk-taking such as sexual risks	be vulnerable to violence, be sexually constrained, have limited freedom of movement and input into decision-making
	speed, drink/drug drive and be involved in traffic accidents	be coerced into sex with potential risk of infection or pregnancy
	conform to expectations about masculine appearance leading to risks of use of steroids to enhance muscularity and body manipulation such as penis enlargement	conform to expectations about feminine appearance leading to exposure to toxins in creams, risks of plastic surgery, body dissatisfaction and body manipulation such as breast enlargement
Access to healthcare	demonstrate strength in times of sickness, be excluded from maternal and child care	care for the sick and prioritise needs of others, especially children, over their own health
	avoid seeking treatment for infection if they have had sex with a man, especially where homosexuality is a crime	have limited access due to lack of money, transport, power, permission from a gatekeeper such as a husband or older woman, shame or stigma
Gender-biased healthcare systems	receive better healthcare	be stereotyped as fragile and over-emotional, have physical symptoms attributed to psychological causes, receive inferior care such as less screening and less aggressive treatment for cardiovascular disease
	be in professions that are male-coded with superior status and pay e.g. surgeons and physicians	be in professions that are female-coded with inferior status and pay, e.g. nurses and midwives
Gender-biased health research, institutions and data collection		be carrying out domestic work, which is not included within occupational health research based on paid occupations
		be excluded or under-represented in clinical research, findings from men are generalised to women which have caused harm to women

Source: Heise *et al.* (2019).

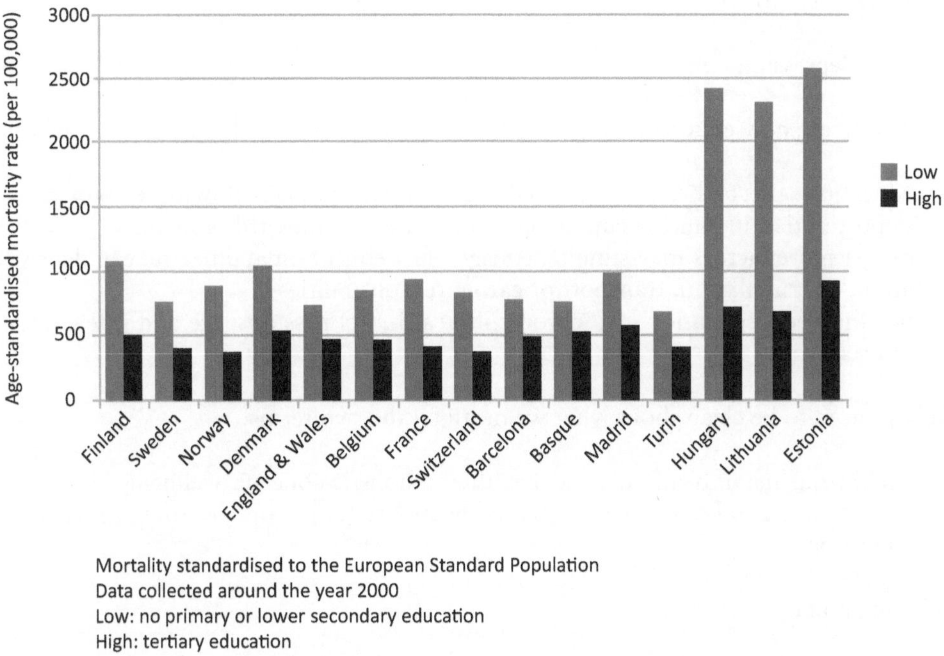

Figure 3.8 Mortality from all causes among the low and high educated men in some European countries

Source: adapted from Mackenbach *et al*, 2015 p.209

and less

- fruit and vegetable consumption
- physical activity

(Forster *et al.*, 2018)

Davies and colleagues (2018) studied 390,412 adults born in England. They compared those who had left school before 1972, when most children left school at 15 years, to those who had left school later, when the law changed the school-leaving age to 16 years. Those who had longer education

- had higher income
- were taller
- were thinner
- scored higher on intelligence tests
- drank more alcohol
- watched less television
- exercised less

and were less likely to

- have high blood pressure, diabetes, heart attacks, strokes
- die early
- smoke or had ever smoked

and more likely to

- have depression

Understanding how education may influence inequalities in health is complex because

- education affects health, e.g. qualifications are associated with employment opportunities, income, occupational exposures and standard of living
- one or more factors may simultaneously affect education and health, e.g. deprivation, discrimination, transport or caring responsibilities
- health affects education, e.g. chronic ill health, sickness absence and side effects of treatment

We also need to be clear about what we mean by the two terms:

- health, e.g. age of death, disease, health as a holistic concept, wellbeing
- education, e.g. school-leaving age, qualifications, quality of education, process of education

Thinking point:

> Consider the pathways for how a good or poor educational experience may affect people's lifelong health.

Hahn and Truman (2015) reviewed a wide range of evidence and concluded that there are three main pathways that link education to health outcomes in adulthood.

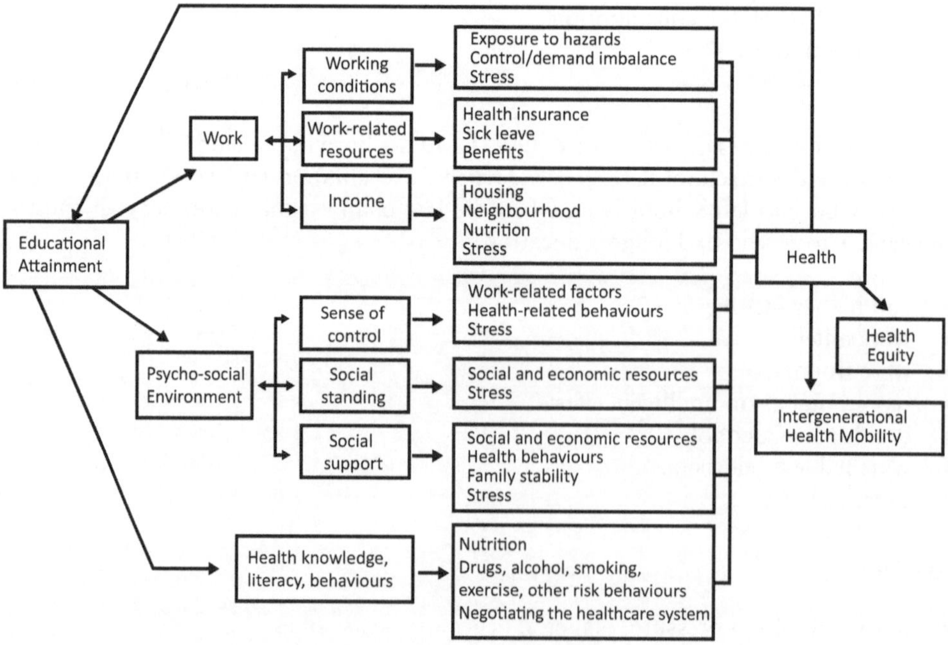

Figure 3.9 Pathways from education to health
Source: adapted from Hahn and Truman, 2015 p.21

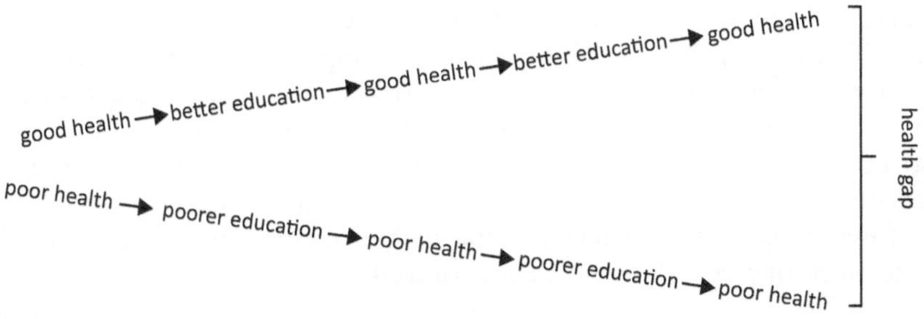

Figure 3.10 Education, health and the health gap

- Psycho-social environment, which includes an individual's social standing, social support and sense of control
- Work, where an individual may achieve income, satisfaction and access to health-related resources
- Health-related behaviours, linked to health-related knowledge and literacy. These may protect an individual from health risks and enable them to negotiate the healthcare system.

Adult health directly affects the health of the next generation, biologically, psychologically and socially. Good or poor health is associated with better or worse educational attainment. Generations of people can continue along an upward or a downward trend, thus increasing or decreasing inequalities in health across the population (Figure 3.10). For many, this is inequitable. The right to education is enshrined in the UK Human Rights Act 1998 and Sustainable Development Goal 4: To ensure inclusive and equitable quality education and promote lifelong learning opportunities for all (UN General Assembly, 2015).

Income

Economic inequality means inequalities due to people's wealth and income. Wealth refers to an individual's material resources such as property, savings and investments; income refers to money received by individuals such as salaries, wages and rent. Marmot (2010) explains how people's income influences the neighbourhood in which they live, the quality of their homes, fuel for heating and cooking, the quality of food and access to amenities and social activities. Income enables choice, and it provides security for unanticipated crises such as illness. Low income is associated with poor health because it affects education and employment, as well as deprivation. This is discussed further in chapter 4.

Occupation and socio-economic position

People who work in some jobs experience worse health than those in other jobs (Bambra, 2011; 2014). Poorer health and shorter lives are more prevalent among manual and/or the lower paid jobs because workers experience

- greater exposure to physical hazards, e.g. exposure to dangerous chemicals or lead, noise, shift work, heavy lifting
- high demands/stress and low control

Among older men, having a physically demanding workload is a risk factor for job loss, often because the physical expectations of the role are more than the man's physical capacity (Sewdas *et al.*, 2019). Those who are unemployed/workless report poorer health than those in paid work (Bambra, 2011; 2014) and there is a strong association between unemployment, poor mental health and suicide (Nordt *et al.*, 2015).

Jobs are grouped into occupations. An occupation provides a reasonable indicator of income, education and living conditions. It is a more rounded measure of someone's standard of living than a single characteristic such as income. It is also recorded on birth and death certificates, along with cause of death.

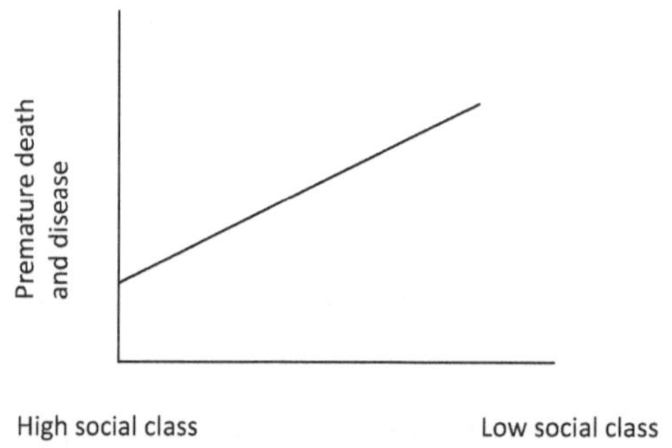

Figure 3.11 The historical relationship between social class based occupation, premature death and disease

Table 3.6 The National Statistics Socio-economic Classification (NS-SEC) (based on SOC 2010)

NS-SEC analytic class	*Examples of occupations*
1 Higher managerial, administrative and professional occupations	Directors of public health, senior police officers, environmental health professionals, dentists, psychologists, university lecturers
2 Lower managerial, administrative and professional occupations	Physiotherapists, occupational therapists, nurses, midwives, youth and community workers, housing officers
3 Intermediate occupations	Paramedics, dental technicians, fire fighters, medical secretaries, nursing assistants, call-centre operatives
4 Small employers and own account workers	Farmers, gardeners, bricklayers, carpenters, driving instructors, childminders
5 Lower supervisory and technical occupations	Electricians, plumbers, cleaners, water and sewerage plant operatives, bakers
6 Semi-routine occupations	fitness instructors, receptionists, cooks, care workers, dental nurses, shop assistants
7 Routine occupations	weavers, butchers, bar staff, leisure-park attendants, hospital porters
8 Never worked and long-term unemployed	

Source: ONS (2010).

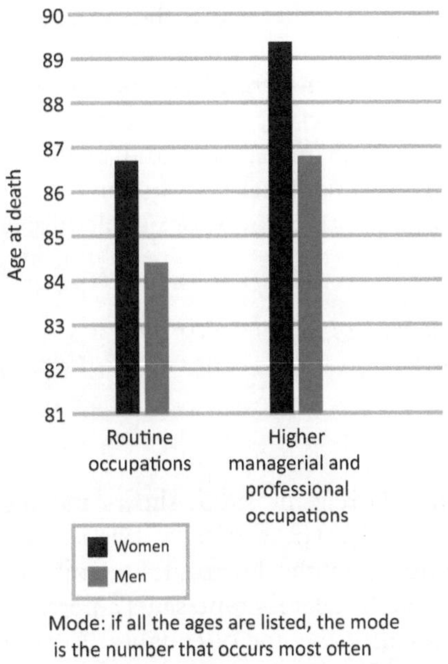

Figure 3.12 Modal age of death for men and women in England and Wales 2007 to 2011 according to socio-economic position

Source: ONS, 2017c

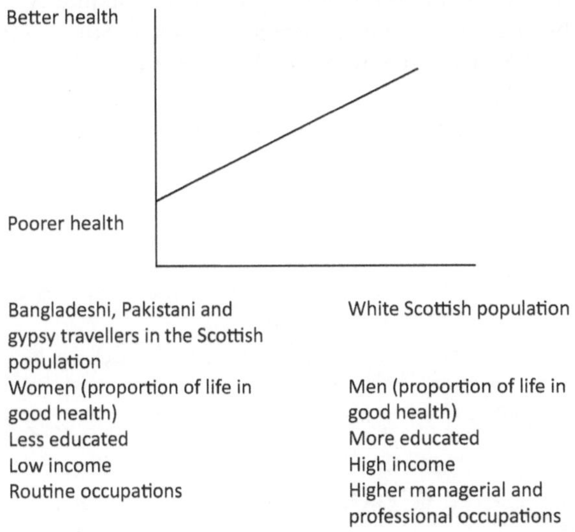

Figure 3.13 Examples of the social gradient of health between people

The UK National Statistics Socio-economic Classification (NS-SEC) of occupations replaced Social Class based on Occupation in 2000. Until then, research into health inequalities had used the term social class to refer to people in certain groups of occupations. In 1980, the Black Report (Black *et al.*, 1982) showed that people in the lower social classes, working in manual occupations, suffered more disease and earlier death than those in higher social class occupations (Figure 3.11).

Today, the NS-SEC groups occupations into eight *non-hierarchical* socio-economic categories (Table 3.6). Figure 3.12 shows that the social gradient exists when we compare age of death for people who work in high managerial and professional occupations to those who work in routine occupations. Figure 3.13 summarises the inequalities in health that we find when we compare the groups of people discussed in this section.

Inequalities in health are found between groups of people according to their ethnicity, gender, education, income, occupation and socio-economic position.

Unequal societies

The Lorenz curve, developed by the economist Lorenz in 1905, shows income or wealth inequality within a population (Figure 3.14). The vertical *y*-axis shows the cumulative income or wealth of the population and the horizontal *x*-axis shows cumulative percentage of the population. A line at 45 degrees represents a perfect distribution of income within a population and is called the line of equality. A value of 20% on the *y* axis and 45% on the *x* axis means that 45% of the population controls 20% of the population's total income.

The Gini coefficient is a way of showing inequality in income/wealth with a number between nought and one, where nought represents perfect equality and all people/households have equal income. A number one shows that only one individual/household has all the income. The higher the number, the greater the inequality. The Gini index expresses the same, but as a percentage. Recent data show South Africa 63%, United States of America 41.1%, United Kingdom 34.8%, Sweden 28.8% and Slovenia 24.2% (The World Bank, 2019).

Wilkinson and Pickett (2009) combined the following into a single index of health and social problems:

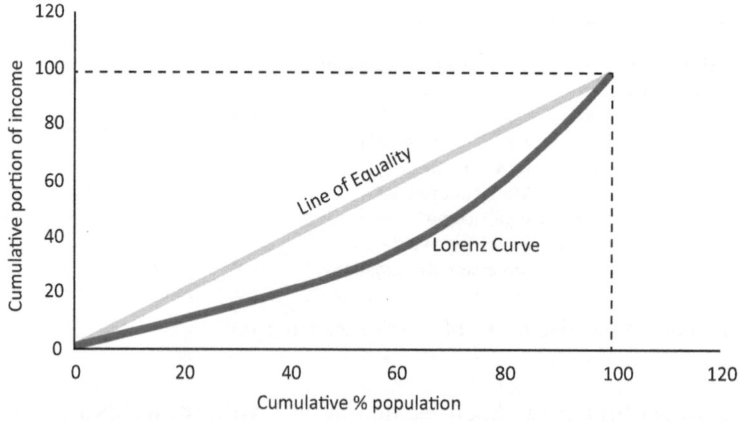

Figure 3.14 Lorenz curve

- trust
- mental illness
- life expectancy
- infant mortality
- obesity
- educational performance
- teenage births
- homicides
- imprisonment
- social mobility

They studied the relationship between the index and average income across the world and found that the amount of health and social problems are

- *not* related to the average income of a country
- worse in countries that are more unequal in other ways

In summary, countries with greater inequalities of income/wealth have a higher Gini coefficient/index and they have more health and social problems compared to others.

Pickett and Wilkinson (2015) conclude:

> The evidence that large income differences have damaging health and social consequences is strong and in most countries inequality is increasing.
>
> (p.316)

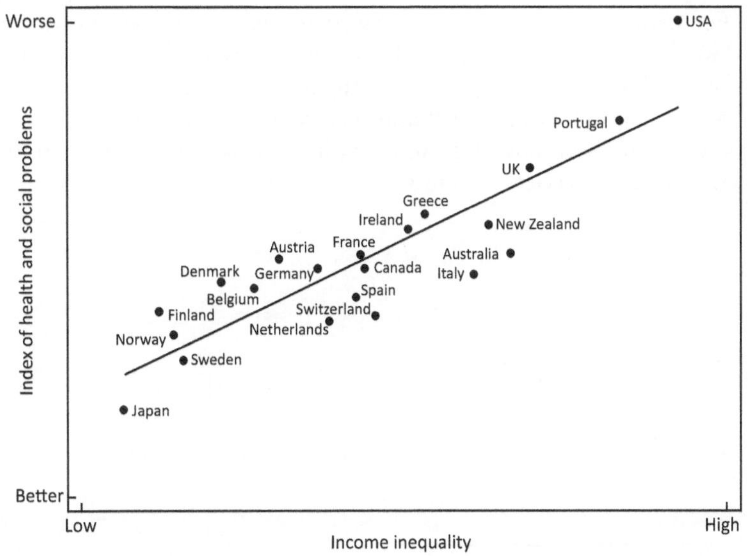

Figure 3.15 Health and social problems are closely related to inequality among rich countries

Source: Wilkinson and Pickett, 2009 p.20. Reproduced with permission from Penguin Random House UK.

Thinking point:

> Go back to Table 3.1 and compare world ranking according to wealth per person with the data in Figure 3.15. What does this tell us about wealth, inequality and health?

Inequalities in income within a country are associated with poor outcomes in the form of

- premature death
- obesity
- infant mortality
- homicides
- poorer educational attainment
- imprisonment
- distrust
- low social mobility

and are most strongly associated with poor outcomes related to

- mental disorders
- teenage births
- drug use (opiates, cocaine, cannabis, ecstasy and amphetamines)
- child wellbeing

(Pickett and Wilkinson, 2015)

Understanding why inequalities in income have adverse consequences is the subject of much study. For example, it is noted that Sweden has a very long history of a highly developed welfare state providing healthcare, pensions, worker protection and education regardless of income. Current theories suggest that in more equal societies qualities such as sharing, cooperation, trust and reciprocity are important. In a more hierarchical society, status becomes more important, it is associated with material resources, it promotes status anxiety and individualism (Forster *et al.*, 2018).

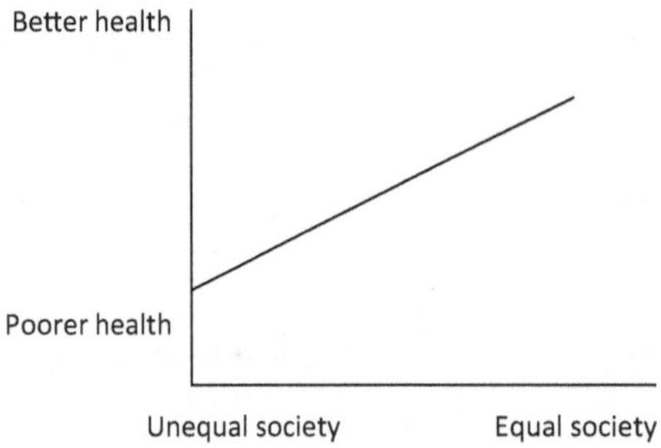

Figure 3.16 The social gradient in health between equal and unequal societies

Concern about inequality, itself, being a direct and indirect cause of poor health for everyone is why the United Nations included it as Sustainable Development Goal 10: Reduce inequality within and among countries (UN General Assembly, 2015).

An unequal society results in worse health and social outcomes than a more equal one.

Social exclusion and vulnerable communities

Some people's social position is so weak that they are at the lowest end of the social gradient. Their money, power and resources are so low that that they have much worse experiences of health, and earlier death rates, compared to the population average. They may be disadvantaged due to where they live, their ethnicity, gender, education, income or occupation, but they also have additional and multiple challenges. They often report being unheard, ignored or stigmatised by others. We describe these vulnerable communities as being socially excluded from mainstream society. They include

- the homeless
- those with very low income/living in poverty
- the unemployed
- people with disabilities
- those who misuse drugs and other substances
- prisoners
- those with certain illnesses including mental disorders
- sex workers
- prisoners
- the lesbian, gay, bisexual, transgender, queer community
- young teenage pregnant women and mothers
- teenage runaways who often become homeless

Aldridge and colleagues (2018) analysed studies carried out in 38 high-income countries about people who had a history of homelessness, sex work, imprisonment or a substance use disorder excluding cannabis or alcohol. This combined socially excluded group were 10 times more likely to die at an earlier age compared to the population average. Men were 7.9 times and women were 11.9 times more likely to die early. Their early deaths were due to a range of, and a combination of, conditions including overdoses, infectious diseases, cancer, liver disease, heart problems, respiratory diseases and accidents.

Intersectionality

Kimberlé Crenshaw (1989) introduced the theory of intersectional feminism, which argued that black women were subject to overlapping systems of discrimination and oppression due to their ethnicity, sexuality and economic background. Her work underlines the importance of not seeing individuals through the lens of just one identity such as their ethnicity, gender, sexuality or education, but through the multiple identities we all have, and then understanding that vulnerability can be the result of multiple disabling social forces working together.

For example, many trans people are also the homeless, the abused and the ones who are excluded from a welcoming education or healthcare system. In one study,

- 41% experienced a hate crime because of their gender identity
- 28% faced domestic abuse from a partner
- 25% had experienced homelessness
- 36% of trans university students had experienced negative comments or behaviour from staff
- 40% adjusted their clothes due to fear of discrimination or harassment
- 41% said healthcare staff lacked understanding of their needs

(Bachmann and Gooch, 2018)

Many people with disabilities are also unemployed and living in poverty. One study found

- less than half of disabled adults were in employment compared with 80% of non-disabled adults.
- disabled adults earned less per hour compared to non-disabled adults
- more disabled people lived in poverty or were materially deprived than non-disabled people.
- 18.4% of disabled people (16–64) were living in food poverty compared to 7.5% of non-disabled
- on average, men with mental health conditions died 20 years earlier than the general population
- on average, women with mental health conditions died 13 years earlier than the general population

(EHRC, 2017)

The Equality and Human Rights Commission (2017) conclude:

> Negative attitudes towards disabled people remain prominent in Britain, and people with a mental health condition, learning disability or memory impairment remain particularly stigmatised.
>
> (EHRC, 2017 p.12)

Rickard and Donkin (2018) report that people with learning disabilities die 15 to 20 years earlier, on average, compared to the general UK population. They cite the underlying social causes as unemployment, low income, poor housing, social isolation, loneliness, bullying and abuse. Crenshaw (1989) argues:

> The goal ... should be to facilitate the inclusion of marginalized groups for whom it can be said: 'When they enter, we all enter.'
>
> (p.167)

People who are particularly vulnerable and become excluded from mainstream society suffer much worse health than the general population.

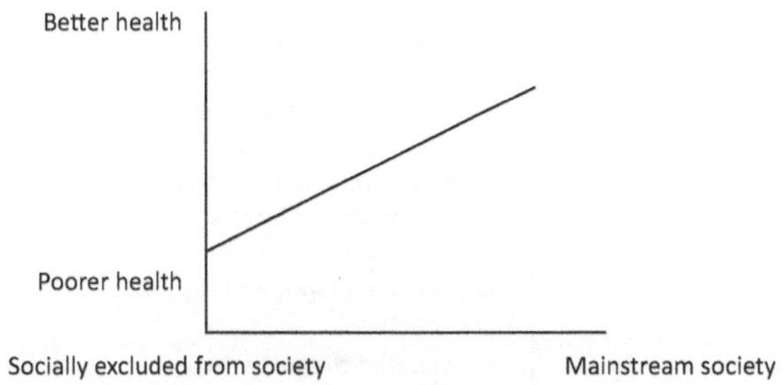

Figure 3.17 The social gradient in health between the socially excluded and mainstream society

Causes of inequalities in health

Social determinants of health inequality and inequity

Inequalities in health arise because of differences in people's daily living conditions. Those with more power, money and resources live and work in better conditions, have better health and a longer life (Marmot, 2010; WHO, 2010). People achieve more power, money and resources if they have a high socio-economic position, which is strongly determined by their ethnicity, gender, education, income and occupation (Figure 3.18).

Socio-economic position reflects and determines people's

- material circumstances, which include their physical environment such as housing, working conditions and neighbourhood, and economic circumstances such as income and access to goods and services
- psychosocial factors, which include stressors caused by negative life events such as bereavement, lack of social support or isolation
- health-related behaviours and biological factors, such as smoking, alcohol consumption and sedentary behaviour, and their biological impact such as high blood pressure. It also includes the influence of genes

(WHO, 2010)

The health system, that is both public health and healthcare, has a role to play. It can

- encourage equal access to care
- promote collaboration to improve the health of citizens such as improving transport so that people can access care
- invest in the early detection of illness, rehabilitation and support with social reintegration
- encourage people to participate in and influence their health system
- use its influence to improve the social determinants of illness and health inequity

(WHO, 2010)

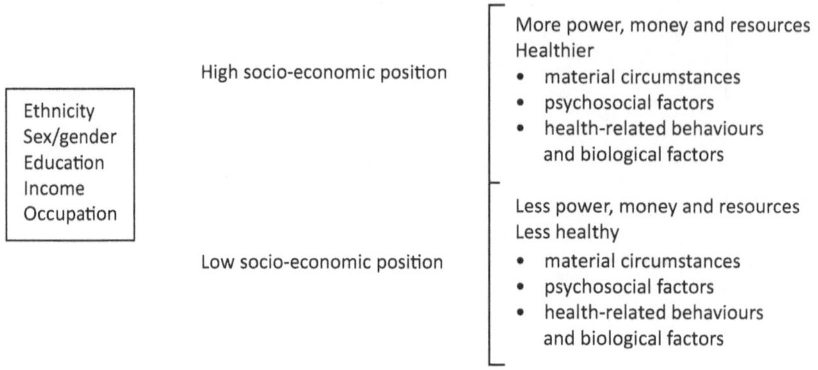

Figure 3.18 Social determinants lead to health inequalities

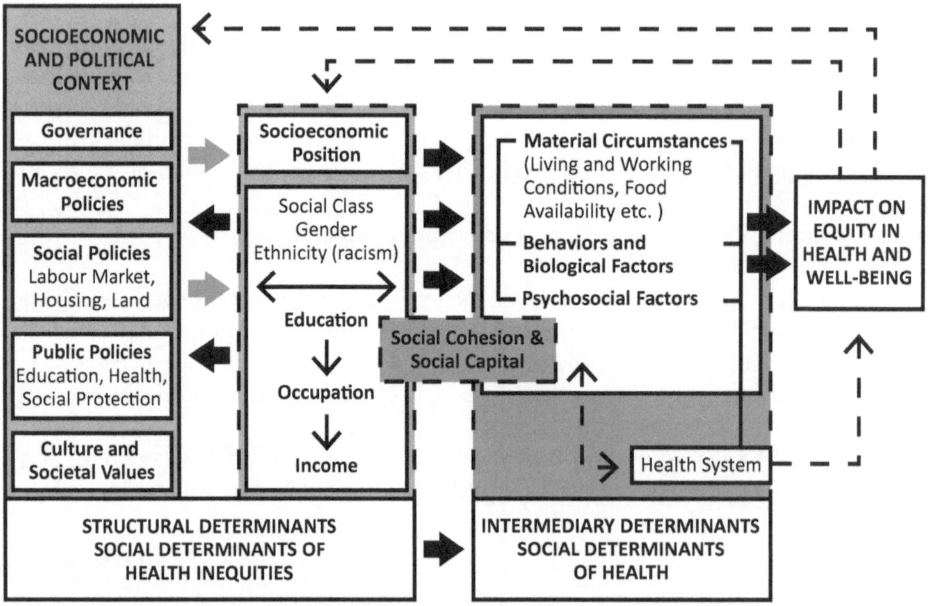

Figure 3.19 Commission on the Social Determinants of Health Conceptual Framework

Source: World Health Organization, 2010 p.6. Reproduced with permission from the World Health Organization.

These social determinants of health are influenced by the ways in which a society organises itself and makes decisions. The wider social, political and cultural context shapes whether power, money and resources are equally or unequally distributed. For example,

- governance and its processes, e.g. how a society defines a population's needs, patterns of discrimination, how much people are encouraged to participate in the governance of a society, whether the administration of public affairs is transparent and whether those who run them are accountable and to whom

- macroeconomic policies, e.g. trade, finance and monetary policies
- social policies, e.g. the distribution of land, housing, employment/the labour market and systems of welfare for the poor or vulnerable
- public policies, e.g. how a society manages water, sanitation, education, housing, health services and social care
- culture and societal values, e.g. value placed on religion(s), equality, health, collective responsibility and the distribution of resources

(WHO, 2010)

The World Health Organization's Conceptual Framework (Figure 3.19) indicates how all the social determinants work with one another to produce a society that promotes health inequalities (WHO, 2010). They argue that health equity is a matter of social justice and is linked to human rights. Reducing the health gap, so that groups of people are not destined to more ill health and a shorter life than others, is related to the sort of society in which people want to live.

Life course approach to understanding inequalities in health

The World Health Organization (2010) acknowledged the importance of considering the life course approach alongside their Conceptual Framework. The two are complementary. The life course approach considers the health journey of an individual from their conception to death. It seeks to understand the risk of disease and/or the long-term health effects from

> ... physical or social exposures during gestation, childhood, adolescence, young adulthood and later adult life. The aim is to elucidate biological, behavioural and psychosocial processes that operate across an individual's life course, or across generations, to influence the development of disease risk.
>
> (Kuh *et al.*, 2003 p.778)

The life course approach aims to bring together the social risks and biological risks to health. It contributes to understanding the factors that culminate in a person's socio-economic position and their health, recognising each influences the other. From this, researchers can understand some of the mechanisms that lead to some people having worse heath and shorter lives than others (Table 3.7). Researchers examine

- the causes of ill health that accumulate over time. These can include chains of risks, that is, one disadvantage may lead to another
- the timing of certain exposures or actions. These are either critical periods, limited windows of time in which an exposure could be protective or adverse, or sensitive periods when we are particularly sensitive to being affected (e.g. infancy)
- people's resilience, susceptibility or vulnerability to exposures or the factors that can help to modify or mitigate an exposure

(Kuh *et al.*, 2003)

Marmot (2017) summarises how the social gradient of health runs across the life course. The lower the socio-economic position of young children, the worse they do on tests that measure linguistic, cognitive, social, emotional and behavioural development.

Table 3.7 Life course models

Accumulation of risk model	The accumulation of facts, events, decisions (direct and indirect) that influences health over time.
Chain of risk model	Events are linked together in a chain, e.g. being born into disadvantage puts an individual on a path from which it is difficult to leave.
Critical period model	Analyses when an event happened to a person because some moments of life are particularly 'sensitive' and events will have a greater impact.

Source: Kuh *et al.* (2003).

This gradient in young children can be greatly explained by parenting activities, and it can be reduced by support for parents and families and by reducing child poverty. A child's readiness for school affects their later school performance, and their educational achievement is strongly associated with adult health. Adults' health is directly influenced by their own education, which also influences their income, working and living conditions and psychological processes. Children born into lower socio-economic circumstances are more likely to experience adverse childhood experiences, which can include abuse, neglect and exposure to violence. These adverse experiences are associated with a range of health-damaging behaviours in adulthood such as substance misuse, smoking, under-age sex, domestic violence, and subsequently higher rates of illness which lead to earlier deaths than the general population.

Fair Society Healthy Lives

In November 2008, Professor Sir Michael Marmot undertook a review of evidence to reduce inequalities in health in England. The review was published in 2010 under the title Fair Society Healthy Lives. His two main reference points were

- the Commission on the Social Determinants of Health Conceptual Framework
- the life course approach

The aims of the review were to

- improve health and wellbeing for all
- reduce health inequalities

The two overarching goals were to

- create an enabling society that maximises individual and community potential
- ensure social justice, health and sustainability are at the heart of all policies

Marmot's key messages were

- reducing health inequalities is about fairness and social justice
- action should focus on reducing the social gradient in health

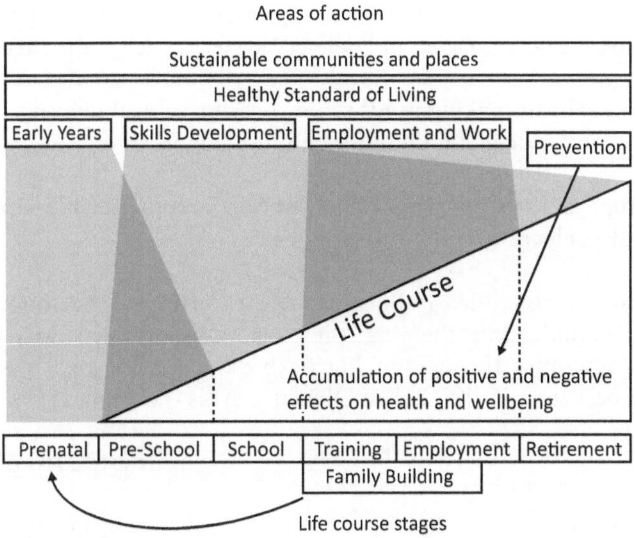

Figure 3.20 Action across the life course

Source: Marmot, M. (2010) Fair society, healthy lives. The Marmot review. H.M. Government: London. Reproduced with permission from UCL Institute of Health Equity.

- health inequalities are the result of social inequalities, and the solutions need action from across all social determinants of health
- the need for proportionate universalism. This means recognising that focusing on the most vulnerable alone will not reduce health inequalities very much. To reduce the steepness of the social gradient in health,

  Actions must be universal, but with a scale and intensity that is proportionate to the level of disadvantage. We call this proportionate universalism.

  (Marmot, 2010 p.15)
- reducing health inequalities will benefit the whole of society in many ways, including economic benefits due to less sickness
- tackling social inequalities in health must go together with tackling climate change. Both are more important measures of a country's success than economic growth
- six objectives for English policy:
  A give every child the best start in life
  B enable all children, young people and adults to maximise their capabilities and have control over their lives
  C create fair employment and good work for all
  D ensure a healthy standard of living for all
  E create and develop healthy and sustainable places and communities
  F strengthen the role and impact of ill health prevention

- national and local government, the National Health Service and private and third-sector organisations, and groups, will need to participate in delivering these national policy objectives. Local policies and delivery systems need to be effective and focused on equity
- Effective participatory decision-making needs to be part of the local delivery, and this depends on empowering local communities and individuals

Marmot illustrates his approach in his diagram of Action across the life course (Figure 3.20). Marmot makes clear:

> Action to reduce health inequalities must start before birth and be followed through the life of the child. Only then can the close links between early disadvantage and poor outcomes throughout life be broken ... For this reason, giving every child the best start in life (Policy Objective A) is our highest priority recommendation.
>
> (Marmot, 2010 p.20)

Health Equity in England

In 2020, Marmot and colleagues reported on the state of health inequalities in England 10 years after Fair Society Healthy Lives (Marmot, 2010). Health Equity in England (Marmot *et al.*, 2020) reinforced the same core recommendations. They commented on the era of austerity that followed the international financial crisis of 2007 to 2008, and cite declines in education, the rise of zero-hours contracts, the rise in unaffordable housing and the rise in the use of food banks as examples of how the social determinants of health had deteriorated in England:

> ... health is getting worse for people living in more deprived districts and regions, health inequalities are increasing and, for the population as a whole, health is declining.
>
> (Marmot *et al.*, 2020 p.149)

> *The social causes of inequalities in health can be traced back to the social, political and cultural contexts in which we live. These affect people's health before they are born, throughout their whole lives and the next generation's. The solutions need to come from all sectors of society and be directed at all stages of people's lives.*

Why health equality matters

Reducing health inequalities matters to Europeans:

> When we change the focus from the individual to the societal level, we lose vast economic, social, and innovative potential for our societies as a result of poor health and health inequalities.
>
> (Forster *et al.*, 2018 p.4)

and to the world:

> Everyone has the right to a standard of living adequate for the health and well-being of himself and of his family ... and the right to security in the event of unemployment, sickness, disability, widowhood, old age or other lack of livelihood beyond his control.
>
> (United Nations, 1948 Article 25 Universal Declaration of Human Rights)

> The existing gross inequality in the health status of the people ... is politically, socially and economically unacceptable and is, therefore, of common concern to all countries.
>
> (WHO, 1978)

> Inequality threatens long-term social and economic development, harms poverty reduction and destroys people's sense of fulfilment and self-worth. This ... can breed crime, disease and environmental degradation ... we cannot ... make the planet better ... if people are excluded from opportunities, services and the chance for a better life.
>
> (United Nations, 2018 p.1)

Equality is important because

> The equality effect can appear magical. In more equal countries, human beings are generally happier and healthier: there is less crime, more creativity, more productivity, more concern over what is ... being produced, and – overall – higher real educational attainment ... Equality means being afforded the same rights, dignity and freedoms as other people. These include the right to access resources, the dignity of being seen as able, and the freedom to choose what to make of your life on an equal footing with others.
>
> (Dorling, 2017 p.11, 12, 13)

Summary

This chapter has

- defined health inequalities, health inequities and the social gradient of health
- provided examples of inequalities in health between places and between people
- presented evidence that unequal societies are associated with poor health and social outcomes
- illustrated the impact of social exclusion for vulnerable people
- explained how social determinants across the life course result in health inequalities
- illustrated why gaining more equality for health matters to the world

Further reading

Marmot, M. (2016) *The health gap. The challenge of an unequal world.* London: Bloomsbury

Wilkinson, R., and Pickett, K. (2019) *The inner level: how more equal societies reduce stress, restore sanity and improve everyone's wellbeing.* London: Penguin

Useful websites

University College London *Institute of Health Equity*. Available at: www.instituteofhealthequity.org/home

Inequality.org. Available at: https://inequality.org

References

Aldridge, R.W., Story, A., Hwang, S.W., Nordentoft, M., Luchenski, S.A., Hartwell, G., Tweed, E.J., Lewer, D., Katikireddi, S.V., and Hayward, A.C. (2018) 'Morbidity and mortality in homeless individuals, prisoners, sex workers, and individuals with substance use disorders in high-income countries: a systematic review and meta-analysis', *The Lancet*, 391, pp.241–250

Bachman, C.L., and Gooch, B. (2018) *LGBT in Britain. Trans report*. London: Stonewall

Bambra, C. (2014) 'Health inequalities, work, and welfare', in Cockerham, W.C., Dingwall, R., and Quah, S.R. (eds) *The Wiley Blackwell Encyclopedia of Health, Illness, Behavior, and Society*. Chichester: Wiley Blackwell, pp.989–992

Bambra, C. (2011) 'Work, worklessness and the political economy of health inequalities', *Journal of Epidemiology & Community Health*, 65(9), pp.746–750

Bhopal, R.S., Gruer, l., Steiner, M.F.C., Millard, A., and Katikireddi, S.V. (2018) 'Mortality, ethnicity, and country of birth on a national scale, 2001–2013: a retrospective cohort (Scottish Health and Ethnicity Linkage Study)', *PLoS Medicine*, 15(3) doi:10.1371/journal.pmed.1002515

Black, D., Morris, J.N., Smith, C., and Townsend, P. (1982) 'The Black Report', in Townsend, P., and Davidson, N. (eds) *Inequalities in health*. London: Penguin, pp.29–213

Clark, D., and Royer, H. (2013) 'The effect of education on adult mortality and health: evidence from Britain', *The American Economic Review*, 103(6), pp.2087–2120

Crenshaw, K. (1989) 'Demarginalizing the intersection of race and sex: a black feminist critique of antidiscrimination doctrine, feminist theory and antiracist politics', *University of Chicago Legal Forum*, 1989(1) Article 8, pp.139–167

Davies, N.M., Dickson, M., Davey Smith, G., van den Berg, G., and Windmeijer, F. (2018) 'The causal effects of education on health outcomes in the UK Biobank', *Nature Human Behaviour*, 2(2) doi:10.1038/s41562-017-0279-y

Dorling, D. (2017) *The equality effect*. Oxford: New Internationalist Publications Ltd.

Equality and Human Rights Commission (2017) *Being disabled in Britain. A journey less equal*. London: Equality and Human Rights Commission

Forster, T., Kentikelenis, A., and Bambra, C. (2018) *Health inequalities in Europe: setting the stage for progressive policy action*. Dublin: Think Tank for Action on Social Change

Hahn, R.A., and Truman, B.I. (2015) 'Education improves public health and promotes health equity', *International Journal of Health Services*, 45(4), pp.657–678

Hassanzadeh, J., Moradi, N., Esmailnasab, N., Rezaeian, S., Bagheri, P., and Armanmehr, V. (2014) 'The correlation between gender inequalities and their health related factors in world countries: a global cross-sectional study', *Epidemiology Research International*, 2014 doi:10.1155/2014/521569

Heise, L., Greene, M.E., Opper, N., Stavropoulou, M., Harper, C., Nascimento, M., and Zewdie, D. (2019) 'Gender inequality and restrictive gender norms: framing the challenges to health', *The Lancet*, 393(10189), pp.2440–2454

Kuh, D., Ben-Shlomo, Y., Lynch, J., Hallqvist, J., and Power, C. (2003) 'Life course epidemiology', *Journal of Epidemiology and Community Health*, 57(10), pp.778–783

Mackenbach, J.P., Kulháanová, I., Menvielle, G., Bopp, M., Borrell, C., Costa, G., Deboosere, P., Esnaola, S., Kalediene, R., Kovacs, K., Leinsalu, M., Martikaenen, P., Regidor, E., Rodriguez-Sanz, M., Strand, B., Hoffmann, R., Eikemo, T.A., Őstergren, O., and Lundberg, O.

(2015) 'Trends in premature mortality: a study of 3.2 million deaths in 13 European countries', *Journal of Epidemiology and Community Health*, 69(3), pp.207–217

Marmot, M. (2010) *Fair society, healthy lives. The Marmot review*. London: H.M. Government

Marmot, M. (2017) 'Social justice, epidemiology and health inequalities', *European Journal of Epidemiology*, 32(9) doi:10.1007/s10654-017-0286-3

Marmot, M., Allen, J., Boyce, J., Boyce, T., Goldblatt, P., and Morrison, J. (2020) *Health equity in England. The Marmot review 10 years on*. London: Institute of Health Equity

McManus, S., Bebbington, P., Jenkins, R., and Brugha, T. (eds) (2016) *Mental health and wellbeing in England: adult psychiatry and morbidity survey 2014*. Leeds: NHS Digital

Ministry of Housing Communities and Local Government (2019) The English indices of deprivation 2019 (IoD2019). Available at: https://assets.publishing.service.gov.uk/government/uploads/system/uploads/attachment_data/file/835115/IoD2019_Statistical_Release.pdf (Accessed 4th December 2019)

Nordt, C., Warnke, I., Seifritz, E., and Kawohl, W. (2015) 'Modelling suicide and unemployment: a longitudinal analysis covering 63 countries,2000–11', *The Lancet Psychiatry*, 2(3), pp.239–245

Office for National Statistics (2010) *Standard occupational classification 2010. Volume 3. The national statistics socio-economic classification (rebased on the SOC2010) user manual*. London: Palgrave Macmillan

Office of National Statistics (2014a) National life tables, UK: 2010 to 2012. Available at: www.ons.gov.uk/peoplepopulationandcommunity/birthsdeathsandmarriages/lifeexpectancies/bulletins/nationallifetablesunitedkingdom/2014-03-21 (Accessed 19th November 2019)

Office of National Statistics (2014b) *Changes in healthy life expectancy (HLE)*. Available at: www.ons.gov.uk/peoplepopulationandcommunity/healthandsocialcare/healthandlifeexpectancies/datasets/changesinhealthylifeexpectancyhle (Accessed 19th November 2019)

Office for National Statistics (2017a) An overview of lifestyles and wider characteristics linked to healthy life expectancy in England: June 2017. Available at: https://bit.ly/3qmOFLU (Accessed 3rd December 2019)

Office for National Statistics (2017b) Health state life expectancies, UK 2014 to 2016. Available at: www.ons.gov.uk/peoplepopulationandcommunity/healthandsocialcare/healthandlifeexpectancies/bulletins/healthstatelifeexpectanciesuk/2014to2016 (Accessed 19th November 2019)

Office for National Statistics (2017c) Most common age at death, by socio-economic position in England and Wales: a 30 years comparison. Available at: www.ons.gov.uk/peoplepopulationandcommunity/healthandsocialcare/healthinequalities/articles/mostcommonageatdeathbysocioeconomicpositionsinenglandandwales/latest (Accessed 29th November 2019)

Office for National Statistics (2018a) *Health state life expectancies by national deprivation deciles, England and Wales: 2014 to 2016*. London: Office for National Statistics

Office for National Statistics (2018b) Health state life expectancies, UK: 2015 to 2017. Available at: www.ons.gov.uk/peoplepopulationandcommunity/healthandsocialcare/healthandlifeexpectancies/bulletins/healthstatelifeexpectanciesuk/2015to2017 (Accessed 12th December 2019)

Office for National Statistics (2019a) What is the difference between sex and gender? Available at: www.ons.gov.uk/economy/environmentalaccounts/articles/whatisthedifferencebetweensexandgender/2019-02-21 (Accessed 19th November 2019)

Office for National Statistics (2019b) Gender identity update. Available at www.ons.gov.uk/methodology/classificationsandstandards/measuringequality/genderidentity/genderidentityupdate (Accessed 20th November 2019)

Office for National Statistics (2019c) Suicides in the UK: 2018 registrations. Available at: www.ons.gov.uk/peoplepopulationandcommunity/birthsdeathsandmarriages/deaths/bulletins/suicidesintheunitedkingdom/2018registrations (Accessed 20th November 2019)

Pickett, K.E., and Wilkinson, R.G. (2015) 'Income inequality and health: a causal review', *Social Science and Medicine*, 128(2015), pp.316–326

Public Health England (2019a) Public health profiles. Available at: https://fingertips.phe.org.uk (Accessed 9th December 2019)

Public Health England (2019b) Tower Hamlets. Local authority health profile 2019. Available at: https://fingertips.phe.org.uk/profile/health-profiles (Accessed 1st April 2020)

Public Health England (2019c) Kensington and Chelsea. Local Authority Health Profile 2019. Available at: https://fingertips.phe.org.uk/profile/health-profiles (Accessed 1st April 2020)

Rickard, W., and Donkin, A. (2018) *A fair, supportive society. Summary report*. London: Institute for Health Equity

Scottish Government (2013) Gypsies/travellers in Scotland: summary of the evidence base, summer 2013. Available at: https://bit.ly/3ojX5BW (Accessed 6th December 2018)

Scottish Government (2015) *Which ethnic groups have the poorest health?* Edinburgh: Scottish Government Statistics

Scottish Government (2018) Ministerial working groups on gypsy/travellers minutes: October 2018. Available at: www.gov.scot/publications/ministerial-working-group-on-gypsy-travellers-minutes-october-2018 (Accessed 6th December 2018)

Sewdas, R., van der Beek, A.J., Boot, C.R.L., D'Angelo, S., Syddall, H.E., Palmer, K.T., and Walker-Bone, K. (2019) 'Poor health, physical workload and occupational social class as determinants of health-related job loss: results from a prospective cohort study in the UK, *BMJ Open*, 9(7) doi:10.1136/bmjopen-2018–026423

The Social Marketing Gateway (2013) *Mapping the Roma community in Scotland. Final report*. Glasgow: The Social Marketing Gateway

The World Bank (2019) Gini index (World Bank estimate). Available at: https://data.worldbank.org/indicator/si.pov.gini (Accessed 14th April 2020)

United Nations (1948) Universal declaration of human rights. Available at: www.un.org/en/universal-declaration-human-rights/ (Accessed 4th December 2019)

United Nations (2018) Reduced inequalities: why it matters. Available at: www.un.org/sustainabledevelopment/wp-content/uploads/2018/01/10.pdf (Accessed 4th December 2019)

United Nations General Assembly (2015) Transforming our world: the 2030 agenda for sustainable development. Available at: www.un.org/ga/search/view_doc.asp?symbol=A/RES/70/1&Lang=E (Accessed 23rd November 2019)

Ventura, L. (2019) *'The worlds' richest and poorest countries 2019', Global Finance, 9th December*. Available at: www.gfmag.com/global-data/economic-data/worlds-richest-and-poorest-countries (Accessed: 9th December 2019)

Wilkinson, R.G., and Pickett, K. (2009) *The spirit level: why more equal societies almost always do better*. London: Allen Lane/Penguin Books

World Health Organization (1978) *Alma -Ata 1978 primary health care*. Geneva: World Health Organization. Available at: www.who.int/publications/almaata_declaration_en.pdf (Accessed 4th December 2019)

World Health Organization (2008) *Closing the gap in a generation: health equity through action on the social determinants of health*. Geneva: World Health Organization

World Health Organization (2010) *A conceptual framework for action on the social determinants of health*. Geneva: World Health Organization

World Health Organization (2018) Social determinants of health. Key concepts. World Health Organization. Available at: www.who.int/social_determinants/thecommission/finalreport/key_concepts/en/ (Accessed 6th December 2018)

World Life Expectancy (2018) World life expectancy. Available at: www.worldlifeexpectancy.com/world-life-expectancy-map (Accessed 9th December 2019)

4 Poverty and health

Elisabetta Corvo and Sally Robinson

Key points

- Introduction
- Defining and measuring poverty
- Poverty in the UK
- Poverty and health
- Reframing poverty in the UK
- Summary

Introduction

This chapter examines the impact of poverty on health. It describes different ways of measuring poverty including current methods used in the UK. We note how poverty may be characterised as low income or broader deprivation; as deep or persistent. The ways in which poverty damages health are many, and we discuss premature death, mental health, food insecurity, education, public transport, housing and homelessness. We conclude with some thoughts about reframing poverty to bring about change.

Defining and measuring poverty

To know how much poverty there is in a population, we need to be able to define and measure it. There are many ways to do this. Subjective poverty is where people perceive themselves to be poor compared to others (Buttler, 2013), but perceptions are personal, difficult to measure and cannot easily be compared across a population. Instead we work with indicators of poverty that can be observed and are relatively straightforward to measure. There are two broad approaches to objectively measuring poverty: unidimensional, where we measure one indicator, and multidimensional, where we measure many (UNECE, 2017).

Unidimensional approaches to poverty

A unidimensional approach means that we measure a single indicator such as food calories or money, as a proxy for poverty. Then we decide where to place the 'poverty line', below which people are living in poverty. Some countries work out the average number of calories eaten per person per day: this measure is called 'food energy intake'. Monetary indicators are about measuring income, expenditure and what can be afforded. Here, we discuss five monetary indicators: absolute poverty, housing costs, basic needs, relative poverty and persistent poverty. We also discuss time poverty.

Absolute poverty/absolute low income

Absolute poverty is where people do not have the minimum necessities to survive, such as food, shelter and clothes. It is about being unable to subsist. Today in the UK, the Government states that individuals are in absolute poverty when they fall below the 'absolute low income'. 'Absolute low income' describes people who are

> ... living in households with income below 60% of the 2010/11 *median, uprated for inflation.
>
> (Francis-Devine *et al.*, 2019 p.4)

These people are living in households where the living standards are the lowest in the country. Over time, absolute poverty in the UK has been steadily reducing for many years (Figure 4.1).

(*median – if everyone's income was put into a hierarchical list, the median is the one in the middle.)

Box 4.1 Absolute poverty in 1950s London

Alan Johnson was a Labour MP who held seven Shadow Cabinet positions including Shadow Chancellor of the Exchequer in 2010. He writes about his childhood with his mother Lily and sister Linda, in the 1950s.

"On cold nights we'd go to bed wearing jumpers with a pile of old coats substituting for blankets. We lived in constant dread of not having a shilling for the meter. Time after time the gas mantles would go out and we'd light candles, or, to be more accurate, night lights – little round blobs of wax, like tiny cakes, that were cheap and portable, requiring no candlesticks.

"Lily's regular 'search for a shilling' would be accompanied by constant pleas for God (in whom she had unquestioning faith) to help her. When she found one, she'd offer up her profound gratitude, eyes tightly shut, face raised to the heavens, or at any rate, to the ceiling, with its dark, damp patches and, in the summer, its covering of flies. We were so used to swarms of flies we didn't register them. Like the trains clanking past at all hours on the line in and out of Paddington, we'd only have noticed them if they'd disappeared.

"With no fridge and the buckets of urine in the bedroom (to avoid having to go out to the yard in the middle of the night), our house was a more attractive venue for the discerning fly than it was for us. There were also cockroaches, beetles and all manner of bugs. During an infestation of earwigs, Linda and I took to stuffing our ears with paper at night – we'd heard that these particular pests liked to crawl into people's ears, intent on eating the brain.

"It is ironic that after leaving home at eighteen, Lily spent almost her entire adult life on the council waiting list ... she regressed from ... electricity to gas, from a bath to a sink, from a garden to a grotty shared yard."

(Source: Johnson, 2013 p.15, 16)

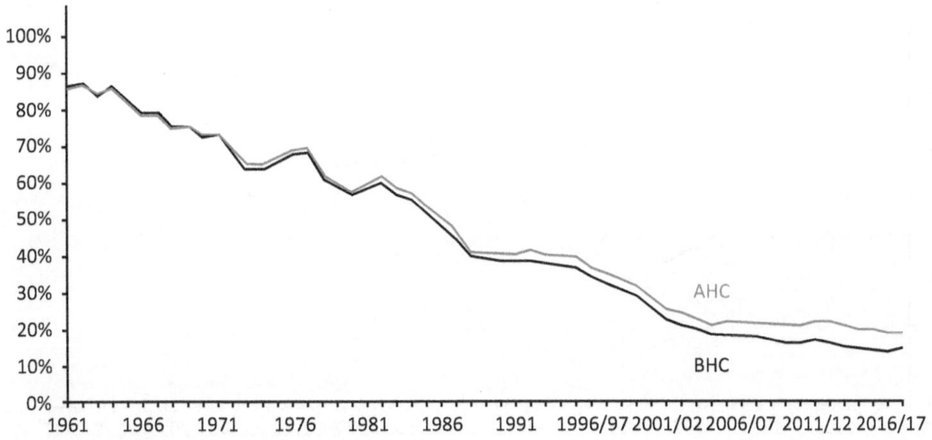

Figure 4.1 Percentage population of Great Britain living in absolute low income (1961 to 2001/02) and of the UK (2002/03 to 2017/18)

Source: Francis-Devine *et al*, 2019 p.10. Reproduced under the terms of Open Parliament Licence v3.0

Housing costs

In the UK, statisticians will often present data about people's income with reference to housing costs, that is rent or mortgages, because these are significant items in a household budget. Figures show Before Housing Costs (BHC) and After Housing Costs (AHC) have been taken out. Generally, the AHC is thought to be more illuminating (Francis-Devine *et al.*, 2019).

Basic needs

In the 1970s, poverty began to be measured in terms of whether people were able to afford to meet their basic needs, which were:

> The minimum consumption needs of a family (i.e. adequate food, shelter and clothing, as well as certain household furniture and equipment); and essential services provided by and for the community at large, such as safe water, sanitation, public transport and health care, education, and cultural facilities.
>
> (UNECE, 2017 p.12)

Relative poverty/relative low income

Unlike absolute poverty, relative poverty considers comparisons with others, shame and social exclusion (Ravaillon, 2016). In the UK, the Government states that individuals are in relative poverty when they fall below the level of 'relative low income' which means people who are

> ... living in a household with income below 60% of the median in that year.
>
> (Francis-Devine *et al.*, 2019 p.4)

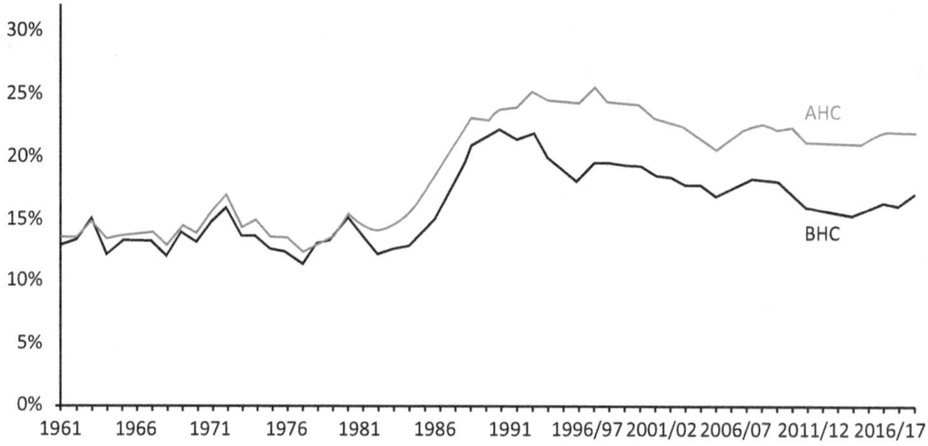

Figure 4.2 Percentage population of Great Britain living in relative low income (1961 to 2001/02) and UK (2002/03 to 2017/18)

Source: Francis-Devine *et al.,* 2019 p.10. Reproduced under the terms of the Open Parliament Licence v3.0

This measure compares those living in households with the lowest income to the rest of the population. Basically, it shows the inequality between low- and middle-income households. In the UK, relative poverty rose markedly during the 1980s (Figure 4.2). In 2017 to 2018, there were 14 million people living in relative poverty (AHC) (Francis-Devine *et al.*, 2019).

Persistent poverty/persistent low income

Persistent poverty is where an individual has experienced relative low income for at least three of the last four years (Francis-Devine *et al.*, 2019). Measuring persistent poverty recognises that being in a state of poverty for long periods is particularly damaging to mental and physical health (Korenman, 1995; Phipps, 2003).

Table 4.1 Rates of UK households in persistent low income from 2012/13 to 2015/16

Type of household	*Before housing costs*	*After housing costs*
No working adults	19%	24%
Social rented	18%	36%
Private rented	10%	25%
Adults with no qualifications	19%	23%
Head of household is Black/African/Caribbean/Black British	14%	29%
Head of household is Asian/Asian British	18%	26%
Children in lone parent families	20%	36%
Three or more children	20%	31%

Source: Francis-Devine *et al.* (2019 p.23).

Wealth

Wealth, or lack of it, may tell us more about poverty than income. Wealth is a measure of savings and investments Some households may have little income but are 'asset rich'. People with wealth tend to have a higher standard of living than their income might suggest (UNECE, 2017). This is because it acts as security against borrowing money and paying later.

Time poverty

Time poverty means that people work long hours. They cannot afford to reduce their work hours because they need the income to keep themselves out of poverty. They are left with very little time for looking after themselves, social care or leisure (UNECE, 2017).

Multidimensional approaches to poverty

Monetary approaches have been criticised as providing only 'indirect' indicators of poverty, and many have supported the move to measuring non-monetary, social indicators. The world has adopted a multidimensional approach in the 2030 Agenda for Sustainable Development (UN, 2015). Here we describe the French sociologist Paugam's work on poverty, the British sociologist Peter Townsend's work on relative deprivation, UK household material deprivation, UK indicators of deprivation and the Social Metrics Commission Poverty Measurement Framework for the UK.

Poverty and society

Paugam's (2001) work captures poverty as part of society. He suggests three types of poverty are experienced in Europe.

- Pauvreté intégrée, integrated poverty, is where people's standard of living is low, but they remain part of their social network and they do not lose status. They may benefit from others in a similar situation, such as through a 'black economy'.
- Marginal pauvreté, marginal poverty, refers to a relatively small group of people who choose to reject society and modern norms of civilisation. This self-excluded group, who do not integrate, are poorly judged by society and they become stigmatised and further excluded.
- Pauvreté disqualifiante, disqualifying poverty, refers to those who suddenly become poor, perhaps due to a personal financial problem, personal loss or wider recession. This group is the most worrying as they experience the shock of a profound change in their lifestyle. They no longer belong to previous social networks, become dependent on social welfare, encounter increasing problems and experience lowered self-esteem. This type of poverty causes society the most anxiety and increases social inequality.

Relative deprivation

Peter Townsend coined the term 'relative deprivation'. He described people as being in poverty when they do not have the resources to access the living conditions, amenities, diet and activities which are customary, or widely approved and encouraged, within the society to which they belong. He explained,

> Their resources are so seriously below those commanded by the average individual or family that they are, in effect, excluded from ordinary living patterns, customs and activities.
>
> (Townsend, 1979 p.31)

Identifying and measuring poverty in terms of deprivation is much more complex than counting money as a proxy indicator. Deciding which resources, items or activities are the most 'customary' or salient to measure, to identify a poverty line and decide who is poor, is a challenge and the subject of much debate.

UK household material deprivation

In the UK, the Government defines households who are materially deprived as those who lack the ability to access key goods and services (Table 4.2). In 2017/2018, 7% of pensioners in the UK experienced material deprivation (Francis-Devine *et al.*, 2019).

UK indicators of deprivation

In the UK, the four nations collect data to indicate the level of deprivation in a place. They focus their data collection on well-chosen features such as the amount of illness, crime and unemployment. If these are high, the place may be described as relatively deprived compared to a place with low levels of illness, crime and unemployment. These features are called the indicators of deprivation and they are grouped under several domain headings. The indicators and domain names differ across the countries, are not directly comparable and are updated regularly (Table 4.3). For example, in England, the 'Health, deprivation and disability' domain includes the indicators: illness, inability to work due to illness or disability and number of life years lost due to early death (MHCLG, 2019a). In Scotland, the 'Health' domain includes the indicators: hospital stays related to alcohol and drugs; emergency hospital stays; prescriptions for anxiety, depression or psychosis; low birth weights and

Table 4.2 Percentage of UK parents who report they want but cannot afford specific goods or services for themselves, 2017 to 2018

Goods and services	*% parents*
One week's holiday away from home not with relatives	38%
Make savings of £10 per month or more	35%
Money to spend on self each week	30%
Replace worn-out furniture	28%
Home contents insurance	20%
Replace broken electrical goods	20%
Money to decorate home	19%
Keep up to date with bills	9%
Keep house warm	7%

Source: Adapted from Francis-Devine *et al.* (2019 p.37).

Table 4.3 Domains of indicators of deprivation across the UK

Scottish index of multiple deprivation	*English indices of deprivation*	*Northern Ireland multiple deprivation measures*	*Welsh index of multiple deprivation*
Income	Income	Income	Income
Employment	Employment	Employment	Employment
Health	Health, deprivation and disability	Health and disability	Health
Education, skills and training	Education, skills and training	Education, skills and training	Education
Crime	Crime	Crime and disorder	Community safety
Geographic access to services	Barriers to housing and services	Access to services	Access to services
Housing			Housing
	Living environment	Living environment	Physical environment

Sources: Scottish Government (2020a); MHCLG (2019a); NISRA (2017); Welsh Government (2019a).

the inability to work due to illness or disability (Scottish Government, 2020a). The collected data from every local community are available on-line. The data help to identify places of greatest need as well as inequalities across each country. Living in a deprived area does not mean all the people living there are deprived, or vice versa.

Box 4.2 The most deprived small area in Wales

Rhyl, Denbighshire, Wales

The area around Rhyl High Street is the most deprived small area in Wales. It is situated within 10 other small areas of deprivation according to measures of income, employment, health, education and community safety. This area of Rhyl has been in the top 50 of the most deprived areas of Wales since 2005. About a fifth of the population are under 16 years old. In 2001, the Census showed that, compared to the Wales average, this part of Rhyl has more rented housing, one-person households, flats/apartments as opposed to a whole house, higher percentage of people from non-white ethnicities and high unemployment.

(Source: Welsh Government 2019b)

Social Metrics Commission Poverty Measurement Framework for the UK

The Social Metrics Commission (SMC) (2018) proposed a new measure of poverty for the UK. It defines poverty as

> The situation where a person's available material resources are insufficient to adequately meet their immediate material needs.
>
> (SMC, 2018 p.20)

The Commission argued that the UK needs to collect data which can illuminate

- who is in poverty
- the nature of the poverty

To identify who is in poverty, the Commission argued that the 'poverty line' should be the result of working through their 'four steps to measuring poverty'. These take into account factors such as

- related individuals in households share resources, and non-related individuals do not
- resources include more than income, but do not include inescapable costs relating to housing, childcare and disability
- the norms in society, e.g. how much others have available to spend
- overcrowding, rough sleeping and norms of living

(SMC, 2018)

Table 4.4 shows the poverty measurement framework. In summary, the Commission's measure of poverty, their 'poverty line', is based on the extent to which an individual's resources can meet their needs, taking into account their inescapable costs of child-care, disability and housing as well as their savings and access to assets. Next, to identify the nature of poverty, the Commission argued we need to understand the depth of those in poverty, how many live in persistent poverty and the lived experience of those in poverty.

Table 4.4 Poverty measurement framework

Understanding who is in poverty	*Understanding more about the nature of the poverty*		
Poverty	Depth of poverty	Persistence of poverty	Lived experience indicators
To measure who is in poverty, follow the four steps to measuring poverty and set the poverty line.	The distance below and the distance just above the poverty line.	Lack of available resources this year and for two of the previous three years.	Mental and physical health, social isolation, low literacy or numeracy, drug or alcohol misuse, trauma, poor spoken English, strained family relationships, barriers to accessing employment, low digital skills.

Source: SMC (2018).

We decide what poverty is, who is living in poverty and understand the experience of being in poverty by measuring one or several indicators. The position of the 'poverty line' is often a political or social decision.

Poverty in the UK

When studying data about poverty, the first task is to note the measure of poverty used. We have presented some data, above, that used income as the measure. Here we present data using the Social Metrics Commission's measure of poverty.

Thinking point:

Compare some of the data in this section, measured using the Social Metrics Commission's measure, with some of the data above, measured using low income.

Poverty rates

Using the Social Metrics Commission's poverty line, in 2017 to 2018 a fifth (22%, 14.3 million) of the UK population were living in poverty. As a proportion of sub-populations, this included 24% of Wales, 22% of England, 28% of London, 20% of Scotland and 20% of Northern Ireland. These 14.3 million people included 8.3 million working-age adults, 4.6 million children and 1.3 million adults of pension age (SMC, 2019). As a proportion of each of these three age groups, the highest rate of poverty was among children (34%). Among the working-age adults in poverty, there was greatest poverty among those in workless families (70%). A fifth of women were in poverty, and 18% of men.

Three-quarters of all those in poverty lived in families with a head of household who was White. As a proportion of ethnic groups, poverty was high among families from ethnic minorities.

- 46% of people in families with a Black head of household
- 37% of people with an Asian head of household
- 19% of people with a White head of household

(SMC, 2019)

Depth of poverty

Out of 14.3 million people in the UK who were in poverty, 31% were in deep poverty. Deep poverty means that their income was at least 50% below the poverty line. More than half (59%) were more than 25% below the poverty line (SMC, 2019).

Persistence of poverty

The Commission found 59% of those living in deep poverty were also living in persistent poverty. Compared to others living in poverty, those who were in persistent poverty were more likely to

- live in a lone-parent family
- be a single adult

Table 4.5 Comparison of some health-related characteristics between UK people in poverty, persistent poverty and those who are not in poverty, 2014/2015 to 2016/2017

Health characteristics	*Proportion of people not in poverty (%)*	*Proportion of people in poverty (%)*	*Proportion of people in persistent poverty (%)*
In a family that includes a disabled child or adult	34%	32%	42%
One or more adults in the family with poor self-reported physical health	21%	23%	29%
One or more adults in the family with poor self-reported mental health	24%	31%	37%
One or more adults in family with low health satisfaction	17%	19%	26%

Source: Adapted from SMC (2019 p.26).

- live in a workless family
- report poor physical and mental health
- live in a family that is behind in paying bills

(SMC, 2019)

The Commission found that poverty, and especially persistent poverty, was more common among families which included someone with a disability or who reported poor health (Table 4.5).

Lived experience of poverty

Compared to those not living in poverty, the Commission found those in poverty were more likely to

- feel unsafe walking home at night
- be less happy living in their neighbourhood
- be in a family where no adult saves
- be in a family that is behind in paying bills
- be in a family where no one has any formal qualifications
- report poor physical and mental health

(SMC, 2019)

Future poverty

In the UK, whether families can get out of poverty, or whether they will continue in poverty and poor children will become poor adults, is determined by

- certainty, whether a factor affects poverty
- strength, how big the effect is
- coverage, how many children are affected

Table 4.6 Relative strength of the factors that influence the amount of time UK families are in poverty

Factor	*Certainty*	*Strength*	*Coverage*
Long-term worklessness and low earnings	High	High	High
Parental qualifications	High	High	High
Family instability	High	Medium	Medium
Family size	High	Medium	Medium
Parental ill health and disability	Medium	Medium	Medium
Drug and alcohol dependency	High	High	Low
Child ill health	Medium	Low	Low
Housing	Low	Low	Medium
Debt	Low	Low	Medium
Neighbourhood	Low	Low	Medium

Source: Adapted from Francis-Devine *et al.* (2019, p.24).

One-fifth of the UK population are living in poverty. Of these, more than half are in deep poverty, and a quarter are in both deep and persistent poverty.

Poverty and health

According to the life course approach, individuals follow a biological and social pathway though their life which shapes their health (Kuh and Ben-Shlomo, 1997). The life course approach sees life as building a stack of paper, where each sheet subtly changes the appearance and texture in a positive or negative way, towards better or poorer health outcomes. Negative aspects of poverty cumulate through life, leading to poorer health, poorer quality of life, more chronic illness and earlier death compared to those who grow up in more affluent circumstances.

The relationship between poverty and health is also cyclical. An example is provided by the British Medical Association (2017), who explain how unemployment and poverty contribute to poor health, chronic disease and mental health problems, each of which increases the likelihood of unemployment. The two become mutually reinforcing. For example, when people cannot afford the price of prescriptions their conditions worsen. Other features of poverty and health which are widely accepted include

- the relationship between an individual's income and health is non-linear, it is more complex
- being exposed to moments of poverty is not as health-damaging as being in persistent poverty
- sudden income shocks, such as an immediate loss of income, have more negative health impacts than the positive benefits for health caused by a positive income shock
- poor health leads to poor income because it impacts on earning capacity and overall opportunities for employment

(Phipps, 2003)

We will discuss the relationship between poverty and premature death, mental health, food insecurity, education, public transport and housing.

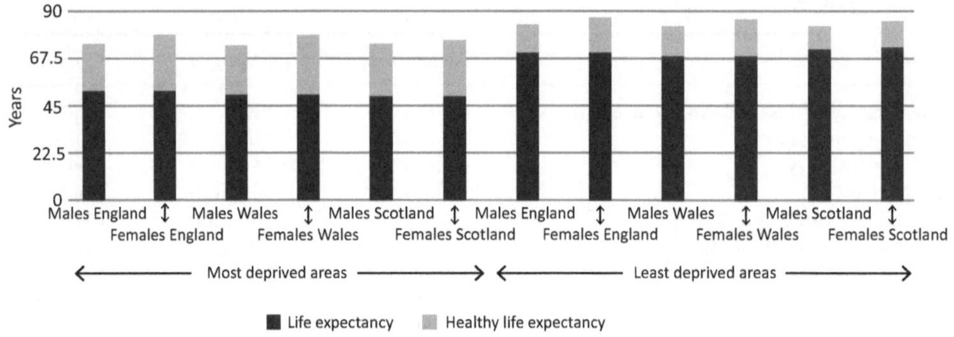

Figure 4.3 Life expectancy and healthy life expectancy in the most and least deprived areas of England, Wales and Scotland, 2015 to 2017

Table 4.7 Causes of mortality that explain the gap in life expectancy between the most and least deprived areas in England, 2014 to 2016

Males	*Most deprived decile*	*Least deprived decile*	*Difference*
Life expectancy	73.9 years	83.3 years	9.4 years
Causes of death that explain the difference of 9.4 years	Heart disease		1 year 6 months
	Dementia and Alzheimers disease		4 months
	Lung cancer		11 months
	Chronic lower respiratory disease		11 months
	Stroke		4 months
	Influenza and pneumonia		4 months
	Prostate cancer		2 weeks
	Colorectal cancer		1 month
	Leukaemia and lymphomas		2 weeks
	Cirrhosis and other liver disease		7 months
	Other		4 years 2 months
Females	*Most deprived decile*	*Least deprived decile*	*Difference*
Life expectancy	78.8 years	86.2 years	7.4 years
Causes of death that explain the difference of 7.4 years	Heart disease		10 months
	Dementia and Alzheimers disease		5 months
	Lung cancer		10 months
	Chronic lower respiratory disease		1 year 5 months
	Stroke		4 months
	Influenza and pneumonia		4 months
	Breast cancer		1 month
	Colorectal cancer		1 month
	Leukaemia and lymphomas		2 weeks
	Urinary disease		1 month 2 weeks
	Other		3 years 3 months

Source: PHE (2019).

Deprivation and premature death

Using the relevant indicators of deprivation for each nation, grouped into domains as shown in Table 4.3, England, Scotland and Wales are each divided into ten deciles. Each decile represents 10% of the population. From this we can identify the places that are the most deprived and least deprived in each country. Figure 4.3 shows both males and females living in areas of least deprivation have longer lives, and live more of their lives in good health, compared to those living in areas of most deprivation (ONS, 2019a).

In England, about a third of the gap in life expectancy between those who live in the most deprived area and those who live in the least deprived area can be explained by heart disease, lung cancer and chronic lower respiratory diseases (Public Health England, 2019) (Table 4.7).

Poverty and mental health

Elliot writes:

> The primary health impacts of economic downturns are on mental health (including the risk of suicide).
>
> (Elliot, 2016 p.9)

Elliot (2016) describes how the global economic crisis of 2007 to 2009 led to many men being made redundant from work, and many women having their wages cut. Those from ethnic minorities and people with disabilities were disproportionately disadvantaged. We know that coping with the stress of job insecurity, unexpected redundancy and the financial, social and emotional impact of losing employment leads to mental health problems. Insecurity and uncertainty encourage low self-esteem and feelings of having little control over one's life and future. Unemployed or poor individuals may experience stigma and shame. We know from studies in the 1980s that when whole communities experience wide-spread unemployment and deprivation, this may be less stigmatising for individuals as they are among the many, but the disadvantages for all accumulate as community resources and the local economy decline. In turn, opportunities for social interaction reduce and people become vulnerable to developing mental health problems.

In summary, everyone's mental health is determined by

> … a wide range of socio-economic factors (… 'social determinants'), which both influence health status and the physical, social and personal resources available for dealing with environmental stressors, satisfying needs and realising potential.
>
> (Elliot, 2016 p.15)

The social determinants of mental health include social, cultural, economic, political factors, living standards, working conditions and social support. All of these can cause poverty and can be worsened by poverty.

Food insecurity

An individual is food-insecure when

> … they lack regular access to enough safe and nutritious food for normal growth and development and an active and healthy life. This may be due to unavailability of food and/or lack of resources to obtain food.
>
> (FAO, 2020)

The Food and Agriculture Organization (2019) explain that food security and insecurity operate along a sliding scale.

- Food security means that people can access the quantity and quality of food that they need, and health is unlikely to be compromised. This can become mild food insecurity when there begins to be some uncertainty about obtaining food.
- Moderate food insecurity means that people are uncertain whether they will be able to access food because it is hard to find, or it is unaffordable. They are forced to compromise the quantity and quality of their diet. Going hungry leads to concerns about undernourishment in the form of too few calories and/or developing deficiencies in specific nutrients. Some people increase their reliance on cheap, highly processed foods which are often high in fat, salt and sugar. These can cause other forms of malnutrition, including obesity, which are associated with the development of chronic diseases that shorten life.
- Severe food insecurity means that food is unavailable to people and they are hungry. At worst, people may have gone without food for days. There is increasing undernutrition across the diet and people's health is at risk. In 2018, 9.2% of the world's population were experiencing severe food insecurity.

Food insecurity includes hunger, food poverty and food malnutrition. The Trussel Trust (2019) found that each phrase can have different connotations in the UK. 'Hunger' may not sufficiently capture that people need premises to cook, pots, pans,

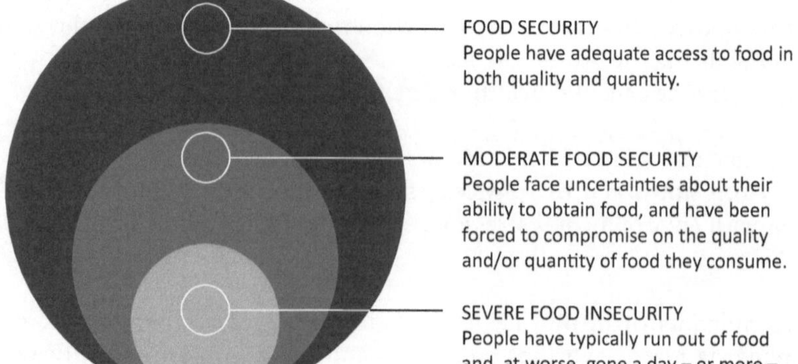

Figure 4.4 Levels of food insecurity
Source: adapted from FAO, 2019 p.5

plates, seasoning and somewhere to sit and eat. 'Food poverty' may be clearer to the public, but 'food insecurity' makes clear that we have people who are not hungry but are very malnourished and getting ill. For some, food poverty is poverty, and the underlying issue is not food but income:

> We do use the term food poverty ... in relation to communicating with the public ... in terms of more technical documents, we would use food insecurity.
>
> (Trussel Trust, 2019 p.20)

> You can start getting side-tracked by food poverty, period poverty, fuel poverty, because it's poverty and poverty is what drives food insecurity ...
>
> (Trussel Trust, 2019 p.20)

In the UK, data collected between 2016 to 2018 indicated that 1.2 million people in the UK were severely food-insecure, that is 1.8% of the population; and 3.7 million people were moderately food-insecure, 5.6% of the population (FAO, 2019). Food insecurity is more often found where families have low income, and especially among those who are unemployed, those who have chronic ill health or those with disabilities (Tarasuk *et al.*, 2013; Loopstra *et al.*, 2019). Food banks provide emergency food for people in need. In 2020, The Trussel Trust were supporting 1,200 food bank centres across the UK. Between April 2018 and March 2019 the Trust provided 1.6 million food bank parcels, each containing three days' food. This represented a 73% increase over the previous five years. The Trust and others (Prayogo *et al.*, 2018) reported that this was because the cost of food rose, wages fell and those eligible for welfare benefits, 'universal credit', received no money for about five weeks.

Food insecurity causes poor health, and where it is found, we can predict that health is likely to worsen (Heflin *et al.*, 2005; Loopstra *et al.*, 2019). The UK's Food Foundation (2019) found that, after housing costs have been met, the poorest tenth of UK households would need to spend about 74% of their income on food if they were to meet the recommendations for healthy eating in the UK outlined in the Eatwell Guide (PHE, 2018). This compares to 6% for the richest tenth of households. Jones and colleagues (2014) carried out an analysis of 94 foods and found the average price of healthy food was more than twice that of unhealthy food, and between 2002 and 2012 the price gap widened.

Table 4.8 Price increases of healthy and less healthy food, UK 2002 to 2012

	Price increase between 2002 to 2012 (£ per 1000 kcals)
All foods	£1.34
Potatoes, bread, rice, pasta and other starchy carbohydrates	£0.13
Fruit and vegetables	£1.73
Dairy and alternatives	£1.07
Beans, pulses, fish, eggs, meat and other proteins	£1.73
Foods and drinks high in fat, salt and sugar	£1.02
Total 'more healthy food'	£1.84
Total 'less healthy food'	£0.73

Source: Adapted from Jones (2014 p.3).

Food is central to people's psychological, social, cultural and spiritual health and their sense of normality. Moderate or severe food insecurity has wider impacts beyond physical health. In high-income countries, the negative effects on people's subjective well-being is stronger than not having income, shelter, housing or employment (FAO, 2019). An international study found that food insecurity is associated with greater prevalence of

- depressive symptoms
- anxiety symptoms
- post-traumatic stress
- psychosocial stress
- self-reported poor mental health
- unspecified common mental disorders

(Tribble *et al.*, 2020)

Education

As we have seen, about a fifth of UK households who experience persistent low income are living with adults with no qualifications (Francis-Devine *et al.*, 2019), but education is more than qualifications. It influences people's chances of living in affluence or poverty and subsequently their health, and vice versa. It

> ... can create opportunities for better health, including social and psychological benefits, better jobs, higher income, greater access to resources, healthier behaviours, and the financial stability to live in healthier neighbourhoods.
>
> (Zimmerman *et al.*, 2018 p.171)

A large study covering 10 years of data from the European Union concluded that the higher the level of education, the higher the income of workers. Education was described as the main social catalyst for improving income, productivity and economic development because

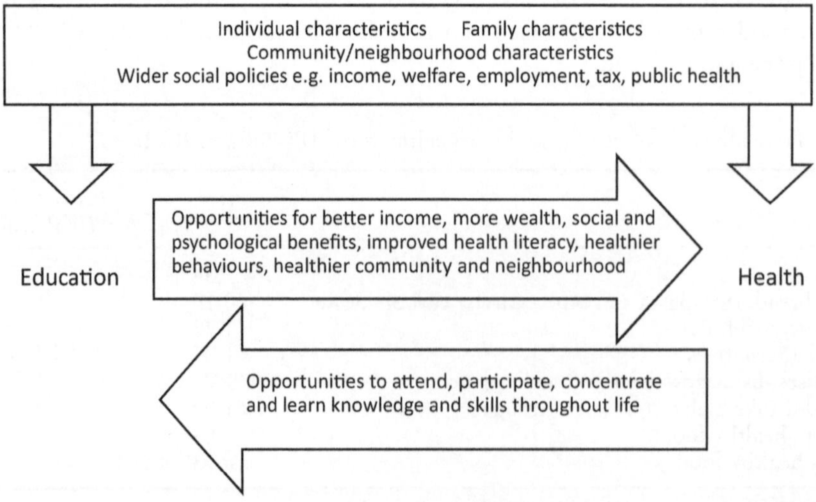

Figure 4.5 The relationship between education and health

> The more educated people, the higher the average level of their costs and fewer people who can be classified as 'poor'… education is the main factor in improving the competitiveness of any country and the wealth of the people.
>
> (Kuznetsova, 2019 p.613)

Education supports the development of a person's personal attributes such as cognitive skills, problem-solving skills and a sense of control over their life which, together, enhance a person's human capital, meaning their value to society (Lochner, 2011; Zimmerman *et al.*, 2018; Brunello *et al.*, 2016). Adults with higher levels of education rate their own health as better than those with less education (Lynch *et al.*, 2016). Education is associated with greater health literacy, the ability to understand and put into practice health-related information. Low health literacy

> … represents a particular challenge to disadvantaged populations, many of whom may possess multiple risk factors for low health literacy.
>
> (Knighton *et al.*, 2017 p.1)

Public transport

Good public transport is crucial to people's health and wellbeing. It is less air and noise polluting than numbers of private vehicles, reduces accidents, decreases community severance, which means it enhances people's mobility, and it encourages greater walking to get to the bus/tram stop or station with subsequent benefits to physical and mental health (van Schalkwyk and Mindell, 2018). Those who are living in poverty are most in need of good public transport to reach schools, healthcare facilities, food outlets and places for recreation.

Lucas (2012) explains when factors which lead to social disadvantage meet factors that lead to transport disadvantage the result is transport poverty (Table 4.9). Being in transport poverty means people are less able to access opportunities, social networks, community resources, goods and services and to participate in local decision making. Together these encourage social isolation and exclusion.

Housing

Having low income means individuals can find it difficult to own, rent or find any permanent place of residence. A substantial part of most people's income goes towards

Table 4.9 Social and transport disadvantages lead to transport poverty

Examples of social disadvantage	*Examples of transport disadvantage*	
Low income No job Low skills Poor health Poor housing	No car Poor public transport services High costs of fares No information Fear of crime e.g personal safety when travelling	*Lead to transport poverty, social isolation and social exclusion*

Source: Lucas (2012).

Table 4.10 Direct and indirect ways that housing can affect health

	Direct	*Indirect*	
	Individual/household		*Neighbourhood*
Hard/physical/material characteristics which affect people's health	Material/physical effects of housing on health including homelessness	Indicates socio-economic position, income, wealth	Built and natural environment, availability of services
		Proximity to services and facilities	
Soft/social/meaningful characteristics which affect people's health	Effect of poor housing on insecurity, shame, anxiety	Culture and behaviours within the household and neighbourhood	
	Feeling of 'home', social status, feeling secure		Community assets, cohesion or fragmentation

Source: Adapted from Shaw (2004 p.398).

accommodation. A house, or other dwelling, should be in good condition, a home, a refuge, a place where people feel protected, safe, at ease and able to be intimate. It is also

> An intermediate structural factor that links broader societal processes and influences with an individual's immediate social and physical environment.
>
> (Rourke, 2012 p.2363)

Shaw (2004) describes how housing has direct and indirect impacts on people's health and wellbeing (Table 4.10). She describes these impacts as

- hard/physical/material; the structure, damp, mould and cold; characteristics associated with respiratory disease, hypothermia, heat, accidents, poisoning and more
- soft/social/meaningful impacts are those characteristics that make people feel ashamed, insecure, unsafe; these could relate to debt, isolation or abuse. In this way, housing is an indicator of people's health, wellbeing and social status
- individual dwellings sit within neighbourhoods of buildings which make up the physical environment, a place of many or few services, and a culture which may be experienced as supportive, fragmented or even hostile

Decent homes

In the UK, a decent home is defined as one that

- meets the minimum standard for housing
- must not contain hazards that present a serious and immediate risk to a person's health and safety
- provides a reasonable degree of thermal comfort
- is in reasonable repair
- has reasonably modern facilities and services

(DCLG, 2006)

In 2018, 18% of homes in England were deemed non-decent, 11% had a hazard that presented a serious and immediate risk to a person's health and safety and 3% had problems with damp. These problems were seen most frequently in the private rented sector (MHCLG, 2019b). Across the UK, households with the lowest income were most commonly living in a non-decent home and experiencing overcrowding, which is associated with greater spread of infections, depression and anxiety (Joseph Rowntree Foundation, 2020).

Fuel poverty

The UK Warm Homes and Energy Conservation Act 2000 defines a person as living in fuel poverty

> ... if he is a member of a household living on a lower income in a home which cannot be kept warm at reasonable cost.

The four nation governments have specific ways in which they assess fuel poverty in populations using measures of average fuel costs and income. Fuel poverty is associated with excess winter deaths. These are the increases in deaths during the winter months, December to March, compared with other months.

The Marmot Review Team (2011) found that living in fuel poverty and a cold home is directly linked to excess deaths from cardiovascular disease, respiratory diseases, influenza and hypothermia, as well as encouraging poor mental health, arthritic and rheumatic symptoms, colds and flu. They also found cold homes indirectly lead to a poor diet, poor dexterity and increased accidents. Older people are more likely to be fuel poor because they spend more time at home. They and others with existing long-term medical conditions are particularly vulnerable. People over 65 years old, and those with medical conditions, are recommended to be in a home heated to at least 18°C during the day and night (PHE, 2014).

Homelessness

Often, poverty per se does not directly cause homelessness, but it is the catalyst that accelerates an accumulation of negative circumstances, some of which may have begun in childhood (Bramley and Fitzpatrick, 2018). There are three types of homelessness.

- Statutory homelessness is defined slightly differently across the UK. It is where people apply to their local authority for help and, if they meet certain criteria, they may be given temporary accommodation
- Rough sleeping is the most visible, where people are sleeping on the streets. Many have mental health or substance misuse problems, and they are at greater risk of violence compared to the rest of the population
- Hidden homelessness is where people don't ask local authorities for help, or they may not meet the statutory homeless criteria. These people may be in bed and breakfast accommodation, in hostels or 'sofa surfing' in the homes of friends or family

(Crisis, 2020)

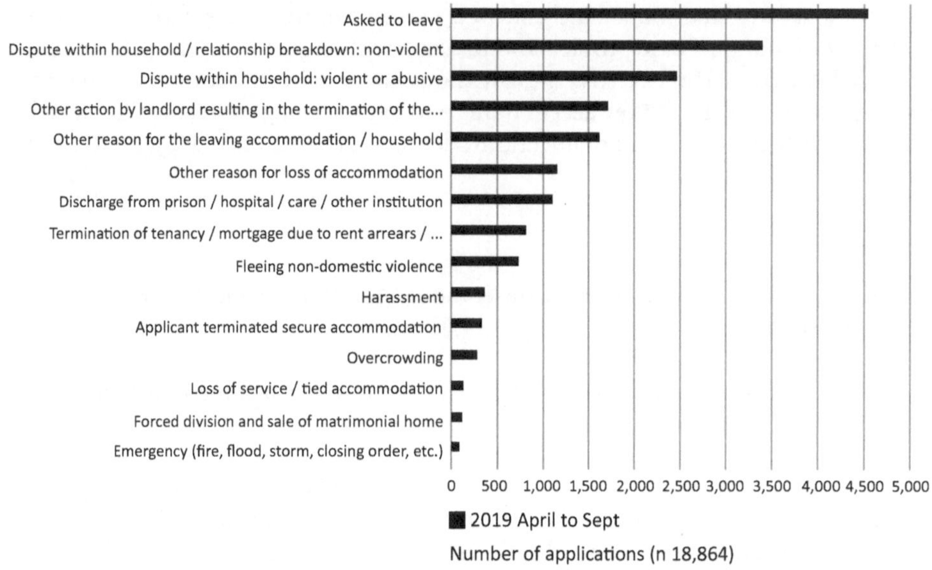

Figure 4.6 Reasons for making a homeless application in Scotland, April to September 2019
Source: adapted from Scottish Government, 2020b p.8

In Scotland, a person is statutory homeless if he/she

> ... has no accommodation in the UK or elsewhere

or if he/she

> has accommodation but cannot reasonably occupy it.

A person is potentially homeless if it is likely that he/she

> ... will become homeless within two months.

A person is intentionally homeless if he/she

> ... deliberately did or failed to do anything which led to the loss of accommodation which it was reasonable for him/her to continue to occupy.
>
> (Scottish Government, 2020b p.31)

In Scotland, between July and September 2019, there were 18,864 applications to the local authority (Scottish Government, 2020b), of which

- 15,542 households were assessed as homeless or threatened with homelessness
- 14,866 households were assessed as unintentionally homeless
- 11,432 households were in temporary accommodation on September 30th

The most common reasons for the making a homeless application were being asked to leave accommodation and disputes (Figure 4.6). Of these, 12,586 applicants recorded a failure to maintain their accommodation (Figure 4.7).

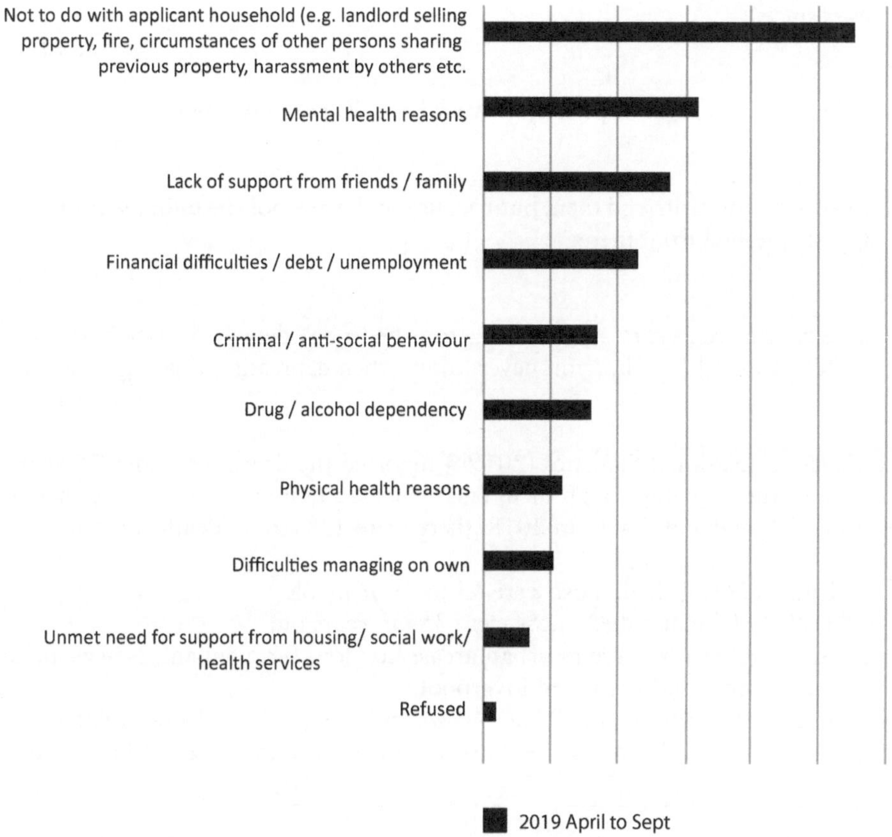

Figure 4.7 Reasons for failing to maintain accommodation in Scotland, April to September 2019 (n = 12,586)

Source: adapted from Scottish Government, 2020b p.9

The charity Shelter spoke to people rough sleeping in England and found the following reasons for their plight (Shelter, 2018):

> I lost my girlfriend last year, I found her dead and I went off the rails a bit. I lost my accommodation ... they gave me 24 hours-notice to leave the premises.
>
> (man, 40s p.18)

Many were unable to get a home for a variety of reasons:

> We can't afford the upfront rent and deposit. You also need a guarantor and a reference. We don't have these things.
>
> (man, 30s, with children 5 and 3 years old p.20)

> Councils do not like single, homeless men, because apparently we can look after ourselves, which is absolute rubbish.
>
> (man, 50s p.19)

> I first slept on the street as soon as I left the Marines and I've been homeless ever since.
>
> (man, 50s p.22)

> When you come out of prison, it's very hard. There's no support.
>
> (man, 40s p.22)

> I was with my girlfriend then, but because of the alcohol she didn't want me there. It just spiralled from there.
>
> (man, 40s p.22)

> Twelve, thirteen years ago, I had a four-bedroom detached place I was paying £1200 [a month] for but you never know when depression is going to strike.
>
> (man, 40s p.23)

The Office for National Statistics (2019b) reported the deaths of under 75-year-olds who were either sleeping rough or in emergency accommodation such as shelters or hostels in England and Wales. In 2018, there were 22% more deaths than in 2017.

- 641 males (88%) died, most were 45 to 49 years old
- 85 (12%) of females died, most were 35–39 years old
- Most (95%) deaths were in urban areas; London, Birmingham, Newcastle upon Tyne, Manchester, Bristol and Liverpool
- People died of drug poisoning (40%), suicide (12%), alcohol-related causes (12%), accidents, heart disease, liver disease, cancer, influenza and pneumonia

Box 4.3 Me, myself and I

Jamie and his wife slept rough on the streets of Manchester for three years. It began when he lost his job as a plasterer. They sold poems and friendship bracelets.

<u>Me myself and I</u>
Sat on the edge of society
Wonderin why am not a priority
What's come of my life an come over me
My life's in tatters can't you see
Beggin at the bank every day
Get a job Get a life people say
I get no benefits Just what people give
To buy food + drink to help me live
I live in the Street a doorway's my bed
People think am thick in the head
It's just me, myself and I
Nobody wants me Do you know why
Don't I deserve to live with a smile
To make my life worth the while.

Jamie Smith
December 2018

There is a mutually reinforcing relationship between increasing poverty and increasing poor health. Both the causes and the outcomes include living in deprivation, mental health problems, food insecurity, poor education, poor housing and transport and fuel poverty. The destination can be homelessness and premature death.

Reframing poverty in the UK

To address the negative impact of poverty on health, the Frameworks Institute (O'Neil *et al.*, 2018), working for the Joseph Rowntree Foundation, carried out research to inform their view of how communicating about poverty needs to be reframed.

1. Understand how the public think about poverty

Common views are that the UK is prosperous; poverty is made by individual choices; our fate is decided by an elitist system and nothing will change. Poverty is dismissed. Show why poverty matters. It is not the past; it is happening now. Most people believe in compassion, justice and protecting each other from harm. We share a moral responsibility to ensure everyone, no matter who they are, has a decent standard of living and the same chances in life.

2. Address poverty head on

The number of those living in relative low income is rising. Many people are struggling and we need to put this right so that everyone can achieve a decent standard of living.

3. Tone down the politics and blaming government

We must all get behind the changes that can reduce poverty.

4. Explain how the economy locks people in poverty

People are having to choose between heating their home, paying their rent or putting food on the table. Rising living costs, low pay and unstable jobs make life a daily struggle. The economy is locking people into poverty and taking away choices.

5. Talk about how welfare benefits loosen poverty's grip

Welfare benefits, such as universal credit, are vital to people who are trying to break through the restrictions within the economy. Public services, such as transport, education and healthcare, are essential to everyone, but most of all to those in most need.

6. Explain how the economy can be redesigned

We need to redesign the economy so that it works well for everyone.

7. Help people see what the facts and stories mean

Translate facts about poverty and stories of people's lives into meaning. In a society that believes in compassion and justice, it is not right to see so many people relying on food banks.

Summary

This chapter has

- described how poverty is defined and measured
- described the characteristics of poverty in the UK
- presented evidence to show how poverty leads to poor health and premature death
- provided examples of the lived experience of poverty
- outlined some ways to reframe the dialogue around poverty in the UK

Further reading

Dalrymple, T. (2010) *Life at the bottom*. Cheltenham: Monday Books

Poole, R., Higgo, R., and Robinson, C.A. (2014) *Mental health and poverty*. Cambridge: Cambridge University Press

Useful websites

Crisis. Available at: www.crisis.org.uk

Joseph Rowntree Foundation. Available at: www.jrf.org.uk

References

Bramley, G., and Fitzpatrick, S. (2018) 'Homelessness in the UK: who is most at risk?', *Housing Studies*, 33(1), pp.96–116

British Medical Association (2017) *Health at a price. Reducing the impact of poverty*. London: British Medical Association

Brunello, G., Fort, M., Schneeweis, N., and Winter-Ebmer, R. (2016) 'The causal effect of education on health: What is the role of health behaviors?', *Health Economics*, 25(3), pp.314–336

Buttler, F. (2013) What determines subjective poverty? An evaluation of the link between relative income poverty measures and subjective economic stress within the EU. Available at: https://horizontal-europeanization.eu/fileadmin/user_upload/proj/horizontal/downloads/pre-prints/PP_HoEu_2013-01_buttler_subjective_poverty_0.pdf (Accessed 30th March 2020)

Crisis (2020) *About homelessness*. Available at: www.crisis.org.uk/ending-homelessness/about-homelessness/ (Accessed 23rd March 2020)

Department for Communities and Local Government (2006) *A decent home: definition and guidance for implementation*. London: Department for Communities and Local Government

Elliott, I. (2016) *Poverty and mental health: a review to inform the Joseph Rowntree Foundation's anti-poverty strategy*. London: Mental Health Foundation

Food and Agriculture Organization of the United Nations (2020) *Hunger and food insecurity*. Available at: www.fao.org/hunger/en/ (Accessed 19th March 2020)

Food and Agriculture Organization (with IFAD, UNICEF, WFP and WHO) (2019) *The state of food security and nutrition in the world 2019*. Rome: Food and Agriculture Organization

Food Foundation (2019) *The broken plate*. Available at: https://foodfoundation.org.uk/wp-content/uploads/2019/02/The-Broken-Plate.pdf (Accessed 20th March 2020)

Francis-Devine, B., Booth, L., and McGuinness, F. (2019) *Poverty in the UK: statistics*. Available at: https://researchbriefings.files.parliament.uk/documents/SN07096/SN07096.pdf (Accessed 20th March 2020)

Heflin, C.M., Siefert, K., and Williams, D.R. (2005) 'Food insufficiency and women's mental health: findings from a 3-year panel of welfare recipients', *Social Science & Medicine*, 61(9), pp.1971–1982

Johnson, A. (2013) *This boy*. London: Transworld

Jones, N.R.V., Conklin, A.I., Suhrcke, M., and Monsivais, P. (2014) 'The growing price gap between more and less healthy foods: analysis of a novel longitudinal UK dataset', *PLoS One*, 9(10) doi:101371/journal.pone.0109343

Joseph Rowntree Foundation (2020) *Non-decent housing and overcrowding*. Available at: www.jrf.org.uk/data/non-decent-housing-and-overcrowding (Accessed 21st March 2020)

Knighton, A.J., Brunisholz, K.D., and Savitz, S.T. (2017) 'Detecting risk of low health literacy in disadvantaged populations using area-based measures', *eGEMs (Generating Evidence & Methods to improve patient outcomes)*, 5(3), pp.7 doi:10.5334/egems.191

Korenman, S., Miller, J.E., and Sjaastad, J.E. (1995) 'Long-term poverty and child development in the United States: results from the NLSY' *Children and Youth Services Review*, 17(1–2), pp.127–155

Kuh, D., and Ben-Shlomo, Y. (eds) (1997) *A lifecourse approach to adult disease*. Oxford: Oxford University Press

Kuznetsova, A. (2019) 'The impact of education on the income of the economically active population in the European Union', Proceedings of the *2nd international conference on education science and social development (ESSD 2019)*. Paris: Atlantis Press

Lochner, L. (2011) *Non-production benefits of education: crime, health, and good citizenship (NBER Working Paper No. w16722)*. Cambridge, MA: National Bureau of Economic Research

Loopstra, R., Reeves, A., and Tarasuk, V. (2019) 'The rise of hunger among low-income households: an analysis of the risks of food insecurity between 2004 and 2016 in a population-based study of UK adults', *Journal of Epidemiology and Community Health*, 73(7), pp.668–673

Lucas, K. (2012) 'Transport and social exclusion: Where are we now?', *Transport Policy*, 20(C), pp.105–113

Lynch, J.L., and von Hippel, P.T. (2016) 'An education gradient in health, a health gradient in education, or a confounded gradient in both?', *Social Science & Medicine*, 154(C), pp.18–27

Marmot Review Team (2011) *The health impacts of cold homes and fuel poverty*. London: Friends of the Earth/Marmot Review Team

Ministry of Housing, Communities and Local Government (2019a) The English indices of deprivation 2019. Available at: https://assets.publishing.service.gov.uk/government/uploads/system/uploads/attachment_data/file/835115/IoD2019_Statistical_Release.pdf (Accessed 13th March 2020)

Ministry of Housing Communities and Local Government (2019b) English housing survey. Headline report 2018–19. Available at https://assets.publishing.service.gov.uk/government/uploads/system/uploads/attachment_data/file/860076/2018-19_EHS_Headline_Report.pdf (Accessed 21st March 2020)

Ministry of Housing, Communities and Local Government (2019c) Statutory homelessness, July to September (Q3) 2019: England. Available at: https://assets.publishing.service.gov.uk/government/uploads/system/uploads/attachment_data/file/873677/Statutory_homelessness_release_Jul-Sep_2019.pdf (Accessed 23rd March 2020)

Morrell-Bellai, T., Goering, P.N., and Boydell, K.M. (2000) 'Becoming and remaining homeless: A qualitative investigation', *Issues in Mental Health Nursing*, 21(6), pp.581–604

National Records of Scotland (2019) *Healthy life expectancy in Scottish areas 2015–2017*. Available at: www.scotpho.org.uk/population-dynamics/healthy-life-expectancy/data/deprivation-deciles (Accessed 16th March 2020)

Northern Ireland Statistics and Research Agency (2017) *Northern Ireland multiple deprivation measures 2017*. Available at: www.nisra.gov.uk/sites/nisra.gov.uk/files/publications/NIMDM17_Description%20of%20Indicators.pdf (Accessed 13th March 2020)

Office for National Statistics (2019a) *Health state life expectancies by national deprivation deciles, England and Wales: 2015 to 2017*. Available at: https://bit.ly/3lBcBYm(Accessed 16th March 2020)

Office for National Statistics (2019b) *Deaths of homeless people in England and Wales: 2018*. www.ons.gov.uk/peoplepopulationandcommunity/birthsdeathsandmarriages/deaths/bulletins/deathsofhomelesspeopleinenglandandwales/2018 (Accessed 24th March 2020)

O'Neil, M., Hawkins, N., Levay, K., Volmert, A., Kendall-Taylor, N., and Stevens, A. (2018) How to talk about poverty in the United Kingdom. *Frameworks Institute*. Available at: http://frameworksinstitute.org/assets/files/PDF_Poverty/JRFUKPovertyMessageMemo2018Final.pdf (Accessed 30th March 2020)

Paugam, S. (2001) 'Les formes contemporaines de la pauvreté et de l'exclusion en Europe', *Etudes Rurales*, 3(159–160), pp.73–95

Phipps, S.A. (2003) *The impact of poverty on health: A scan of research literature*. Ottawa, Canada: Canadian Institute for Health Information.

Prayogo, E., Chater, A., Chapman, S., Barker, M., Rahmawati, N., Waterfall, T., and Grimble, G. (2017) 'Who uses foodbanks and why? Exploring the impact of financial strain and adverse life events on food insecurity', *Journal of Public Health*, 40(4), pp.676–683

Public Health England (2014) *Minimum home temperature thresholds for health in winter – a systematic review*. Available at: https://assets.publishing.service.gov.uk/government/uploads/system/uploads/attachment_data/file/776497/Min_temp_threshold_for_homes_in_winter.pdf (Accessed 24th March 2020)

Public Health England (2018) *The eatwell guide*. London: Public Health England

Public Health England (2019) *Health profile for England*. Available at: www.gov.uk/government/publications/health-profile-for-england-2019 (Accessed 14th March 2020)

Ravallion, M. (2016) 'Toward better global poverty measures', *The Journal of Economic Inequality*, 14(2), pp.227–248.

Rourke, S.B., Bekele, T., Tucker, R., Greene, S., Sobota, M., Koornstra, J., Monette, L., Bacon, J., Bhuiyan, S., Rueda, S., and Watson, J. (2012) 'Housing characteristics and their influence on health-related quality of life in persons living with HIV in Ontario, Canada: results from the positive spaces, healthy places study', *AIDS and Behavior*, 16(8), pp.2361–2373

Scottish Government (2020a) *Scottish index of multiple deprivation 2020: indicators*. Available at: www.gov.scot/publications/scottish-index-of-multiple-deprivation-2020-indicator-data2/ (Accessed 13th March 2020)

Scottish Government (2020b) *Homelessness in Scotland: bi-annual update 1 April to 30 September 2019*. Available at: https://bit.ly/36zNz7N (Accessed 26th May 2020)

Shaw, M. (2004) 'Housing and public health', *Annual Review of Public Health*, 25(1), pp.397–418

Shelter (2018) *On the streets. An investigation into rough sleeping*. Available at: https://bit.ly/3ogoB36 (Accessed 24th March 2020)

Social Metrics Commission (2018) *A new measure of poverty for the UK: The final report of the Social Metrics Commission*. London: Social Metrics Commission

Social Metrics Commission (2019) *Measuring poverty 2019*. London: Social Metrics Commission

Tarasuk, V., Mitchell, A., McLaren, L., and McIntyre, L. (2013) 'Chronic physical and mental health conditions among adults may increase vulnerability to household food insecurity', *The Journal of Nutrition*, 143(11), pp.1785–1793

Tribble, A.G., Maxfield, A., Hadley, C. and Goodman, M. (2020) 'Food insecurity and mental health: a meta-analysis', *The Lancet*, January doi:10.2139/ssrn.3520061

Trussel Trust (2019) *The state of hunger: introduction to a study of poverty and food insecurity in the UK.* Available at: www.trusselltrust.org/wp-content/uploads/sites/2/2019/06/SoH-Interim-Report-Final-2.pdf (Accessed 19th March 2020)

Townsend, P. (1979) *Poverty in the United Kingdom: a survey of household resources and standards of living.* London: Allen Lane/Penguin

United Nations (2015) *Transforming our world: the 2030 agenda for sustainable development.* Available at: www.un.org/ga/search/view_doc.asp?symbol=A/RES/70/1&Lang=E (Accessed 23rd November 2019)

United Nations Economic Commission for Europe (2017) *Guide on poverty measurement.* Available at: www.unece.org/fileadmin/DAM/stats/publications/2018/ECECESSTAT20174.pdf (Accessed 30th March 2020)

van Schalkwyk, M.C.I. and Mindell, J.S. (2018) 'Current issues impacts of transport on health', *British Medical Bulletin*, 125(1), pp.67–77

Warm homes and energy conservation act (2000). Available at: https://www.legislation.gov.uk/ukpga/2000/31/section/1 (Accessed: 30th March 2020)

Welsh Government (2019a) *Welsh index of multiple deprivation (WIMD) 2019. Guidance.* Available at: https://gov.wales/sites/default/files/statistics-and-research/2020-01/welsh-index-multiple-deprivation-guidance.pdf (Accessed 13th March 2020)

Welsh Government (2019b) *Welsh index of multiple deprivation (WIMD) 2019. Results Report.* Available at: https://gov.wales/sites/default/files/statistics-and-research/2020-02/welsh-index-multiple-deprivation-2019-results-report.pdf (Accessed 13th March 2020)

Wunderlich, G.S., and Norwood, J.L. (2006) *Panel to review U.S. department of agriculture's measurement of food insecurity and hunger. Food insecurity and hunger in the United States: an assessment of the measure, and national research council (U.S).* Washington DC: National Academies Press

Zimmerman, E.B., Woolf, S.H., Blackburn, S.M., Kimmel, A.D., Barnes, A.J., and Bono, R.S. (2018) 'The case for considering education and health', *Urban Education*, 53(6), pp.744–773

5 Mental, emotional and spiritual health

Sally Robinson and Athene Lane-Martin

Key points

- Introduction
- Defining mental, emotional and spiritual health
- Disorders and distress
- Social exclusion
- Communities and mental, emotional and spiritual health
- Summary

Introduction

This chapter focuses on those priorities for health promotion and public health that most immediately relate to how we think and feel about ourselves. To introduce key aspects of our inner worlds, we will define mental, emotional and spiritual health. Each has a long and distinctive body of research that contributes to our understanding of health. We provide examples of how these can become unsettled, undermined or disordered through social perceptions, actions or structures. In turn, these can affect our physical health and become wider social concerns that have a major impact on the public's health.

Defining mental, emotional and spiritual health

Mental health

Thinking point:

> Think about the term 'mental health'. How would you would define it and what does it include? If you were defining your own mental health, what might you say?

Mental disorders

Mental disorders are characterised by a combination of abnormal thoughts, emotions, behaviours and relationships with others (WHO, 2019a). This is a broader and more up to date term than 'mental illness', which is strongly associated with the fields of psychiatry and psychology, with an emphasis on a medical diagnosis and medical treatment (Mental Health Foundation, 2019a). As the medical model of health and illness was challenged, as discussed in Chapter 1, and research confirmed that mental disorders were the result of complex interactions between psychological, social and biological factors, so the term 'mental illness' and the significant social stigma associated with it is becoming less used. During the 21st century we have seen the adoption of terms such as 'mental health problems', 'mental ill health' and sometimes simply 'mental health', when mental disorders and their treatment are being discussed. The World Health Organization (2004) argue that this euphemistic language is confusing, and currently use the terms 'mental disorders' or 'mental, behavioural or neurodevelopmental disorders' (WHO, 2019a; 2019b).

Mental disorders are classified in the American Psychiatric Association's Diagnostic and Statistical Manual of Mental Disorders and the World Health Organization's Manual of the International Statistical Classification of Diseases, Injuries and Causes of Death (WHO, 2019b), which outlines 20 categories, some of which are

- neurodevelopmental disorders, e.g. disorders of intellectual development
- schizophrenia and other primary psychotic disorders, e.g. delusional disorder
- mood disorders, e.g. bipolar, recurrent depressive disorder
- anxiety or fear-related disorders, e.g. panic disorder, agoraphobia
- obsessive-compulsive or related disorders, e.g. hypochondriasis
- disorders specifically associated with stress, e.g. post-traumatic stress disorder
- feeding or eating disorders, e.g. anorexia nervosa
- disorders due to substance use or addictive behaviours, e.g. disorder due to use of alcohol
- paraphilic disorders, e.g. voyeuristic disorder
- neurocognitive disorders, e.g. dementia due to Alzheimer disease

Across the world, compared to the rest of the population, people with mental disorders are more likely to be homeless, living in poverty, inappropriately incarcerated, stigmatised, abused, discriminated against and have their human rights violated (WHO, 2013). They experience higher rates of disability and early death due to suicide, accidents, homicide and other physical health problems. People with mental disorders, such as severe and enduring depression, schizophrenia and bipolar disorder, live 10 to 20 years less, on average, compared to the rest of the population. Behaviours that contribute to their early death are substance use (drugs, alcohol and/or smoking), physical inactivity, poor diets and excess weight; and they have high rates of diabetes, cardiovascular disease, cancer, HIV/AIDS and other infectious diseases such as hepatitis B/C and tuberculosis (WHO, 2018).

Mental health problems

The term 'mental health problems' covers the range of negative states of mental health. It includes the more common conditions of poor mental health such as short-term anxiety and depression and the rarer, more severe, mental disorders (Faculty of Public Health and Mental Health Foundation, 2016).

Mental wellbeing

Mental wellbeing or 'positive mental health' is about feeling good and functioning well (FPH/MHF, 2016).

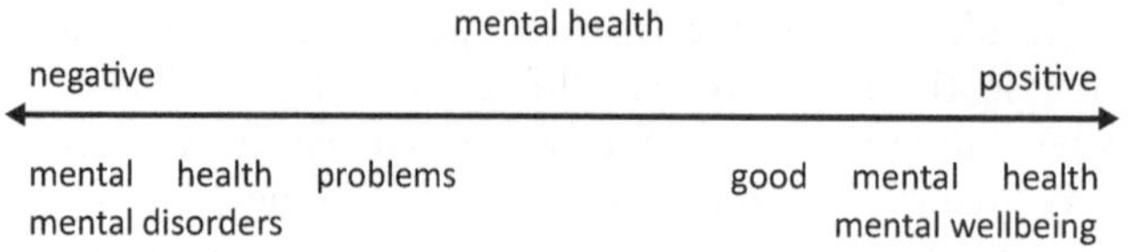

Figure 5.1 Mental health continuum

Mental health

Mental health can be illustrated as a continuum that includes mental disorders, mental health problems and mental wellbeing (Figure 5.1). In public health, the focus is about supporting the social and environmental factors that can help to move people towards positive mental health (FPH/MHF, 2016).

Corey Keyes (2002; 2005; 2007) carried out many research studies that demonstrate how a simple representation of mental health along a single axis, from mental disorder to mental wellbeing, is limited because it fails to show how people's experience of mental health is the sum of two separate but related dimensions; the presence or absence of a mental disorder and the presence or absence of subjective psychological, emotional and social wellbeing, which at best is 'flourishing'. He suggests that psychological wellbeing concerns how we personally evaluate our own functioning and includes self-acceptance, autonomy, positive relationships and having a purpose. Emotional wellbeing concerns feeling positive with life; being in good spirits, as opposed to feeling hopeless. Social wellbeing is achieved when we see society as meaningful and understandable, we feel accepted and integrated into our community, and see it as a place where we can thrive. He describes the absence of subjective wellbeing as 'languishing' in life. Figure 5.2 shows,

A – a person has no mental disorder and feels good about life. Overall, they are mentally healthy and achieve mental wellbeing. Life may throw difficulties in their way and they could move to B.

B – a person has no mental disorder, but they do not feel good about life. Overall, they have moderate or sub-optimal mental health. They are not coping well and if this is sustained they will move to C.

C – a person has a mental disorder and does not feel good about life. Overall, they have poor mental health. With appropriate support, such as medication, therapy and/or lifestyle changes, they may move to D.

D – a person has a mental disorder, but they feel good about life. Overall, they have moderate or sub-optimal mental health. With continued individual and community support, they may achieve a full recovery and move back to A.

In summary,

> Mental health is conceived of as a complete state in which individuals are free of psychopathology and flourishing with high levels of emotional, psychological and social well-being.
>
> (Keyes, 2005 p. 539)

Keyes's work supported the World Health Organization's mission to create an understanding of mental health that included wellbeing. In 2001 they adopted their current definition:

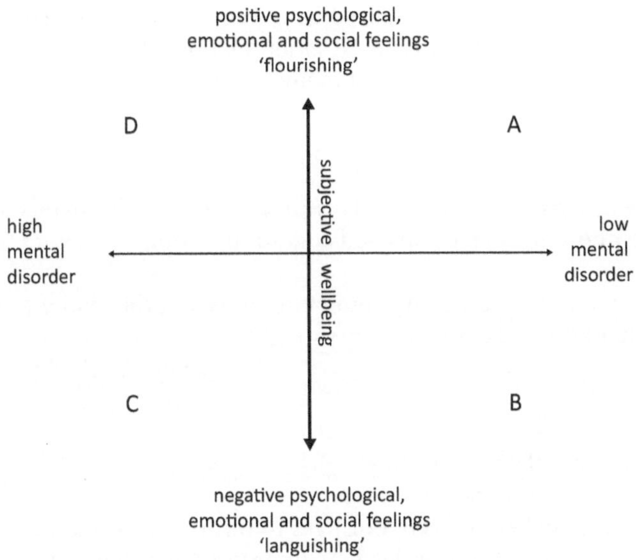

Figure 5.2 Keyes's model of mental health

> Mental health is a state of well-being in which the individual realizes his or her own abilities, can cope with the normal stresses of life, can work productively and fruitfully, and is able to make a contribution to his or her community.
>
> (World Health Organization, 2001, p.1)

The World Health Organization (2004) set out key messages about mental health

- there is no health without mental health; it is an integral part of our health
- mental health is more than the absence of a mental disorder
- mental health and physical health are inextricably linked; neither can exist alone
- mental health is linked to behaviour
- mental health is the foundation for our well-being
- mental, physical and social functioning are interdependent
- mental health is determined by socioeconomic and environmental factors
- mental health is everybody's business

Having 'positive mental health', or mental wellbeing, can protect people from developing mental health problems and consequently some physical health problems (WHO, 2004; FPH/MHF, 2016). Creating mentally healthy people means supporting their psychological, social, emotional, spiritual, socio-economic and environmental health and wellbeing.

Emotional health

There are several related fields of study that illuminate our understanding of emotional health. Weare and Gray (2003) explain how the work of different disciplines and professions culminated in a wide range of terminology to describe a common interest.

These include: social and emotional intelligence, emotional and social literacy, emotional literacy, emotional and social competence, mental health, and emotional and social wellbeing. We will introduce three, emotional intelligence, emotional-social intelligence and emotional literacy, before examining current understandings of emotional health.

Emotional intelligence

Emotional intelligence emerged from psychological research into multiple intelligences and an interest in learning about how emotions and cognition (thought) interact. It is

> The ability to carry out accurate reasoning about emotions and the ability to use emotions and emotional knowledge to enhance thought.
>
> (Mayer *et al.*, 2008 p.507)

It includes

- being able to solve emotion-related problems
- being able to perceive emotions in people's faces
- knowing how to use emotional episodes in our lives to inform our thinking
- understanding the meanings of emotions, such as understanding that sad people may wish to be left alone and angry people may be potentially dangerous
- knowing how to manage our own emotions
- knowing how to manage other people's emotions, such as knowing a sad person is unlikely to accept a party invitation in contrast to a happy person

(Mayer, 2009)

A person's emotional intelligence can predict their relations with other people, their performance in the workplace, their physical and mental wellbeing and therefore it can affect many aspects of their life (Mayer *et al.*, 2008).

Emotional-social intelligence

Bar-On (2006) explains how investigations into the condition alexithymia, the inability to describe, recognise or understand emotions, helped to develop fields of research into emotional awareness, psychological mindedness and emotional-social intelligence. Emotional-social intelligence is

> A cross-section of interrelated emotional and social competencies, skills and facilitators that determine how effectively we understand and express ourselves, understand others and relate to them, and cope with daily demands.
>
> (Bar-On, 2006 p.3)

The elements of social-emotional intelligence which have the strongest impact on our physical health and subjective/self-reported wellbeing are

- self-regard; to accurately perceive, understand and accept oneself
- self-actualisation; to strive to achieve personal goals and actualise one's potential

- stress tolerance; to effectively and constructively manage emotions
- optimism; to be positive, hopeful and look on the brighter side of life
- happiness; to feel content with oneself, others and life in general

(Bar-On, 2012)

Emotional literacy

Claude Steiner defines emotional literacy as 'intelligence with a heart' (Steiner, 2003). It is

> The ability to recognise, understand, handle and appropriately express emotions.
>
> (Sharp, 2001 p.1)

Akbağ and colleagues (2016) explain how low levels of emotional literacy are associated with internalising stress, depression, problems with friendships, poor coping, mental health problems, aggression and violence and, in turn, wider social problems. Opportunities to develop people's emotional literacy, through practising emotional and social skills, is offered within education and counselling/psychotherapy (Liau *et al.*, 2003; Weare and Gray, 2003; Sorin, 2009; Bayne and Thompson, 2018).

Emotional health

There are many definitions of emotional health; for example,

> The ability to recognise emotions such as fear, joy, grief and anger and to express such emotions appropriately. Emotional (or affective) health also means coping with stress, tension, depression and anxiety.
>
> (Scriven, 2017 p.8)

and

> A set of malleable skills and beliefs which shape our feelings, thoughts and behaviour.
>
> (FLTCEH, 2018 p.3)

Family Links: The Centre for Emotional Health (2018) defines emotional health in terms of people's social and emotional functioning, their competences. Emotional health is determined by the interaction between the individual and their environment. The environment can enable or disable our functioning. When this interaction works well, we experience emotional health. In turn, this supports our motivation, resilience, the tools to build positive relationships and mental health.

Table 5.1 shows how our skills, and our beliefs about ourselves and about others, underpin our feelings, thoughts and behaviour. These are grouped as the seven emotional assets, strengths, which are associated with emotionally healthy individuals and emotionally healthy workplaces.

Table 5.1 Emotional health assets and their characteristics

	Emotional health asset	*Related concepts*	*Characteristics of an emotionally healthy individual*	*Characteristics of an emotionally healthy workplace*
Beliefs	Self beliefs The set of beliefs we hold about our self-identity, including our skills, abilities and sense of value and worth.	Feeling valued Feeling competent	Has a positive self identity. Has a stable sense of competence. Has a stable self-worth.	Ensures employees feel valued.
	Self agency The set of beliefs we hold about our capacity to influence our lives and wider environment.	Autonomy Influence/a voice	Recognises that they have choices about how they act. Can self motivate. Recognises that they can influence their lives and wider environment.	Enables choice and autonomy.
	Beliefs about others The set of beliefs we hold about others, including how trustworthy they are and how they will respond to us.	Trust Acceptance Belonging	Can trust others. Accepts others. Believes others will respond positively towards them.	Creates a psychologically safe culture.
Awareness	Self awareness Our awareness of our own thoughts, feelings and behaviours.	Self reflection Reflective practice	Is aware of their thoughts, feelings and behaviours. Can accurately reflect on their thoughts, feelings and behaviours and the impact they have.	Encourages self reflection.
	Social awareness Our awareness of the thoughts and feelings of others, and the impact our behaviour may have.	Empathy Compassion	Is aware of the thoughts and feelings of other people. Is aware of the impact their behaviour has on others.	Fosters compassion.
Management	Self regulation Our ability to manage our thoughts, feelings and behaviours.	Managing emotions Cognitive reframing	Can manage their thoughts, feelings and behaviours in positive and constructive ways.	Supports healthy self regulation.
	Relationship skills Our ability to form and maintain positive relationships with others.	Communication Team work Conflict resolution	Can communicate effectively. Can work collaboratively towards shared goals. Can manage and resolve conflict in healthy ways.	Develops relationship skills.

Source: Adapted from FLTCEH (2018 p.13, p.24).

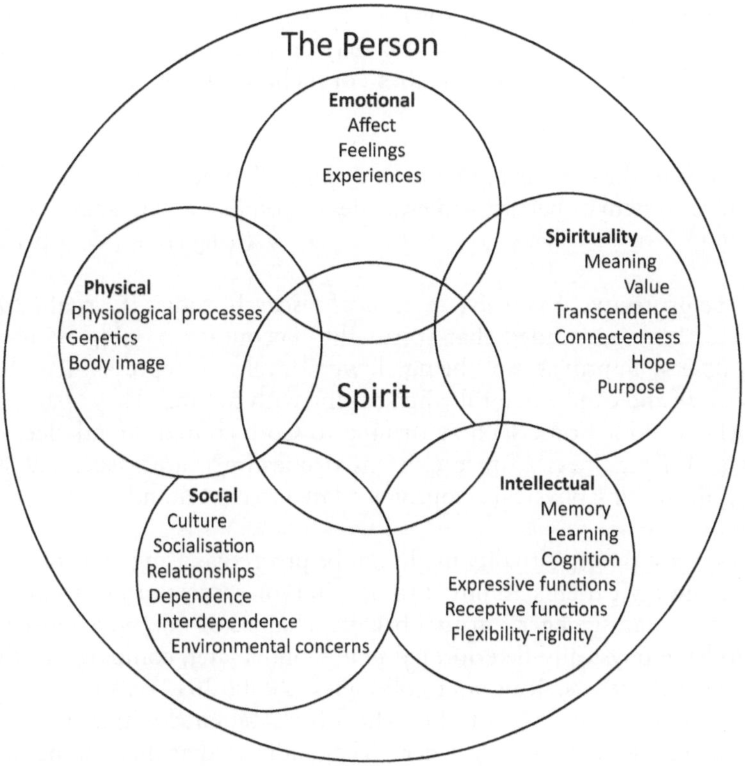

Figure 5.3 Model of a person
Source: adapted from Swinton, 2001 p.36

Spiritual health

Before defining spiritual health, we will outline the meanings of spirit, spirituality and religion.

Spirit

Swinton (2001) puts spirit at the core of a person. He suggests that the spirit cannot be directly observed, but a person's spirituality is revealed in their thoughts, language and behaviours. He argues that the spiritual cannot be separated from the physical, intellectual, emotional and social aspects of a person.

Spirituality and religion

Fisher (2011) writes that spirituality and religion are sometimes used interchangeably, but they are also distinct, overlapping constructs. He argues that spirituality concerns an individual's awareness of the existence and experience of their inner feelings and beliefs, and a recognition of how these give meaning, purpose and value to their life. Spirituality helps individuals to be at peace with themselves, to love their neighbour, to love God (if this is meaningful to them), and to live in harmony with the environment. For some, spirituality may involve an encounter with God, or another transcendent reality, and this may occur within the context of an organised religion; for others, spirituality does not include a belief in the supernatural. King and colleagues suggest:

> Religion pertains to the outward practice of a spiritual understanding and/or the framework for a system of beliefs, values, codes of conduct and rituals.
> (King *et al.*, 1999 p.1292)

Spirituality may be protective. Extensive reviews of research studies (Cornah, 2006; Tabei *et al.*, 2016) have concluded that spirituality encourages coping with, and recovery from, illness; improves well-being; lowers levels of depression; reduces anxiety; lowers stress and can be helpful when coping with trauma. They also report that religious beliefs and actions, such as turning to God, church attendance, religious openness and a readiness to face existential questions, are associated with reducing anxiety, decreasing physical symptoms related to cancer and recovery from trauma.

Other studies suggest that spirituality might not be protective. King and colleagues (1999) found that among patients admitted to hospital for cardiac or gynaecological conditions, those who had stronger spiritual beliefs, religious or not, were more than twice as likely to have physically deteriorated nine months later, compared to those who did not have such beliefs. King and colleagues (2009; 2013) also found that people who have a spiritual approach to life which is not situated within a religious framework are vulnerable to mental disorders. They indicate that this finding might be partly explained by religious people being less likely to use recreational drugs and alcohol.

Spiritual health

Fisher (2011) defines spiritual health as

> A dynamic state of being, shown by the extent to which people live in harmony.
> (Fisher, 2011 p.20)

He argues that our spiritual health concerns the quality of our relationships within four domains. The

- personal domain is where one relates to oneself about the meaning, purpose and values of life. It is our search for self-identity and self-worth
- communal domain concerns the quality of our relationships with others. It includes morality, culture, religion, and expressions of love, trust, hope, forgiveness and faith in humanity
- environmental domain is about nurturing and having a sense of unity with the environment, perhaps including a sense of awe
- transcendental domain is about our relationship with someone/something beyond the human level, perhaps a cosmic force, an ultimate concern or a transcendent reality. It might inspire adoration and worship

Each domain has a knowledge (head) aspect and an inspirational (heart) aspect. When the relationships within and between the domains are of good quality and integrated, Fisher argues that we achieve wholeness and health. In the same way that Swinton (2001) argues that the spiritual cannot be separated from other aspects of a person, Fisher argues that the spiritual cannot be separated from the physical, mental, emotional and social dimensions of health.

> *Mental health, emotional health and spiritual health are inter-dependent dimensions of our health. They affect, and are affected by, our physical and social health, and the wider socio-economic and environmental context in which we live.*

Disorders and distress

Many aspects of life can challenge people's mental, emotional and spiritual health and cause a range of disorders and distress. Here we discuss some of the more common ones.

Stress

Stress is a natural physical and emotional reaction that helps to keep people alert and protect them from danger. Symptoms of acute stress include rapid breathing, trembling, awareness of the heart beating rapidly, muscle tension, sweating and gastro-intestinal discomfort. These symptoms relate to the body's readiness to 'fight, flight or freeze'. The body activates its sympathetic nervous system, the heart rate and blood pressure rise, and the body produces a surge in adrenaline and cortisol. After the event, the body activates its parasympathetic nervous system to return the body back to rest and its normal functions.

People who experience chronic stress may feel overwhelmed, irritable, exhausted, have difficulty in concentrating and experience pain. The body is in a constant state of high alert, with raised heart rate and blood pressure causing wear and tear throughout the cardiovascular system (McEwen, 2008). Persistently raised cortisol leads to low-grade chronic inflammation which is associated with fatigue, depression, pain, the breakdown of muscle and bone, inflammatory autoimmune diseases such as arthritis, and it can interfere with a person's ability to accurately appraise new situations, perhaps seeing them as fearful or threatening (Hannibal and Bishop, 2014). Chronic stress is associated with health-damaging behaviours such as smoking, eating too much, poor sleep and drinking excess alcohol (McEwen, 2008). Chronic stress alone does not cause cardiovascular disease, but where individuals already have early markers of the disease, stress can trigger the disease and encourage its progression (Kivimäki and Steptoe, 2018).

Segerstrom and O'Conner (2012) explain stress in three ways; focusing on the environment, the appraisal or the response. Stress can be

- about a physical or psychological stressor in the environment, such as heat, injury, a diagnosis, medical treatment, role changes such as becoming a mother, or a loss of resources such as a job
- experienced when a person appraises the demand placed upon them, such as a threat, and balances this against their own personal resources. In this conceptualisation, the same stressor will affect people differently

- the internal distress caused by a stressor. For example, an event may make one person feel mildly irritated, and another very angry

Preventing chronic stress, or ameliorating it, reflects its multiple causes. Some researchers have drawn attention to having low control and high stress in work environments, while others focus on people's early life experiences, their genes or their coping strategies (Bosma *et al.*, 1997; McEwen, 2008; Segerstrom and O'Connor, 2012). Mental disorders associated with stress include post-traumatic stress disorder, prolonged grief disorder and disinhibited social engagement disorder (WHO, 2019a).

Trauma

Traumatic events are

> ... shocking and emotionally overwhelming situations that may involve actual or threaten death, serious injury, or threat to physical integrity.
>
> (ISTSS, 2019)

The body's response to trauma is the same as for stress, but in this case the stressor is extremely threatening or horrific, and the individual may develop a disorder such as post-traumatic stress disorder which is characterised by

- re-experiencing the traumatic event, and the strong emotions of fear and horror, in the form of intrusive memories, flashbacks or nightmares
- avoiding thinking about the event or related activities and situations
- hypervigilance such as a heightened awareness of potential threat
- symptoms which last for several weeks and interfere with the person's ability to function in normal life

(WHO, 2019a)

Adverse childhood experiences (ACEs) are traumatic and stressful psychosocial conditions that are out of a child's control. They tend to co-occur and often persist over time, causing chronic, 'toxic', stress responses (Kelly-Irving *et al.*, 2013; Barr, 2017). ACEs include

- emotional abuse
- physical abuse
- sexual abuse
- emotional neglect
- physical neglect
- domestic violence/mother treated violently
- household substance misuse
- household mental disorders
- criminality/household member in prison
- separation/divorce

The more ACEs a person experiences in childhood, the stronger the risk, in adulthood, that they will experience

- depression
- stress disorders, post-traumatic stress disorder
- suicide attempts/self-directed violence
- borderline personality disorder
- hallucinations
- poor health-related quality of life
- intimate partner violence
- early initiation of sexual activity, multiple sexual partners and sexually transmitted infections
- unintended pregnancies and teenage pregnancy
- alcohol misuse
- smoking and early initiation of smoking
- drug misuse
- physical inactivity
- overweight/obesity
- frequent headaches
- disability
- autoimmune diseases
- cancer
- chronic obstructive pulmonary disease (COPD)
- foetal death
- cardiovascular disease
- liver disease
- type 2 diabetes

(Felitti *et al.*, 1998; Barr, 2017; Holman *et al.*, 2016; Hughes *et al.*, 2017; Deschênes *et al.*, 2018; CDC, 2020)

Anxiety

The Mental Health Foundation defines anxiety as

> A feeling of unease, worry or fear which, when persistent and impacting on daily life may be a sign of an anxiety disorder.
>
> (Mental Health Foundation, 2019b)

Psychological symptoms of anxiety include restlessness, a feeling of being 'on-edge' or 'dread', difficulty with concentrating and sleeping, and irritability. Physical symptoms may include a dry mouth, being short of breath, a fast heart rate, sweating and dizziness. Some anxiety in response to challenging events is normal; it can promote healthy caution and can be motivational. Chronic anxiety can become distressing, affecting daily life such as avoiding places, people or situations.

In Wales, more than 14,000 people were asked, "On a scale where 0 is 'not at all anxious' and 10 is 'completely anxious' overall how anxious did you feel yesterday?" (Figure 5.4).

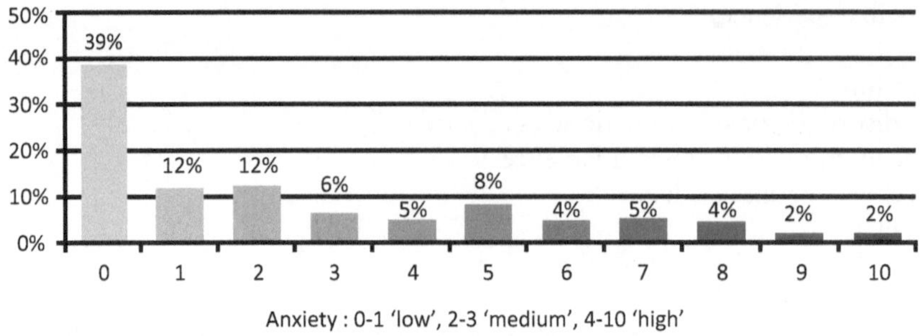

Figure 5.4 Responses to 'anxiety yesterday' question

Source: Statistics for Wales, 2015 p.8. Reproduced under the terms of the Open Government Licence v3.0

Anxiety disorders can cause long-term distress for the individual and their families, and significant long-term disability. They often occur alongside depression or substance misuse. They include

- generalised anxiety disorder; characterised by more than six months of excessive worry, heightened tension, irritability, and poor concentration and sleeping
- social anxiety disorder; a fear of social situations that involve interaction, observation and performance which is out of proportion to the actual situation
- post-traumatic stress disorder; pervasive distress caused by a stressful or exceptionally threatening event or situation
- panic disorder; recurring, unforeseen panic attacks followed by persistent worrying about having another
- obsessive-compulsive disorder; unwanted intrusive thoughts or images and repetitive behaviours or mental acts that a person feels driven to perform
- body dysmorphic disorder; preoccupation with an imagined defect in a person's own appearance. It is characterised by time-consuming behaviours such as camouflaging and seeking reassurance

(NICE, 2005; NICE, 2014)

Depression

We can all have days when we feel a little low in mood, slightly unhappy or just not wanting to get up and face the day. These are feelings of sadness, which are normal responses to life's challenges. This is not depression. Depression, sometimes called 'clinical depression', is a mental disorder characterised by a depressed mood and/or a loss of pleasure in most activities (NICE, 2011). It may be mild, moderate or severe depending on the number, severity and duration of symptoms. Severely depressed people find it almost impossible to get through daily life.

Depression is a symptom within postnatal depression, bipolar disorder and seasonal affective disorder. Depression often presents with anxiety. Some populations, such as those who receive social care, are particularly vulnerable to depression and anxiety.

Table 5.2 Symptoms of depression

Psychological symptoms	*Physical symptoms*	*Social symptoms*
constant sadness no enjoyment no motivation hopelessness helplessness tearful irritable guilt-ridden anxious low self-esteem suicidal thoughts thoughts about self-harming	speaking more slowly than usual moving more slowly than usual changes in weight changes in appetite changes in appearance lack of energy unexplained aches and pains constipation loss of libido disturbed sleep changes to menstrual cycle	not doing well at work avoiding friends avoiding social activities neglecting hobbies and interests difficulties in home and family life

Source: NHS (2016).

Table 5.3 Depression and anxiety in England and regions

	Depression: recorded prevalence (percentage of adult population 2017/2018)	*Depression and anxiety prevalence (percentage of adult respondents to GP Patient Survey 2016/2017)*	*Percentage of social care users reporting depression and anxiety (2017/2018)*
England	9.9%	13.7%	54.4%
Surrey	8.9%	10.4%	52.6%
Middlesborough	8.9%	18.6%	52.1%
Cornwall	8.7%	13.6%	55.5%

Source: Public Health England (2019).

Loss and bereavement

Loss is painful because it is something out of people's control, and we like to feel in control of what happens to us. People experience loss when a negative event leads to a change in their situations, relationships and ways of viewing the world. Some losses are personal such as the loss of one's hearing, some are interpersonal such as the ending of a friendship, some are material such as losing a job and some are intangible such as losing self-worth. Bereavement is a loss due to death. Loss can be particularly agonising if it is not understood by others or if the loss relates to something that is taboo and there is no support.

Thinking point:

> List some of the losses that you have experienced in your life and reflect on how you felt and behaved. How did they change how you viewed yourself and the world?

Grief is what we call the collective signs and symptoms of loss, and it is influenced by culture, ethnicity, spirituality and an individual's personal coping strategies. Acute grief is often intense. Over time, grief becomes integrated into the person's life.

Table 5.4 Symptoms of grief in bereavement

Acute grief	*Integrated grief*
Intense yearning, sorrow, emotional pain. Physical symptoms like heart palpitations, butterflies in the stomach, yawning, dizziness/fogginess	Symptoms emerge intermittently
Feelings of disbelief, difficulty comprehending the death	Comprehension of the reality and consequences of death A mix of emotions with bittersweet positive emotions usually dormant
Insistent distracting thoughts of the deceased, trouble focusing attention, forgetfulness	Thoughts and memories of the deceased are accessible but not preoccupying
Loss of sense of self or sense of purpose and belonging, and feeling aimless, incompetent, without feelings of wellbeing	Restoration of sense of self and sense of purpose and belonging; feelings of competence and wellbeing
Feeling disconnected from other people and ongoing life	Interest and engagement in life and other people are re-established; happiness seems possible

Source: Adapted from Shear *et al.* (2017).

Among older people, the death of a spouse is a major loss because widowhood requires the individual to cope with significant emotional loss alongside the loss of the behavioural, social and economic environment that the couple once shared. This double loss can suppress the immune system. There is an association between poor physical health and greater levels of grief and depression; each may exacerbate the other, and the outcome is an increased risk of death (Utz *et al.*, 2012).

Suicide

Every year, across the world, there are 800,000 deaths from suicide and it is the second leading cause of death among 15 to 29 year olds (WHO, 2019c). Many more attempt suicide. In the UK, the Office for National Statistics (ONS) defines suicide as

> Death from intentional self-harm for persons aged 10 and over, and deaths caused by injury or poisoning where the intent was undetermined for those aged 15 and over.
>
> (ONS, 2019)

The ONS reported 6,507 suicides in 2018, of which three-quarters were among men. Male suicides significantly increased from 2017. Deaths by suicide are certified by coroners. In England and Wales the standard of proof recently changed from 'criminal standard' (beyond reasonable doubt) to the lower 'civil standard' (balance of probabilities), and this might have led to an increase in the recording of suicides. Northern Ireland and Scotland have slightly different recording practices.

Table 5.5 UK age-standardised rates of suicide, 2018

Jurisdiction	*Suicide rate per 100,000 people*
Northern Ireland	18.6
Scotland	16.1
Wales	12.8
England	10.3

Sources: ONS (2019); NISRA (2019).

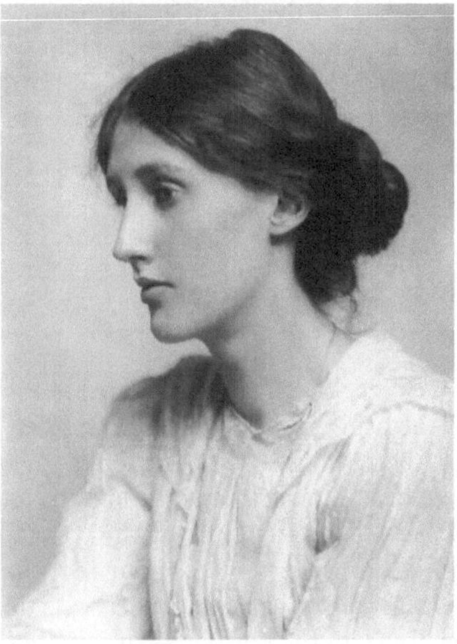

Figure 5.5 Portrait of Virgina Woolf, British author and feminist, 1902

Source: George Charles Beresford https://commons.wikimedia.org/wiki/File:George_Charles_Beresford_-_Virginia_Woolf_in_1902_-_Restoration.jpg

Suicidal feelings and action are often caused by

- addiction or substance abuse
- adjusting to a big change, such as retirement or redundancy
- being in prison
- bereavement
- bullying
- cultural pressure such as a forced marriage
- discrimination towards lesbian, gay, bisexual, transgender, intersex people
- discrimination towards refugees, migrants or prisoners
- domestic abuse
- doubts about one's own sexual or gender identity
- feeling inadequate or a failure

- isolation or loneliness
- long-term physical pain or illness
- losing a loved one to suicide
- mental health problems such as depression
- money problems or homelessness
- pregnancy, childbirth or postnatal depression
- sexual or physical abuse
- the end of a relationship

(Mind, 2019; WHO, 2019c)

Suicidal feelings and thoughts are often expressed as hopelessness and helplessness; 'no point in going on'. Quite often people do not wish to die, but they do not want to carry on living with the physical pain or emotional trauma that they are facing. This can be very difficult for the friends and family left behind who experience not only the loss of someone important, but often feelings of guilt and sadness that they should have noticed or done something different.

Box 5.1 Virginia Woolf's suicide note to her husband, 28th March 1941

Dearest,

I feel certain I am going mad again. I feel we can't go through another of those terrible times. And I shan't recover this time. I begin to hear voices, and I can't concentrate. So I am doing what seems the best thing to do. You have given me the greatest possible happiness. You have been in every way all that anyone could be. I don't think two people could have been happier till this terrible disease came. I can't fight any longer. I know that I am spoiling your life, that without me you could work. And you will I know. You see I can't even write this properly. I can't read. What I want to say is I owe all the happiness of my life to you. You have been entirely patient with me and incredibly good. I want to say that – everybody knows it. If anybody could have saved me it would have been you. Everything has gone from me but the certainty of your goodness. I can't go on spoiling your life any longer.

I don't think two people could have been happier than we have been.

A UK survey reported the effects of sudden bereavement on 3,400 young adults (Pitman *et al.*, 2016). In the four years since the loss, 45% had experienced suicidal thoughts, 6% had attempted suicide, 31% experienced symptoms of depression. Those who were both bereaved by suicide and felt stigmatised by it were more likely to attempt suicide themselves, drop out of a job or course and describe poor social functioning compared to those bereaved by sudden natural causes.

> *Chronic stress, trauma, anxiety and depression can have very distressing effects on people's mental, emotional and spiritual health. They can lead to death from their physical consequences or suicide.*

Social isolation and loneliness

Social isolation is

> A state in which the individual lacks a sense of belonging socially, lacks engagement with others, has a minimal number of social contacts and they are deficient in fulfilling and quality relationships.
>
> (Nicholson, 2009 p.1346)

Loneliness is

> ... not about being alone, but a subjective experience of feeling isolation ... it is often overlooked ... because our social norms praise independence and self-reliance ... But when loneliness sets in long enough to create a persistent, self-reinforcing loop of negative thoughts and sensations, it can wear us down ...
>
> (Farmer and Edwards, 2014 p.34)

People aged 50 years and over living in England are more likely to be often lonely if they:

- have no one to open up to when they need to talk
- are in poor health
- are widowed
- are unable to do what they want
- feel as if they do not belong in their neighbourhood
- live alone

and this is not due to their age, gender or how often they meet with other people (Age UK, 2018).

Loneliness and social isolation are associated with physical health problems that cause earlier death than the rest of the population. In Denmark, a study found that social isolation was associated with 60% to 70% increased mortality from all causes, irrespective of socioeconomic circumstances, mental health disorders and lifestyles; and having no partner further increased mortality (Laugesen *et al.*, 2018). In Ireland, a study showed those who reported feeling lonely, rather than being alone, were more likely to die earlier from all causes (O'Súilleabháin *et al.*, 2019). However, it should be noted that it is difficult to disentangle whether the isolation and/or feeling lonely causes early death or whether those who are vulnerable, perhaps with a health problem that limits their lives, are more likely to report being isolated and lonely (Liu and Floud, 2017).

> *Stress, trauma, anxiety, depression, loss and bereavement can lead to social isolation and loneliness which, itself, may contribute to early death.*

Social exclusion

Humans are naturally social animals. Social contact is vital for learning, bonding and fulfilling a deep need to belong. From early infancy, experiments show babies and children become distressed when experiencing even small interruptions in social contact

(Over, 2016). Having social relationships, social identities and positive experiences in groups, what we might call collectively 'social inclusion', seems to protect people from developing mental health problems (van Bergen *et al.*, 2018). Quite simply,

> A person is a person because of other people.
>
> (Popay *et al.*, 2008 p.2)

Social exclusion,

- is driven by unequal power relationships
- is dynamic; exclusion affects people in different ways and to different degrees over time
- is multidimensional; exclusion happens within economic, political, social and cultural spheres, and at different levels from individual, household, group, community, country and world
- ruptures relationships between people and within society. It leads to a lack of social protection, social participation, social integration and power
- results in unequal access to resources, capabilities and rights, which lead to inequalities in health

(Popay *et al.*, 2008; Khan *et al.*, 2015)

Reasons for social exclusion include: beliefs, religion, ethnicity, race, caste, decent, sexual orientation, age, gender, disability, HIV status, mental disorders, migrant status, culture, poverty, criminality, homelessness and where someone lives.

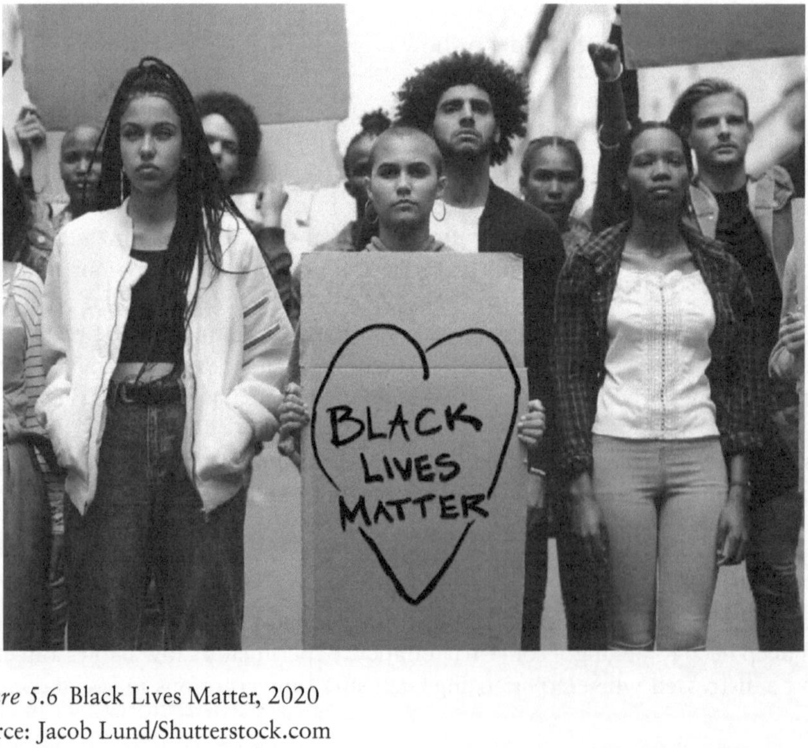

Figure 5.6 Black Lives Matter, 2020
Source: Jacob Lund/Shutterstock.com

Prejudice, stigma and discrimination

Once people internalise the inferior labels placed on them by society, they experience being inferior, having no voice and being deprived, and they put a limit on what they can expect, what they can do and what they can achieve (Khan *et al.*, 2015). Prejudice and stigma often drive the discrimination that can lead to social exclusion.

- Prejudice means "An unfair or unreasonable opinion or feeling, especially when formed without enough thought or knowledge".
- Stigma is "A strong feeling of disapproval that most people in society have about something, especially when this is unfair".
- Discrimination is "Treating a person or particular group of people differently, especially in a worse way from the way in which you treat other people, because of their skin colour, sex, sexuality etc".

(Cambridge Dictionary, 2020)

Social exclusion is disadvantaging groups of people from succeeding in society, and it can be fuelled by prejudice, stigma and discrimination.

Stigma and mental health problems

In a large survey in England (Time to Change, 2008), 87% of people who had a mental health problem requiring support from health and/or social services said that stigma and discrimination were pervasive and had a negative impact on their lives. The figure was higher for women, those living with severe mental disorders, those who were gay, lesbian or bisexual, those who had additional disabilities and those of middle age. Carers from black and ethnic communities, and those with a disability themselves, reported higher levels of stigma and discrimination.

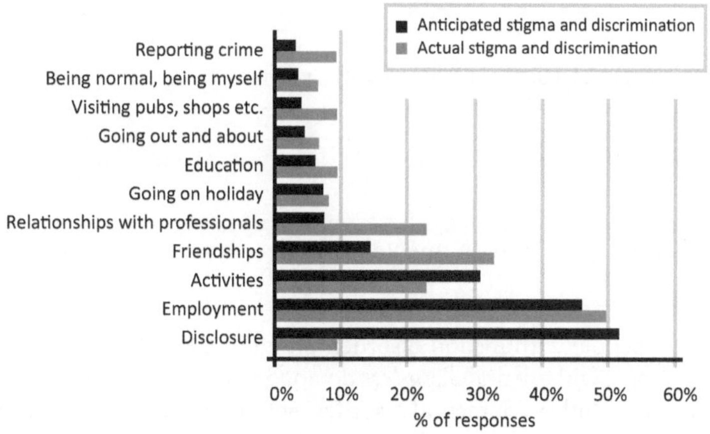

Figure 5.7 What mental health service users stop or fear doing because of stigma and discrimination (n = 3,699)

Source: adapted from Time to Change, 2008 p.7

Box 5.2 Attitudes towards mental health problems in the South Asian community in Harrow, north west London

People with mental health problems and carers living in Harrow were invited to a consultation group to discuss stigma and discrimination. Nearly all described their ethnicity as Indian, with a few describing themselves as Pakistani, Sri Lankan, Asian and one as 'mixed Asian and white'. The key findings were:

Shame, fear and secrecy

> "People are afraid [of mental health problems] they are afraid they might become contaminated or tarnished with the same brush."

The causes of mental health problems are often misunderstood

> "They think there is no need to go to the doctor – the doctor won't do anything."

The family can be both caring and isolating

> "In our culture, we do not throw our children out."
>
> "He doesn't go out so he doesn't have the chance to do something irrational or look out of place. If he doesn't go out, you're not going to see what his behaviour's like. So his brother, mum and dad don't want him to go out because they don't want to be talked about."

Social pressure to conform

> "To associate with someone with mental health problems might be an issue for the rest of the community. It wouldn't actually look good."

People with mental health problems are not valued

> "If someone knows [about my illness], think I have an issue, I've noticed they say hello, but just walk away, they don't look at my face – they go and talk to other friends and leave me out of it."

Marriage prospects can be damaged

> "If someone is suffering from mental health, the whole family becomes tarnished."

(Source: Time to Change, 2010. Reproduced with permission from Time to Change)

People's prejudice against people with mental disorders seems to be primarily underpinned by:

- fear/avoidance, e.g. people with mental disorders should be avoided
- malevolence, e.g. people with mental disorders do not deserve sympathy or support
- authoritarianism, e.g. people with mental disorders should be controlled by others
- unpredictability, e.g. people with mental disorders have unpredictable behaviours

(Kenny *et al.*, 2018)

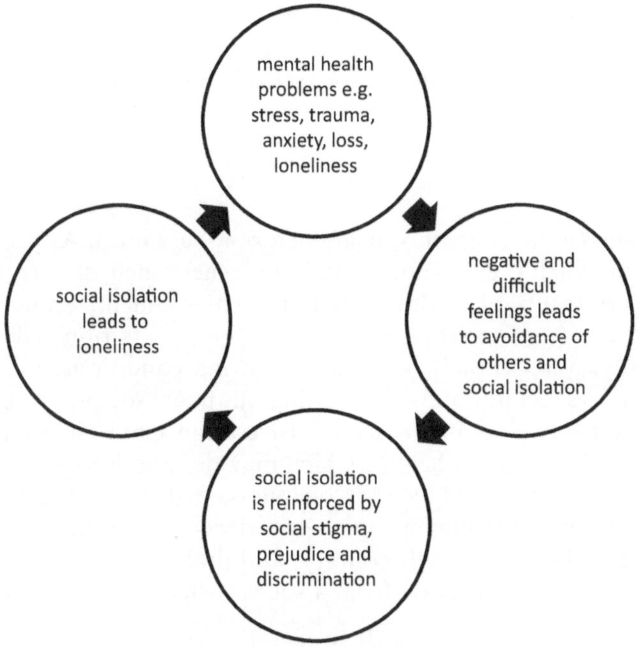

Figure 5.8 The cycle of mental health problems and loneliness

It is worth noting that research shows people with severe mental disorders are more likely to be victims of violent and non-violent crime than perpetrators (Khalifeh *et al.*, 2015; de Vries *et al.*, 2019).

The stigma associated with mental health problems can increase social isolation and therefore loneliness. Loneliness is both a cause and consequence of mental health problems and/or social isolation (Figure 5.8).

> *Those with mental health problems are particularly vulnerable to stigma, prejudice and discrimination, which encourages social isolation, loneliness and social exclusion.*

For those with mental disorders, requiring support, there is a recognised lack of parity across the UK between mental health services and physical health services. This is discriminatory. In England, an independent mental health taskforce (IMHT, 2016) reported that people with severe mental disorders are at risk of dying 15 to 20 years earlier than the general population, partly due to poor mental health contributing to poor physical health, yet the funding lags far behind that which goes into physical care. They reported the following as being most vulnerable to developing a mental health problems

- black, Asian and minority ethnic people (BAME)
- those who have had contact with the criminal justice system
- lesbian, gay, bisexual and transgender people
- those with disabilities

The independent task force noted that those in BAME households are more likely to live in poorer and overcrowded conditions, which increase the risks of developing a mental health problem. A holistic approach to the care of people with mental disorders acknowledges the importance of social inclusion for recovery and the prevention of future health problems.

Inequalities in health

Inequalities in health, discussed in Chapter 3, begin before we are born. As people grow, the social context in which they live powerfully influences their quality and length of life. Social determinants of health include the environment, economy, culture, agriculture, services (e.g. health, social care, water, sanitation, education), the local community, and people's working and living conditions. People are disadvantaged by adverse childhoods and living in poor socio-economic conditions, including unsafe/divided communities. Distress can manifest itself as poor mental, emotional and/or spiritual health, which may develop into a mental health problem. This can be compounded by loss, loneliness, stigma and discrimination. Collectively, these factors undermine people's confidence, erode their social-emotional competences, destabilise their self-concept, and drain the meaning and purpose from their lives until they withdraw from a society which is withdrawing from them.

Compared to the rest of the population, those with mental disorders are much more likely to

- be living in poverty
- be homeless
- live alone
- live in less safe neighbourhoods
- be in prison
- be unemployed
- collect state benefits
- be socially isolated
- have less access to healthy food
- have less access to healthy activities
- have physical health conditions
- die earlier

(Gov.UK, 2018; NHS Health Scotland, 2017)

> *We need a holistic approach to preventing and quickly intervening in the factors that affect our mental, emotional and spiritual health because the causes of deterioration and potential death are often within the society in which we live.*

Communities and mental, emotional and spiritual health

Figures 5.9 and 5.10 illustrate ways in which communities can encourage mental, emotional and spiritual distress or provide nurture to support good mental, emotional

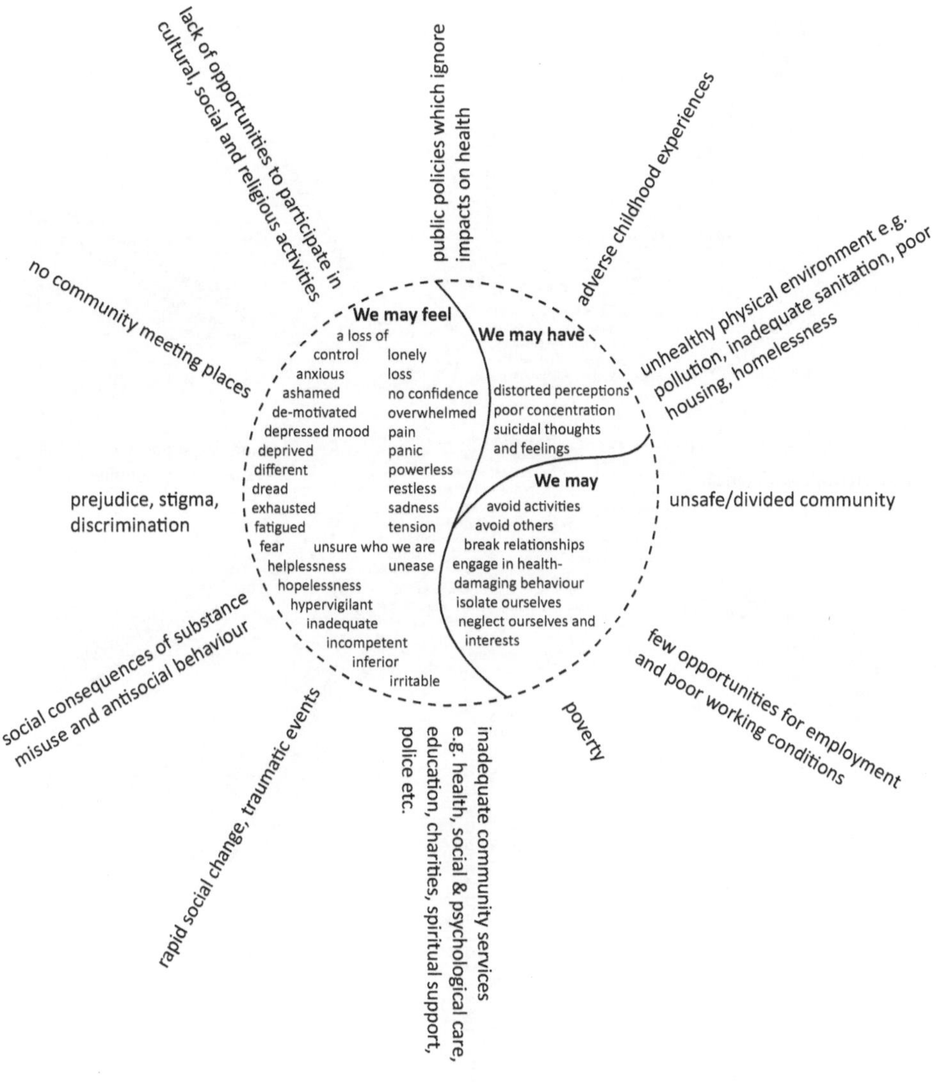

Figure 5.9 Mental, emotional and spiritual distress in a harsh society

and spiritual health. The clock face symbolises how these social factors accumulate with time and through people's life courses.

Summary

This chapter has

- defined and described mental health, emotional health and spiritual health
- described examples of people's distress and mental disorders, and shown how these can lead to physical illness and death

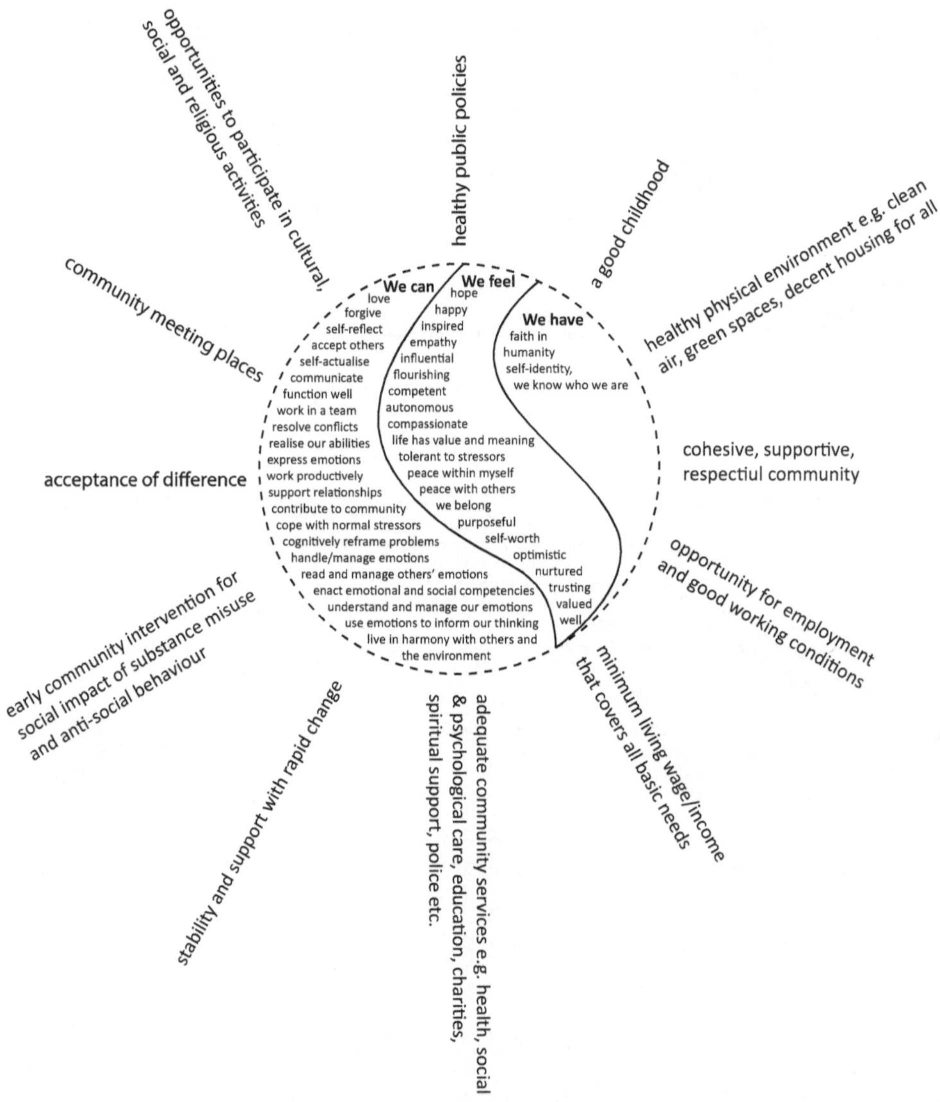

Figure 5.10 Mental, emotional and spiritual health within a nurturing society

- explained how society contributes to and exacerbates poor mental, emotional and spiritual health through stigma, discrimination and social exclusion
- illustrated how disadvantage can be fuelled by additional social determinants of health
- argued why people and communities play an important role in supporting people's mental, emotional and spiritual health

Further reading

Culliford, L. (2011) *The psychology of spirituality. An introduction.* London: Jessica Kingsley
Felman Barrett, L. (2018) *Handbook of emotions.* 4th edn. New York: Guildford Press
Filer, N. (2019) *The heartland: finding and losing schizophrenia.* London: Faber and Faber

Useful websites

Mental Health UK. Available at: https://mentalhealth-uk.org

World Health Organization *Preventing suicide at work: information for employers, managers and employees.* Available at: www.youtube.com/watch?v=C0iQLEwABpc&list=PL9S6xGsoqIBXrjS3UWKPXlo29PWI4X7Ez&index=3

World Health Organization/Matthew Johnstone *I had a black dog, his name was depression.* Available at: www.youtube.com/watch?v=XiCrniLQGYc

References

Age UK (2018) All the lonely people: loneliness in later life. Available at: www.ageuk.org.uk/globalassets/age-uk/documents/reports-and-publications/reports-and-briefings/loneliness/loneliness-report_final_2409.pdf (Accessed 17th December 2019)

Akbağ,M., Küçüktepe, S.E., and Özmercan, E.E. (2016) 'A study on emotional literacy scale development', *Journal of Education and Training Studies*, 4(5), pp.85–91

Bar-On, R. (2006) 'The Bar-On model of emotional-social intelligence', *Psicotherma*, 18, supl., pp.13–25

Bar-On, R. (2012) 'The impact of emotional intelligence on health and wellbeing', in Di Fabio, A. (ed) *Emotional intelligence – new perspectives and applications.* London: Intech Open, pp.29–50

Barr, D.A. (2017) 'The childhood roots of cardiovascular disease disparities', *Mayo Clinic Proceedings*, 92(9), pp.1415–1421

Bayne, H.B., and Thompson, S.K. (2018) 'Helping clients who have experienced trauma gain emotional literacy', *Journal of Creativity in Mental Health*, 13(2), pp.231–242

Bosma, H., Marmot, M.G., Hemingway, H., Nicholson, A.G., Brunner, E., and Stansfield, A. (1997) 'Low job control and risk of coronary heart disease in Whitehall II (prospective cohort) study', *BMJ*, 314(7080), pp.558–565

Cambridge Dictionary (2020) *Cambridge Dictionary.* Available at: https://dictionary.cambridge.org/dictionary/english/ (Accessed 16th April 2020)

Centres for Disease Control and Prevention (2020) *Adverse childhood experiences (ACEs).* Available at: www.cdc.gov/violenceprevention/acestudy/index.html (Accessed 5th September 2020)

Cornah, D. (2006) *The impact of spirituality on mental health.* London: Mental Health Foundation

de Vries, B., van Busschbach, J.T., van der Stouwe, E.C.D., Aleman, A., van Dijk, J.J.M., Lysaker, P.H., Arends, J., Nijman, S.A., and Pijnenborg, G.H.M. (2019) 'Prevalence rate and risk factors of victimization in adult patients with a psychotic disorder: a systematic review and meta-analysis', *Schizophrenia Bulletin*, 45(1), pp.114–126

Deschênes. S.S., Graham, E., Kivimäki, M., and Schmitz, N. (2018) 'Adverse childhood experiences and the risk of diabetes: examining the roles of depressive symptoms and cardiometabolic dysregulations in the Whitehall II cohort study', *Diabetes Care*, 41(10), pp.2120–2126

Faculty of Public Health and Mental Health Foundation (2016) *Better mental health for all. A public health approach to mental health improvement.* London: Faculty of Public Health and Mental Health Foundation

Family Links: The Centre for Emotional Health (2018) *Emotional health at work: why it matters and how you can support it.* London: Family Links: The Centre for Emotional Health and Institute for Public Policy Research

Farmer, J., and Edwards, P. (2014) 'The most terrible poverty: loneliness and mental health', in *Alone in the crowd: loneliness and diversity.* Campaign to End Loneliness/Calouste Gulbenkian Foundation, pp.34–38. Available at: www.campaigntoendloneliness.org/wp-content/uploads/CEL-Alone-in-the-crowd.pdf (Accessed 17th December 2019)

Felitti, V.J., Anda, R.F., Nordenberg, D., Williamson, D.F., Spitz, A.M., Edwards, V., Koss, M.P., and Marks, J.S. (1998) 'Relationship to childhood abuse and household dysfunction to many of the leading causes of death in adults', *American Journal of Preventive Medicine*, 14(4), pp.245–258

Fisher, J. (2011) 'The four domains model: connecting spirituality, health and well-being', *Religions*, 2(1), pp.17–18

Gov.UK (2018) *Health matters: reducing health inequalities in mental illness.* Available at: www.gov.uk/government/publications/health-matters-reducing-health-inequalities-in-mental-illness/health-matters-reducing-health-inequalities-in-mental-illness (Accessed 17th December 2019)

Hannibal, K.E., and Bishop, M.D. (2014) 'Chronic stress, cortisol dysfunction, and pain: a psychoneuroendocrine rationale for stress management in pain rehabilitation', *Physical Therapy*, 94(12), pp.1816–1825

Holman, D.M., Ports, K.A., Buchanan, N.D., Hawkins, N.A., Merrick, M.T., Metzler, M., and Trivers, K.F. (2016) 'The association between adverse childhood experiences and risk of cancer in adulthood: a systematic review of the literature', *Pediatrics*, 138(Suppl 1), S81–S91 doi:10.1542/peds.2015-4268L

Hughes, K., Bellis, M.A., Hardcastle, K.A., Sethi, D., Butchart, A., Mikton, C., Jones, L., and Dunne, M.P. (2017) 'The effect of multiple childhood experiences on health: a systematic review and meta-analysis', *Lancet Public Health*, 2, e356–366 doi:10.1016/S2468-2667(17)30118-4

Independent Mental Health Taskforce (2016) *The five year forward view for mental health. NHS England.* Available at: www.england.nhs.uk/wp-content/uploads/2016/02/Mental-Health-Taskforce-FYFV-final.pdf (Accessed 17th December 2019)

International Society for Traumatic Stress Studies (2019) '*What is traumatic stress?*' Available at: www..org/public-resources/what-is-traumatic-stress.aspx (Accessed 15th December 2019)

Kelly-Irving, M., Lepage, B., Dedieu, D., Bartley, M., Blane, D., Grosclaude, P., Lang, T., and Delpierre, C. (2013) 'Adverse childhood experiences and premature all-cause mortality', *European Journal of Epidemiology*, 28(9), pp.721–734

Kenny, A., Bizumic, B., and Griffiths, K.M. (2018) 'The prejudice towards people with mental illness (PPMI) scale: structure and validity', *BMC Psychiatry*, 18(1) doi:10.1186/s128888-018-1871-z

Keyes, C.L.M. (2002) 'The mental health continuum: from languishing to flourishing in life', *Journal of Health and Social Behavior*, 43(June), pp.207–222

Keyes, C.L.M. (2005) 'Mental illness and/or mental health? Investigating axioms of the complete state model of health', *Journal of Consulting and Clinical Psychology*, 73(3), pp.539–548

Keyes, C.L.M. (2007) 'Promoting and protecting mental health as flourishing' *American Psychologist*, 62(2), pp.95–108

Khalifeh, H., Johnson, S., Howard, L.M., Borschmann, R., Osborn, D., Dean, K., Hart, C., Hogg, J., and Moran, P. (2015) 'Violent and non-violent crime against adults with severe mental illness', *British Journal of Psychiatry*, 206(4), pp.275–282

Khan, S., Combaz, E., and McAslan Fraser, E. (2015) *Social exclusion: topic guide.* Revised edn. Birmingham: Governance and Social Development Resource Centre, University of Birmingham

King, M., Marston, L., McManus, S., Brugha, T., Meltzer, H., and Bebbington, P. (2013) 'Religion, spirituality and mental health: results from a national study of English households', *British Journal of Psychiatry*, 202(1), pp.68–73

King, M., Speck, P., and Thomas, A. (1999) 'The effect of spiritual beliefs on outcome from illness', *Social Science & Medicine*, 48(9), pp.1291–1299

King, M., Weich, S., Nazroo, J., and Blizard, R. (2009) 'Religion, mental health and ethnicity. EMPIRIC – a national survey of England', *Journal of Mental Health*, 15(2), pp.153–162

Kivimäki, M., and Steptoe, A. (2018) 'Effects of stress on the development and progression of cardiovascular disease', *Nature Reviews Cardiology*, 15(4), pp.215–229

Laugesen, K., Baggesen, L.M., Schmidt, S.A.J., Glymour, M.M., Lasgaard, M., Milstein, A., Sørensen, H.T., Adler, N.E., and Ehrenstein, V. (2018) 'Social isolation and all-cause mortality: a population-based cohort study in Denmark', *Scientific Reports*, 8(1) doi:10.1038/s41598-018-22963-w

Liau, A.K., Liau, A.W., Teoh, G.B.S., and Laiau, M.T. (2003) 'The case for emotional literacy: the influence of emotional intelligence on problem behaviours in Malaysian secondary school students', *Journal of Moral Education*, 32(1), pp. 51–66

Liu, B., and Floud, S. (2017) 'Unravelling the association between social isolation, loneliness, and mortality', *The Lancet Public Health*, 2 doi:10.1016/S2468-2667(17)30090–7

Mayer, J. (2009) 'What emotional intelligence is and is not', *Psychology Today*, 21st September. Available at: www.psychologytoday.com/us/blog/the-personality-analyst/200909/what-emotional-intelligence-is-and-is-not (Accessed 17th December 2019)

Mayer, J.D., Roberts, R.D., and Barsade, S.G. (2008) 'Human abilities: emotional intelligence', *Annual Review of Psychology*, 59, pp.507–536

McEwen, B.S. (2008) 'Central effects of stress hormones in health and disease: understanding the protective and damaging effects of stress and stress mediators', *European Journal of Pharmacology*, 583(2–3), pp.174–185

Mental Health Foundation (2019a) *Terminology*. Available at www.mentalhealth.org.uk/a-to-z/t/terminology (Accessed 17th December 2019)

Mental Health Foundation (2019b) *Anxiety*. Available at: www.mentalhealth.org.uk/a-to-z/a/anxiety (Accessed 17th December 2019)

Mind (2019) *Why do I feel suicidal?* Available at: www.mind.org.uk/information-support/types-of-mental-health-problems/suicidal-feelings/causes-of-suicidal-feelings/?o=6813#.XcW5SeRCd9A (Accessed 17th December 2019)

National Health Service (2016) *Symptoms. Clinical depression*. Available at: www.nhs.uk/conditions/clinical-depression/symptoms (Accessed December 17th 2019)

National Institute for Health and Care Excellence (2005) *Obsessive-compulsive disorder and body dysmorphic disorder: treatment*. Available at: www.nice.org.uk/guidance/cg31 (Accessed 17th December 2019)

National Institute for Health and Care Excellence (2011) *Depression in adults. Quality standard [QS8]*. Available at: www.nice.org.uk/guidance/qs8 (Accessed 17th December 2019)

National Institute for Health and Care Excellence (2014) *Anxiety disorders. Quality standard [QS53]*. Available at: www.nice.org.uk/guidance/qs53 (Accessed 17th December 2019)

Nicholson, N.R. (2009) 'Social isolation in older adults: an evolutionary concept analysis', *Journal of Advanced Nursing*, 65(6), pp.1342–1352

NHS Scotland (2017) *Mental health*. Available at: www.healthscotland.scot/media/1626/inequalities-briefing-10_mental-health_english_nov_2017.pdf (Accessed 17th December 2019)

Northern Ireland Statistics and Research Agency (2019) *Suicide statistics*. Available at: www.nisra.gov.uk/publications/suicide-statistics (Accessed 17th December 2019)

Office for National Statistics (2019) *Suicides in the UK: 2018 registrations*. Available at: www.ons.gov.uk/peoplepopulationandcommunity/birthsdeathsandmarriages/deaths/bulletins/suicidesintheunitedkingdom/latest (Accessed 18th December 2019)

O'Súilleabháin, P.S., Gallagher, S. and Steptoe, A. (2019) 'Loneliness, living alone, and all-cause mortality: the role of emotional and social loneliness in the elderly during 19 years of follow-up', *Psychosomatic Medicine*, 81(6), pp.521–526

Over, H. (2016) 'The origins of belonging: social motivation in infants and young children', *Philosophical Transactions of the Royal Society of London. Series B, Biological Sciences*, 371(1686) doi:10.1098/rstb.2015.0072

Pitman, A., Osborn, D., Rantell, K., and King, M. (2016) 'Bereavement by suicide as a risk factor for suicide attempt: a cross-sectional national UK-wide study of 3,432 young bereaved adults', *BMJ Open*, 6 doi:10.1136/bmjopen-2015–009948

Popay, J., Escorel, S., Hernandez, M., Johnston, H., Mathieson, J., and Rispel, L. (on behalf of the WHO Social Exclusion Knowledge Network) (2008) *Understanding and tackling social exclusion*. Available at: www.who.int/social_determinants/knowledge_networks/final_reports/sekn_final%20report_042008.pdf?ua=1 (Accessed 17th December 2019)

Public Health England (2019) *Public health profiles*. Available at: https://fingertips.phe.org.uk © crown copyright (Accessed 17th December 2019)

Scriven, A. (2017) *Ewles and Simnett's promoting health. A practical guide*. 7th edn. London: Elsevier

Segerstrom, S.C., and O'Connor, D.B. (2012) 'Stress, health and illness: four challenges for the future', *Psychology and Health*, 27(2), pp.128–140

Sharp, P. (2001) *Nurturing emotional literacy*. London: David Fulton

Shear, M.K., Muldberg, S., and Periyakoil, V. (2017) 'Supporting patients who are bereaved', *BMJ*, 358 doi 10.1136/bmuj.j2854

Sorin, R. (2009) 'Teaching emotional literacy', in Bhatnagar, M. (ed) *Emotional literacy: concept, application and experiences*. Hyderabad: ICFAI University Press, pp.43–52

Statistics for Wales (2015) *Statistical Bulletin. National Survey for Wales. Well-being in 2013–14 and 2014–15*. Available at: https://gov.wales/sites/default/files/statistics-and-research/2019-05/national-survey-wales-well-being-2013–15.pdf (Accessed 18th December 2019)

Steiner, C. (2003) *Emotional literacy; intelligence with a heart*. 2nd edn. Chicago: Personhood Press

Swinton, J. (2001) *Spirituality and mental health care*. London: Jessica Kingsley

Tabei, S.Z., Zarei, N., and Joulaei, H. (2016) 'The impact of spirituality on health', *Shiraz E-Medical Journal*, 17(6) e39053 doi:10.17795/semj39053

Time to Change (2008) *Stigma shout. Service user and carer experiences of stigma and discrimination* Available at: www.time-to-change.org.uk/sites/default/files/Stigma%20Shout.pdf (Accessed 18th December 2019)

Time to Change (2010) *Family matters. A report into attitudes towards mental health problems in the South Asian community in Harrow, North West London*. Available at: www.time-to-change.org.uk/sites/default/files/imce_uploads/Family%20Matters.pdf (Accessed 17th December 2019)

Utz, R.L., Caserta, M., and Lund, D. (2012) 'Grief, depressive symptoms, and physical health among recently bereaved spouses', *Gerontologist*, 52(4), pp.460–471

van Bergen, A.P.L., Wolf, J.R.L.M., Badou, M., de Wilde-Schutten, K., IJzelenberg, W.I., Schreurs, H., Carlier, B., Hoff, S.J.M., and van Hemert, A.M. (2018) 'The association between social exclusion or inclusion and health in EU and OECD countries: a systematic review, *European Journal of Public Health*, 29(3), pp.575–582

Weare, K., and Gray, G. (2003) *What works in developing children's emotional and social competence and wellbeing?* London: Department for Education and Skills

World Health Organization (2001) *The world health report 2001. Mental health: new understanding, new hope*. Geneva: World Health Organization

World Health Organization (2004) *Promoting mental health: concepts, emerging evidence, practice: summary report*. Geneva: World Health Organization

World Health Organization (2013) *Mental health action plan 2013–2020.* Geneva: World Health Organization

World Health Organization (2018) *Management of physical health conditions in adults with severe mental disorder.* WHO Guidelines. Geneva: World Health Organization

World Health Organization (2019a) *Mental health: mental disorders.* Available at: www.who.int/mental_health/management/en/ (Accessed 17th December 2019)

World Health Organization (2019b) *International statistical classification of diseases and related health problems 11th revision (ICD-11).* Available at: https://icd.who.int/browse11/l-m/en (Accessed 17th December 2019)

World Health Organization (2019c) *Suicide: fact sheet.* Available at: www.who.int/news-room/fact-sheets/detail/suicide (Accessed 17th December 2019)

Part II

Health-related behaviours

Part II

6 Sexual health

Rajeeb Kumar Sah and Sally Robinson

Key points

- Introduction
- Defining sexual health
- Sexually transmitted infections
- Unintended pregnancy and abortion
- Sexual violence
- Sociocultural aspects of sexual health
- Positive sexual health: sexual rights and relationships
- Summary

Introduction

This chapter explains why sexual health is a priority for health promotion and public health. It begins by defining sexual health and noting how it is understood as a holistic concept. It examines negative aspects of sexual health including sexually transmitted infections, unintended pregnancy, abortion and sexual violence. It explains how sociocultural dimensions influence individuals' sexual attitudes and behaviours. The chapter concludes by arguing that positive sexual health includes sexual rights and relationships; it is an important aspect of human life that contributes towards the positive health and wellbeing of individuals, families and communities.

Defining sexual health

People's understanding of health and wellbeing, including sexual health, has evolved over time. In 1948, the World Health Organization defined health as:

> A state of complete physical, mental and social well-being and not merely the absence of disease or infirmity.
>
> (p.1)

If health is not merely the absence of disease, then sexual health cannot be limited to the absence of sexually transmitted infections. It needs to include physical, mental and social dimensions, such as sexual rights and relationships. In 1974, the World Health Organization held a meeting about education and treatment in the context of human sexuality. They recognised that human sexuality, particularly the right to sexual information and the right to pleasure, was important to the health and well-being of individuals. They defined sexual health as:

> The integration of the somatic, emotional, intellectual, and social aspects of sexual being, in ways that are positively enriching and that enhance personality, communication, and love.
>
> (WHO, 1975 p.6)

This definition communicated a positive approach, by making clear that sexual health was something that enhanced life and personal relationships and was not merely about procreation or sexual ill-health. During the 1990s, sexual health was often discussed as part of reproductive health, particularly family planning or pregnancy (UN, 1995). In recent years, this approach has been increasingly questioned, as most sexual activity is not directly associated with pregnancy but relates to sexual lifestyles and relationships. Even when discussing pregnancy and contraception, it seems important to take the same holistic approach which applies to all aspects of sexual health.

The pandemic of human immunodeficiency virus (HIV) was instrumental in advancing understanding of sexual health. In 2002, the World Health Organization convened a group of global experts to discuss the challenges that HIV presented. The group reaffirmed sexual health as an important and integral aspect of human development and it published revised definitions of sexual health and related concepts in 2006, with further updates in 2010 (WHO, 2006; 2010). The group articulated a view that sexual health includes physical health, mental wellbeing, sexual rights and positive, autonomous, respectful and pleasurable sexual experiences. Sexuality and relationships should be experienced freely without violence, coercion or discrimination. This holistic approach is increasingly adopted across health promotion and public health research, campaigns and policies across the world.

Box 6.1 Working definitions of sexual health and related concepts

"**Sexual health** is a state of physical, emotional, mental and social well-being in relation to sexuality; it is not merely the absence of disease, dysfunction or infirmity. Sexual health requires a positive and respectful approach to sexuality and sexual relationships, as well as the possibility of having pleasurable and safe sexual experiences, free of coercion, discrimination and violence. For sexual health to be attained and maintained, the sexual rights of all persons must be respected, protected and fulfilled.

"**Sex** refers to the biological characteristics that define humans as female or male. While these sets of biological characteristics are not mutually exclusive, as there are individuals who possess both, they tend to differentiate humans as males and females. In general use in many languages, the term sex is often used to mean 'sexual activity', but for technical purposes in the context of sexuality and sexual health discussions, the above definition is preferred.

"**Sexuality** is a central aspect of being human throughout life and encompasses sex, gender identities and roles, sexual orientation, eroticism, pleasure, intimacy and reproduction. Sexuality is experienced and expressed in thoughts, fantasies, desires, beliefs, attitudes, values, behaviours, practices, roles and relationships.

While sexuality can include all of these dimensions, not all of them are always experienced or expressed. Sexuality is influenced by the interaction of biological, psychological, social, economic, political, cultural, ethical, legal, historical, religious and spiritual factors.

"**Sexual rights** embrace certain human rights that are already recognized in international and regional human rights documents and other consensus documents and in national laws. The fulfilment of sexual health is tied to the extent to which human rights are respected, protected and fulfilled. Rights critical to the realization of sexual health include:

- the rights to life, liberty, autonomy and security of the person
- the rights to equality and non-discrimination
- the right to be free from torture or from cruel, inhumane or degrading treatment or punishment
- the right to privacy
- the rights to the highest attainable standard of health (including sexual health) and social security
- the right to marry and to found a family and enter into marriage with the free and full consent of the intending spouses, and to equality in and at the dissolution of marriage
- the right to decide the number and spacing of one's children
- the rights to information, as well as education
- the rights to freedom of opinion and expression, and
- the right to an effective remedy for violations of fundamental rights.

"The application of existing human rights to sexuality and sexual health constitute sexual rights. Sexual rights protect all people's rights to fulfil and express their sexuality and enjoy sexual health, with due regard for the rights of others and within a framework of protection against discrimination."

(Source: WHO, 2006 p.5; 2010 p.3, 4. Reproduced with permission from the World Health Organization)

Sexual health is a holistic concept which includes physical, mental and social dimensions including respectful relationships and sexual rights.

Sexually transmitted infections

Sexually transmitted infections are a major public health concern because, if left undiagnosed and untreated, they may cause further complications such as infertility, pelvic inflammatory disease, cancer, ectopic pregnancy and chronic abdominal pain. As well as the personal impact on the health of individuals, they incur significant costs to healthcare services and to the socioeconomic circumstances of individuals, families and communities through their impact on employment, income and social activities.

Sexually transmitted infections are caused by bacteria, viruses or parasites. Many are asymptomatic, but the most common symptoms are dysuria (painful urination); an unusual discharge from the vagina, penis or anus; rashes, lumps, sores, itching,

Table 6.1 Pathogens which cause the most common sexually transmitted infections

Bacteria	*Viruses*	*Parasites*
Chlamydia (*Chlamydia trachomatis*)	Herpes (herpes simplex)	Pubic lice (crabs)
Gonorrhoea (*Neisseria gonorrhoeae*)	Genital warts (human papilloma virus)	Scabies
Syphilis (*Treponema pallidum*)	Human immunodeficiency virus (HIV)	Trichomoniasis
	Hepatitis B	

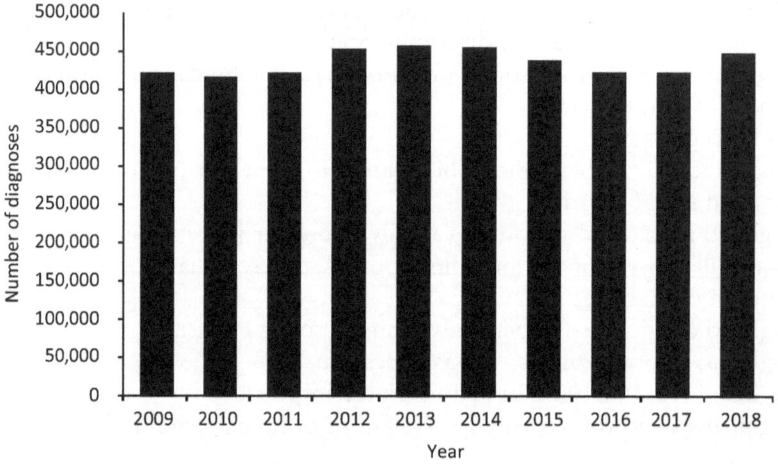

Figure 6.1 Number of new diagnoses of sexually transmitted infections, England 2009 to 2018
Source: PHE, 2019a p.4. Reproduced under the terms of the Open Government Licence v3.0

or skin growth around the genitals. In males, additional symptoms may include testicular pain, and in females, vaginal bleeding between periods or post-coital bleeding.

In England, data from 2018 showed a total of 447,694 diagnosed sexually transmitted infections, which was an increase of 5% on the previous year (PHE, 2019a) (Figure 6.1). Of these, chlamydia was the most common (49% of all new sexually transmitted infections), followed by first-episode genital warts (13%), gonorrhoea (13%) and genital herpes (8%). Young heterosexuals aged 15 to 24 years, people from Black and minority ethnic groups, and gay, bisexual and other men who have sex with men are at higher risks of contracting sexually transmitted infections compared to the rest of the population.

Chlamydia

Chlamydia is a sexually transmitted bacterial infection caused by the *Chlamydia trachomatis* bacterium. It is the most commonly diagnosed, curable, sexually transmitted infection in the UK. In 2018, there were 218,095 new cases of chlamydia in England, an increase of 6% from the previous year (PHE, 2019a). At the same time, 2017 to 2018, there was a 4% rise in chlamydia infections in Scotland and a 6%

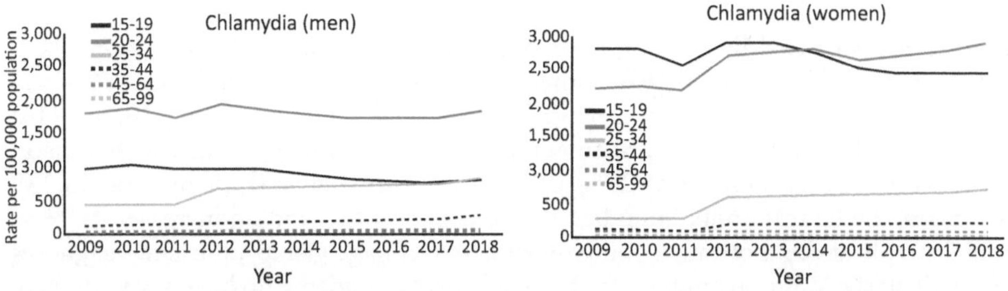

Figure 6.2 Rates of newly diagnosed chlamydia by sex and age, England 2009 to 2018
Source: PHE, 2019a p.6. Reproduced under the terms of the Open Government Licence v3.0

rise in Northern Ireland (Cameron *et al.*, 2019; PHA, 2019). The data in Wales are collated differently and comparing April to September 2017 with the same period in 2018 rates of chlamydia fell by 2% (PHW, 2019). Chlamydia affects both men and women across all age groups, but it is particularly prevalent among sexually active young people.

The chlamydia bacteria can be transferred from one mucous site to another via the eyes, throat, anus, urethra, cervix, vagina or penis. Most people are asymptomatic in the early stage of infection. When signs or symptoms occur, it is usually one or two weeks after exposure. The most common symptoms for men are

- pain or a burning sensation during urinating
- watery discharge from penis
- pain or tenderness in the testicles

and for women

- pain or a burning sensation during urinating
- vaginal discharge
- heavy periods
- bleeding between periods
- pain in the lower abdomen during or after sex

Infection during pregnancy may cause severe respiratory infections or conjunctivitis in new born babies.

A diagnosis of chlamydia can be made from a urine test or by taking a swab of the affected area. The infection is easily treated with antibiotics. It is advised not to have sexual intercourse for a week and all sexual partners for the past three months should be contacted for screening and treatment. If left untreated, it may persist for years and cause severe complications such as infertility, ectopic pregnancy and pelvic inflammatory disease.

Free testing for chlamydia is available from the UK's National Health Services and home test kits. England has a National Chlamydia Screening Programme which recommends that all sexually active people under 25 years old should be tested every time they change sexual partner, or annually if with the same partner (PHE, 2018a).

Gonorrhoea

Gonorrhoea is caused by *Neisseria gonorrhoeae*, a Gram-negative diplococcus bacterium. In 2018, compared to 2017, infection rates rose by 26% in England, 24% in Scotland and 30% in Northern Ireland (PHE, 2019a; Cameron *et al.*, 2019; PHA, 2019). In Wales, comparing April to September 2017 with the same six months in 2018, there was an increase of 29% (PHW, 2019). In England, there were 56,259 new cases, the largest annual number reported since 1978 and an increase of 249% from 2009. It affects both men and women across all age groups, but new diagnoses are particularly common among gay, bisexual and other men who have sex with men.

Gonorrhoea is transmitted through unprotected vaginal, oral or anal sexual contact, by sharing contaminated sex toys, or by other forms of non-penetrative sexual activity. The bacteria can affect the throat, genital or rectal areas, and is transferred from one mucous site to another. It can also infect people's eyes, joints, urethra, cervix, prostate and other pelvic organs. An infected woman can pass it to her baby during childbirth, causing blindness in the baby.

Almost half of women will have no symptoms, but common symptoms for women include

- yellow or green vaginal discharge
- heavy periods or bleeding between periods
- vulvar swelling
- painful vaginal intercourse

One in 10 infected men will have no symptoms, but common symptoms for men include

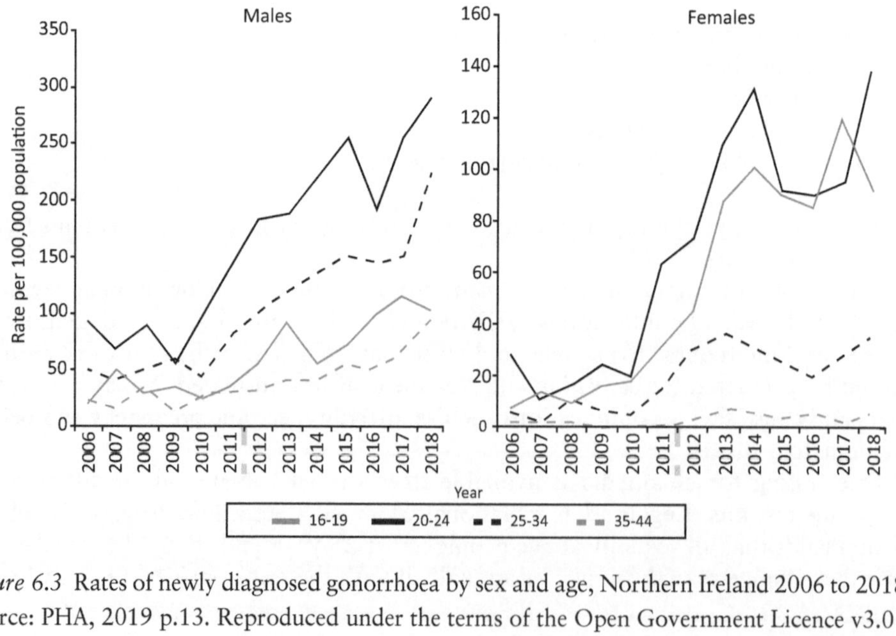

Figure 6.3 Rates of newly diagnosed gonorrhoea by sex and age, Northern Ireland 2006 to 2018
Source: PHA, 2019 p.13. Reproduced under the terms of the Open Government Licence v3.0

- yellow or clear discharge from the penis
- pain in testicles or scrotum
- inflammation or swelling of foreskin

Both men and women may have

- painful urination
- anal discharge
- itching
- bleeding or pain during anal intercourse or bowel movements

Gonorrhoea is diagnosed by a urine test or from a swab of the infected area. If tested positive, the individual and their partner need to undergo treatment, usually a single dose of an antibiotic tablet or injection. It is advised not to have sexual intercourse for a week after treatment and all sexual partners for the past three months should be contacted for screening and treatment. In 2018, there were cases of infection with *Neisseria gonorrhoeae* that were resistant to the antibiotics ceftriaxone and azithromycin, used as front-line drugs for treatment, so future treatment is likely to become more challenging.

Syphilis

Syphilis is a bacterial infection caused by *Treponema pallidum*. In 2018, compared to 2017, syphilis infection rates rose by 5.5% in England, 14% in Scotland and 72% in Northern Ireland (PHE, 2019b; Cullen *et al.*, 2019; PHA, 2019). In Wales, comparing six months in 2017 with the same period in 2018, rates rose by 32% (PHW, 2019). In England, the 7,541 new cases represented the largest annual number reported

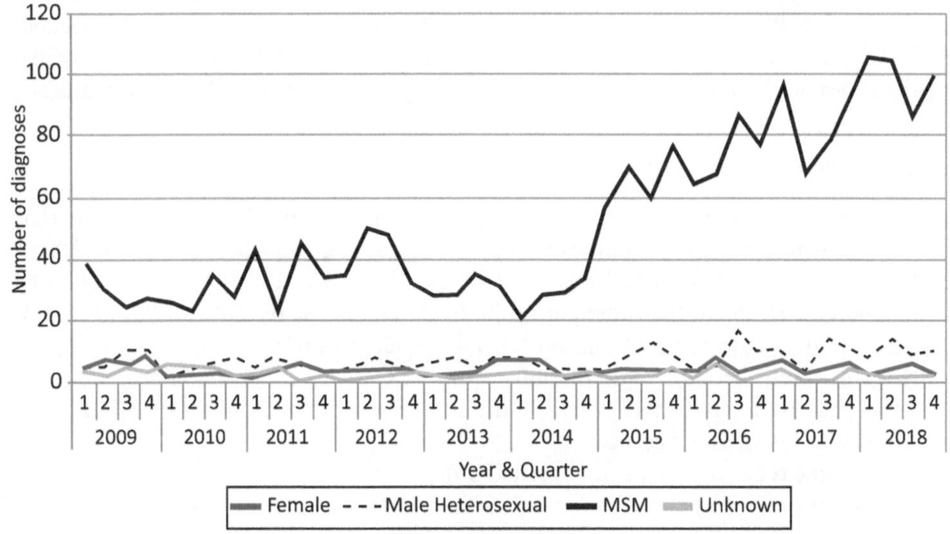

Figure 6.4 Number of new diagnoses of syphilis by sex and sexual orientation, Scotland 2009 to 2018

Source: Cullen *et al*, 2019 p.3. Reproduced under the terms of the Open Government Licence v3.0

since 1949. Across the UK, men who have sex with men (MSM) make up over three-quarters of all cases.

Syphilis is a chronic, systemic infection characterised by periods of active clinical manifestation interrupted by periods of latency. It is usually transmitted through sexual contact, but it can be passed from mother to baby during pregnancy (*congenital syphilis*). The bacteria spread from person to person through painless sores, small cuts in the skin or mucous membranes.

Based on the time after exposure, syphilis is classified into 'early infectious' and 'late non-infectious' syphilis. The early infectious syphilis is defined as the first two years of the infection and comprises primary and secondary syphilis.

- Primary syphilis, within the first 90 days of infection
  A person has a painless 'chancre' that looks like an ulcer with a clearly defined oval or round outline. It normally appears on the penis, vagina, anus, buttocks, lips, tonsils or hands. It is highly contagious and if untreated will spread to other parts of the body.
- Secondary syphilis, six to 12 weeks from infection
  The chancre will have disappeared and the person develops a symmetrical rash on the face, trunk, limb, palms of the hands and soles of the feet. The rash may disappear and person becomes asymptomatic entering the latent phase but the symptoms may reappear over a period of weeks or months. The latent period is classified as 'early latent' if syphilis is less than two years old and 'late latent' if it is more than two years old. If left untreated, syphilis enters the third stage.
- Tertiary or late non-infectious syphilis
  This final stage is reached if the person has not been treated and the bacteria have reached the musculoskeletal, cardiovascular and neurological systems, leading to paralysis, memory loss and antisocial behaviour.

Syphilis is diagnosed from a blood test and a swab from any sore. It is treated with antibiotics, but if it has progressed to later stages, specific treatments may be needed. In the UK, all pregnant women are screened for syphilis, and self-testing kits, which require a 'pin prick' blood sample to be posted to a laboratory for analysis, are available.

Genital herpes

Genital herpes is caused by *herpes simplex virus* types 1 and 2, the same virus that causes cold sores. In 2018, compared to 2017, rates of genital herpes rose by 3% in England and 8% in Northern Ireland (PHE, 2019a; PHA, 2019). Comparing April to September 2017 with the same period in 2018, rates rose by 26% in Wales (PHW, 2019). The latest data for Scotland report 3,420 cases in 2014 (HPS, 2015). It is generally transmitted through vaginal, anal or oral sex, or by sharing contaminated sex toys. It is passed through small cracks in the skin or via the mucous membranes in the mouth, vagina, urethra or rectum.

Most people remain asymptomatic, but some people may develop symptoms within two to 14 days after exposure to the virus. The general symptoms are

- flu-like
- feeling unwell

- tiredness
- fever
- headache
- swollen glands
- pains in the lower back, groin and down the legs

Genital herpes presents as small painful blisters or sores that may cause itching or tingling in the genital or anal area. It may be painful to urinate and there may be a vaginal discharge. There is no cure for genital herpes but using antiviral medicine can usually control the symptoms. Individual sores will take around five to 10 days to heal. The recurrence of infection and outbreaks are common.

Genital warts

Genital warts are caused by the *human papilloma virus* (HPV). HPV has over 100 different variants that can affect various parts of the body. There are over 30 different types of HPV that live around the genital and anal areas, but most genital warts are caused by *HPV type 6* and *HPV type 11*. Genital warts are the most common viral sexually transmitted infection in the UK. In 2018, compared to 2017, the rates decreased by 3% in England and 10% in Northern Ireland (PHE, 2019a; PHA, 2019). Data from Scotland are currently unavailable. In Wales, comparing April to September 2017 with the same period in 2018, rates decreased by 9% (PHW, 2019). The decrease in rates has been mostly among girls who have received the quadrivalent HPV vaccine at the age of 12 to 13 years.

Genital warts are generally transmitted through vaginal or anal intercourse, sharing contaminated sex toys and rarely through oral sex. HPV may spread through skin-to-skin contact. Most people remain asymptomatic without any visible warts. If genital warts appear, they are usually benign bumps or small fleshy skin growths on or around the genital or anal area. Genital warts are usually painless, and may present some redness or itching with occasional bleeding. Diagnosis is made by visual inspection. Treatments vary according to the shape, size and number of warts, and include ointments (cream or liquid), cryotherapy, surgery or laser treatment.

Human immunodeficiency virus (HIV)

Human immunodeficiency virus (HIV), like most viruses, needs a host cell where it replicates to survive. In humans, the host cell for HIV is part of the immune system which protects the body from infections. HIV invades the 'cluster of differentiation 4 (CD4)' cells, also called T helper cells. As it destroys these cells, the normal processes of protection cease and the immune system gradually weakens. The body is increasingly unable to fight against everyday infections and diseases. Individuals become vulnerable to opportunistic infections such as tuberculosis and pneumonia; this develops into a condition known as acquired immunodeficiency syndrome (AIDS).

In 2018, there were an estimated 96,300 people living with diagnosed HIV in the UK, and 7,500 were thought to be undiagnosed (O'Halloran, 2019). There has been a continued decline in new HIV diagnoses among heterosexual men and women over the past decade and, recently, a sharp decline in new diagnoses among gay and bisexual men.

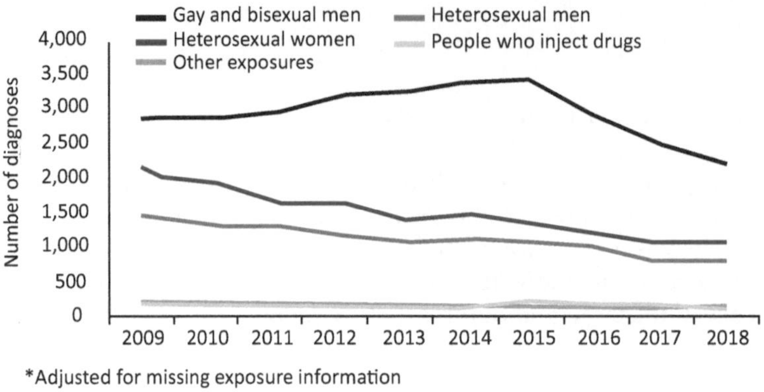

Figure 6.5 New diagnoses of HIV by exposure group, UK 2009 to 2018
Source: O'Halloran, 2019 p.17. Reproduced under the terms of the Open Government Licence v3.0

HIV is transmitted through

- sexual contact – most HIV is usually contracted through unprotected sexual intercourse through infected semen, vaginal fluids or contact with mucous membranes
- blood-borne infection – particularly amongst injecting drug users through sharing needles or syringes
- vertical transmission – less commonly, HIV may be transmitted through the placenta from mother to baby during gestation, via cervical secretions or blood at delivery, or through breast milk

HIV is not transmitted through hugging, kissing, shaking hands, sharing dishes, mosquito bites, saliva, tears and sweat, or through the air. HIV is rarely passed through oral sex and through blood transfusions.

People with HIV mostly remain asymptomatic in the initial stages, but typically symptoms appear two to six weeks after infection. Common symptoms are

- flu-like symptoms
- sore throat
- fever
- aching limbs
- ulceration in mouth or genitals

The diagnosis of HIV is made through a saliva or blood test. HIV self-testing uses a sample of saliva or a small spot of blood from the finger. The blood test is the most accurate. In the UK, HIV testing is free through the National Health Service and all pregnant women are offered a blood test as part of their routine antenatal screening.

Although there is no cure for HIV infection, a person can live with it and have a near normal life span. In 2018, about 103,800 people were thought to be living with HIV in the UK. Of these, 93% were diagnosed; 97% of those diagnosed were receiving antiretroviral treatment and 97% of those receiving treatment were virally suppressed

(O'Halloran, 2019). This means the UK has continued to exceed the United Nations 90:90:90 targets which are; 90% of people living with HIV to be diagnosed; 90% of the people diagnosed receive antiretroviral drug therapy; and 90% of the people receiving the antiviral drugs are virally suppressed and unable to pass on the infection (UNAIDS, 2014). The decline in new cases of HIV infection is due to intensified HIV testing, improvements in the uptake of antiretroviral therapy and the availability of a daily pill for those who do not have HIV but are in a high-risk population (PrEP).

Sexually transmitted infections are a major public health concern, particularly for young people, Black and minority ethnic populations, gay, bisexual and other men who have sex with men, and people living in deprived areas where rates are higher.

Unintended pregnancy and abortion

Pregnancies that occur when there is no desire for children at that time (mistimed) or at any time (unwanted) are called unintended or unplanned pregnancies (Santelli *et al.*, 2013). Both terms are used interchangeably. These pregnancies have the potential to impact women's lives negatively and, as such, they are a key indicator of a population's health. In England, 45% of total pregnancies are unintended or are associated with ambivalent feelings (PHE, 2018b). This is the second highest rate in the developed world after the United States of America (Bexhell *et al.*, 2016).

Some of the key risk factors for unintended pregnancies include being a young age, being single, having lower educational attainment, living in poverty, smoking and substance misuse. Unintended pregnancies are associated with greater adverse health and socioeconomic outcomes for women and children than pregnancies that are planned (Wellings *et al.*, 2013). For women, these include late antenatal care, antenatal and postnatal depression, physical and sexual violence, relationship breakdown and obstetric complications. Children born as a result of unintended pregnancies are more likely to have low birthweights, are less likely to be breastfed, have poorer physical and mental health, and tend to do less well in cognitive tests. Unintended pregnancies can restrict the opportunities for women to improve their livelihood and perpetuate cycles of poverty. In these ways, unintended pregnancies are widely seen as both a cause and a consequence of socioeconomic inequalities.

Unintended pregnancies may result from either non-use of contraception at the time of conception or inconsistent or incorrect use of contraception (Teuton *et al.*, 2016). The use of contraception, in principle, should prevent up to 99% of unintended pregnancies. Most types of contraception in the UK are available for free. The use of the oral contraceptive pill and condoms, although popular, contribute to most unintended pregnancies due to poor compliance by the users. Long-acting reversible contraception is generally more effective than other forms of contraception and the use of emergency contraception, in the form of the 'morning after pill' or intrauterine device (IUD), can also reduce unintended pregnancies.

Many unintended pregnancies end in abortion, which is the termination of pregnancy by the removal of a foetus or embryo from the womb (Glasier and Wellings, 2012). In 2018, nearly 1 in 4 babies in England and Wales were aborted (DHSC, 2019). Most abortions were performed citing the risk to the mental health of the pregnant woman, which indicates these pregnancies were unintended. Abortion, in varying circumstances, is legal and safe in many parts of the world but in countries where abortions are illegal, unintended pregnancies lead to unsafe abortions which put pregnant women at risk of long-term illness or death.

Box 6.2 Unsafe abortions

An unsafe abortion is one where a pregnancy is terminated by people who do not have the appropriate skills and/or it takes place in an environment which does not meet minimum medical standards. Across the world, between 2010 and 2014, there were about 25 million unsafe abortions each year. Of these, a third were performed with untrained people using dangerous, invasive methods. About half of all unsafe abortions take place in Asia and 29% in Africa; 62% of the world's unsafe abortion-related deaths occur in Africa.

The harms of unsafe abortions include

- incomplete abortion, where not all the pregnancy tissue is removed
- infection
- haemorrhage (heavy bleeding)
- perforation of the uterus
- physical damage to other tissues and organs due to instruments such as glass or knitting needles

(Source: WHO, 2019)

On 31st March 2020, the law in Northern Ireland was changed to allow women to access abortion services in the rest of the UK without committing a criminal offence. Until that point, there had been a near-blanket ban on abortions. Sarah Ewert was denied an abortion despite a scan showing that her foetus would not survive. She took her case to court, arguing that the law in Northern Ireland breached her human rights, and won. The decision remains contentious with the 'pro-life' groups who argue that the right to life is a human right that applies to all, including unborn babies.

Table 6.2 Examples of global abortion laws

Criteria for abortion	*Examples of countries*
On request, with varying limits to the gestational timing	USA, Canada, Uruguay, South Africa, Mozambique, Nepal, France, Spain, Sweden, Russian Federation, China, Australia, Turkey
For social or economic reasons (including reasons below)	Great Britain, Ethiopia, Zambia, Finland, India, Japan, Taiwan
To preserve health only	Peru, Argentina, Algeria, Chad, Zimbabwe, Saudi Arabia, Poland, Thailand, Pakistan, New Zealand
To save a woman's life only	Mexico, Brazil, Nigeria, Libya, Iran, Myanmar, Indonesia, Bangladesh, United Arab Emirates
Prohibited altogether	Nicaragua, Dominican Republic, Mauritania, Egypt, Iraq, Congo, Philippines, Jamaica, Sierra Leone

Source: Centre for Reproductive Rights (2020).

Table 6.3 Abortion laws in Great Britain and Northern Ireland

Great Britain	*Northern Ireland*
Abortion Act 1967 (amended by the Human Fertilisation and Embryology Act 1990)	The Abortion (Northern Ireland) Regulations 2020
Medically supervised abortion is allowed	
up to 24 weeks and when continuance of pregnancy would involve greater risk than if the pregnancy was terminated, of injury to the physical or mental health of the pregnant woman or any existing children of her family	up to 12 weeks unconditionally
when is necessary to prevent grave permanent injury to the physical or mental health of the pregnant woman	up to 24 weeks when continuing pregnancy would risk physical or mental injury to the woman that is greater than the risk of terminating the pregnancy
when there is substantial risk that if the child were born it would suffer mental or physical abnormalities as to be seriously handicapped	with no time limit when there is substantial impairment to the foetus, including when death is likely before or shortly after birth
	with no time limit when there is risk of serious permanent injury or death to the woman that is (i) greater than the risk of termination and (ii) when necessary to prevent serious mental or physical harm, including during birth

Sources: Amnesty International UK (2019); BPAS (2013).

> *Unintended pregnancies can impact women's lives negatively through unsafe abortions, poor physical and mental health, and by restricting opportunities to improve their livelihood, which may perpetuate cycles of poverty.*

Sexual violence

Sexual violence is a violation of human rights. Sexual violence has been defined in the World Report on Violence and Health as:

> Any sexual act, attempts to obtain a sexual act, or acts to traffic for sexual purposes, directed against a person using coercion, harassment or advances made by any person regardless of their relationship to the victim, in any setting, including but not limited to home and work.
>
> (Jewkes *et al.*, 2002 p.149)

Coercion is central to sexual violence. It covers a spectrum that ranges from physical force, blackmail, intimidation or threats of job loss and physical harm. It may also occur when a person is unable to give consent, for example, while asleep, intoxicated, drugged or incapable of understanding the situation. Sexual violence can take place in many forms, for example, rape, sexual harassment, sexual abuse, sexual exploitation, forced marriage, female genital mutilation, and denying the right to protect against pregnancy or sexually transmitted infections in different circumstances and in various settings (Jewkes *et al.*, 2002). Rape is one of the gravest forms of sexual violence. The UK Sexual Offences Act 2003 defines rape as the intentional penetration of the vagina, anus or mouth of another person with a penis, without their consent.

Box 6.3 Coercive control

Coercive control became illegal in England and Wales in 2015 under the Serious Crime Act.

"Coercive control is when a person, with whom you are personally connected, repeatedly behaves in a way which makes you feel controlled, dependent, isolated or scared."

It includes

- isolation from family and friends
- control of personal finances
- monitoring daily activities
- repeatedly putting someone down, name calling, telling an individual that they are worthless
- threats to harm or kill an individual, or a loved one such as their child
- threats to publish information about an individual without their consent
- damaging property or contents
- being forced to participate in criminal or abusive activities

(Source: Rights of Women, 2016)

The Crime Survey for England and Wales, for the year ending September 2019, estimated 2.9% of adults aged 16 to 59 years had been victims of sexual assaults in the last year (ONS, 2020). Women were nearly four times as likely as men to have experienced sexual assault. Most sexual violence cases remain unreported, and less than one in five victims of rape or assault reported their experiences due to associated risks of embarrassment and humiliation in reporting the case (ONS, 2018). Reporting is more limited among women from Black, Asian and minority ethnic (BAME) groups due to embarrassment and humiliation, and because females are expected to maintain the pride and honour of the family (Sah, 2017).

Sexual violence transgresses the sexual rights of the victim and is rooted in gender inequality. While both men and women are at risk of experiencing sexual violence, women and girls are much more likely to be the victims and men the perpetrators, often someone known and even trusted such as a family member, colleague, friend, partner or ex-partner (Dartnall and Jewkes, 2013). Sexual violence seems more likely in the context of younger age, alcohol and drug consumption, economic difficulties, early sexual initiation, sexual submissiveness and patriarchal norms. People with a childhood history of physical, sexual or emotional abuse, an unsupportive family environment and involvement in intimate partner violence are at higher risk of sexual violence, and they are also likely to become perpetrators (Garcia-Moreno *et al.*, 2012).

Sexual violence presents severe consequences for the physical and psychological health of the victims, including an increased risk of sexually transmitted infections, unintended pregnancy, abortion, gynaecological disorders and emotional trauma such as anxiety, depression, suicide attempts and social phobias (Bott, 2010). Sexual violence towards women disempowers them, making it harder for them to negotiate safe sex, the use of contraception and access to sexual health services; they become increasingly vulnerable and at risk of poor sexual health (Jewkes *et al.*, 2002).

Box 6.4 Reflections on a sexual assault

In her early days as a hospital doctor, Elizabeth cared for Katie, who was admitted to the intensive care unit. Katie had been found in her partner's flat, raped and beaten unconscious. As the medical team examined Katie's wounds, the unspoken questions included "How did this happen?" and "Has she taken drugs?" In summary, Elizabeth wondered whether Katie was, in some way, responsible for what had happened. Five months later, Elizabeth asked herself the same question, but this time she was the patient.

Elizabeth was sexually assaulted and raped one morning by a stranger, and she was taken by ambulance to her hospital. The man was arrested. As the criminal justice system moved along, Elizabeth's own struggle remained private and silent to all but a few. She feared the judgement of others. Would they think her responsible? Alternatively, she feared their pity. She lost her confidence, no longer trusted her instincts and her relationships floundered. Only within the walls of the hospital did she feel safe. When she attended court, she felt she was letting down her work colleagues, but couldn't explain. She felt voiceless and marginalised. She tried to ignore her own feelings and needs by working long hours. Attending to the patients' needs was something she could control and manage. She told herself that if her patients could find the strength for another round of chemotherapy, then she could cope with another day in court where the intimidation of the defence lawyer made her feel that she was on trial.

"In hindsight, I appreciate the medical consequences of sexual assault are enduring ... I was unaware how [it] can affect long-term physical and emotional well-being. Consequences include ... feelings of helplessness, depression, fears of intimacy, post-traumatic stress disorder and even suicide" (p.78).

Elizabeth reflects that the wounds of sexual assault flourish in atmospheres of shame and stigma. Years after her rape, she wondered why no professional had ever asked her to provide a sexual violence history. When she asked a colleague why not, she said, "You do not look like a victim of sexual violence".

(Source: Volkmann, 2017)

In the UK, when sexual violence is reported to the police, an investigation will normally be launched. However, if the victim decides not to go through the investigation process because of embarrassment, humiliation or other reasons, they may decide to contact a support organisation such as a Rape Crisis service. They provide national helplines to support victims of sexual violence.

> *Coercive control is a key aspect of sexual violence, which can take many forms. Women disproportionately fall victim to sexual violence which may have long term severe impacts on their physical and psychological health and wellbeing.*

Sociocultural aspects of sexual health

Social and cultural factors often work together to influence people's sexual behaviour, as well as their access to sexual health services. From a social constructionist viewpoint, individuals' sexual behaviour is constructed through the various discourses/communications that are embedded into the social and cultural fabric of their lives. These include their socioeconomic situation, interpersonal interactions, social networks, peers, family traditions, moral values, cultural influences, religious beliefs, the media and the provision of sex education (Rao *et al.*, 2012; Sah, 2017). Individuals are exposed to these social and cultural factors to different degrees and in different ways, which influences their risks of experiencing a sexually transmitted infection, an unintended pregnancy, an abortion or sexual violence (Malarcher, 2010).

Sexual attitudes and behaviours

The sexual attitudes and behaviours of the British population have changed significantly over recent decades. In Britain, the age at first sexual intercourse has decreased, the number of sexual partners for women has increased and attitudes towards same-sex relationships have become more positive (Mercer *et al.*, 2013). Same-sex marriage became legal in the UK under The Marriage (Same Sex Couples) Act 2013 and the Northern Ireland (Executive Formation etc.) Act 2019. In the UK, the number of same-sex couples increased by 50% between 2015 and 2018, and the number of cohabitating families increased by 25.8% between 2008 and 2018 (ONS, 2019b). Sexual attitudes towards pre-marital sex, cohabiting couples and having children outside of marriage are becoming increasingly accepting and they are seen as 'normal'. In April 2020, the UK Prime Minister Boris Johnson and his partner Carrie Symonds became the first unmarried couple to reside in 10 Downing Street and to have a child.

People's attitudes towards sex and sexuality are guided by the peculiar sociocultural norms of different societies. The British National Survey of Sexual Attitudes and Lifestyles (NATSAL – 3) found that sexual behaviours differ across ethnic groups within the British population (Wayal *et al.*, 2017). For example, compared to the rest of the population, the youngest average age of sexual debut was among Black Caribbean men and women, and the oldest was among those who described themselves as Indian. In terms of sexual competence at sexual debut, the survey found the lowest among the Black Caribbean respondents and highest among the Indian respondents. Sexually transmitted infections were higher among Black Caribbean men and mixed-ethnicity women, and emergency contraception was reported most frequently by Black Caribbean women.

Box 6.5 What factors explain the differences in sexual outcomes across different ethnic groups?

Dr Sonali Wayal and her colleagues wanted to understand if known determinants of health, and health inequalities, influenced different sexual health outcomes across different ethnic groups. They examined

- socio-economic factors, e.g. marital status, socio-economic status, academic qualifications
- mental health, e.g. depressive symptoms
- substance use, e.g. smoking, alcohol, drugs
- sexual outcomes, e.g. diagnosis of a sexually transmitted infection, use of emergency contraception

They hypothesised

- socio-economic factors influence mental health and substance use. In turn these influence sexual behaviours
- together, socio-economic factors, mental health, substance use and sexual behaviours lead to certain sexual outcomes
- socio-economic factors, mental health and substance use may directly or indirectly explain the different sexual health outcomes across ethnic groups

Their findings supported their hypothesis to an extent, they but did not fully explain all the differences in sexual outcomes across different ethnic groups.

(Source: Wayal *et al.*, 2017)

Cultural and religious norms

Religion is an important aspect of culture, and culture may influence religious beliefs (Barry *et al.*, 2010). Cultural norms surrounding gender roles and religious affiliation play an important role in shaping an individual's sexual attitudes and behaviours. In turn, these are also shaped by the social and cultural context in which they live, such as the religious values, beliefs and practices of their parents and family, and the cultural beliefs of their peer groups and the wider neighbourhood (Sah, 2017). All major religions have some proscriptions regarding sex and sexuality, but they can be interpreted differently depending on the sex and religious affiliation of the individual (Adamczyk and Hayes, 2012). Sometimes the exaggeration of cultural norms or preconceptions relating to a religion can present false perceptions and representations about a community (Sinha *et al.*, 2007).

Today, culture is less localised and increasingly globalised because of the international flow of ideas, people, capital and information. The changes in politics, culture and economics bring multifaceted changes to the sexual health of a population (Altman, 2003). Political changes have allowed new social structures to develop, and people to more freely express their sexual identities and lifestyles. Cultural changes have broadened people's understanding of sexual identity and sexual behaviour in ways that often conflict with traditional norms. Economic changes have allowed people to organise their lives in new ways and they have contributed toward the commodification of sex and sexuality through prostitution and pornography.

Internet and digital media

The rapid increase in the availability and accessibility of digital media and a steady increase in access to the internet have extended opportunities for people to engage with online content associated with sex, sexuality and sexual lifestyles. In 2019, 87% of all British adults used the internet daily, 79% accessed the internet via mobile phone or a smartphone, 71% of women and 64% of men used social networking, and 68% of women and 59% of men looked for health-related information online (ONS, 2019a). The high uptake and use of social networking sites, online dating applications, text messaging, webpages and location-based social media mobile applications (apps) have dramatically changed interpersonal sexual communications (Kesten *et al.*, 2019; Wadham *et al.*, 2019).

Many people access pornography online, either intentionally or accidentally, which can lead to unnecessary worries or unrealistic expectations about 'normal' sexual behaviour (Bailey *et al.*, 2015). Pornography provides the least esteemed and least convincing depiction of real relationships, sex and sexuality (Segal, 2003). Braun-Courville and Rojas (2009), in their cross-sectional survey at a health centre, reported that exposure to internet pornography was associated with high-risk sexual behaviours such as multiple sexual partners, an increased number of lifetime sexual partners, substance use during sexual activity and unprotected sex. Lo and Wei (2005), in a survey of Taiwanese adolescents, found that exposure to internet pornography was associated with greater acceptance of sexually permissive attitudes and behaviour, even after accounting for gender, age, religion and exposure to traditional media pornography. Pornography makes unachievable assumptions about gender norms and sexual practices, in contrast to the sexual realities of 'real' people. Although the impact of online pornography on the sexual health and wellbeing of the population remains uncertain, it should not be used as a guide to real-life sexual experiences or as a primary source for sexual health information or education (Lim *et al.*, 2016).

Digital media can also provide valuable opportunities to raise awareness about sexual health and the availability of sexual health services within the community and clinical settings (Nadarzynski *et al.*, 2017; Gabarron and Wynn, 2016). For example, SH:24 works in partnership with the National Health Service in England and Wales to provide quick, discreet and completely confidential free online sexual health advice, infection testing, contraception and remote clinical support.

> *The sexual health of the population is determined by a complex web of interrelated factors. Sexual attitudes and behaviours are shaped by the various social and cultural factors in which people are born, grow, live and work.*

Thinking point:

> Consider some of the challenges to achieving positive, holistic sexual health amongst people from diverse social and cultural backgrounds.

Positive sexual health: sexual rights and relationships

Most people will engage in some form of sexual relationship at some point in their lives. In most cases, people are told what not to do rather than their sexual rights within a relationship. Richardson (2000) describes sexual rights in terms of sexual practice, sexual identity and sexual relationships. Sexual practice includes performing various sexual acts to achieve pleasurable sexual experiences without fear, violence or social constraints. Sexual identity is about rights to self-definition, self-expression and self-realisation. Rights in sexual relationships include the right to consensual sexual practice and opportunities to freely choose sexual partners that can be publicly recognised.

Dixon-Mueller and colleagues (2009) argue that people need to understand their own sexual rights and responsibilities, and to respect the rights of others. They propose a 'conceptual framework for sexual ethics of equal rights and responsibilities' which includes

- sexual relationships and the right to choose one's partner
- sexual expression and the right to seek pleasure
- sexual consequences and the right to cooperation from one's partner
- sexual harm and the right to protection
- sexual health and the right to information, education and health services

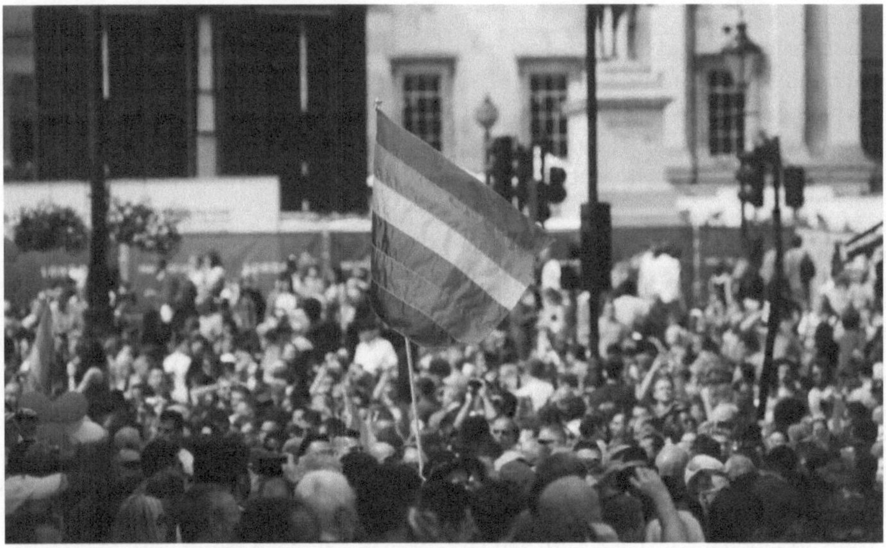

Figure 6.6 London's gay pride parade wave the rainbow flag to symbolise diversity
Source: Bikeworldtrave/Shutterstock.com

From this perspective, the authors suggest that every individual has the right to make their own decisions about their own sexual development, which will contribute to their sexual practice, identity and relationships. Any deviance from this sexual norm will result in sexual harassment, abuse, violence, rape or forced marriage.

Sexual rights are generally understood as the formal and informal application of human rights to the domain of sex, sexuality and sexual relationships. Sexual rights refer to the sexual freedom of individuals, their autonomy, integrity and dignity, as well as to the equal rights of others, especially their sexual partners. Rights include speaking openly without feeling shame or guilt, having a sexual voice, having choices about sexual engagement, being asked for consent and opportunities to withdraw consent. They include being treated with respect and ensuring that sexual activity remains consensual. Equal rights, mutual respect, consent and shared responsibilities apply to all sexual partners regardless of their sex, sexual orientation, gender identity, marital status, and other personal or social characteristics.

> *Sexual health requires a positive and respectful approach to human sexuality and relationships, and an understanding of the complex factors that shape human sexual behaviour. To achieve this, it is paramount for people to understand their sexual rights.*

Summary

This chapter has

- described current understandings of sexual health
- provided examples of negative and positive sexual health outcomes
- explained how sexual violence and unintended pregnancies can negatively impact women's lives
- discussed how sexual attitudes and behaviour are partly influenced by socio-economic and lifestyle factors arising from the social and cultural contexts in which people are born, live and work
- argued that positive sexual health is about experiencing sexual rights and taking a positive and respectful approach to human sexuality and relationships

Further reading

French, K. (ed) (2009) *Sexual health*. Chichester: John Wiley and Sons

Wellings, K., Mitchell, K., and Collumbien, M. (eds) (2012) *Sexual health: a public health perspective*. Maidenhead: Open University Press

Useful websites

Avert. Global information on information and education on HIV and AIDS. Available at: www.avert.org

British Association for Sexual Health and HIV. Available at: www.bashh.org

Brook. Available at: www.brook.org.uk

Family Planning Association. Available at: www.fpa.org.uk

SH:24 Sexual health 24 hours a day. Available at: https://sh24.org.uk/
Terrence Higgins Trust. Available at: www.tht.org.uk/

References

Adamczyk, A., and Hayes, B.E. (2012) 'Religion and sexual behaviours: understanding the influence of Islamic cultures and religious affiliation for explaining sex outside of marriage', *American Sociological Review*, 77(5), pp.723–746

Altman, D. (2003) 'Globalisation, political economy and HIV/AIDS', in Weeks, J., Holland, J., and Waites, M. (eds) *Sexualities and society: a reader*. Cambridge: Polity Press, pp.186–194

Amnesty International UK (2019) *Abortion in Ireland and Northern Ireland*. Available at: www.amnesty.org.uk/abortion-rights-northern-ireland-timeline (Accessed 23rd April 2020)

Bailey, J., Mann, S., Wayal, S., Hunter, R., Free, C., Abraham, C., and Murray, E. (2015) 'Sexual health promotion for young people delivered via digital media: a scoping review', *Public Health Research*, 3(13), pp.1–119

Barry, C., Nelson, L., Davarya, S., and Urry, S. (2010) 'Religiosity and spirituality during the transition to adulthood', *International Journal of Behavioral Development*, 34(4), pp.311–324

Bexhell, H., Guthrie, K., Cleland, K., and Trussell, J. (2016) 'Unplanned pregnancy and contraceptive use in Hull and East Yorkshire', *Contraception*, 93(3), pp.233–235

Bott, S. (2010). 'Sexual violence and coercion: implications for sexual and reproductive health', in Malarcher, S. (ed) *Social determinants of sexual and reproductive health*. Geneva: World Health Organization, pp.133–157

Braun-Courville, D.K., and Rojas, M. (2009) 'Exposure to sexually explicit web sites and adolescent sexual attitudes and behaviors', *Journal of Adolescent Health*, 45(2), pp.156–162

British Pregnancy Advisory Service (2013) *Britain's abortion law. What it says, and why*. Available at: www.reproductivereview.org/images/uploads/Britains_abortion_law.pdf (Accessed 29th April 2020)

Cameron, R.L., Cullen, B.L., Wallace, L.A., Glancy, M.E., Shepherd, J., Templeton, K., and Goldberg, D.J. (2019) *Surveillance report. Genital chlamydia and gonorrhoea infection in Scotland: laboratory diagnoses 2009–2018*. Health Protection Scotland/Public Health Scotland

Centre for Reproductive Rights (2020) *The world's abortion laws*. Available at: https://reproductiverights.org/worldabortionlaws?category[294]=294 (Accessed 22nd April 2020)

Cullen, B.L., Wallace, L.A., Cameron, R., Nicholson, D., Glancy, M., and Goldberg, D.J. (2019) *Surveillance report. Syphilis in Scotland 2018: update*. Health Protection Scotland/Public Health Scotland

Dartnall, E., and Jewkes, R. (2013) 'Sexual violence against women: the scope of the problem', *Best Practice and Research Clinical Obstetrics and Gynaecology*, 27(1), pp.3–13

Department of Health and Social Care (2019) *Abortion statistics, England and Wales: 2018*. Available at: https://assets.publishing.service.gov.uk/government/uploads/system/uploads/attachment_data/file/808556/Abortion_Statistics__England_and_Wales_2018__1_.pdf (Accessed 23rd April 2020)

Dixon-Mueller, R., Germain, A., Fredrick, B., and Bourne, K. (2009) 'Towards a sexual ethics of rights and responsibilities', *Reproductive Health Matters*, 17(33), pp.111–119

Gabarron, E., and Wynn, R. (2016) 'Use of social media for sexual health promotion: a scoping review', *Global Health Action*, 9(1) doi.org/10.32193

Garcia-Moreno, C., Mitchell, K., and Wellings, K. (2012) 'Sexual violence', in Wellings, K., Mitchell, K., and Collumbien, M. (eds) *Sexual health: a public health perspective*. Maidenhead: Open University Press, pp.47–58

Glasier, A., and Wellings, K. (2012) 'Unplanned pregnancy', in Wellings, K., Mitchell, K., and Collumbien, M. (eds) *Sexual health: a public health perspective*. Maidenhead: Open University Press, pp.33–46

Health Protection Scotland (2015) *HPS weekly report*, 49(2015/24). Available at: https://hpspubsrepo.blob.core.windows.net/hps-website/nss/2757/documents/1_genital%20herpes%20annual%20report%202014.pdf (Accessed 21st April 2020)

Jewkes, R., Sen, P., and Garcia-Moreno, C. (2002) 'Sexual violence', in Krug, E., Dahlberg, L., Mercy, J.A., Zwi, A.B., and Lozano, R. (eds) *World report on violence and health*. Geneva: World Health Organization, pp.147–181

Kesten, J.M., Dias, K., Burns, F., Crook, P., Howarth, A., Mercer, C.H., Rodger, A., Simms, I., Oliver, I., Hickman, M., and Hughes, G. (2019) 'Acceptability and potential impact of delivering sexual health promotion information through social media and dating apps to MSM in England: a qualitative study', *BMC Public Health*, 19(1236) doi.org/10.1186/s12889-019-7558-7

Lim, M.S., Carrotte, E.R., and Hellard, M.E. (2016) 'The impact of pornography on gender-based violence, sexual health and well-being: what do we know?', *Journal of Epidemiology and Community Health*, 70(1), pp.3–5

Lo, V.H., and Wei, R. (2005) 'Exposure to internet pornography and Taiwanese adolescents' sexual attitudes and behaviour', *Journal of Broadcasting and Electronic Media*, 49(2), pp.221–237

Malarcher, S. (ed) (2010) *Social determinants of sexual and reproductive health: informing future research and programme implementation*. Geneva: World Health Organization

Mercer, C.H., Tanton, C., Prah, P., Erens, B., Sonnenberg, P., Clifton, S., Macdowall, W., Lewis, R., Field, N., Datta, J., and Copas, A.J. (2013) 'Changes in sexual attitudes and lifestyles in Britain through the life course and over time: findings from the National Surveys of Sexual Attitudes and Lifestyles (Natsal)', *The Lancet*, 382(9907), pp.1781–1794

Nadarzynski, T., Morrison, L., Bayley, J., and Llewellyn, C. (2017) 'The role of digital interventions in sexual health', *Sexually Transmitted Infections*, 93(4), pp.234–235

Office for National Statistics (2018) Sexual offending: victimisation and the path through the criminal justice system. Available at: www.ons.gov.uk/peoplepopulationandcommunity/crimeandjustice/articles/sexualoffendingvictimisationandthepaththroughthecriminaljusticesystem/2018-12-13#how-prevalent-are-sexual-offences (Accessed 23rd April 2020)

Office for National Statistics (2019a) Internet access – households and individuals, Great Britain: 2019. Available at: www.ons.gov.uk/peoplepopulationandcommunity/householdcharacteristics/homeinternetandsocialmediausage/bulletins/internetaccesshouseholdsandindividuals/2019 (Accessed 20th April 2020)

Office for National Statistics (2019b) Families and households in the UK: 2018. Available at: www.ons.gov.uk/peoplepopulationandcommunity/birthsdeathsandmarriages/families/bulletins/familiesandhouseholds/2018 (Accessed 28th April 2020)

Office for National Statistics (2020) Crime survey for England and Wales. Crime in England and Wales: year ending September 2019. Available at: www.ons.gov.uk/peoplepopulationandcommunity/crimeandjustice/bulletins/crimeinenglandandwales/yearendingseptember2019 (Accessed 23rd April 2020)

O'Halloran, C., Sun, S., Nash, S., Brown, A., Croxford, S., Connor, N., Sullivan, A.K., Delpech, V., and Gill, O.N. (2019) *HIV in the United Kingdom: towards zero HIV transmissions by 2030. 2019 report*. London: Public Health England

Public Health Agency (2019) *Sexually transmitted infection surveillance in Northern Ireland 2019. An analysis of data for the calendar year 2018*. Available at: www.publichealth.hscni.net/sites/default/files/2019-08/STI%20surveillance%20report%202019.pdf (Accessed 21st April 2020)

Public Health England (2018a) National chlamydia screening programme standards. 7th ed. Available at: https://assets.publishing.service.gov.uk/government/uploads/system/uploads/attachment_data/file/759846/NCSP_Standards_7th_edition_update_November_2018.pdf (Accessed 22nd April 2020)

Public Health England (2018b) Health matters: reproductive health and pregnancy planning. Available at: www.gov.uk/government/publications/health-matters-reproductive-health-and-pregnancy-planning/health-matters-reproductive-health-and-pregnancy-planning (Accessed 22nd April 2020) (Accessed 28th April 2020)

Public Health England (2019a) Sexually transmitted infections and screening for chlamydia in England, 2018. Available at: https://assets.publishing.service.gov.uk/government/uploads/system/uploads/attachment_data/file/806118/hpr1919_stis-ncsp_ann18.pdf (Accessed 22nd April 2020) (Accessed 28th April 2020)

Public Health England (2019b) *Addressing the increase in syphilis in England: PHE action plan, June 2019*. Available at: https://assets.publishing.service.gov.uk/government/uploads/system/uploads/attachment_data/file/806076/Addressing_the_increase_in_syphilis_in_England_Action_Plan_June_2019.pdf (Accessed 23rd April 2020)

Public Health Wales (2019) Sexual health in Wales surveillance scheme (SWS) quarterly report, January 2019 (data to end September 2018). Available at: www.wales.nhs.uk/sitesplus/documents/888/Quarterly%20Report_Jan2019_v1.pdf (Accessed 28th April 2020)

Rao, T.S.S., Gopalakrishnan, R., Kuruvilla, A., and Jacob, K.S. (2012) 'Social determinants of sexual health', *Indian Journal of Psychiatry*, 54(2), pp.105–107

Richardson, D. (2000) 'Constructing sexual citizenship: theorizing sexual rights', *Critical Social Policy*, 20(1), pp.105–135

Rights of Women (2016) Coercive control and the law. London. Available at: https://rightsofwomen.org.uk/wp-content/uploads/2016/03/ROW--Legal-Guide-Coercive-control-final.pdf (Accessed 22nd April 2020)

Sah, R.K. (2017) Positive sexual health: an ethnographic exploration of social and cultural factors affecting sexual lifestyles and relationships of Nepalese young people in the UK. PhD thesis. Canterbury Christ Church University. Available at: https://bit.ly/36EgXtx (Accessed 30th May 2020)

Santelli, J., Rochat, R., Hatfield-Timajchy, K., Gilbert, B.C., Curtis, K., Cabral, R., Hirsch, J.S., and Schieve, L. (2003) 'The measurement and meaning of unintended pregnancy', *Perspectives on sexual and reproductive health*, 35(2), pp.94–101

Segal, L. (2003) 'Only the literal: the contradictions of anti-pornography feminism', in Weeks, J., Holland, J., and Waites, M. (eds) *Sexualities and society: a reader*. Cambridge: Polity Press, pp.95–104

Sinha, S., Curtis, K., Jayakody, A., Viner, R., and Roberts, H. (2007) ' "People make assumptions about our communities": sexual health amongst teenagers from black and minority ethnic backgrounds in East London', *Ethnicity and Health*, 12(5), pp.423–441

Teuton, J., Johnston, R., and Windsor, S. (2016) *Outcomes framework and supporting evidence for the pregnancy and parenthood in young people strategy in Scotland*. Edinburgh: NHS Health Scotland

UNAIDS (2014) *90-90-90. An ambitious treatment target to help end the AIDS epidemic. Joint United Nations Programme on HIV/AIDS*. Available at: www.unaids.org/sites/default/files/media_asset/90-90-90_en.pdf (Accessed 21st April 2020)

United Nations (1995) *Report of the international conference on population and development. Cairo, 5–13 September 1994*. New York: United Nations

Volkmann, E.R. (2017) 'Silent survivors', *The Annals of Family Medicine*, 15(1), pp.77–79

Wadham, E., Green, C., Debattista, J., Somerset, S., and Sav, A. (2019) 'New digital media interventions for sexual health promotion among young people: a systematic review'. *Sexual health*, 16(2), pp.101–123

Wayal, S., Hughes, G., Sonnenberg, P., Mohammed, H., Copas, A.J., Gerressu, M., Tanton, C., Furegato, M., and Mercer, C.H. (2017) 'Ethnic variations in sexual behaviours and sexual health markers: findings from the third British national survey of sexual attitudes and lifestyles (Natsal-3)', *The Lancet Public Health,* 2(10), e458–472 doi:10.1016/S2468-2667(17)30159-7

Wellings, K., Jones, K.G., Mercer, C.H., Tanton, C., Clifton, S., Datta, J., Copas, A.J., Erens, B., Gibson, L.J., Macdowall, W., and Sonnenberg, P. (2013) 'The prevalence of unplanned pregnancy and associated factors in Britain: findings from the third national survey of sexual attitudes and lifestyles (Natsal-3)', *The Lancet*, 382(9907), pp.1807–1816

World Health Organization (1948) *Constitution of the World Health Organisation.* Available at: http://apps.who.int/gb/bd/PDF/bd47/EN/constitution-en.pdf?ua=1 (Accessed 20th April 2020)

World Health Organization (1975) *Education and treatment in human sexuality: the training of health professionals.* Geneva: World Health Organization

World Health Organization (2006) *Defining sexual health: report of a technical consultation on sexual health, 28–31 January 2002.* Geneva: World Health Organization

World Health Organization (2010) *Developing sexual health programmes: a framework for action.* Geneva: World Health Organization

World Health Organization (2019) Preventing unsafe abortion. Available at: www.who.int/news-room/fact-sheets/detail/preventing-unsafe-abortion (Accessed 22nd April 2020)

7 Physical inactivity and health

Gail Sheppard

Key points

- Introduction
- The rise of physical inactivity and sedentary behaviour
- Physical inactivity, sedentary behaviour and health
- Economic costs of physical inactivity and sedentary behaviour
- Measuring physical inactivity, activity and sedentary behaviour
- Current levels of physical inactivity and sedentary behaviour in the UK
- UK physical activity guidelines
- Benefits of increasing physical activity and reducing sedentary behaviour
- Summary

Introduction

This chapter explains how inactivity and sedentary behaviour have risen over time, and why they are collectively an important public health priority. The chapter discusses how they contribute to non-communicable diseases, early death and costs to the economy. It will describe how inactivity and sedentary behaviour are measured and how recent surveys, such as UK travel surveys, show that the population is moving less and less. The chapter outlines the UK guidelines for activity and reducing sedentary behaviour, and concludes with an overview of the evidence that shows how physical activity protects against disease and early death, and promotes good health.

It is important to set out what we mean by inactivity and sedentary behaviour.

- Inactivity means not doing enough physical activity; a person is not meeting the amount of physical activity that is recommended for good health
- Sedentary behaviour means sitting, lying or reclining whilst awake

(Tremblay *et al.*, 2017)

Sometimes 'physical inactivity' is used as an umbrella term for both, and sometimes researchers use the term 'physical inactivity' or 'sedentary behaviour' very deliberately.

The rise of physical inactivity and sedentary behaviour

Since the Stone Age, over two million years ago, there has been a significant shift away from humans surviving by being physically active hunter-gatherers. Over time,

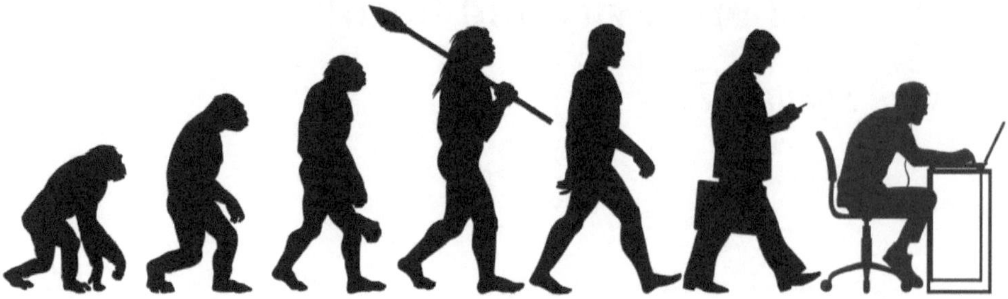

Figure 7.1 From movement for survival to an inactive lifestyle
Source: Uncle Leo/Shutterstock.com

improvements in agriculture and technology have led to people becoming increasingly inactive and more sedentary. This is known as the *physical activity transition* (Katzmarzyk and Mason, 2009).

Levels of physical inactivity have steadily increased over the past century. International research shows people's work-related inactivity has risen since the 1970s, and between 2001 and 2016 inactivity in high-income countries rose from a prevalence of 31.6% to 36.8% (Knuth and Hallal, 2009; Guthold *et al.*, 2018). This is twice as much inactivity as we see in low-income countries. We have also seen a shift towards more sedentary behaviours, such as sitting to travel, work and play. Some argue,

> In view of the prevalence, global reach, and health effect of physical inactivity, the issue should be appropriately described as *pandemic*, with far-reaching health, economic, environmental, and social consequences.
>
> (Kohl *et al.*, 2012 p.294)

Reasons for the rise in physical inactivity and sedentary behaviour

Katzmarzyk and Mason (2009) explain the world's population has become increasingly dense, and by 2008, for the first time ever, more people lived in urban areas rather than rural ones. Traditional rural life comprises small-scale farming and the use of bicycles and walking; urban living means using machines, a transport system, an organised labour force and the development of a very different social and economic environment. It can be characterised as one where many people earn money from industry and service-based occupations, desk-based work is common, domestic activities are light and leisure time is spent watching television or interacting with a computer. In summary, inactivity has grown because

- urbanisation fuels and is fuelled by economic growth
- mechanised labour-saving devices in the workplace and home have proliferated
- built environments are conducive to motor vehicles and to perceptions that the environment is less safe for activities such as walking
- the environment has led to changes in people's norms and expectations, the general social climate

Together these developments have decreased people's everyday moderate activity, increased sedentary behaviour and made vigorous activity rarely necessary.

> *Over centuries humans have undergone a physical activity transition leading to a rise in physical inactivity and sedentary behaviour.*

Physical inactivity, sedentary behaviour and health

Early studies into physical activity/inactivity and cardiovascular disease

In the mid-twentieth century, three seminal research studies introduced the idea that inactivity may be a cause of cardiovascular disease and activity may protect health. The London Transport Workers Study in the 1950s was one of the first contemporary research studies to suggest a connection between inactivity and cardiovascular disease. Professor Jeremy Morris and his colleagues studied those who worked on London buses and found that those who sat for most of the time, the bus drivers, had more heart attacks than the active bus conductors who climbed up and down the bus steps many times during the working day, even when both groups were matched for age (Morris *et al.*, 1953).

The Harvard Alumni Study (Paffenbarger *et al.*, 1978) researched 17,000 ex-college students aged 35 to 74 years old. They found those who were less active had experienced more heart attacks than those who were more active. Men whose activity, comprising walking, stair climbing and strenuous sport, burnt less than 2,000 calories

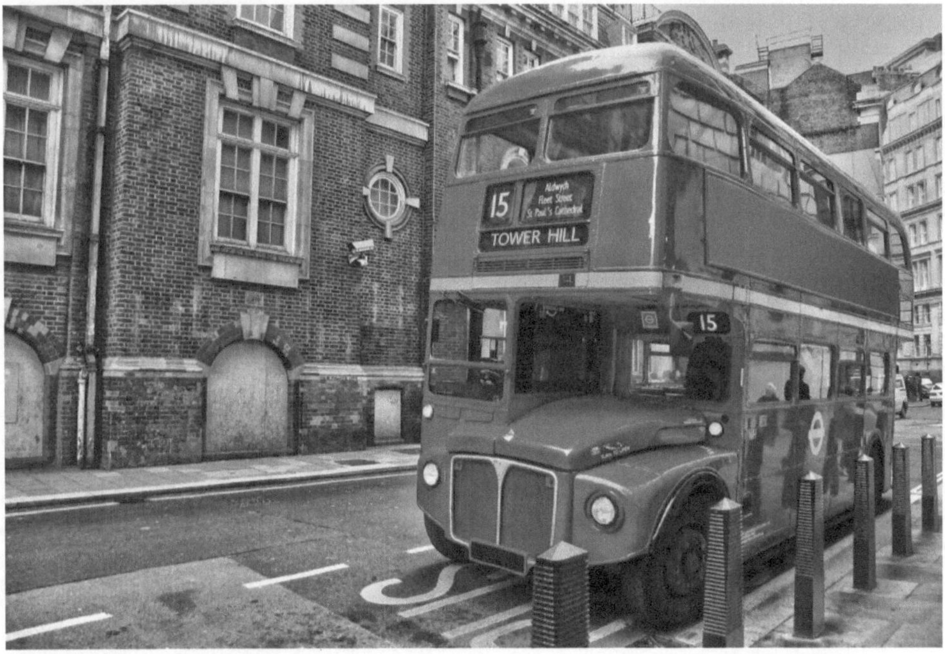

Figure 7.2 A typical London bus in the 1950s
Source: Delpixel/Shutterstock.com

per week were 64% more likely to have a heart attack than those whose activity was greater. The Framingham Heart Study, a series of long-term multigenerational studies into the factors that contribute to cardiovascular disease, included research into physical activity and found more death from cardiovascular disease among inactive than active men and women (Kannel and Sorlie 1979).

Over the next 50 years, research in this field vastly increased (Lee *et al.*, 2012). Researchers questioned whether the benefits to health were due to the presence of activity, and how much activity, or whether the harms to health were due to the presence of inactivity, and how much inactivity. From this emerged a new branch of work into the health impacts of time spent with almost no activity at all, sedentary behaviour.

Physical inactivity, sedentary behaviour and early death

Across the world, physical inactivity is one of the leading causes of death, responsible for five million deaths every year (Kohl *et al.*, 2012). In the UK, it is thought to cause one in six deaths and one in 10 premature deaths (British Heart Foundation, 2017). One of the earliest studies to investigate this phenomenon was the College Alumni Study, which investigated whether activity prolonged life (Paffenbarger *et al.*, 1986). Between 1962 and 1978 researchers followed 16,936 men for between 12 and 16 years and found that those who undertook more walking, stair climbing and sports, burning over 2,000 calories per week, lived longer than those who did not, independent of their smoking, high blood pressure or body weight. For example, of those who entered the study at age 50 to 54 years old, 69.9% of the active men were living at 80 years old compared to 59.8% of the relatively inactive men.

In 2011, Thorp and colleagues reviewed a wide range of studies that examined sedentary behaviour, often measured in terms of time spent sitting, TV viewing time and other screen-viewing time. Overall, there appeared to be an association between sedentary behaviour, increases in weight gain and early death. Chau and colleagues (2013) reviewed research published between 1989 and 2013 and concluded that high amounts of daily sitting time were associated with increased early death from all causes. They estimated sitting caused a 2% increase in risk of early death, and this increased by 5% for each hour when adults sat for more than seven hours per day. The relationship between sitting and early death has also been found by Ekelund and colleagues (2016), who noted that people who watched TV for more than three hours per day died early, regardless of how much physical activity they did. Katzmarzyk (2014) followed 16,586 Canadian adults, aged between 18 and 90 years old, over about 12 years. Data were collected on the amount of time spent standing and cause of death. Of interest, their results showed that, unlike sitting, standing was not associated with early death.

Physical inactivity, sedentary behaviour and disease

Physical inactivity and sedentary behaviour are associated with premature death because they are harmful to the human body, and they encourage the development of common non-communicable diseases (Healy *et al.*, 2011; Biswas *et al.*, 2015).

Table 7.1 Non-communicable diseases attributable to physical inactivity in the UK, 2012

Disease	*Attributable risk (%)*
Colon cancer	18.7%
Breast cancer	17.9%
Type 2 diabetes	13.0%
Coronary heart disease	10.5%
All premature deaths	16.9%

Source: Lee *et al.* (2012).

Muscular skeletal conditions

Daneshmandi *et al.* (2017) studied office workers and found that those who sat for an average six and a half hours per day reported lower back (53%), neck (53%) and shoulder (52%) pain. The authors explain that when sitting, the spine deviates from its normal S-shaped curve, which causes greater pressure on the spine and less pressure on the lower limbs. When we stand, the spine returns to its normal shape and the lower limbs take more of the body's weight. Sitting means we are not using muscles in our legs and buttocks, which can lead to muscle atrophy. Atrophy means the muscle shortens and weakens. One outcome is that the hip joints are poorly supported, resulting in pain and limping. In turn, pain discourages muscle use and a downward cycle begins (Amaro *et al.*, 2007; Tamura *et al.*, 2019). Sitting also puts stress on the other muscles and the spine. For example, the longer we sit, the more likely we are to slouch, causing prolonged muscle contraction and pressure on the joints around the neck and lower back which eventually leads to pain (Kwon *et al.*, 2018).

Type 2 diabetes

Muscle atrophy is associated with insulin resistance. Insulin enables the cells of the body to take in glucose from the blood. Many of these cells are muscle cells, so when muscles are atrophied there are fewer muscle cells to take in the glucose and more of it remains in the blood. This is a type of insulin resistance (Cleasby *et al.*, 2016). Without enough glucose, the body's metabolism is affected and people can develop prediabetes or type 2 diabetes. Also, the excess glucose in the bloodstream irritates the blood vessel linings, and this may contribute to cardiovascular disease (Carter *et al.*, 2017).

Weight gain and obesity

Physical inactivity and sedentary behaviour contribute to weight gain because low levels of activity use few calories from food and drink (Table 7.2). The excess is stored as increased body fat, unless someone is also eating a low-calorie diet. Excess body weight is strongly associated with osteoarthritis, where the protective cartilage around the ends of bones wears down, causing painful, stiff, swollen joints. This occurs in both weight-bearing and non-weight bearing joints, which suggests that arthritis and weight may be more complex than simply the mechanical load on a

Table 7.2 The activity equivalence of 10 calorie-dense food and drinks

Food type	*Approximate calories*	*Time needed to 'walk off' the calories (medium walking 3–5 mph)*	*Time needed to 'run off' the calories (slow running 5 mph)*
Can of sugary soft drink (330 ml)	138 kcals	26 minutes	13 minutes
Standard chocolate bar	229 kcals	42 minutes	22 minutes
Chicken and bacon sandwich	445 kcals	1 hour 22 minutes	42 minutes
Quarter of a large pizza	449 kcals	1 hour 23 minutes	43 minutes
Medium mocha coffee	290 kcals	53 minutes	28 minutes
Packet of crisps	171 kcals	31 minutes	16 minutes
Packet dry roasted peanuts (50 g)	296 kcals	54 minutes	28 minutes
Iced cinnamon roll	420 kcals	1 hour 17 minutes	40 minutes
Bowl of cereal	172 kcals	31 minutes	16 minutes
Blueberry muffin	265 kcals	48 minutes	25 minutes

Source: Royal Society for Public Health (2016). Reproduced with permission from RSPH.

joint (Bliddal *et al.*, 2014). In turn, arthritis limits people's physical activity, which contributes to weight gain. Overweight and obesity are strongly associated with an increased risk of developing cardiovascular disease and cancer (WCRF/AICR, 2018; Hingorani *et al.*, 2020).

Cardiovascular disease

Carter and colleagues (2017) describe some current thinking about why sedentary behaviour is associated with cardiovascular disease. They explain how sitting slows down the rate of blood flow, especially in the legs and feet, and alters the shear rate, which is the rate at which the blood is 'worked' as it flows through the body. A high shear rate is where flow is fast and the vessel diameter is small. Sitting is associated with a reduced shear rate. Sitting is also associated with affecting the healthy function of the endothelium. Endothelium is the thin membrane that lines the blood vessels and the heart; it is important for regulating blood clotting and the relaxation of blood vessels.

Dempsey and colleagues (2018) present some theories about why sitting may lead to high blood pressure. For example, they explain that the seated posture creates bends and constrictions in the major blood vessels of the lower limbs, especially under the thighs, and this interferes with normal blood flow and the normal regulation of blood pressure. Blood pressure may also be raised due to changes in the endothelium and the shear rate, which encourage the blood vessels to constrict and the blood pressure to rise.

Another risk factor for developing cardiovascular disease is high levels of low density lipoproteins (LDL) in blood cholesterol. LDLs are associated with developing atherosclerosis, the blocking of arteries with fatty plaque. Lipoprotein lipase is an enzyme located inside the blood vessel wall which helps to breaks down the fatty part of LDL. Researchers think that lipoprotein lipase is suppressed when an individual is sedentary and muscles are not contracting (Hamilton *et al.*, 2007; Bergouignan *et al.*, 2011).

Cardiorespiratory fitness measures how well the body takes oxygen and delivers it to the organs, tissues and muscles of the body during physical activity. It reflects the functional ability of the circulatory and respiratory systems. Sitting is associated with low levels of cardiorespiratory fitness, which means a person is at higher risk of developing cardiovascular disease, including strokes and heart failure (Carter *et al.*, 2017).

Metabolic syndrome is a combination of risk factors for cardiovascular disease and type 2 diabetes, including high blood cholesterol, high blood glucose, high blood pressure, abdominal fat and a high waist measurement. All these risk factors are increased with longer periods of sitting, independent of body weight, body fat or occupation (Hamilton *et al.*, 2007; Nam *et al.*, 2016).

Cancer

Research into understanding how inactivity and sedentary behaviour may encourage cancer is in its early stages. Current research suggests that physical activity seems to protect the body and prevent some cancers, but some of the research is conflicting (Tatjana *et al.*, 2019).

Physical inactivity, sedentary behaviour and mental health problems

Some research studies suggest that physical inactivity and/or sedentary behaviour is associated with mental health problems. For example, Sanchez-Villegas and colleagues (2008) followed 10,000 Spanish university students over six years and found that those who were more sedentary, and spent more time looking at screens, had an increased risk of developing a mental health disorder such as depression, bipolar, anxiety or stress. Another study of Scottish adults found that about a quarter of the 3,920 participants who completed a questionnaire spent at least four hours a day watching television or engaged in other screen viewing. The researchers found that these participants obtained poorer mental health scores compared to other participants who engaged in less screen time (Hamer *et al.*, 2010). Teychenne and colleagues (2015) carried out a review of published studies and found that greater time spent being sedentary and time spent sitting were both associated with greater anxiety. The studies indicated that this may be explained by changes in the central nervous system, disturbances in sleep, the impact of sedentary behaviour on the metabolic functions of the body and the lack of physical activity which is associated with reduced anxiety, or it may be due to sedentary behaviours being associated with increased solitude. They also note that those with symptoms of anxiety may choose to engage in sedentary behaviours as a way of coping with their anxiety. One of the challenges for this area of research is disentangling whether a deterioration in mental health leads to greater sedentariness or vice versa.

The experience of being sedentary

Rawlings and colleagues (2019) examined 30 research studies which examined people's experiences of being sedentary and the reasons for their decisions. They concluded that sedentary behaviour is influenced by

> ... a complex interaction between individual, environmental and socio-cultural factors. Micro and macro pressures are experienced at different life stages and in the context of illness; these shape individuals' beliefs and behaviour related to sedentariness. Knowledge of sedentary behaviour and associated health consequences appears limited in adult populations ...
>
> (Rawlings *et al.*, 2019 p.1)

They found that people are sedentary because of

- the home environment and parenting styles, sometimes being told to 'not to overdo it' or 'read a book' as a child
- feeling inadequate compared to peers during school sports, so turning to more pleasurable sedentary activities
- perceptions of 'slowing down' in older age, sedentary group activities being linked to social and cognitive benefits
- perceptions that older adults 'should rest'
- illness, fatigue, pain and depression
- perceptions that sedentariness will protect against further poor health
- a disinterest in active pursuits, it is 'easy' or 'lazy'
- environmental barriers that discourage walking such as crime
- limitations of time, work-life balance and money
- a lack of social support to be active
- socio-cultural norms such as being 'entitled to sit after having raised a family'

and because

- studying requires long periods of sitting, a belief that education is more important than healthy activity
- employment incudes commuting, long working hours, sitting at a desk, sitting in meetings and fatigue
- it contributes to a preferred self-image, enjoyment and self-reward for a 'hard day at work'

Thinking point:

> Having looked at this list of reasons for why people spend time being sedentary, draw up a list of the social, cultural, environmental and individual factors that encourage people to be physically active in their everyday lives. How do the two lists compare?

Economic costs of physical inactivity and sedentary behaviour

Physical inactivity and sedentary behaviour place an economic burden on societies. This comprises direct costs, such as healthcare, and indirect costs, such as sick leave

Table 7.3 Costs of physical inactivity, 2013

	Cost per year (US dollars)
Global cost to international healthcare systems	$53 billion
Global costs to productivity	$13.7 billion
Total costs to the UK	$2 billion
Total costs to United States of America	$27 billion

Source: Ding *et al.* (2016).

Table 7.4 Costs of physical inactivity-related disease to UK healthcare, 2006 to 2007

Inactivity-related disease	*Cost per year (£million)*
Cardiovascular disease	£659
Colorectal cancer	£65
Breast cancer	£54
Type 2 diabetes	£158

Source: Adapted from Scarborough *et al.* (2011 p.532).

from work and loss of productivity to business. The burden of physical inactivity-related disease over a lifetime can be measured in disability-adjusted life-years (DALYs), the number of years of healthy life that have been lost. Globally, this totals 13.4 million years (Ding *et al.*, 2016).

> *Since the 1950s, research has linked physical inactivity and then sedentary behaviour to disease, death and possibly to poor mental health. Yet socio-cultural and environmental factors continue to encourage sedentary behaviour, costing the UK millions of pounds in healthcare.*

Measuring physical inactivity, activity and sedentary behaviour

We often measure people's activity/inactivity by asking people to

- self-report their activity
- keep a diary of their activity
- use a pedometer, which measure footsteps
- use an accelerometer, which counts speed and distance

The Health Survey for England is an example of a national survey which collects data on activity/inactivity. It uses the Short-Form International Physical Activity Questionnaire (IPAQ) and reports people who recorded less than 30 minutes of moderate to vigorous physical activity per week as being 'inactive' and those reporting more than 30 minutes per week, as 'active' (NHS Digital, 2019). These data are used by many health organisations, but it is worth noting that many researchers do not define inactivity in this way; instead they define inactivity as that which does not meet the recommendations for health. In the UK, these are the Chief Medical Officers' Physical Activity Guidelines (DHSC, 2019a).

Sedentary behaviour is often measured by

- total sitting time, reported in hours and minutes
- recall of sitting during the previous week
- time spent watching TV
- time spent sitting at work

Strain and colleagues (2019) compared how the four nations of the UK are collecting activity/inactivity and sedentary behaviour data (Table 7.5). Despite the UK having

Table 7.5 Surveys that report on physical activity/inactivity and sedentary behaviour, UK

UK nation	*Surveys*	*Commissioners*
England	Active Lives Survey Health Survey for England	Sport England Department of Health and Social Care
Northern Ireland	Health Survey for Northern Ireland Continuous Household Survey	Department of Health Several government departments and agencies
Scotland	Scottish Health Survey	The Scottish government
Wales	National Survey for Wales	Welsh government

Source: Adapted from Strain *et al.* (2019 p.3).

uniform Physical Activity Guidelines (DHSC, 2019a), they found differences in the data-collection methods of surveys which make accurate UK data and cross-nation comparisons difficult.

Current levels of physical inactivity and sedentary behaviour in the UK

Physical inactivity

In 2017, the British Heart Foundation reported about 39% of UK adults did not meet the recommendations outlined in the UK Physical Activity Guidelines, meaning that about 20 million adults were physically inactive (BHF, 2017) (Table 7.6). As people age, they become more inactive (Figure 7.3). In Wales, Scotland and England

- women are more inactive than men across all age groups
- people who live in the most deprived areas are the most inactive, and those who live in the more affluent areas are the least inactive
- people who have disabilities or those with long-term conditions are more inactive than others
- there are limited data about ethnicity, but it seems inactivity is highest in the Asian (excluding Chinese) communities in England (Figure 7.4) and Scotland

(Welsh Government, 2019; McLean and Dean, 2020; Sport England, 2019)

Sedentary behaviour

In 2017, the British Heart Foundation reported that the average person in the UK spent about 78 days sitting each year, with men sitting more than women. In Scotland and England sedentary behaviour has been generally stable over time. Figure 7.5 shows people in England are sedentary for about 4.75 hours per day during the week and 5.2 hours per day at weekends (Scholes, 2017). People in Scotland are sedentary for about 5.25 hours per day during the week and 6 hours at weekends (McLean and Dean, 2020). Men are more sedentary than women. In Northern Ireland, 44% of respondents to a survey in 2016 to 2017 spent over four hours per day being sedentary on weekdays (DH, 2017).

Table 7.6 Levels of adult physical inactivity across the UK

		Percentage adults who are physically inactive	*Number of women who are physically inactive*	*Number of men who are physically inactive*
England	North West	47%	1,510,000	1,130,000
	North East	42%	570,000	330,000
	West Midlands	40%	1,040,000	770,000
	London	40%	1,610,000	1,060,000
	Yorkshire and Humber	40%	1,050,000	670,000
	East Midlands	39%	840,000	620,000
	East of England	37%	980,000	770,000
	South West	35%	950,000	600,000
	South East	34%	1,410,000	960,000
England		39%	9,900,000	6,900,000
Northern Ireland		46%	370,000	280,000
Wales		42%	600,000	430,000
Scotland		37%	930,000	690,000

Source: Adapted from BHF (2017 p.4).

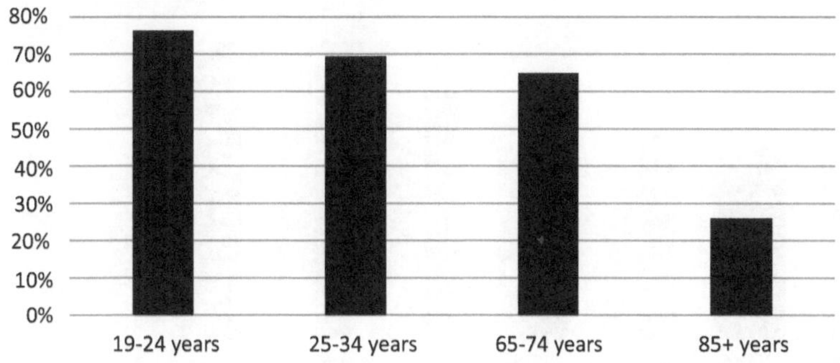

Figure 7.3 Percentage of adults meeting the recommended levels of activity by age, England 2016 to 2017

Source: PHE, 2018

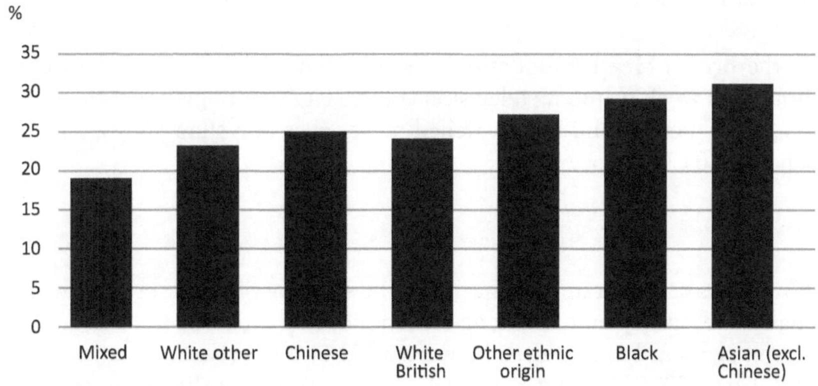

Figure 7.4 Percentage of inactivity by ethnicity, England 2018 to 2019

Source: adapted from Sport England, 2019 p.11

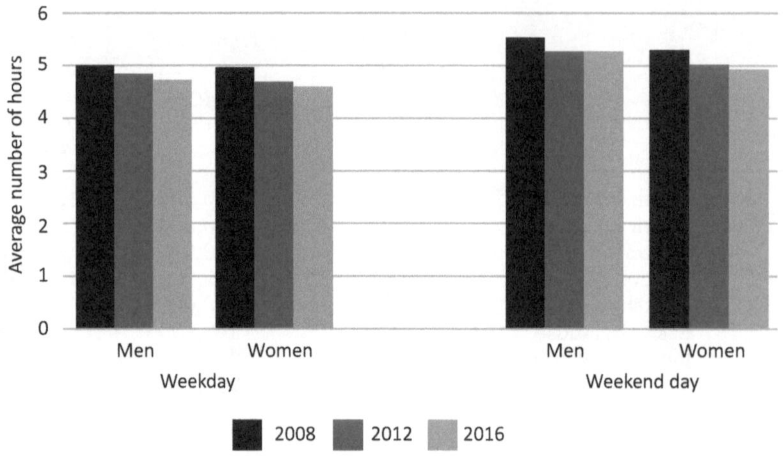

Figure 7.5 Average time spent being sedentary, England 2008, 2012 and 2016
Source: Scholes, 2017 p.31. Reproduced under the terms of the Open Government Licence v.3.0

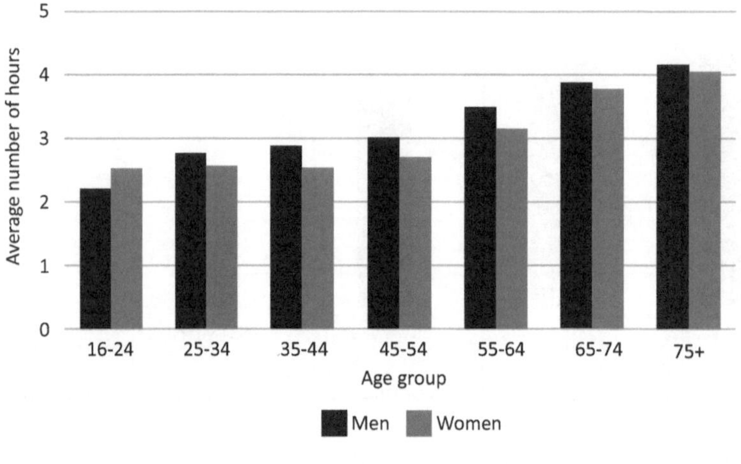

Figure 7.6 Average time spent watching TV at the weekend by age in England, 2016
Source: Scholes, 2017 p.28. Reproduced under the terms of the Open Government Licence v.3.0

In 2017, the British Heart Foundation reported that each person in the UK spent about 30 hours per week watching television (BHF, 2017). In England, at the weekend during 2016, older people and men watched more television than younger adults or women (Scholes, 2017) (Figure 7.6).

Travel

Trends in how we travel illustrate how inactivity and sedentary behaviour have increased. The National Travel survey monitors long-term trends in travel. The total distance travelled per person per year has increased between 1972 to 1973 (Great Britain) and 2018 (England only) by 46% (Evans *et al.*, 2019). We are travelling longer distances over longer periods of time, largely because of the greater ownership and use of cars.

Table 7.7 Comparisons of average travel distance, time and trips per person/per year, 1972 to 1973 (Great Britain) and 2018 (England)

	Great Britain 1972/1973	*England 2018*	*Percentage change*
Average miles travelled per person per year	4,476 miles	6,530 miles	+46%
Average hours spent travelling per person per year	353 hours	377 hours	+7%
Average number of trips per person per year	956 trips	986 trips	+3%

Source: Evans *et al.* (2019).

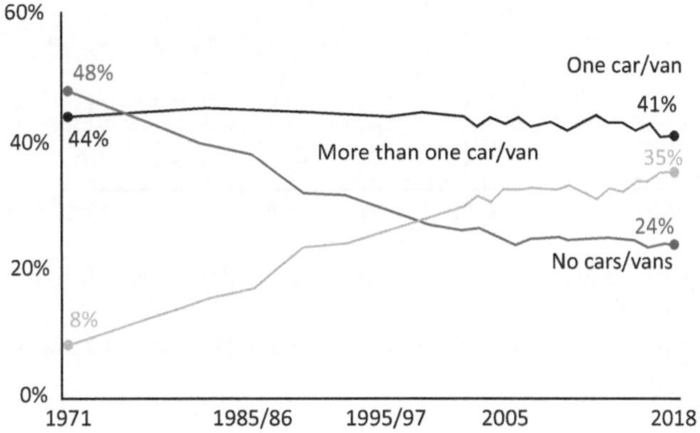

Figure 7.7 Percentage of households with access to a car, 1971 to 1988 (Great Britain) and 1989 to 2018 (England)

Source: Evans et al, 2019 p.11. Reproduced under the terms of the Open Government Licence v.3.0

Data from Great Britain between 1971 and 1988 and England between 1989 and 2018 show a 35% increase in households owning more than one car or van (Evans *et al.*, 2019) (Figure 7.7). Data from Great Britain between 1975 and 1988 and England between 1997 and 2015 show the average number of walking trips, per person, decreased (DT, 2018) (Figure 7.8). By 2018, people in England spent approximately one hour per day travelling; this included 36 minutes in a car, 12 minutes on public transport, 12 minutes walking and two minutes using other private transport such as bicycles. Only 3% of the average distance travelled was by walking and 1% by cycling (Evans *et al.*, 2019).

Physical activity and sedentary behaviour can be measured in different ways, which makes comparisons difficult, but data from across the UK consistently show levels of physical inactivity and sedentary behaviour are too high for good health.

UK Physical Activity Guidelines

We have noted that being physically inactive is defined as not meeting the levels of activity recommended for health. The World Health Organization updated its recommendations in 2020 (WHO, 2020) to support its Global Action Plan on Physical

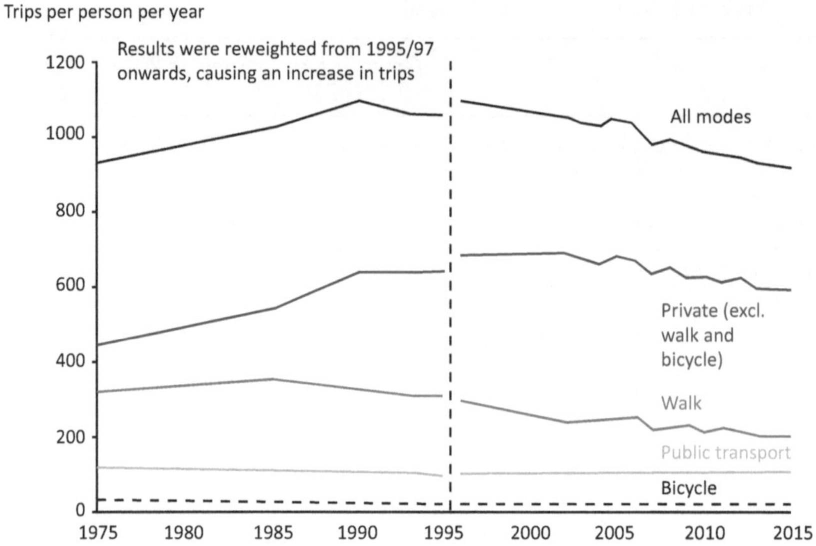

Figure 7.8 Trips per person/per year by mode of transport, 1975 to 1996 (Great Britain) and 1997 to 2015 (England)

Source: Department of Transport, 2018a p.5. Reproduced under the terms of the Open Government Licence v.3.0

Activity 2018 to 2030 (WHO, 2018). The UK recommendations were published as the Physical Activity Guidelines in 2019. Both

- promote activity for health. The UK recommendations clarify the frequency, intensity, type and time of activities that are needed for good health. People who do not meet these recommendations are defined as physically inactive
- encourage a reduction in sedentary behaviour

(WHO, 2018; DHSC, 2019a)

UK guidelines for promoting activity

The UK Physical Activity Guidelines (Table 7.8) were developed to guide policy-makers and to support those who work with individuals and communities to increase levels of physical activity, to promote health and prevent disease. They take a life course perspective, making recommendations for all ages. The Chief Medical Officers of the four UK nations state:

> If physical activity were a drug, we would refer to it as a miracle cure, due to the great many illnesses it can prevent and help treat.
>
> (DHSC, 2019a p.3)

Intensity of physical activity

The intensity of activity refers to how hard a person must work. This is often illustrated as a physical activity continuum (Figure 7.10).

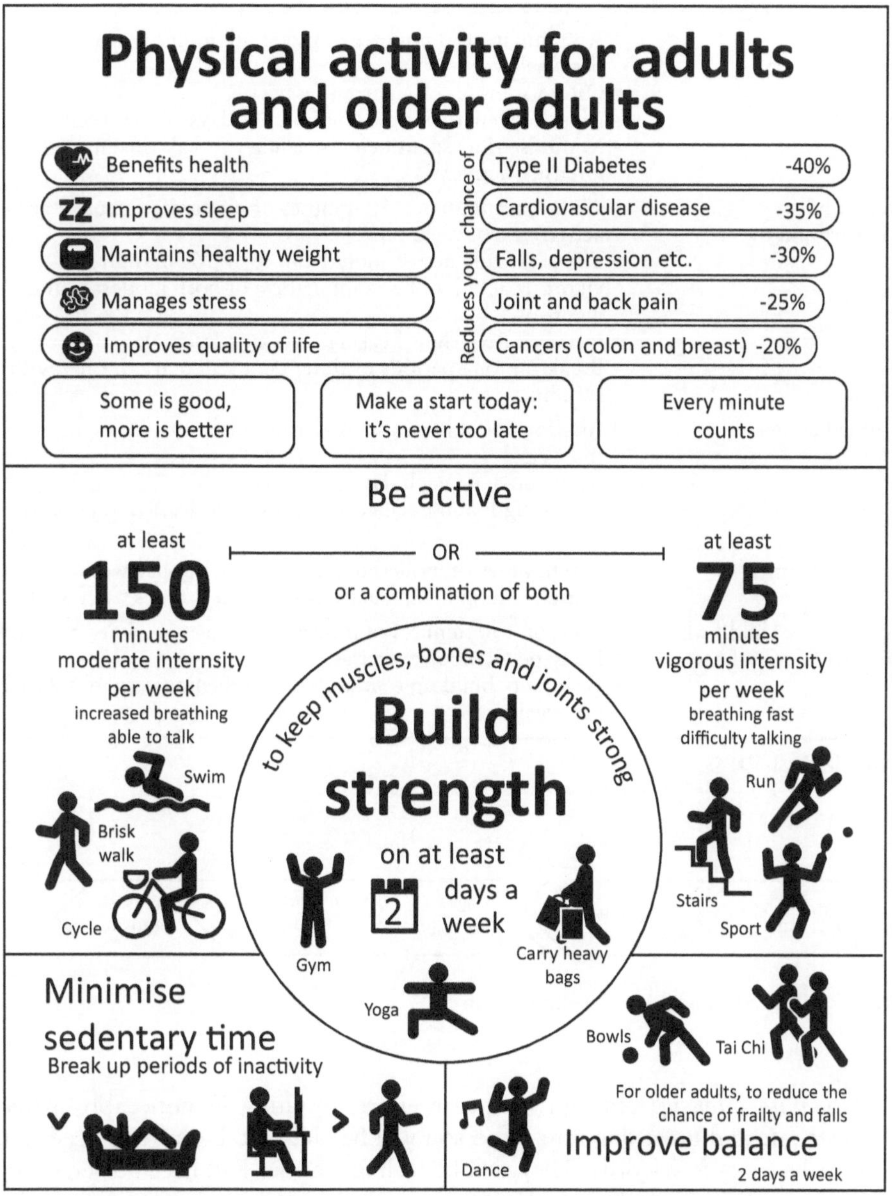

Figure 7.9 Physical activity for UK adults and older adults: 19 years and over
Source: DHSC, 2019a. Reproduced under the terms of the Open Government Licence v.3.0

The four main types of intensity are sedentary, light, moderate and vigorous.

- *Sedentary* means a lack of movement during an individual's waking hours, including being seated
- *Light intensity* can include standing or walking slowly. Light activity will not increase the heart rate too much and the person will still be able to talk freely

Table 7.8 UK Chief Medical Officers' Physical Activity Guidelines

Adults (19 to 64 years)	• Accumulate 150 minutes of moderate-intensity activity per week • OR 75 minutes of vigorous activity • Muscle strengthening activities on 2 days of the week • Minimise time spent being sedentary, break this up with light intensity activity
Older adults (65 years and over)	• Aim to accumulate 150 minutes of moderate-intensity aerobic activity each week. • Those already active should aim to add 75 minutes of vigorous activity or a combination of both moderate and vigorous. • Incorporate weight-bearing activities daily. • Break up long periods of time spent sedentary, if only with standing.
Disabled adults	• Aim for 150 minutes of moderate-intensity activity over the week. • Keep active on each day of the week. • Do strength and balance activities on at least 2 days of the week.
Pregnant women	• 150 minutes of moderate-intensity activity per week. • Muscle-strengthening activities at least 2 times each week.
Women after childbirth (birth to 12 months)	• Aim for 150 minutes of moderate-intensity activity per week. • Daily pelvic-floor exercises. • Gradually build up to muscle-strengthening activities 2 times per week.

Source: DHSC (2019a).

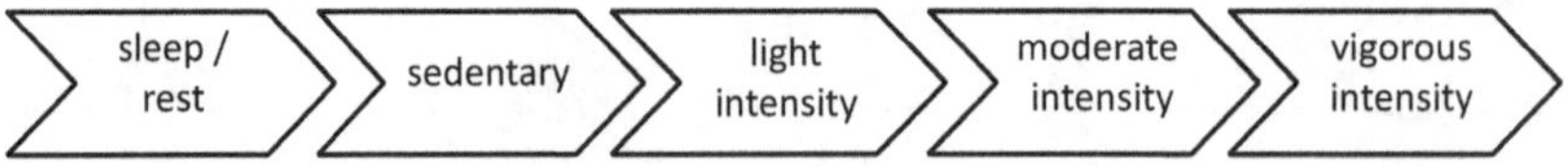

Figure 7.10 The physical activity continuum

- *Moderate intensity* requires moderate effort, resulting in noticeably increased heart rate and breathing rate. A person will be able to talk but will need to take breaths every few words. They will be feeling warmer and may be perspiring or sweating. Examples of moderate activity are brisk walking, gardening and household activities
- *Vigorous intensity* requires a lot more effort than moderate-intensity activity. A person will not be able to hold a conversation easily and their heart and breathing rates will be significantly increased

Not all activities activate the same response in each individual. An activity which is vigorous for one person may be light or moderate for another, depending on their fitness level, age and mobility status. Generally, activity should be at *moderate intensity* for it to be health enhancing.

UK guidelines for reducing sedentary behaviour

The UK Chief Medical Officers' Physical Activity Guidelines advise:

> Adults should aim to minimise the amount of time spent being sedentary, and when physically possible should break up long periods of inactivity with at least light physical activity.
>
> (DHSC, 2019a p. 30)

They do not give further details but an expert statement, commissioned by Public Health England, advises office-based employers and employees to reduce sitting during the working day (Buckley *et al.*, 2015). It recommends

- during each working day long periods of time spent sitting should be broken up with regular periods of standing
- all desk-based employees should start to replace sitting with two hours of standing time and light activity, building up to a total of four hours during the working day
- workplaces should incorporate opportunities for employees to discuss areas of lifestyle behaviour (stress management, smoking cessation, physical activity, diet, alcohol) as regular activities
- employees should provide opportunities for the use of adaptable desks where the employee has the choice between sitting or standing during the working day

Thinking point:

> Consider whether a person can be described as both physically active and sedentary.

> *The UK recommendations for physical activity and sedentary behaviour provide evidence-based practical guidance for the general population to increase their activity for good health*

Benefits of increasing physical activity and reducing sedentary behaviour

Physical activity can help to protect against disease and early death, and it can help to maintain and improve people's mental and emotional health and wellbeing.

Protection against disease

Physical activity helps to prevent weight gain and to maintain a healthy weight (Leskinen *et al.*, 2009), which reduces the risks of developing obesity, type 2 diabetes, metabolic syndrome and cardiovascular disease. It also protects against cancer and musculoskeletal problems.

Type 2 diabetes

Physical activity can help to prevent and to control type 2 diabetes because it helps to prevent weight gain and it helps to regulate blood sugar (glucose). The contraction of muscles during an acute bout of activity encourages the body to use up the glucose in the blood. Regular moderate-intensity activity encourages this process even at rest (Colberg *et al.*, 2010). Insulin resistance is where the body does not use its insulin correctly, to deal with blood glucose. Physical activity reduces insulin resistance and enhances insulin sensitivity (Bird and Hawley, 2017).

Metabolic syndrome

Physical activity seems to protect against developing metabolic syndrome (Ekelund *et al.*, 2007; Healy *et al.*, 2008; Sisson, 2010). Metabolic syndrome is when someone has a cluster of risk factors including obesity, high waist circumference, type 2 diabetes, poor glucose regulation, insulin resistance, high blood pressure and high blood cholesterol. They are vulnerable to developing type 2 diabetes and cardiovascular disease. Physical activity strengthens the heart, which reduces high blood pressure, helps to control the 'bad' LDL blood cholesterol and increases the 'good' HDL blood cholesterol.

Cardiovascular disease

Physical activity reduces cardiovascular disease, including heart disease and stroke, by up to 35% (BHF, 2017). The risk factors for developing cardiovascular disease include those features associated with metabolic syndrome as well as stress, a poor diet, smoking and physical inactivity. Research shows that physical activity

- can help with stress management
- is associated with healthier dietary behaviours
- can provide a distraction to those people undergoing smoking cessation and counters the life-limiting effects of smoking
- removes the risk factor of inactivity

(Sharon-David and Tenebaum, 2017; Joo *et al.*, 2019; Bize *et al.*, 2010)

Cancer

Regular physical activity reduces the risk of developing cancer and the risk of death from cancer (Schmid and Leitzmann, 2014; Lahart *et al.*, 2015; Li *et al.*, 2015). Physical activity has been found to reduce the risk of lung, breast, uterine and colon cancers (Hardman and Stensil, 2009; Islami *et al.*, 2018; Schmid *et al.*, 2014; Liu *et al.*, 2015). For example, research carried out in workplaces found that people who were more active in their daily work were less likely to develop colon cancer than those who spent most of their working day sitting down (Lee *et al.*, 1991; Slattery *et al.*, 1997). Researchers think that this is due to the positive effects of physical activity on the biochemical processes of the body, levels of immunity and weight management (Hardman and Stensel, 2009). Among individuals who have cancer, physical activity appears to help with fatigue and improve survival rates, cardiorespiratory and muscular fitness, body composition and wellbeing (Stevinson *et al.*, 2017).

Osteoporosis

Regular physical activity can delay, or minimise, musculoskeletal changes that naturally occur with age. These include a decrease in height, muscle wasting and reduced flexibility of the joints. Keeping active with age has been found to slow down the decrease in muscle mass (Raguso *et al.*, 2006). More than three million people in the UK are diagnosed with osteoporosis, a condition of 'brittle bones' which particularly affects post-menopausal women (International Osteoporosis Foundation, 2018). Weight-bearing and strength and resistance exercises help to maintain and increase bone density, which prevents the development of osteoporosis. In those with osteoporosis, these exercises increase bone density and reduce falls and therefore the number of fractures (Benedetti *et al.*, 2018; Howe *et al.*, 2011; Giangregorio *et al.*, 2014).

Promotion of mental and emotional health

Several studies have suggested that physical activity is associated with lower levels of depression and anxiety in differing populations. For example, Tyson and colleagues (2010) researched students at the University of Gloucestershire and found those with the highest levels of physical activity were also those with lower levels of anxiety and depression. McIntyre and colleagues (2019) studied 1,932 women aged 45 years and older who had been diagnosed with chronic disease, and found those who were more physically active had less severe depressive symptoms and better health-related quality of life.

Physical activity is also associated with positive emotions. For example, in Australia, Pasco and colleagues (2011) carried out research with a sample of 276 women and found that higher levels of regular physical activity were associated with positive emotions such as interest, excitement, enthusiasm and alertness. Reed and Buck (2009) reviewed 105 studies, yielding a sample size of over 9,800 participants, and found that regular aerobic activity results in moderate increases in positive emotions. In addition, research studies have found that regular physical activity can help with concentration, memory, self confidence and general improvements in mental health and quality of life (Biddle *et al.*, 2015; DHSC, 2019a).

Physical activity may help with mental and emotional health because of a range of physiological biochemical and psychosocial influences. Activity may provide

- a distraction from the stresses of everyday life
- opportunities for social interaction
- a sense of achievement
- positive emotional experiences as a by-product

(Faulker and Sparkes, 1999; Crone, 2007; Fogarty and Happell, 2005)

The message for most people is:

> Keep active, that doesn't mean to say you've got to play tennis or golf … but keep the body moving even if it's doing a bit of gardening for half an hour every day and make it every day, walk for your paper, don't get in the car …
>
> (Norfolk man aged between 75 and 80 years; Guell *et al.*, 2016 p.4)

Summary

This chapter has

- explained the reasons for the rise in physical inactivity and sedentary behaviour and how each is defined and measured in different ways
- discussed how inactivity and sedentary behaviour negatively impact health and increase the risks of early death
- outlined the economic costs of an inactive and sedentary population
- described the current levels of inactivity and sedentary behaviour in the UK, using travel as an example
- outlined the UK recommendations for physical activity and reducing sedentary behaviour
- described how increasing physical activity and reducing sedentary behaviour protects against disease and promotes good health

Further reading

Biddle, S.J.H., Mutrie, N., and Gorely, T. (2015) *Psychology of physical activity: determinants, wellbeing and interventions.* 2nd edn. London: Routledge

Leitzmann, M.F., Jochem, C., and Schmid, D. (eds) (2018) *Sedentary behaviour epidemiology.* New York: Springer

Zhu, W., and Owen, N (2017) *Sedentary behaviour and health.* Champaign, IL: Human Kinetics

Bouchard, C., Blair, S.N., and Haskell, W.L. (2012) *Physical activity and health.* 2nd edn. Champaigne, Illinois: Human Kinetics

Useful websites

British Heart Foundation. Available at: www.bhf.org.uk

University of Cambridge Centre for Diet and Activity Research. Available at: www.cedar.iph.cam.ac.uk

Sedentary Behaviour Research Network. Available at: www.sedentarybehaviour.org

References

Amaro, A., Amado, F., Duarte, J.A., and Appell, H.J. (2007) 'Gluteus medius muscle atrophy is related to contralateral and ipsilateral hip joint osteoarthritis', *International Journal of Sports Medicine*, 12(28), pp.1035–1039

Benedetti, M.G., Furlini, G., Zati, A., and Mauro, G.L. (2018) 'The effectiveness of physical exercise on bone density in osteoporotic patients', *BioMed Research International*, 2018(4) doi:10.1155/2018/4840531

Bergouignan, A., Rudwill, F., Simon, C., and Blanc, S. (2011) 'Physical inactivity as the culprit of metabolic inflexibility: evidence from bed-rest studies', *Journal of Applied Physiology*, 111(4), pp.1201–2011

Biddle, S.J.H., Mutrie, N., and Gorely, T. (2015) *Psychology of physical activity: determinants, well-being and interventions.* 3rd edn. London: Routledge

Bird, S.R., and Hawley, J.A. (2017) 'Update on the effects of physical activity on insulin sensitivity in humans', *BMJ Open Sport and Exercise Medicine*, 2(1) doi.10.1136/bmjsem-2016-000143

Biswas, A., Oh, P.I., Faulkner, G.E., Bajaj, R.R., Silver, M.A., Mitchell, M.S., and Alter, D.A. (2015) 'Sedentary time and its association with risk for disease incidence, mortality, and hospitalization in adults: a systematic review and meta-analysis', *Annals of Internal Medicine*, 162(2), pp.123–132

Bize, R., Willi, C., Chiolero, A., Stoianov, R., Payot, S., Locatelli, I., and Cornuz, J. (2010) 'Participation in a population-based physical activity programme as an aid for smoking cessation: a randomised trial', *Tobacco Control*, 19(6), pp.488–494

Bliddal, H., Leeds, A.R., and Christensen, R. (2014) 'Osteoarthritis, obesity and weight loss: evidence, hypotheses and horizons – a scoping review, *Obesity Reviews*, 15(7), pp.578–586

British Heart Foundation (2017) Physical inactivity and sedentary behaviour. Report 2017. www.bhf.org.uk/informationsupport/publications/statistics/physical-inactivity-report-2017 (Accessed 7th June 2020)

Buckley, J.P, Hedge, A., Yates, T., Copeland, R.J., Loosemore, M., Hamer, M., Bradley, G., and Dunstan, D.W. (2015) 'The sedentary office: a growing case for change towards better health and productivity. An expert statement on the growing case for change towards better health and productivity', *British Journal of Sports Medicine*, 49(21) doi:10.1136/bjsports-2015–094618

Carter, S., Hartman, Y., Holder, S., Thijssen, D.H., and Hopkins, N. (2017) 'Sedentary behaviour and cardiovascular disease risk: mediating mechanics', *Exercise, Sport Sciences Review*, 45(2), pp.80–86

Chau, J.Y., Grunseit, A.C., Chey, T., Stamatakis, E., Brown, W.J., Matthews, C.E., Bauman, A.E., and van der Ploeg, H.P. (2013) 'Daily sitting time and all-cause mortality: a meta-analysis', *PlosOne*, 8(11) doi.10.1371/journal.pone.0080000

Cleasby, M.E., Jamieson, P.M., and Atherton, P.J. (2016) 'Insulin resistance and sarcopenia: mechanistic links between common co-morbidities', *Journal of Endocrinology*, 229(2), R67–R81 doi:10.1530/JOE-15–0533

Colberg, S.R., Sigal, R.J., Fernhall, B., Regensteiner, J.G., Blissmer, B.J., Rubin, R.R., Chasan-Taber, L., Albright, A.L., Braun, B., and American College of Sports Medicine, American Diabetes Association (2010) 'Exercise and type 2 diabetes: the American college of sports medicine and the American diabetes association: joint position statement', *Diabetes Care*, 33(12), pp.2692–2696

Crone, D. (2007) 'Walking back to health: a qualitative investigation into service users' experiences of a walking project', *Issues in Mental Health Nursing*, 28(2), pp.167–184

Daneshmandi, H., Choobineh, A., Ghaem, H., and Karimi, M. (2017) 'Adverse effects of prolonged sitting behaviour on the general health of office workers', *Journal of Lifestyle Medicine*, 7(2), pp. 69–75

Dempsey, P.C., Larsen, R.N., Dunstan, D.W., Owen, N., and Kingwell, B.A. (2018) 'Sitting less and moving more', *Hypertension*, 72(5), pp.1037–1046

Department for Transport (2018) Analyses from the national travel survey 2016. Available at: https://assets.publishing.service.gov.uk/government/uploads/system/uploads/attachment_data/file/674568/analysis-from-the-national-travel-survey.pdf (Accessed 6th June 2020)

Department of Health (2017) *Health survey Northern Ireland trend tables*. Belfast: Department of Health

Department of Health and Social Care (2019a) UK chief medical officers' physical activity guidelines. Department of Health and Social Care/Welsh Government/Department of Health/Scottish Government. Available at: https://assets.publishing.service.gov.uk/government/uploads/system/uploads/attachment_data/file/832868/uk-chief-medical-officers-physical-activity-guidelines.pdf (Accessed 5th June 2020)

Department of Health and Social Care (2019b) *Physical activity guidelines: infographics*. Available at: www.gov.uk/government/publications/physical-activity-guidelines-infographics (Accessed 5th June 2020)

Ding, D., Lawson, K.D., Kolbe-Alexander, T.L., Finkelstein, E.A., Katzmarzyk, P.T., van Mechelen, W., and Pratt, M. (2016) 'The economic burden of physical inactivity: a global analysis of major non-communicable diseases', *The Lancet*, 388(10051), pp.1311–1324

Ekelund, U., Griffin, S.J., and Wareham, N.J. (2007) 'Physical activity and metabolic risk in individuals with a family history of type 2 diabetes', *Diabetes Care*, 30(2), pp.337–342

Ekelund, U., Steene-Johannessen, J., Brown, W.J., Wang Fagerland, M.W., Owen, N., Powell, K.E., Bauman, A., and Lee, I.M. (2016) 'Does physical activity attenuate, or even eliminate, the detrimental association of sitting time with mortality? A harmonised meta-analysis of data from more than 1 million men and women', *The Lancet*, 388(10051), pp.1302–1310

Evans, A, Kelly, A., and Slocombe, M. (2019) National travel survey: England 2018. Department for Transport. Available at: https://assets.publishing.service.gov.uk/government/uploads/system/uploads/attachment_data/file/823068/national-travel-survey-2018.pdf (Accessed 5th June 2020)

Faulkner, G., and Sparkes, A. (1999) 'Exercise as a therapy for schizophrenia: an ethnographic study', *Journal of Sport and Exercise Psychology*, 21(1), pp. 52–69

Fogarty, M., and Happell, B. (2005) 'Exploring the benefits of an exercise program for people with schizophrenia: a qualitative study', *Issues in Mental Health Nursing*, 26(3), pp.341–351

Giangregorio, L.M., Papaioannou, A., Macintyre, N.J., Ashe, M.C., Heinonen, A., Shipp, K., Wark, J., McGill, S., Keller, H., Jain, R., Laprade, J., and Cheung, A.M. (2014) 'Too fit to fracture: exercise recommendations for individuals with osteoporosis or osteoporotic vertebral fracture', *Osteoporosis International*, 25(3), pp.821–835

Guel, C., Shefer, G., Griffin, S., and Ogilvie, D. (2016) ' "Keeping your body and mind active": an ethnographic study of aspirations for healthy ageing', *BMJ Open*, 6(1) doi:10.1136/bmjopen-2015–009973

Guthold, R., Stevens, G.A., Riley, L.M., and Bull, F.C. (2018) 'Worldwide trends in insufficient physical activity from 2001 to 2016: a pooled analysis of 358 population-based surveys with 1.9 million participants', *The Lancet*, 6(10) doi.org/10.1016/S2214-109X(18)30357-7

Hamer, M., Stamatakis, E., and Mishra, G.D. (2010) 'Television- and screen-based activity and mental well-being in adults', *American Journal of Preventive Medicine*, 38(4), pp.375–380

Hamilton, M.T., Hamilton, D.G., and Zderic, T.W. (2007) 'Role of low energy expenditure and sitting in obesity, metabolic syndrome, type 2 diabetes, and cardiovascular disease', *Perspectives in Diabetes*, 56(11), pp.2655–2667

Hardman, A.E., and Stensel, D.J. (2009) *Physical activity and health. The evidence explained*. 2nd edn. London: Routledge

Healy, G.N., Wijndaele, K., Dunstan, D.W., Shaw, J.E., Salmon, J., Zimmet, P.Z., and Owen, N. (2008) 'Objectively measured sedentary time, physical activity, and metabolic risk: the Australian diabetes, obesity and lifestyle study (AusDiab)', *Diabetes Care*, 31(2), pp.369–371

Healy, G.N., Matthews, C.E., Dunstan, D.W., Winkler, E.A.H., and Owen, N. (2011) 'Sedentary time and cardio-metabolic biomarkers in US adults: NHANES 2003–06', *European Heart Journal*, 32(5), pp.590–597

Hilton, C., Trigg, R., and Minniti, A. (2015) 'Improving the psychological evaluation of exercise referral: psychometric properties of the exercise referral quality of life scale', *Health Psychology Open*, 2(2) doi:10.1177/2055102915590317

Hingorani, A.D., Finan, C., and Schmidt, A.F. (2020) 'Obesity causes cardiovascular diseases: adding to the weight of evidence', *European Heart Journal*, 41(2), pp.227–230

Howe, T.E., Shea, B., Dawson, L.J., Downie, F., Murray, A., Ross, C., Harbour, R,T., Caldwell, L.M., and Creed, G. (2011) 'Exercise for preventing and treating osteoporosis in postmenopausal women', *Cochrane Database of Systematic Reviews*, Issue 7 doi:10.1002/14651858.CD000333.pub2

International Osteoporosis Foundation (2018) *Broken bones, broken lives: a roadmap to solve fragility fracture crisis in Europe*. Nyon: International Osteoporosis Foundation

Islami, F., Sauer, A.G., Miller, K.D., Siegel, R.L., Fedewa, S.A., Jacobs, E.J., McCullough, M.L., Patel, A.V., Ma, J., Soerjomafaram, I., Flanders, W.D., Brawley, O.W., Gapstur, S.M., and Jemal, A. (2018). 'Proportion and number of cancer cases and deaths attributable to potentially modifiable risk factors in the United States', *CA: A Cancer Journal for Clinicians*, 68(1), pp.31–54

Joo, J., Williamson, S.A., Vazquez, A.I., Fernandez, J.R., and Bray, M.S. (2019) 'The influence of 15-week exercise training on dietary patterns among young adults', *International Journal of Obesity*, 43(9), pp.1681–1690

Kannel, W.B., and Sorlie, P. (1979) 'Some health benefits of physical activity. The Framingham study', *Archives of Internal Medicine*, 139(8), pp.857–861

Katzmarzyk, P.T. (2014) 'Standing and mortality in a prospective cohort of Canadian adults', *Medicine and Science in Sport and Exercise Science*, 46(5), pp.940–946

Katzmarzyk, P.T., and Mason, C. (2009) 'The physical activity transition', *Journal of Physical Activity and Health*, 6(3), pp.269–280

Kohl, H.W., Craig, C.L., Lambert, E.V., Inoue, S., Alkandari, J.R., Leetongin, G., and Kahlmeier, S (2012) 'The pandemic of physical inactivity: global action for public health', *The Lancet*, 380(9838), pp.294–305

Knuth, A.G., and Hallal, P.C. (2009) 'Temporal trends in physical activity: a systematic review', *Journal of Physical Activity and Health*, 6(5) doi.org/10.1123/jpah.6.5.548

Kwon, Y., Kim, J.., Heo, J., Jeon, H., Choi, E., and Eom, G. (2018) 'The effect of sitting posture on the loads at cervico-thoracic and lumbosacral joints', *Technology and Health Care*, 26(1), pp.409–418

Lahart, I.M., Metsios, G.S., Nevill, A.M., and Carmichael, A.R. (2015) 'Physical activity, risk of death and recurrence in breast cancer survivors: a systematic review and meta-analysis of epidemiological studies', *Acta Oncologica*, 54(5), pp.635–654

Lee, I.M., Paffenbarger, R.S., and Hsieh, C.C. (1991) 'Physical activity and the risk of developing colorectal cancer among college alumni', *Journal of the National Cancer Institute*, 83(18), pp.1324–1329

Lee, I., Shiroma, E.J., Lobelo, F., Puska, P., Blair, S.N., Katzmarzyk, P.T., and Lancet physical activity series working group (2012) 'Effect of physical inactivity on major non-communicable diseases worldwide: an analysis of burden of disease and life expectancy', *The Lancet*, 380(9838), pp.219–229

Leskinen, T., Sipilä, S., Alen, M., Cheng, K.H., Pietilainen, K.H., Usenius, J.-P., Suominen, H., Kovanen, V. Kainulainen, H., Kaprio, J., and Kujala, U.M. (2009) 'Leisure-time physical activity and high-risk fat: a longitudinal population-based twin study', *International Journal of Obesity*, 33(11), pp.1211–1218

Li, T., Wei, S., Shi, Y., Pang, S., Qin, Q., Yin, J., Deng, Y., Chen, Q., Wei, S., Nei, S., and Liu, L. (2015) 'The dose-response effect of physical activity on cancer mortality: findings from 71 prospective cohort studies', *British Journal of Sports Medicine*, 50(6), pp.372–378

Liu, L., Shi, Y., Li, T., Qin, Q., Yin, J., Pang, S., Nie, S., and Wei, S. (2015) 'Leisure time physical activity and cancer risk: evaluation of the WHO's recommendation based on 126 high-quality epidemiological studies', *British Journal of Sports Medicine*, 50(6), pp.372–378

McIntyre, E., Lauche, R., Frawley, J., Sibbritt, D., Reddy, P., and Adams, J. (2019) 'Physical activity and depression symptoms in women with chronic illness and the mediating role of health-related quality of life', *Journal of Affective Disorders*, 252 June, pp.294–299

McLean, J., and Dean, L. (2020) *The Scottish Health Survey. 2018 edition, amended February 2020, volume 1*. Edinburgh: The Scottish Government

Morris, J.N., Heady, J.A., Raffle, P.A., Roberts, C.G., and Parks, J.W. (1953) 'Coronary heart disease and physical activity of work', *Lancet*, 265(6795), pp.1053–1057

Nam, J.Y., Kim, Y., Cho, K.H., Choi, Y., Choi, J., Shin, J., and Park, E. (2016) 'Associations of sitting time and occupation with metabolic syndrome in South Korean adults: a cross sectional study', *BMC Public Health*, 16(1) doi:10.1186/s12889-016-3617-5

NHS Digital (2019) Health survey for England 2018. Adult's health-related behaviours. Available at: https://files.digital.nhs.uk/B5/771AC5/HSE18-Adult-Health-Related-Behaviours-rep-v3.pdf (Accessed 4th June 2020)
Paffenbarger, R.S., Wing, A.L., and Hyde, R.T. (1978) 'Physical activity as an index of heart attack risk in college alumni', *American Journal of Epidemiology*, 108(3), pp.161–175
Paffenbarger, R., Hyde, R., Wing, A.L., and Hsieh, C. (1986) 'Physical activity, all-cause mortality, and longevity of college alumni', *The New England Journal of Medicine*, 314(10), pp.605–613
Pasco, J.A., Jacka, F.N., Williams, L.J., Brennan, S.L., Leslie, E., and Berk, M. (2011) 'Don't worry, be active: positive affect and habitual physical activity', *Australian and New Zealand Journal of Psychiatry*, 45(12), pp.1047–1052
Public Health England (2018) Physical activity data tool: statistical commentary, April 2018. Available at: www.gov.uk/government/publications/physical-activity-data-tool-april-2018-update/physical-activity-data-tool-statistical-commentary-april-2018 (Accessed 7th March 2020).
Raguso, C.A., Kyle, U., Kossovsky, M.P., Roynette, C., Paoloni-Giacobino, A., Didier, H., Genton, L., and Pichard, C. (2006) 'A 3-year longitudinal study on body composition changes in the elderly: role of physical exercise', *Clinical Nutrition*, 25(4), pp.573–580
Rawlings, G.H., Williams, R., Clarke, D.J., Perry, M., Fitzsimons, C., Mead, G., Birch, K.M., Carter, G., English, C., Farrin, A., Holloway, I., Lawton, R., Patel, A., and Forster, A. (2019) 'Exploring adults' experiences of sedentary behaviour and participation in non-workplace interventions designed to reduce sedentary behaviour: a thematic synthesis of qualitative studies', *BMC Public Health*, 19(1) doi:10.1186/s12889-019-7365-1
Reed, J., and Buck, S. (2009) 'The effect of regular aerobic exercise on positive-activated affect: a meta-analysis', *Psychology of Sport and Exercise*, 10(6), pp.581–594
Royal Society for Public Health (2016) *Introducing "activity equivalent" calorie labelling to tackle obesity*. Available at: www.rsph.org.uk/uploads/assets/uploaded/26deda5b-b3b7-4b15-a11bea931dabf041.pdf (Accessed 7th June 2020)
Sanchez-Villegas, A., Ara, I., Guillen-Grima, F., Bes-Rastrollo, M., Varo-Cenarruzabeitia, J.J., and Martinez-Gonzalez, M.A. (2008) 'Physical activity, sedentary index and mental disorders in the SUN cohort study', *Medicine and Science in Sports and Exercise*, 40(5), pp.827–834
Scarborough, P., Bhatnagar, P., Wickramasinghe, K.K., Allender, S., Foster, C., and Rayner, M. (2011) 'The economic burden of ill health due to diet, physical inactivity, smoking, alcohol and obesity in the UK: an update to 2006–2007 NHS costs', *Journal of Public Health*, 33(4), pp.527–535
Schmid, D., and Leitzmann, M.F. (2014) 'Association between physical activity and mortality among breast cancer and colorectal survivors: a systematic review and meta-analysis', *Annals of Oncology*, 25(7), pp.1293–1311
Schmid, D., Steindorf, K., and Leitzmann, M.F. (2014) 'Epidemiologic studies of physical activity and primary prevention of cancer', *Deutsch Zeitschrift Fur Sportmedizin*, 65, pp.5–10
Scholes, S. (2017) Health survey for England 2016. Physical activity in adults. Health and Social Care Information Centre. Available at: http://healthsurvey.hscic.gov.uk/media/63730/HSE16-Adult-phy-act.pdf (Accessed 4th June 2020)
Sharon-David, H., and Tenebaum, G. (2017) 'The effectiveness of exercise interventions on coping with stress: research synthesis', *Studies in Sport Humanities*, 22, pp.19–29
Sisson, S.B., Camhi, S.M., Church, T.S., Tudor-Locke, C., Johnson, W.D. and Katzmarzyk, P.T. (2010) 'Accelerometer-determined steps/day and metabolic syndrome', *American Journal of Preventive Medicine*, 38(6), pp.575–582
Slattery, M.L., Edwards, S.L., Ma, K.N., Friedman, G.D., and Potter, J.D. (1997) 'Physical activity and colon cancer: a public health perspective', *Annals of Epidemiology*,7(2), pp.137–145

Sport England (2019) Active lives. Adult survey. May 18/19 report. Available at: https://bit.ly/37ClRWW (Accessed 4th June 2020)

Stevinson, C., Campbell, A., Cavill, N., and Foster, J. (2017). Physical activity and cancer: a concise evidence review. Macmillan Cancer Support. Available at: www.macmillan.org.uk/_images/the-importance-physical-activity-for-people-living-with-and-beyond-cancer_tcm9-290123.pdf (Accessed 6th June 2020)

Strain, T., Milton, K., Dall, P., Standage, M., and Mutrie, N. (2019) 'How are we measuring physical activity and sedentary behaviour in the four home nations of the UK? A narrative review of current surveillance measures and future directions', *British Journal of Sports Medicine*, 19 doi:10.1136/bjsports-2018–100355

Tamura, K., Takao, M., Hamada, H., Sakai, T., and Sugano, N. (2019) 'Does muscle atrophy correlate with muscle weakness in unilateral hip disease?' *Orthopaedic Proceedings*, 101-B(4). Available at: https://online.boneandjoint.org.uk/doi/abs/10.1302/1358-992X.2019.4.130#:~:text=Most%20of%20patients%20with%20unilateral,the%20patient%20with%20hip%20disorders (Accessed 24th June 2020)

Tatjana, K., and Muensterer, O. (2019) 'Sedentary behaviour, exercise, and cancer development', *International Journal of Surgery Oncology*, 4(6) doi:10.1097/IJ9.0000000000000078

Teychenne, M., Costigan, S.A., and Parker, K. (2015) 'The association between sedentary behaviour and risk of anxiety: a systematic review', *BMC Public Health*, 15(513) doi:10.1186/s12889-015-1843-x

Thorp, A.A., Owen, N., Neuhaus, M., and Dunstan, D.W. (2011) 'Sedentary behaviors and subsequent health outcomes in adults: a systematic review of longitudinal studies, 1996–2011', *American Journal of Preventive Medicine*, 41(2), pp.207–215

Tremblay, M.S., Aubert, S., Barnes, J.D., Saunders, T.J., Carson, V., Latimer-Cheung, A.E., Chastin, S.F.M., Altenburg, T.M., Chinapaw, M.J.M., and SBRN terminology consensus project participants (2017) 'Sedentary Behavior Research Network (SRBN) – terminology consensus project process and outcome', *International Journal of Behavioral Nutrition and Physical Activity*, 14(1) doi:10.1186/s12966-017-0525-8

Tyson, P., Wilson, K., Crone, D., Brailsford, R., and Laws, K. (2010) 'Physical activity and mental health in a student population', *Journal of Mental Health*, 19(6), pp.492–499

Welsh Government (2019) Statistical bulletin. National Survey for Wales 2018–19: adult lifestyle. Available at: https://gov.wales/sites/default/files/statistics-and-research/2019-06/national-survey-for-wales-april-2018-to-march-2019-adult-lifestyle-534.pdf (Accessed 4th June 2020)

World Cancer Research Fund/American Institute for Cancer Research (2018) *Body fatness and weight gain and the risk of cancer*. London: World Cancer Research Fund International

World Health Organization (2018) *Global action plan on physical activity 2018–2030. More active people for a healthier world*. Geneva: World Health Organization

World Health Organization (2020) *WHO guidelines on physical activity and sedentary behaviour*. Geneva: World Health Organization

8 Diet and health

Sally Robinson

Key points

- Introduction
- Public health nutrition
- Energy
- Macronutrients and health
- Micronutrients and health
- Food and health
- Preventing diet-related disease and promoting good health
- Food-based guidelines for healthy eating
- Healthy eating in context
- Summary

Introduction

This chapter will examine how public health nutrition can help to prevent non-communicable diseases and support good health. It will describe the roles of macro and micronutrients as well as food groups. It shows how nutritionists bring together a wide range of evidence to protect and promote good health.

Public health nutrition

Public health nutrition is concerned with the promotion of good health through nutrition and the primary prevention of nutrition-related illness. It is a multi-disciplinary subject drawing on research from nutritional science and social science. It comprises understanding the nutritional content of foods and drinks; analysing people's diets; understanding research into the health effects of different foods and nutrients; understanding people's eating patterns and eating choices; and making realistic recommendations.

Nutritional content of foods and drinks

Dr Elsie Widdowson was one of the first women to graduate from Imperial College London. As a chemist, she worked on understanding the nutritional content of fruits, vegetables and nuts (Nichols, 2003). In 1933, while studying for her postgraduate

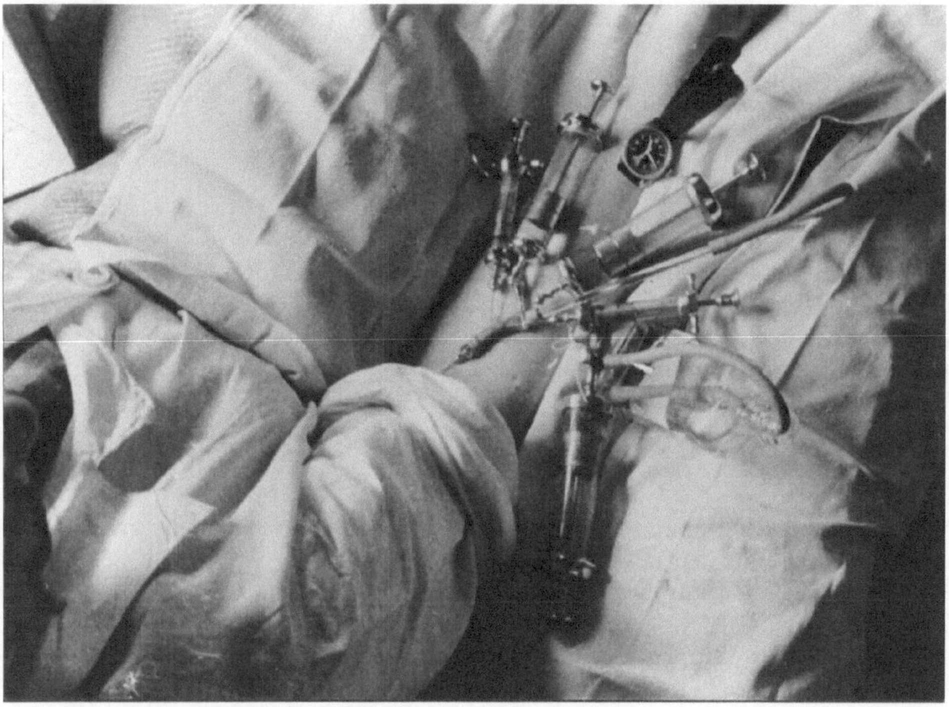

Figure 8.1 Dr Elsie Widdowson injecting herself with solutions of iron, calcium and magnesium
Source: Wellcome Collection made available under Creative Commons Attribution 4.0 International licence https://creativecommons.org/licences/by/4.0/

diploma in dietetics at King College London, she met Dr Robert McCance, a medical doctor, physiologist and biochemist, in the kitchens at St Bartholomew's Hospital. Over decades, they pioneered the science of nutrition, often experimenting on themselves. They produced the first comprehensive compendium of the chemical/nutritional composition of foods in 1940. It continues to be updated by the Royal Society of Chemistry and, in their honour, it is now called McCance and Widdowson's Composition of Foods (PHE/FSA, 2015). It is available as a detailed on-line data set (PHE, 2015). The British Nutrition Foundation (2019a) has developed a simple user-friendly version.

The UK's diet: what we are eating

The National Diet and Nutrition Survey collects information about the dietary habits and nutritional status of the UK population. We can compare what the UK is eating measured against recommendations for healthy eating (Bates *et al.*, 2014, 2016; Roberts *et al.*, 2018). People are eating

- too much free sugar
- too much saturated fat
- too much salt

- some men are eating too much red and processed meat
- too little dietary fibre
- too little oily fish
- too little fruit and vegetables
- too little vitamin D, calcium, folate and iron
- about the right amount of total fat

Dietary Reference Values (DRVs): what we should be eating

UK Dietary Reference Values (DRVs) are recommendations for a healthy diet based on the best evidence to date. They are goals for populations, not for individuals nor for those who require a special diet due to poor health. Table 8.1 shows examples, such as half our daily calories should come from carbohydrates and no more than a third should come from fat.

Energy

We need energy for all bodily functions and activities. How much energy a person needs from their food depends on their age, weight, sex and levels of physical activity. Energy is stored and transported in a molecule called adenosine triphosphate (ATP). Glycogen contains many of these molecules along with glucose. Glucose also stores chemical energy. We store glycogen in body cells, especially in the liver and muscles. When these stores are full, excess glucose is stored as fat in the body's adipose tissue. When we need immediate energy, glycogen is broken down to release glucose which is metabolised (chemically changed) to release energy. When glycogen stores are depleted, we break down and metabolise the body's fat and protein to release energy.

We measure energy in kilocalories (kcals). In everyday language, we often shorten kilocalories to the word 'calories'. The number of 'calories' in our food and drink depends on how many grams of carbohydrate, protein, fat and alcohol are present.

1 gram of carbohydrates provides 3.75 kcals of energy
1 gram of protein provides 4 kcals of energy
1 gram of fat provides 9 kcals of energy
1 gram of alcohol provides 7 kcals of energy

Table 8.1 Examples of UK Dietary Reference Values

Percentage of energy (kcals), based on population average	
Total fat	Not more than 35% (33% if alcohol in the diet)
of which saturated fat	Not more than 11% (10% if alcohol in the diet)
Trans fat	Not more than 2%
Total carbohydrate	50% (47% if alcohol in the diet)
of which free sugars	Not more than 5%
Dietary fibre	30 grams for adults
Salt	Not more than 6 grams for adults

Source: PHE (2016).

People of different ages, sexes and activity levels require a different number of 'calories' per day. An average man needs about 2,500 'calories', and an average woman needs about 2,000 (PHE, 2016).

Macronutrients and health

Macronutrients comprise protein, carbohydrates and fats.

Protein

As protein is the building material for the whole body, it is essential for growth and repair. In the UK, most people obtain plenty of protein from meat, milk, milk products such as cheese and yoghurt, and cereals such as wheat, rice and cereal products (Bates *et al.*, 2014). Proteins are made up of amino acids. When we eat protein, it is digested/broken down into amino acids which are absorbed into the blood stream. These amino acids can re-form to make the type of protein, such as skin or hair, the body needs. The diet needs to contain a good range of amino acids to do this.

Complementation

Complete proteins are found in foods and drinks from animal sources, such as meat, fish, eggs and milk. They contain all the essential amino acids that the body needs. Incomplete proteins are those from vegetable sources, such as beans, cereals and nuts, and they frequently do not contain all the amino acids that the body needs. For example, lentils do not contain the amino acid methionine. For those who do not eat animal proteins, it is important to eat a good variety of vegetable-based protein at the same meal, to increase the likelihood that the absent amino acids in one food are present in another.

Those who don't eat animal proteins need to complement vegetable proteins.

Carbohydrates

Carbohydrates provide the body with its preferred source of energy in the form of glucose. In the UK, it is recommended that half of the calories eaten should come from carbohydrates. This allows half for the other essential nutrients. Both less than this and more than 55% have been associated with greater risk of early death (Seidelmann *et al.*, 2018). In the UK, people obtain most of their carbohydrates from starchy foods such as cereals and cereal products, vegetables and potatoes, and sugary foods such as drinks, fruit, table sugar and confectionary (Bates *et al.*, 2014). Carbohydrates include sugars, starches and dietary fibre.

Sugars

All sugars and starches are digested and absorbed as single sugar molecules: glucose, galactose and fructose. These are absorbed into the blood stream at different rates, measured as their glycaemic index, on their journey to be stored as glycogen or fat, and used for energy. We find natural sugars in the cells of fruits, vegetables, dairy products and some grains, and in general these do not present health concerns.

Free sugar comprises

- all types of table sugar (brown, white, caster, cane and icing), which we add to drinks, recipes and foods for sweetness
- honey and syrups
- all types of sugar added to products by the food industry, in processed foods
- sugar that is mechanically crushed out through the cell walls of fruits and vegetables, for example unsweetened fruit juices and smoothies

Free sugar is a health concern because

- the UK population is consuming far too much
- it has no nutrients, only calories
- it is strongly associated with tooth decay
- it is contributing to the UK obesity epidemic
- regular consumption of sugary drinks is associated with type 2 diabetes

(SACN, 2015)

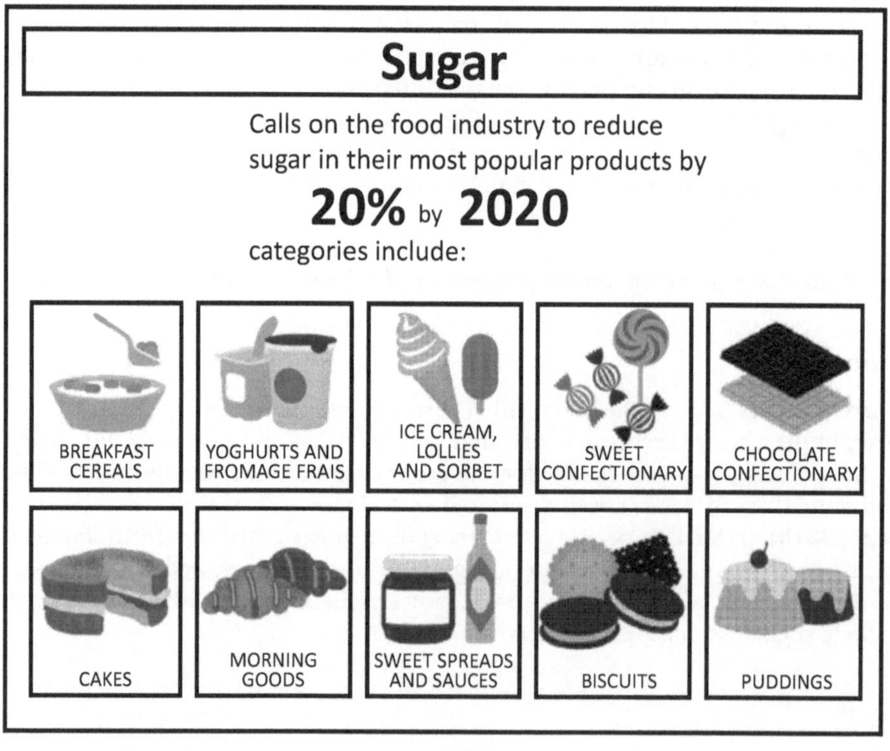

Figure 8.2 Public Health England calls on the food industry to reduce sugar
Source: PHE, 2018 p.1. Reproduced under the terms of the Open Government Licence v3

In 2018, the UK Government introduced a tax on soft drinks and Public Health England is working with the food industry to reduce sugar in products by 20% by 2020.

Starches

Starchy foods include flour, bread, pasta, rice, potatoes and pulses. When consumed, some starch is digested and breaks down into individual sugar molecules that are absorbed into the blood stream; resistant starch is not digested and is classified as a type of dietary fibre.

Dietary fibre

There is no universal definition of dietary fibre. Generally, it comprises the non-digestible carbohydrates, which means they are neither digested nor absorbed into the blood from the small intestine. They remain unchanged until they reach the large intestine. Foods that are high in dietary fibre include wheat, rice, maize, fruit, vegetables, oats, barley and rye. Wholegrains are natural seeds containing dietary fibre, germ and associated nutrients. Refined grains, such as white flour or white rice, have had the fibre removed. Research shows,

- diets high in dietary fibre, particularly cereal fibre and wholegrains, are associated with less
  - cardiovascular disease, specific heart-related events and stroke
  - type 2 diabetes
  - constipation
  - bowel cancer
- diets high in dietary fibre from fruit, vegetables and pulses are associated with less constipation
- vegetable dietary fibre is associated with fewer heart-related events, but not fruit dietary fibre
- the fibre in oats helps to lower harmful low-density lipoprotein (LDL) blood cholesterol and reduces blood pressure

(SACN, 2015)

Reynolds and colleagues (2019) reviewed many studies comparing the health of people who ate high-fibre and low-fibre diets. When people ate a high-fibre diet, containing 25 to 29 grams per day, they were less likely to die early from cardiovascular disease, type 2 diabetes or bowel cancer. Higher intakes could give even greater protection.

> *For a healthier population, the UK needs to eat less free sugar and more dietary fibre and wholegrains.*

Fats

The fat in butter, spreads, oil and lard is called 'visible' fat. We might be less aware of the 'invisible' fat within food such as cakes and pastry. Fat contributes to flavour and contains the fat-soluble vitamins A, D, E and K. It is calorie dense, and therefore very 'fattening'. In the UK, people obtain most of their fat from meat, cereals, cereal products, which include biscuits and pastries, milk and milk products (Bates *et al.*, 2014). The body can break down the fats we eat into fatty acids and glycerol and, like protein, it can remake the types of fat that the body needs.

Box 8.1 Cholesterol

Blood cholesterol

Once inside the body, all types of fat are called lipids. Lipids include very small fat molecules called triglycerides and cholesterol.

- Cholesterol is an essential component of every cell membrane. We need it for synthesising bile acids, some hormones and vitamin D
- Cholesterol is mostly made in the liver and carried in the blood (blood cholesterol) by proteins, at which point we call them lipoproteins
- Low-density lipoproteins (LDL) deliver cholesterol to tissues
- High-density lipoproteins (HDL) transfer cholesterol to the liver
- Both LDL and HDL contribute to measures of total blood cholesterol, and high total cholesterol is strongly associated with cardiovascular disease
- LDLs become part of the plaque that clogs up arteries
- HDLs are seen as 'protective' because we know that, in populations, low average levels of HDL in the blood are associated with greater cardiovascular disease
- LDLs can be increased or decreased by the diet
- HDLs can potentially be enhanced by physical activity, but research is unclear
- The 'total blood cholesterol to HDL cholesterol ratio' is often used to assess the risk of cardiovascular disease
- Blood 'cholesterol-raising' foods include those that are high in saturated fats such as processed meats
- Blood 'cholesterol-lowering' foods include fruit, vegetables and oats

Dietary cholesterol

We eat cholesterol in the diet.

- Foods which have a high cholesterol content are those of animal origin
- If we eat a lot or a little dietary cholesterol, the liver will compensate and make less or more accordingly
- Eating dietary cholesterol has very little effect on people's blood cholesterol unless they have certain health conditions
- The general population do not need to restrict foods containing dietary cholesterol

Types of fat in the diet include saturated, unsaturated, trans and essential.

Saturated fats

Saturated fats are usually solid at room temperature, such as butter and lard. Most saturated fats in the British diet come from meat, cereals/cereal products, milk and milk products (Bates *et al.*, 2014). They raise harmful LDL blood cholesterol which contributes to atherosclerosis and cardiovascular disease. Reducing saturated fats reduces cardiovascular disease and coronary heart disease events, and they improve the 'total cholesterol: HDL cholesterol ratio' (SACN, 2019).

> *Saturated fat, not dietary cholesterol, is strongly associated with raising blood cholesterol.*

Palm oil and coconut oils contain high quantities of saturated fat. The demand for palm oil by the food industry has led to mass de-forestation which is associated with global warming.

Unsaturated fats

Unsaturated fats are usually liquid at room temperature. Monounsaturated and polyunsaturated fats are found in vegetable oils, fish and fish oils, and some fat spreads, nuts, seeds and avocados. Reducing saturated fats and replacing them with monounsaturated and/or polyunsaturated fats lowers harmful LDL cholesterol, but polyunsaturated fats are better for controlling blood sugar as well (SACN, 2019).

> *People in the UK are eating about the right amount of total fat but too much saturated fat which needs to be replaced with unsaturated fats.*

Trans fats

Most trans fats are formed when the food industry adds hydrogen to an oil to make it a hard spread like margarine. In turning the liquid unsaturated fats into solid saturated fats, some fats are malformed into trans fats. Trans fats raise LDL cholesterol. They are also associated with a wide range of health concerns beyond cardiovascular disease, such as breast cancer, pregnancy-related risks, disorders of the nervous system and diabetes (Dhaka *et al.*, 2011). No more than 2% of calories should come from trans fats and, largely due to changes in food processing, the average UK diet contains much less than this (Roberts *et al.*, 2018).

Essential fats

Essential fats are those which the body cannot make from other fats. We must have these in the diet to be healthy. Omega 6 fats are unsaturated, eaten widely, and found in seeds, most vegetable oils, poultry, eggs and nuts. Omega 3 fats are unsaturated and found in oily fish.

Both omega 6 and omega 3 fats compete for the same enzymes to make them work, and so too much omega 6 prevents the benefits of omega 3. The UK diet is high in

Table 8.2 Types of fats

	Percentage saturated fat	*Percentage monounsaturated fat*	*Percentage polyunsaturated fat*
Almond oil	9	73	18
Sunflower oil	11	20	69
Corn oil	13	29	57
Olive oil (refined)	14	75	11
Olive oil (extra virgin)	14	75	11
Olive oil (light)	15	42	44
Sesame oil (light)	15	42	44
Margarine (soft)	20	47	33
Goose fat	35	52	13
Lard	41	47	12
Ghee	65	25	5
Butter	68	28	4
Margarine (hard)	80	14	6

omega 6 and low in omega 3, and this imbalance is associated with cardiovascular disease, cancer, inflammatory and autoimmune diseases and impacts on brain development (Simopoulos, 2010; Zivkovic *et al.*, 2011). The diet can be rebalanced by eating more oily fish such as mackerel, kippers, salmon, sardines and trout.

Heated fats

Heating fats to high temperatures, and re-heating them, encourages the development of unhealthy trans fats and saturated fats, as well as volatile aldehydes which are toxic (Harinageswara *et al.*, 2010; Bhardwaj *et al.*, 2016). Saturated animal fats such as goose fat, lard and butter are more chemically stable, and recommended for deep fat, extensive frying and baking.

People in the UK need to eat more oily fish.

Micronutrients and health

Micronutrients comprise vitamins and minerals. These are essential in small quantities to maintain health. Vitamins are either water-soluble or fat-soluble. We need to eat the water-soluble vitamins B and C daily, as they cannot be stored in the body. Fat-soluble vitamins A, D, E and K can be stored in the body and therefore eating excess quantities can be toxic. Minerals include calcium, magnesium, iron, sodium, chloride, zinc, copper, selenium, manganese, chromium and iodine.

Rickets, osteomalacia and osteoporosis

Vitamin D and calcium work together to make and maintain strong bones. Osteomalacia and rickets are conditions characterised by having soft, weak bones that bend and break. Both are caused by deficiencies in calcium and/or vitamin D. Deficiency of vitamin D in pregnant mothers is associated with deficiency in their infants, who have a high risk of developing rickets (Dawodu and Wagner, 2007).

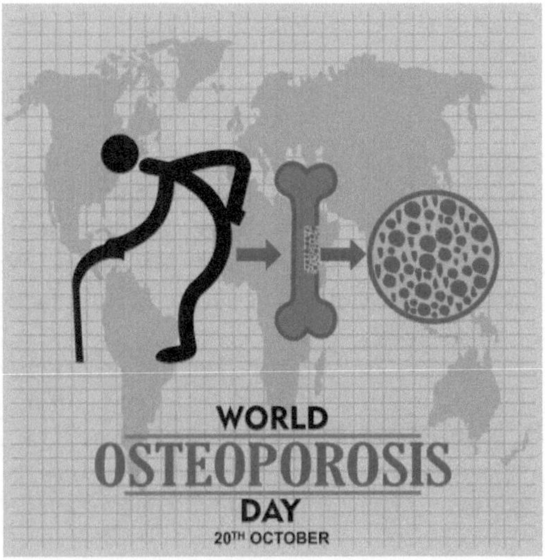

Figure 8.3 World Osteoporosis Day 20th October
Source: Haryadi CH/Shutterstock.com

Osteoporosis means having soft/brittle/porous bones because hormonal changes cause bones to lose their calcium. It is important for females to maximise their bone density before their mid-twenties to prevent osteoporosis at menopause, when oestrogen falls. Osteoporosis affects 200 million women worldwide, 21.8% of over-fifties in the UK, and it is the commonest cause of fragility fractures (International Osteoporosis Foundation, 2018).

In the UK, many people across all age groups are eating too little vitamin D (Roberts *et al.*, 2018). The daily recommendation (DRV) for everyone over a year old is 10 micrograms (μg) (SACN, 2016). Supplements are recommended from October to March, and all year for those with darker skins, pregnant women, breastfeeding mothers, older people and anyone whose skin has little exposure to sun due to covering up with clothes or sunscreen.

Folate, megaloblastic anaemia and neural tube defects

Folate is one of the many B vitamins, B9. Being deficient in folate, or vitamin B12, can cause megaloblastic anaemia. Abnormally large and immature blood cells are unable to carry oxygen around the body efficiently, so people feel very tired and may have a sore tongue, mouth ulcers, weak muscles, disturbed vision and psychological difficulties. Folate deficiency during pregnancy is associated with the development of neural-tube defects, such as spina bifida, in unborn babies.

In the UK, about three-quarters of teenage and adult women of childbearing age do not eat enough folate (Roberts *et al.*, 2018). Women are advised to take 400 micrograms of folic acid, the synthetic version of folate, daily for three months prior to pregnancy and for three months after pregnancy is confirmed (PHE, 2018b). Some countries have fortified their flour with folic acid. About half of all UK pregnancies are unplanned, and the Scientific Advisory Committee on Nutrition (2017) has recommended flour fortification for the UK.

Iron-deficiency anaemia

Iron-deficiency anaemia is the most common anaemia in the world, affecting about a quarter of pregnant women and 14% of non-pregnant women in the UK (NICE, 2018). We need iron to make the red blood cells that carry oxygen around the body. A deficiency leads to a lack of oxygen and symptoms such as shortness of breath, fatigue, heart palpitations and a pale/grey complexion. Iron is lost during menstruation and at times of growth, including pregnancy.

Dietary iron comes from animal sources, haem iron, and from vegetable sources, non-haem iron. The body absorbs haem iron from red meat, offal such as liver and poultry reasonably well. Non-haem iron is less well absorbed, and comes from pulses, fortified breakfast cereals, dark-green leafy vegetables, tofu, nuts, seeds and dried fruit. To increase the absorption of non-haem iron we are advised to

- eat it with a food or drink that contains vitamin C
- eat it with some food containing haem iron
- cook or soak nuts and seeds before eating

Deficiencies in vitamin D, folate and iron are common in the UK.

Dietary supplements

Most people who take vitamin or mineral supplements do not need them if they are eating a reasonably varied diet. The risks are

- they can be a waste of money
- some can be toxic if not taken carefully
- some might interact with medicine
- pregnant women should not take fish liver oil because liver contains large amounts of vitamin A which can harm unborn babies
- vitamin E should be avoided by those with cardiovascular disease
- effervescent vitamin drinks can be very high in salt

(British Dietetic Association, 2016a)

Those who may benefit from supplements include

- vegans, who do not eat any animal products, should consider taking vitamin B12, riboflavin (B2), omega 3, iron, vitamin D and calcium
- women of childbearing age who may become pregnant should take 400 micrograms of folic acid daily, and continue for three months into pregnancy
- pregnant women and those who have an infant under one year might benefit from 'healthy start' vitamins containing folic acid, vitamin C and vitamin D
- people who have health conditions may be recommended to take a supplement by a registered dietician or medical doctor

- vitamin D supplements of 10 micrograms (μg) are recommended for those with darker skins, pregnant women, breastfeeding mothers, older people, and for everyone at times when the skin is not exposed to much sun

Vitamins and mineral supplements are helpful for certain people. More is not better. Some can be toxic if taken in large quantities.

Antioxidants

A healthy body produces free radicals as part of its normal cellular processes. We also absorb excess free radicals from air pollution, ozone, radiation, cigarette smoke, sunlight and certain chemicals. Excess free radicals damage cells and tissues through a process called oxidative stress. Atoms normally contain electrons, negative charges, in pairs to keep them balanced. Free radicals have one or more unpaired electrons, so they snatch electrons from other atoms, which causes damage. Oxidative stress leads to low-grade inflammation which is associated with a range of health conditions. Antioxidants can donate electrons to free radicals and stop the damage. They include

- phytochemicals such as flavonoids and carotenoids. These are within the yellow/red/orange pigments of fruit and vegetables
- vitamin C
- vitamin E
- selenium

There is much ongoing research into antioxidants and disease prevention. Their role seems promising in scientific research studies and observational studies. However, when generally healthy people with no known nutritional deficiencies are asked to take supplements for large population studies such as clinical trials, the evidence shows an unclear mix of benefits, no effect or harm (Hajhashemi *et al.*, 2010; Biswas, 2016).

Antioxidants appear to be health-enhancing, but there is no clear evidence for taking antioxidant supplements to prevent disease.

Salt

Salt is sodium chloride. Sodium is vital to a healthy fluid balance inside the body. If we lose salt through sweating in hot weather or diarrhoea we get a headache and become dehydrated, fatigued and nauseous. This can progress to a medical emergency.

Salt is often high in processed foods. High sodium/salt intakes are strongly associated with

- high blood pressure
- stomach cancer

(WHO, 2012; WCRF/AICR, 2018a)

The World Health Organization (2012) has set a maximum target of 5 grams of salt per day. The UK recommendation is 6 grams per day, about a teaspoon, and the food industry is being strongly encouraged to reduce the salt in processed foods.

Table 8.3 Salt and food labels (per 100g of food)

	High	*Medium*	*Low*
Salt	More than 1.5 grams	0.3 to 0.5 grams	0 to 0.3 grams
Sodium	More than 0.6 grams	0.1 to 0.6 grams	0 to 0.1 grams

Source: Adapted from British Dietetic Association (2020).

Food and health

Processed foods

The food industry makes processed foods and drinks from substances derived from foods and additives. They are durable, convenient, accessible, very palatable, highly profitable and ready to heat, drink or eat. As well as being high in salt, these foods are usually high in energy (calories), free sugars and fat, and low in dietary fibre. They are highly advertised, often as snacks, and are less satiating (filling) than natural foods, making it easy to over-consume. The UK eats the highest amount of ultra-processed foods in Europe, about half of all food purchases, which is directly contributing to the UK obesity epidemic (Moneiro *et al.*, 2018). Consumers need to know:

> ... most manufactured food products have been carefully designed and tested by a team of food engineers and focus groups to ensure they 'optimize palatability to ensure profitability' ..."If you find that optimum point in a set of ingredients ... you may be well on your way to converting that array of chemicals and physical substrates into a successful product," ... one that we buy again and again, one we consume independent of hunger or health. And often, that success can be traced to just three ingredients: sugar, fat, and salt.
>
> (Kimble, 2015 p.22)

Red and processed meat

Red meat is a source of complete protein, iron, zinc and vitamin B12. In the UK, men aged 65 to 75 are eating more than the recommended 70 grams of red and processed meat (Roberts *et al.*, 2018). High consumption of red and processed meat is associated with

- weight gain
- cardiovascular disease, largely because of its saturated fat content and its association with weight gain
- type 2 diabetes, because of weight gain
- bowel cancer

Processed meat such as sausages and bacon is a greater concern than red meat alone because it

- can contain four times as much sodium as unprocessed meat and is more strongly associated with cardiovascular disease
- contains carcinogenic, cancer-causing, chemicals due the processes of curing or smoking. (This can apply to smoked fish also.) It is very strongly associated with bowel cancer.

(Bronzato and Durante, 2017; WCRF/AICR, 2018b)

High-temperature cooking, such as frying, grilling and barbecuing of meat or fish, can produce carcinogenic chemicals, but the evidence for their association with stomach cancer is limited (WCRF/AICR, 2018b). In the UK, men aged 65 to 75 are eating more than the recommended 70 grams of red and processed meat (Roberts *et al.*, 2018).

> *Processed foods are associated with high blood pressure, stomach cancer and obesity.*

Fruit and vegetables

Fruit and vegetables reduce the risks of premature death from all causes, cardiovascular disease and cancers. They reduce blood cholesterol and blood pressure, enhance the health of blood vessels and support the immune system (Steinmetz and Potter, 1991; Macready *et al.*, 2014).

A study by Aune and colleagues (2017) found,

- apples, pears, berries, citrus fruits, cooked vegetables, cruciferous vegetables (e.g. broccoli, cabbage and cauliflower), potatoes, green leafy vegetables and salads were associated with less premature death from all causes
- apples, pears, citrus fruits, cruciferous vegetables, green leafy vegetables, tomatoes and beta-carotene-rich (yellow/orange/red pigments) and vitamin C-rich fruit and vegetables (e.g. citrus fruits, berries, tomatoes, green vegetables) were associated with less cardiovascular disease
- cruciferous vegetables and vitamin C-rich fruit and vegetables were associated with less cancer

When compared to eating none, Aune and colleagues found that the more portions of fruit and vegetables eaten per day, the more we prevent early death.

- Two to three portions per day was associated with a 13% reduced risk of cardiovascular disease, 4% reduced risk of cancer and 15% reduced risk of early death
- Ten portions a day was associated with 28% reduced risk of cardiovascular disease, 13% reduced risk of cancer and 31% reduced risk of early death

The average UK adult eats about four portions of fruit and vegetables a day (Bates *et al.*, 2016; Roberts *et al.*, 2018).

> *Many people in the UK need to eat less processed foods, especially processed meat, and more fruit and vegetables.*

Preventing diet-related disease and promoting good health

We have discussed preventing rickets, osteomalacia, osteoporosis, megaloblastic and iron-deficient anaemia and neural tube defects. Here, we outline how diet helps in the prevention of other major non-communicable diseases, disease prevention in pregnancy and the promotion of mental health and wellbeing.

Low-grade inflammation

When cells of the body are injured, as they are in the very early stages of disease, they set off an inflammation response as part of the body's defences. Sometimes this inflammatory response does not 'switch off', leading to chronic low-grade inflammation. This inflammation is associated with a range of chronic diseases including cardiovascular disease, cancer arthritis and type 2 diabetes (Lobo *et al.*, 2010; Singh *et al.*, 2015). The concept of an 'anti-inflammatory' diet continues to be researched (Minihane *et al.*, 2015). There is some evidence to suggest that it might look like a Mediterranean diet (Casas *et al.*, 2014).

Cardiovascular disease

To help prevent cardiovascular disease eat plenty of

- cereal-based dietary fibre including wholegrains and oats
- polyunsaturated and monounsaturated fats, e.g. olive oil
- omega 3 unsaturated fats, e.g. oily fish/fish oil
- fruit and vegetables

Also, minimise sedentary behaviour and be more physically active.

The following should be minimised

- saturated fats, e.g. red and processed meat, high-fat dairy foods and milk, lard and butter
- trans fats, e.g. processed food and fried 'takeaways'
- salt, e.g. processed food

Replacing saturated fat with unsaturated fat, but not carbohydrate, is important (SACN, 2019).

Type 2 diabetes

The dietary prevention of type 2 diabetes is through decreasing weight and sugary drinks, and increasing dietary fibre, fruit and vegetables.

Weight

Excess weight significantly increases people's chances of developing type 2 diabetes as the extra body fat prevents the body from being able to use insulin and control blood sugar (WHO, 2016).

Sugary drinks

Regularly drinking sugary soft drinks is associated with a greater risk of developing type 2 diabetes (Wang *et al.*, 2015; SACN, 2015; Imamura *et al.*, 2016; Drouin-Chartier *et al.*, 2019). A full understanding of the reasons is still lacking, but the drinks cause a dramatic increase in blood sugar followed by an associated rapid increase in insulin. Avoiding them can also reduce the risk of weight gain.

Dietary fibre

Diets that are high in dietary fibre, particularly cereal fibre and wholegrains, are associated with less type 2 diabetes (SACN, 2015).

Fruit and vegetables

Diets that are high in fruit and vegetables are associated with less type 2 diabetes (Zheng *et al.*, 2020).

Glycaemic index and glycaemic load

Blood sugar is the amount of glucose travelling in the bloodstream. After eating and drinking, the body's blood glucose rises. The pancreas releases insulin, which causes the glucose to leave the blood and travel to the cells. This keeps blood glucose levels within the range needed to keep the blood vessels healthy.

Although the body prefers to use carbohydrates for supplying its blood glucose and energy, it can break down proteins and fats, and chemically change them to become blood glucose when needed. It can also retrieve glucose from the glycogen stores in the liver and muscles if needed. Blood glucose does not come from carbohydrates alone but starches and sugars, the digestible carbohydrates, have the most impact.

Glycaemic index (GI) is a measure of how quickly blood glucose rises after eating a quantity of carbohydrates. Glycaemic load (GL) is a measure of both the glycaemic index and the amount of carbohydrate in a food. Eating foods, or drinks, with both a high GI and GL can promote rapid rises in blood glucose, exaggerating the insulin response, leading to low blood glucose and hunger (Bell and Sears, 2003; Bellisle *et al.*, 2007).

- A diet that has a high glycaemic index and a high glycaemic load is associated with greater risk of type 2 diabetes (SACN, 2015) and endometrial cancer (WCRF/AICR, 2018a)
- As glucose levels are not solely determined by carbohydrate intake, the evidence about the health benefits of a low GI/GL diet is not yet confirmed (SACN, 2015)
- Replacing saturated with polyunsaturated fats helps to sustain and control blood glucose levels (SACN, 2019)
- We need regular carbohydrates, from wholegrains, fruit, vegetables and pulses, to maintain concentration, energy levels and stable blood glucose levels

Table 8.4 Glycaemic index and glycaemic loads of food and drink

	Weight	*Carbohydrate*	*Glycaemic index*	*Glycaemic load*	
Lentils	150 grams	23 grams	38	9	Low
Peanuts	50 grams	6 grams	14	1	Low
Apple juice	240 grams	29 grams	52	12	Medium
Whole-grain bread	30 grams	14 grams	62	9	Medium
Popcorn	20 grams	11 grams	72	8	High
Cornflakes	30 grams	26 grams	92	24	High

Source: Adapted from Bell and Sears (2003 p. 360).

Cancer

To prevent cancer, we are advised to

- avoid being overweight as body fatness increases the risk of many cancers
- eat a diet rich in wholegrains, vegetables, fruit and pulses
- limit the consumption of 'fast foods' and processed foods high in fat, starches or sugars
- limit red meat and eat little, if any, processed meat
- limit sugary drinks because they contribute to weight gain and high glycaemic load is a cause of endometrial cancer
- limit alcohol; it is best to avoid alcohol completely
- avoid taking supplements, focus on a healthy diet
- breastfeed for the first six months as it helps to prevent breast cancer in mothers
- achieve a healthy diet through food and drink rather than supplements

Also, minimise sedentary behaviour and be more physically active.

(WCRF/AICR, 2018a)

Disease prevention in pregnancy

Pregnant women need to take care with

- raw meats, poultry and shellfish which could cause salmonella
- soft ripened cheeses, blue cheeses, pate, soft ice cream, which could cause listeria
- food that is not heated through properly or out of date could cause listeria
- shark marlin, swordfish or high quantities of tinned tuna are linked to contaminants such as mercury
- foods that contain high quantities of retinol (vitamin A), such as liver and fish liver oils, which can harm the unborn baby
- caffeine, which can cause miscarriage and low birth weight

(British Dietetic Association, 2016b)

Cognitive impairment and dementias

The Scientific Advisory Committee on Nutrition (2018) examined evidence pertaining to the prevention of cognitive impairment or dementias, including Alzheimer's disease. The committee recommended a Mediterranean diet.

Mental health and wellbeing

Advice for keeping mentally well includes

- following healthy eating guidelines such as a 'Mediterranean-style diet', not only for optimum physical health, mood and brain function, but because it is the type of diet associated with better sleep
- eating foods containing iron, vitamins B1, B3 or B12, folate or selenium because deficiencies are associated with tiredness, low mood and depression
- keeping blood sugar levels stable, maintain energy levels, concentration, and prevent cravings by eating breakfast and then eating regular wholegrains, fruit, vegetables and beans through the day
- consuming some caffeine can help to counter tiredness and promote being alert; however, too much caffeine can cause headaches, irritability and insomnia. Avoid 'energy' drinks which can be very high in caffeine

(British Dietetic Association, 2017; St-Onge *et al.*, 2016; Mamalaki *et al.*, 2018)

Food-based guidelines for healthy eating

Food-based guidelines are a way of presenting the best nutritional evidence to people in terms of their everyday food and drink.

Mediterranean diet

There is no single 'Mediterranean diet', but generally it includes

- a high intake of fruit, vegetables, nuts, legumes and wholegrains
- moderate intakes of fish/oily fish, poultry, eggs and fermented dairy products such as cheese and yoghurt
- small amounts of red meat, processed meat and sugary foods
- frequent but moderate amounts of wine, especially red wine, with meals

It is

- high in fat (40–50% of daily calories)
- low in saturated fats (about 8%)
- high in monounsaturated fats (15–25%), mostly from olive oil
- high in omega 3 fats and low in omega 6 fats

(Casas *et al.*, 2014)

Eatwell Guide

The Eatwell Guide (PHE, 2018b; 2018c) presents food-based guidelines for the four nations of the UK (Figures 8.5 to 8.12). The Guide is similar to a Mediterranean diet. It sets realistic, not perfect, goals for disease prevention and health promotion.

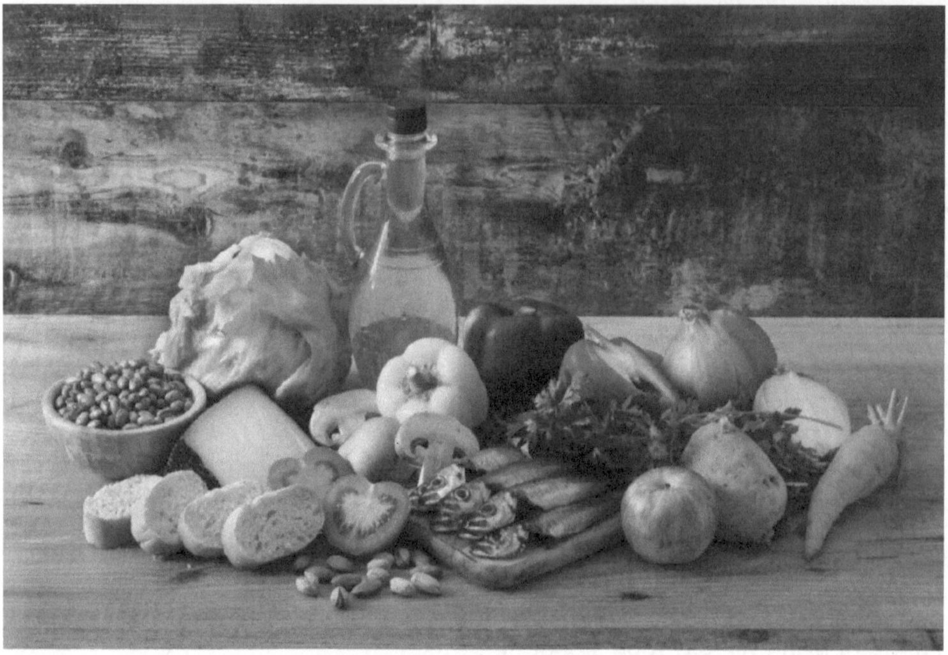

Figure 8.4 A Mediterranean diet
Source: Etorres/Shutterstock.com

Sustainable healthy eating

In 1967, Martin Luther King Jr spoke about all of life being interrelated, how every person is mutually dependent on others:

> And before you finish eating breakfast in the morning, you've depended on more than half the world.
>
> (Martin Luther King, Jr.)

A large international study into diet and future sustainable food systems for health recommended that the world needs to move towards a flexitarian diet, which is a plant-based diet including a little meat. The authors recommended a diet called the planetary health diet, shown in Figure 8.13. It comprises

- mostly vegetables, fruits, wholegrains, legumes (includes alfalfa and pulses), nuts and unsaturated oils
- low to moderate amounts of seafood and poultry
- no or very low red meat, processed meat, free sugar, refined grains and starchy vegetables

(Willett *et al.*, 2019)

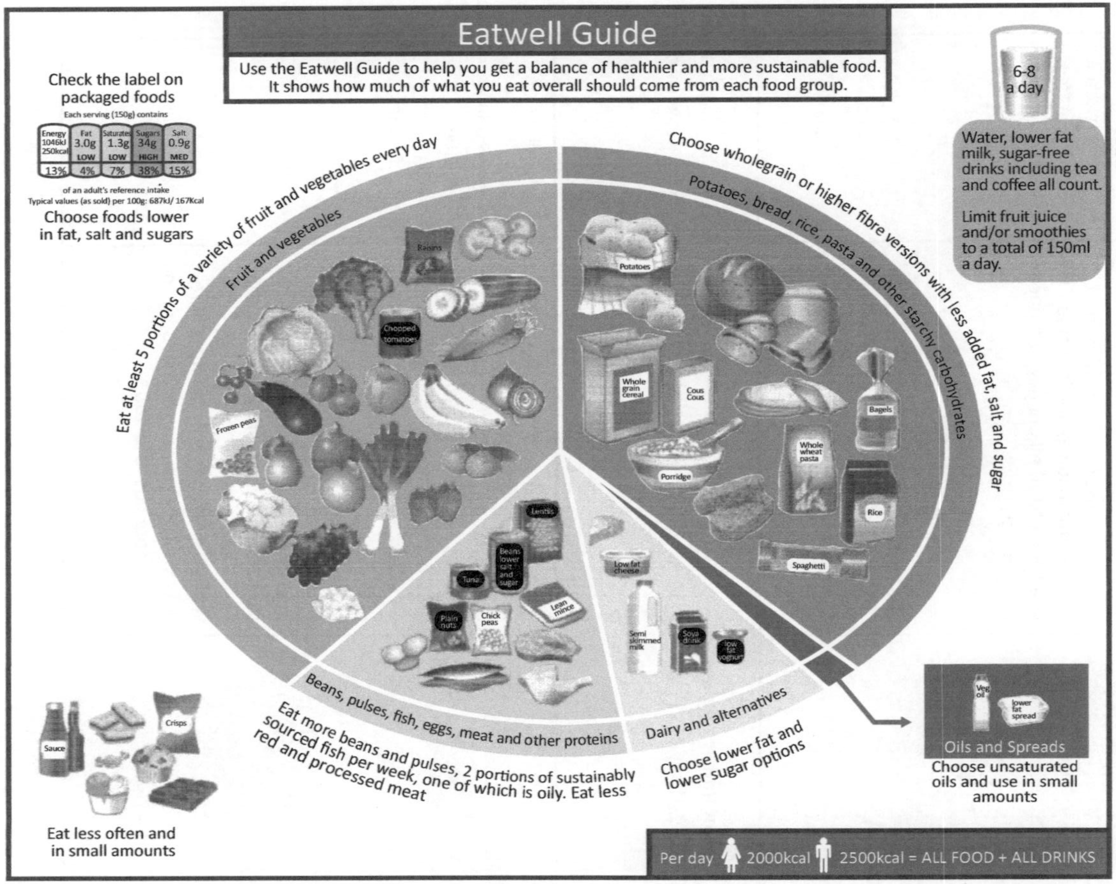

Figure 8.5 Eatwell Guide

Source: PHE in association with the Welsh Government, Food Standards Scotland and the Food Standards Agency in Northern Ireland, 2018c p.5. Reproduced under the terms of the Open Government Licence v3

<table>
<tr>
<td>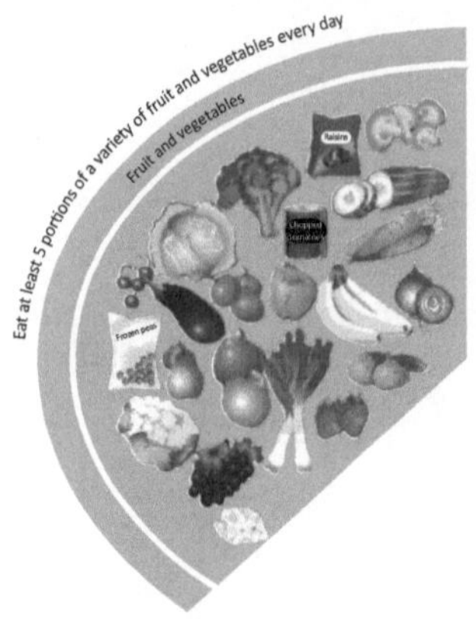
</td>
<td>Eat at least 5 portions of a variety of fruit and vegetables every day.

A portion is 80 grams or a handful.

Limit the consumption of 100% fruit and vegetable juices and/or smoothies to a total of 150 ml per day to reduce tooth decay.</td>
<td>Good sources of:

• vitamin C
• beta carotene
• folate
• carbohydrates (sugar, starch, dietary fibre)</td>
</tr>
</table>

Figure 8.6 Fruit and vegetables

Source: PHE, 2018b; BNF, 2019b. Reproduced under the terms of the Open Government Licence v3

<table>
<tr>
<td>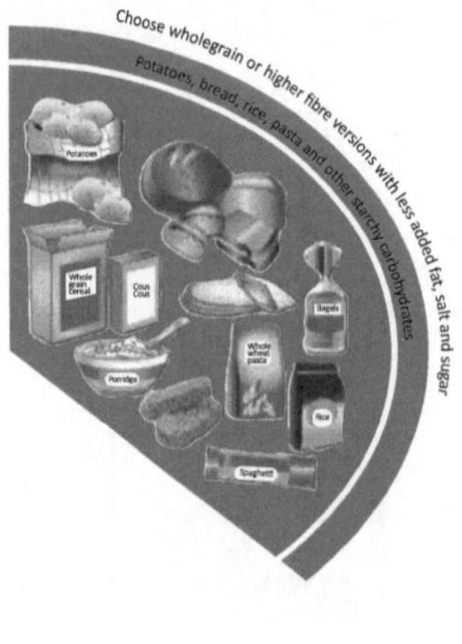
</td>
<td>Base meals around potatoes, bread, rice, pasta or other starchy carbohydrates. Choose wholegrain versions such as whole wheat pasta, brown rice, or simply leaving the skins on potatoes.

Eat 3 to 4 portions per day. A portion is 3 handfuls of cereal, 2 slices of medium bread, 2 cupped hands of cooked pasta, a fist sized baked potato.

Wholegrain foods contain more fibre than white or refined starchy food, and often more nutrients too.</td>
<td>Good sources of:

• dietary fibre
• calcium
• iron
• B vitamins</td>
</tr>
</table>

Figure 8.7 Potatoes, bread, rice, pasta and other starchy carbohydrates

Source: PHE, 2018b, BNF, 2019b. Reproduced under the terms of the Open Government Licence v3

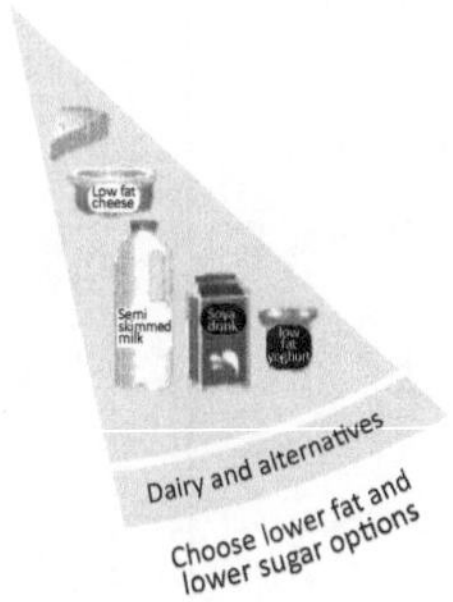	Eat 2 to 3 portions of dairy and alternatives per day. A portion is 3 teaspoons of low fat soft cheese, small pot of yoghurt, half a glass of semi-skimmed milk for cereal, 'two thumbs' of hard cheese. Choose lower fat and lower sugar options. When buying dairy alternatives like soya drinks, go for unsweetened, calcium-fortified versions.	Good sources of: • protein • vitamins A and B12 • calcium

Figure 8.8 Dairy and alternatives

Source: PHE, 2018b, BNF, 2019b. Reproduced under the terms of the Open Government Licence v3

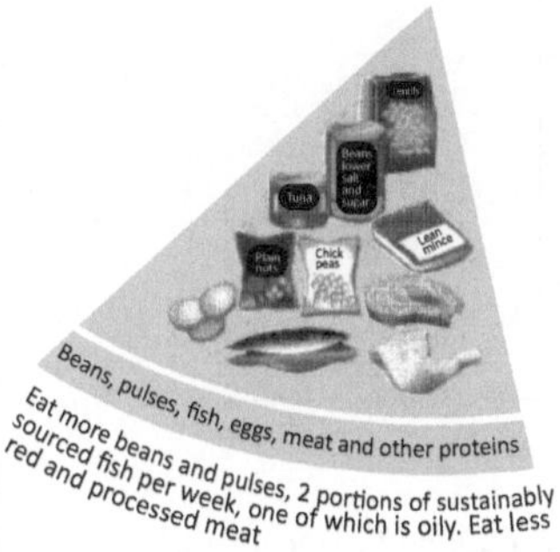	Eat 2 to 3 portions of beans, pulses, fish, eggs, meat and other proteins. Include 2 portions of fish every week, one of which should be oily. Oily fish includes salmon, sardines, mackerel and kippers. A portion is 2 boiled eggs, grilled chicken breast, half 'a hand' of cooked salmon, 2 tablespoons houmous, 200g baked beans. Beans, peas and lentils (which are all types of pulses) are good alternatives to meat because they are naturally very low in fat, and high in fibre, protein, vitamins and minerals. On average eat no more than 70 grams of red and processed meat a day. Processed meat includes sausages, bacon, cured meats and reformed meat products. Some types of meat are high in fat, particularly saturated fat, choose lean cuts and avoid frying.	Good sources of: • protein • B vitamins • iron • selenium • zinc Oily fish are a good source of: • omega 3 fats • vitamin A • vitamin D • protein • calcium

Figure 8.9 Beans, pulses, fish, eggs, meat and other proteins

Source: PHE, 2018b, BNF, 2019b. Reproduced under the terms of the Open Government Licence v3

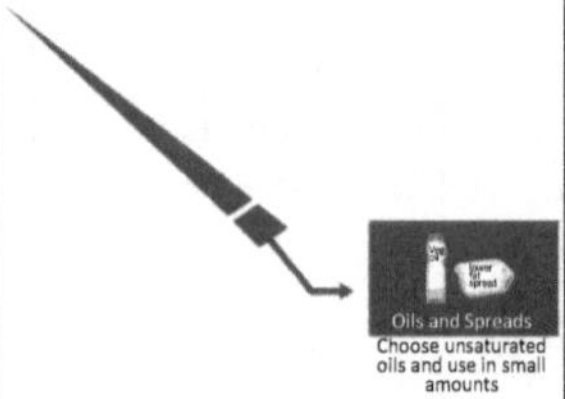	Choose unsaturated oils and spreads and eat in small amounts. Although some fat in the diet is essential, generally we are eating too much saturated fat. Unsaturated fats are healthier fats that are usually from plant sources and in liquid form as oil. This includes vegetable oil, rapeseed oil and olive oil; as well as spreads made from these oils. All types of fat are high in energy and should be limited in the diet.	Good sources of: • unsaturated fats • energy • vitamin A • vitamin D • vitamin E • vitamin K

Figure 8.10 Oil and spreads
Source: PHE, 2018b, BNF, 2019b. Reproduced under the terms of the Open Government Licence v3

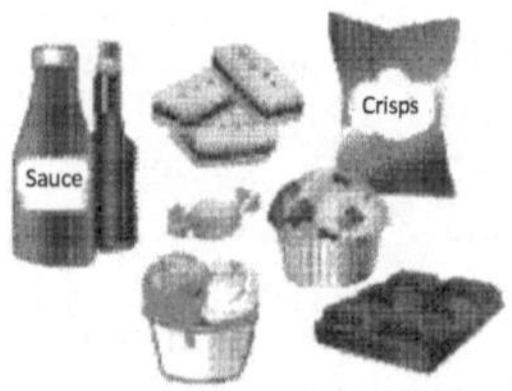	Eat less often and in small amounts. This includes products such as chocolate, cakes, biscuits, full-sugar soft drinks, butter, cream and ice-cream. These foods are not needed in the diet and so if included, should only be consumed infrequently and in small amounts. Check the label and avoid foods which are high in fat, salt and sugar.	Good sources of: • free sugar • saturated fat • energy

Figure 8.11 Foods high in fat, salt and sugar
Source: PHE, 2018b, BNF, 2019b. Reproduced under the terms of the Open Government Licence v3

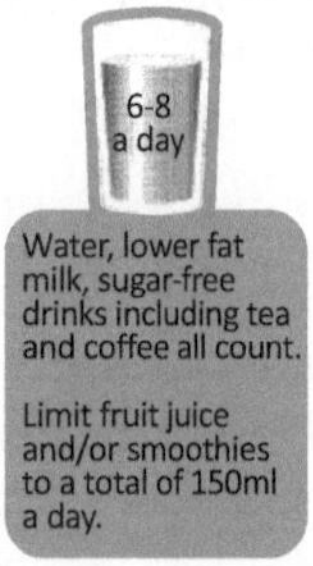	Drink 6-8 cups/glasses of fluid a day. Water, low fat milk and sugar-free drinks including tea and coffee all count. 100% fruit and vegetable juices and smoothies also count towards total fluid consumption. As they are a source of free sugars these should be limited to 150 ml per day. Swap sugary soft drinks for diet, sugar-free or no added sugar varieties.

Figure 8.12 Hydration
Source: PHE, 2018b, BNF, 2019b. Reproduced under the terms of the Open Government Licence v3

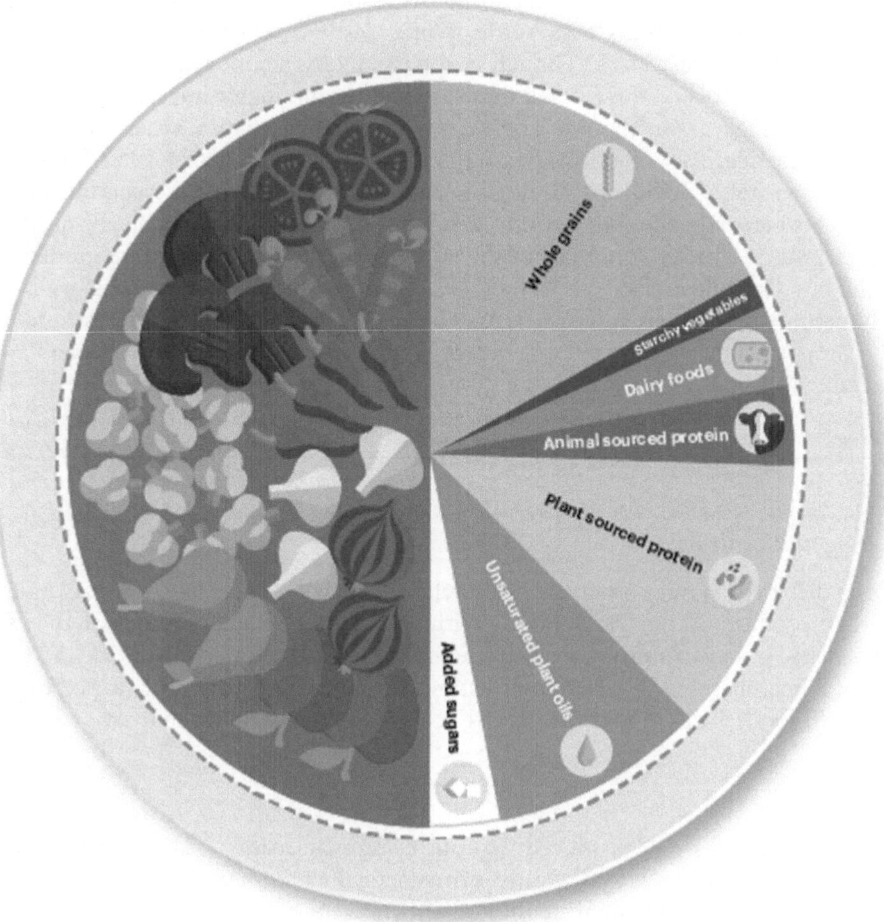

Figure 8.13 The planetary health diet

Source: EAT Foundation (2019) Healthy diets from sustainable food systems. Food planet health. Summary report of the EAT-lancet commission. Available at: https://eatforum.org/content/uploads/2019/01/EAT-Lancet_Commission_Summary_Report.pdf. (Accessed 24th October 2019)

Healthy eating in context

Box 8.2 The supermarket

"Before I can reach a row of refrigerators labelled 'PURE & WHOLESOME', I am pulled into an aisle full of yoghurts, cheeses, and puddings – the pull is unexplainable but explicit – so I follow this urge up DAIRY CHOICES and swing ... left at the end. Before I turn into FROZEN CHOICES, I survey the end-aisle display facing me. It holds a disparate assortment of frozen foods; Green Giant baby brussels sprouts with butter, White Castle frozen cheeseburgers, and DiGiorno Rising Crust Pizza. Though it appears like someone with a particular set of munchies stocked this freezer, these are high-profit, highly advertised items, likely to be bought ... on impulse. These items are not bought; rather they are *sold*.

"... Today aggressive food marketing is all but assumed, but in 1957 Vance Packard [wrote], "Buying psychologists have teamed up with merchandising experts to persuade the wife to buy products she may not particularly need or even want ... today's shopper in the supermarket is more and more guided by the buying philosophy ... I WANT IT." ... These hidden persuasions gradually became more overt ... advertisements ... promise to generate interest – to help shoppers buy exactly what retailers want them to buy ... 'loss leaders', discounted specials ... get you in the door to buy more expensive items."

(Source: Kimble, 2015 p.18–19)

Marketing and health claims

Food and drink companies often use health claims, such as 'sugar free', on packaging to sell their produce. In the UK, working within health labelling and food safety laws (Gov.UK, 2019), they can promote characteristics such as organic, probiotics and fortification. Sometimes health claims can distract the consumer from other aspects of a product. No food, drink or diet can 'detox', this is the function of the liver.

Organic

Organic food includes that produced without using man-made fertilisers, pesticides, growth regulators, livestock feed additives or genetically modified organisms. There is little difference in the nutritional quality of organic versus non-organic food (Smith-Spangler *et al.*, 2012), but organic may have higher levels of antioxidants and fewer pesticide residues (Baranski *et al.*, 2014).

Box 8.3 Orthorexia

" 'Organic' is now a brand like any other, and as with all brands, it has the potential to mislead ... some food shoppers invest all their hopes, viewing it as a guarantee that the food in question is morally spotless, gastronomically perfect and entirely, reassuringly safe. But there is no such thing as perfect food and the drive to find it can make people slightly unhinged. A new condition has been diagnosed in affluent modern societies: orthorexia or a fixation with righteous eating. Unlike anorexics, orthorexics do not particularly want to get thin; they only want to eat the healthiest, most ecologically sound food possible. The drive to do so, however, may push them to cut out first one food group and then another, until they are subsisting on an extremely limited and socially isolating diet."

(Source: Wilson, 2008 p.307)

Probiotics

The human intestine contains bacteria, fungi, protozoa, viruses and Archaea, collectively called intestinal microbiota. A diversity of microbiota is thought to protect people's health. Among the microbiota we have good and potentially harmful bacteria. Low diversity and harmful bacteria are counteracted by eating 'friendly' bacteria which, when added to food as a supplement, are called probiotics. Lockyer (2017) examined the many health claims associated with probiotics. She explains that while Estonia, Italy, Germany, Poland and Spain recommend probiotics in the diet, the European Food Safety Authority (EFSA) does not because their scientists do not believe the evidence is sufficiently clear. Lockyer concludes that there is some evidence that certain strains might help with mild gastro-intestinal symptoms or in reducing the duration of a cold, but more research is needed.

Box 8.4 Boosting the microbiome

Professor Tim Spector's research suggests the microbiota have a major influence on people's immune system, propensity for illness and allergies, metabolism, weight, appetite and mood. However, he does not recommend we achieve this by dietary supplements. He argues we need to encourage diversity and good bacteria by eating

- as wide a variety of fruit and vegetables as possible
- dietary fibre, more than 40 g per day
- plenty of high-fibre vegetables such as leeks, onions and artichokes which contain inulin
- plenty of sources of polyphenols, e.g. nuts, seeds, berries, brassicas (e.g. broccoli), olive oil, tea and coffee
- fermented foods, e.g. kefir, unsweetened yoghurt

avoiding

- snacking between meals, to allow the microbiome to rest
- sweeteners, e.g. aspartame, sucralose, saccharine
- dietary supplements; focus on eating diverse foods
- antibiotics and non-essential medicines
- large amounts of alcohol
- being obsessed by hygiene

and spend more time

- in the countryside and gardening
- stroking animals
- close to a lean person (strangely, microbiota from a lean animal can reverse obesity in another)

(Source: Spector, 2020)

Fortified foods

Food fortification is the process of adding nutrients to food. Iron and B vitamins are often added to breakfast cereals. In the UK, margarine must be fortified with vitamin A and D by law to make margarine nutritionally comparable with butter and protect the population's health.

Functional foods and super foods

Functional food is one that claims to deliver an enhanced nutritional benefit. It might be formulated around a single ingredient such as a probiotic. Superfood is a marketing term. All food is 'super' if it supplies what the body needs for good health. Both functional and superfoods promote the idea that we can take individual foods to achieve health like we take medicine: an attractive marketing ploy. Some functional foods can be helpful in certain circumstances, but nutrition is not medicine and the overall balance of the whole diet is much more important than any individual food or drink.

Challenges for public health nutrition

Research

Research into diet and health is complex because diets contain multiple nutrients eaten in varied combinations. Diet is only one part of a person's lifestyle.

Thinking point:

> Nadia is a vegetarian who eats plenty of fruit, vegetables, bread, cheese, crisps and chocolate. She mostly drinks coffee and wine. She smokes occasionally and has a stressful job.
>
> Nadia is diagnosed with high blood cholesterol and high blood pressure. Which item from her lifestyle is the cause?

It is very difficult to separate out one food or nutrient and conclusively argue that it had one effect. Individual research studies focussing on one factor are never conclusive, though they sometimes make media headlines. Public health nutrition, guidance for the population, is never based on a single research study. 'Behind the headlines' is a web site that critiques health-related news stories in the UK (www.nhs.uk/news).

Guidelines

National guidelines, such as the UK's Eatwell Guide, are not entirely about the ideal diet. They are tempered by an understanding of the national culture, current eating habits and realistic goals. For example, in the UK five fruit and vegetables a day is an ambitious goal for the population, even though research suggests that more would be better.

Population versus individual

Public health nutrition advice is based on what seems to be most health-promoting for the population. It cannot claim to meet the exact needs of an individual person with their personal biology, lifestyle and circumstances.

Nanny state versus individual choice

In a democracy, governments have a duty to protect the public's health whilst also supporting economies which rely on the food industry and respecting personal choices.

Food is life

Although this chapter has focussed on the nutritional value of the diet, it is important to recognise that food and drink are more than nutrients, they are fundamental for life and for security. What people eat reflects something of their social, psychological, religious, cultural, political and environmental values and priorities (Webb, 2012). For example, in the UK, those with higher incomes tend to have healthier diets (Bates *et al.*, 2019). The giving of food is often an expression of love.

Thinking point:

> Consider all the reasons why you eat what you eat.

Table 8.5 Religion and diet

Religion	*Common dietary custom*	*Foods that are avoided*
Buddhist	Vegetarian or vegan	
Hindu	Vegetarian	Beef
Jehovah's Witness		Foods containing blood such as black pudding
Judaism	Kosher lamb, beef, poultry and fish (with fins and scales). Kosher means foods selected and prepared according to rules of the Jewish religion.	Pork Shellfish Seafood without fins and scales
Muslim	Halal beef, lamb, poultry and fish (with fins and scales). Halal means animals are killed according to Muslim law.	Pork Shellfish Seafood without fins and scales
Pagan	Vegetarian	Meat from animals that are not humanely treated
Rastafarian	Some may be vegetarian	Pork Some fish
Seventh Day Adventist	Vegetarian or vegan	
Sikh	Vegetarian	Beef Halal or kosher meat Some do not eat pork

Source: PHE (2016).

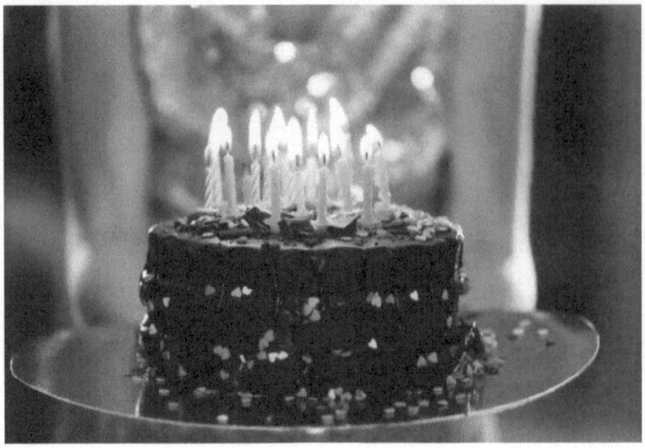

Figure 8.14 Food as an expression of love
Source: Pixel-Shot/Shutterstock.com

Summary

This chapter has

- described the aims and scope of public health nutrition
- explained how nutrients and food contribute to non-communicable diseases and to good health and wellbeing
- provided the evidence that underpins food-based guidelines for healthy eating
- indicated how nutrition and healthy eating need to be seen in the wider context of people's lives

Further reading

Webb, G. (2020) *Nutrition. Maintaining and improving health.* 5th edn. London: CRC Press

Useful websites

British Dietetic Association. Available at: www.bda.uk.com
British Nutrition Foundation. Available at: www.nutrition.org.uk
Scientific Advisory Committee on Nutrition (SACN). Available at: www.gov.uk/government/groups/scientific-advisory-committee-on-nutrition

References

Aune, D., Giovannucci, E., Boffetta, P., Fadnes, L.T., Keum, N.N, Norat, T., Greenwood, D., Riboli, E., Vatten, L.J., and Tonstad, S. (2017) 'Fruit and vegetable intake and the risk of cardiovascular disease, total cancer and all-cause mortality – a systematic review and dose-response meta-analysis of prospective studies', *International Journal of Epidemiology*, 46(3), pp.1019–1056

Baranski, M., Srednicka-Tober, D., Volakakis, N., and Seal, C. (2014) 'Higher antioxidant and lower cadmium concentrations and lower incidence of pesticide residues in organically grown crops: a systematic literature review and meta-analysis', *British Journal of Nutrition*, 112(5), pp.794–811

Bates, B., Lennox, A., Prentice, A., Bates, C., Page, P., Nicholson, S., and Swan, G. (eds) (2014) *National diet and nutrition survey. Results from year 1–4 (combined) of the rolling programme (2008/2009–2011/2012)*. London: Public Health England

Bates, B., Cox, L., Nicholson, S., Page, P., Prentice, A., Steer, T., and Swan, G. (eds) (2016) *National diet and nutrition survey. Results from years 5 and 6 (combined) of the rolling programme (2012/2013–2014)*. London: Public Health England

Bates, B., Collins, D., Cox, L., Nicholson, S., Page, P., Roberts, C., Steer, T., and Swan, G. (eds) (2019) *National diet and nutrition survey. Years 1 to 9 of the rolling programme (2008/2009–2016/2017): time trend and income analysis*. London: Public Health England

Bell, S.J., and Sears, B. (2003) 'Low-glycemic-load diets: impact on obesity and chronic diseases', *Critical Reviews in Food Science and Nutrition*, 43(4), pp.357–377

Bellisle, F., Dalix, A.M. De Assis, M.A., and Kupek, E. (2007) 'Motivational effects of 12-week moderately restrictive diets with or without special attention at the glycaemic index of foods', *British Journal of Nutrition*, 97(4), pp.790–798

Bhardwaj, S., Passi, S.J., Misra, A., Pant, K.K., Anwar, K., Pandey, R.M., and Kardam, V. (2016) 'Effect of heating/reheating of fats/oils, as used by Asian Indians, on trans fatty acid formation', *Food Chemistry*, 212, pp.663–670

Biswas, S.K. (2016) 'Does the interdependence between oxidative stress and inflammation explain the antioxidant paradox?' *Oxidative Medicine and Cellular Longevity*, 2016(12), pp.1–9 doi: 10.1155/2016/5698931

British Dietetic Association (2016a) Food fact sheet: supplements. Available at: www.bda.uk.com/foodfacts/supplements.pdf (Accessed 26th October 2019)

British Dietetic Association (2016b) Food fact sheet: pregnancy. Available at: www.bda.uk.com/foodfacts/Pregnancy.pdf (Accessed 26th October 2019)

British Dietetic Association (2017) Food fact sheet: food and mood. Available at: www.bda.uk.com/foodfacts/foodmood.pdf (Accessed 26th October 2019)

British Dietetic Association (2020) Salt: food fact sheet. Available at: www.bda.uk.com/resource/salt.html (Accessed 26th April 2020)

British Nutrition Foundation (2019a) Food a fact of life: explore food. Available at: http://explorefood.foodafactoflife.org.uk/ (Accessed 26th October 2019)

British Nutrition Foundation (2019b) Find your balance. Available at: hwww.nutrition.org.uk/healthyliving/find-your-balance.html (Accessed 21st October 2019)

Bronzato, S., and Durante, A. (2017) 'A contemporary review of the relationship between red meat consumption and cardiovascular risk', *International Journal of Preventative Medicine*, 8(40) doi:10.4103/ijpvm.IJPVM_206_16

Casas, R., Sacanella, E., and Estruch, R. (2014) 'The immune protective effect of the Mediterranean diet against chronic low-grade inflammatory diseases', *Endocrine, Metabolic and Immune Disorders-Drug Targets*, 14(4), pp.245–254

Dawodu, A., and Wagner, C.L. (2007) 'Mother-child vitamin D deficiency: an international perspective', *Archives of Disease in Childhood*, 92(9), pp.737–740

Dhaka, V., Gulia, N., Ahlawat, K.S., and Khatkar, B.S. (2011) 'Trans fats – sources, health risks and alternative approach – a review', *Journal of Food Science and Technology*, 48(5), pp.534–541

Drouin-Chartier, J., Zheng, Y., Li, Y., Malik, V., Pan, A., Bhupathiraju, S.N., Tobias, D.K., Manson, J.E., Willett, W.C., and Hu, F.B. (2019) 'Changes in consumption of sugary beverages and artificially sweetened beverages and subsequent risk of type 2 diabetes: results from three large prospective U.S. cohorts of women and men', *Diabetes Care*, 42(12), pp.2181–2189

EAT Foundation (2019) Healthy diets from sustainable food systems. Food planet health. Summary report of the EAT-lancet commission. Available at: https://eatforum.org/content/uploads/2019/01/EAT-Lancet_Commission_Summary_Report.pdf (Accessed 24th October 2019)

Gov.UK (2019) Food labelling and packaging. Available at: www.gov.uk/food-labelling-and-packaging (Accessed 26th October 2019)

Hajhashemi, V., Vaseghi, G., Pourfarzam, M., and Abdollahi, A. (2010) 'Are antioxidants helpful for disease prevention?' *Research in Pharmaceutical Sciences*, 5(1), pp.1–8

Harinageswara, R.K., Fullana, A., Sidhu, S., and Carbonell-Barrachina, A.A. (2010) 'Emissions of volatile aldehydes from heated cooking oils', *Food Chemistry*, 120(1), pp.59–65

Hu, Y., Ding, M., Sampson, L. Willett, W.C., Mason, J.E., Want, M., Rosner, B., Hu, F.B and Sun, S. (2020) 'Intake of whole grain foods and risk of type 2 diabetes: results from three prospective cohort studies', *BMJ*, 370 doi:10.1136/bmj.m2206

Imamura, F., O'Connor, L., Ye, Z., Mursu, J., Hayashino, Y., Bhupathiraju, S.N., and Forouhi, N.G. (2016) 'Consumption of sugar sweetened beverages, artificially sweetened beverages, and fruit juice and incidence of type 2 diabetes: systematic review, meta-analysis, and estimation of population attributable fraction', *British Journal of Sports Medicine*, 50(8), pp.496–504

International Osteoporosis Foundation (2018) *Broken bones, broken lives: a roadmap to solve the fragility fracture crisis in Europe.* Nyon: International Osteoporosis Foundation

Kimble, M. (2015) *Unprocessed.* New York: William Morrow

Lobo, V., Patil, A., Phatak, A., and Chandra, N. (2010) 'Free radicals, antioxidants and functional foods: impact on human health', *Pharmacognosy Review*, 4(8), pp.118–126

Lockyer, S. (2017) 'Are probiotics useful for the average consumer?', *Nutrition Bulletin*, 42, pp.42–48

Macready, A.L., George, T.W., Chong, M.F., Alimbetov, D.S., Jin, Y., Spencer, J.P., Kennedy, O.B., Tuohy, K.M., Minihane, A.M., Gordon, M.H., Lovegrove, J.A., and FLAVURS Study Group (2014) 'Flavonoid-rich fruit and vegetables improve microvascular reactivity and inflammatory status in men at risk of cardiovascular disease – FLAVURS: a randomised controlled trial', *American Journal of Clinical Nutrition*, 99(3), pp.479–489

Mamalaki, E., Anasasiou, C.A., Ntanasi, E., Tsapanou, A., Kosmidis, M.H., Dardiotis, E., Hadjigeorgiou, G.M., Sakka, P., Scarmeas, N., and Yannakoulia, M. (2018) 'Associations between the Mediterranean diet and sleep in older adults: results from the hellenic longitudinal investigation of aging and diet study', *Geriatrics and Gerontology International*, 18, pp.1543–1548

Minihane, A.M., Vinoy, S., Russell, W.R., Baka, A., Roche, H.M., Tuohy, K.M., Teeling, J.L., Blaak, E.E., Fenech, M., Vauzour, D., McArdle, H.J., Kremer, B.H.A., Sterkman, L., Vafeiadou, K., Benedetti, M.M., Williams, C.M., and Calder, P.C. (2015) 'Low-grade inflammation, diet composition and health: current evidence and its translation', *British Journal of Nutrition*, 114(7), pp.999–1012

Moneiro, C.A., Moubarac, J., Levy, R.B., and Canella, D.S. (2018) 'Household availability of ultra-processed foods and obesity in nineteen European countries', *Public Health Nutrition* 21(Special Issue 1), pp.18–26

National Institute for Health and Care Excellence (NICE) (2018) *Anaemia – iron deficiency.* Available at: https://cks.nice.org.uk/anaemia-iron-deficiency#!backgroundSub:2 (Accessed 26th October 2019)

Nichols, B.L. (2003) 'Icie Macy and Elsie Widdowson: pioneers of child nutrition and growth', *The Journal of Nutrition*, 133, pp.3690–3692

Public Health England (2015) McCance and Widdowson's composition of foods integrated dataset. Available at: www.gov.uk/government/publications/composition-of-foods-integrated-dataset-cofid (Accessed 26th October 2019)

Public Health England (2016) *Government dietary recommendations*. London: Public Health England

Public Health England (2018a) *The problem with sugar*. London: Public Health England

Public Health England (2018b) *A quick guide to the government's healthy eating recommendations*. London: Public Heath England

Public Health England (2018c) *The eatwell guide*. London: Public Health England

Public Health England/Food Standards Agency (2015) *McCance and Widdowson's the composition of foods*. 7th edn. London: Royal Society of Chemistry

Reynolds, A., Mann, J., Cummings, J., Winter, N., Mete, E., and Morenga L.T. (2019) 'Carbohydrate quality and human health: a series of systematic reviews and meta-analyses', *The Lancet*, 393(10170), pp.434–445

Roberts, C., Steer, T., Maplethorpe, N., Cox, L., Meadows, S., Nicholson, S., Page, P., and Swan, G. (2018) *National diet and nutrition survey. Results from years 7 and 8 (combined) of the rolling programme (2014/15 to 2015/16)*. London: Public Health England

Scientific Advisory Committee on Nutrition (SACN) (2015) *Carbohydrates and health*. London: The Stationery Office

Scientific Advisory Committee on Nutrition (2016) Vitamin D and health. Available at: www.gov.uk/government/publications/sacn-vitamin-d-and-health-report (Accessed 26th October 2019)

Scientific Advisory Committee on Nutrition (2017) Update on folic acid. Available at: www.gov.uk/government/publications/folic-acid-updated-sacn-recommendations (Accessed 26th October 2019)

Scientific Advisory Committee on Nutrition (2018) SACN statement on diet, cognitive impairment and dementias. Available at: www.gov.uk/government/publications/sacn-statement-on-diet-cognitive-impairment-and-dementia (Accessed 26th October 2019)

Scientific Advisory Committee on Nutrition (2019) Saturated fats and health. London. Available at: https://assets.publishing.service.gov.uk/government/uploads/system/uploads/attachment_data/file/814995/SACN_report_on_saturated_fat_and_health.pdf (Accessed 26th October 2019)

Seidelmann, S.B., Claggett, B., Cheng, S. Henglin, M., Shah, A., Steffen, L.M., Folsom, A.R., Rimm, E.B., Willett, W.C., and Solomon, S.D. (2018) 'Dietary carbohydrate intake and mortality: a prospective cohort study and meta-analysis', *Lancet Public Health*, 3(9) e419-e428 doi.org/10.1016/S24242468-2667(18)30135

Simopoulos, A.P. (2010) 'The omega-6/omega-3 fatty acid ratio: health implications', *OCL – Oilseeds and Fats, Crops and Lipids*, 17(5), pp.267–275

Singh, R., Devi, S., and Gollen, R. (2015) 'Role of free radical in atherosclerosis, diabetes and dyslipidaemia: larger-than-life', *Diabetes Metabolism Research and Reviews*, 31(2), pp.113–126

Smith-Spangler C., Brandeau, M.L., Hunter, G.E., Bavinger, J.C., Pearson, M., Eschbach, P.J., Sundaram, V., Lie, H., Schirmer, P., Stave, C., Olkin, I., and Bravata, D.M. (2012) 'Are organic food safer or healthier than conventional alternatives? A systematic review', *Annals of Internal Medicine*, 157(5), pp.348–366

Spector, T. (2020) *'15 tips to boost your gut microbiome', Science Focus*. Available at: www.sciencefocus.com/the-human-body/how-to-boost-your-microbiome/ (Accessed 24th August 2020)

St-Onge, M., Mikic, A., and Pietrolungo, C.E. (2016) 'Effects of diet on sleep quality', *Advances in Nutrition*, 7(5), pp.938–949

Steinmetz, K.A., Potter, J.D. (1991) 'Vegetables, fruit and cancer. II. Mechanisms', *Cancer Causes Control*, 2(6), pp.427–442

Wang, M., Yu, M., Fang, L., and Hu R. (2015) 'Association between sugar-sweetened beverages and type 2 diabetes: a meta-analysis', *Journal of Diabetes Investigation*, 6(3), pp.360–366

Webb, G. (2012) *Nutrition. Maintaining and improving health*. 4th edn. London: Hopper Arnold

Willett, W., Rockström, J., Loken, B., *et al.* (2019) 'Food in the Anthropocene: the EAT-Lancet commission on healthy diets from sustainable food systems', *The Lancet*, 393(10170), pp.447–492

Wilson, B. (2008) *Swindled*. London: John Murray

World Cancer Research Fund/American Institute for Cancer Research (2018a) *Diet, nutrition, physical activity and the prevention of cancer. A global perspective*. London: World Cancer Research Fund International

World Cancer Research Fund/ American Institute for Cancer Research (2018b) *Meat, fish and dairy products and the risk of cancer*. London: World Cancer Research Fund International

World Health Organization (2012) *Guideline: sodium intake for adults and children*. Geneva: World Health Organization

World Health Organization (2016) *Global report on diabetes*. Geneva: World Health Organization

Zheng, J., Sharp, S.J., Imamura, F., *et al* (2020) 'Association of plasma biomarkers of fruit and vegetable intake with incident type 2 diabetes: EPIC-InterAct case-cohort study in eight European countries', *BMJ*, 370 doi:10.10.1136/bmj.m2194

Zivkovic, A.M., Telis, N., and German, J.B. (2011) 'Dietary omega-3 fatty acids aid in the modulation of inflammation and metabolic health', *California Agriculture*, 65(3), pp.106–111

9 Tobacco and health

Sally Robinson

Key points

- Introduction
- Tobacco
- Smoking tobacco
- Vaping tobacco
- Smokeless tobacco
- Non-tobacco products
- Benefits of quitting tobacco
- Summary

Introduction

Tobacco, a harmful substance that causes disease and early death, is marketed and sold around the world by a powerful tobacco industry. Smoking, smokeless and heated tobacco products are toxic to the human body. This chapter outlines how the industry gained and maintains its influence. It explains how tobacco harms health and causes early death and describes the role of nicotine as an addictive substance but one that can be helpful when trying to quit using tobacco. The chapter describes the pros and cons of non-tobacco products such as electronic cigarettes (e-cigarettes). It concludes with an overview of how quitting tobacco benefits health.

Tobacco

The tobacco epidemic is

> … one of the biggest public health threats the world has ever faced.
>
> (WHO, 2019a)

Tobacco companies promote and sell tobacco to be burnt and smoked, to be heated and inhaled, to be sniffed or to be chewed. Across the world, each year, seven million deaths are caused by the direct use of tobacco and 1.2 million are caused by non-smokers being exposed to second-hand smoke (WHO, 2019a). Each year, the consequences of consuming tobacco cost the world two trillion dollars in healthcare and loss of productivity due to people being unable to work (ACS/VS, 2019).

The tobacco industry

Ravenholt (1990) describes the history of tobacco as a global death march. Tobacco plants, grown in North and South America, were used as medicine by the Native Americans. In the 1580s Sir Walter Raleigh colonised the area named Virginia and helped to popularise pipe smoking at the English court of Queen Elizabeth I. Portuguese traders carried tobacco to India, Africa, Japan and China; Spanish traders took it to the Philippines and European merchants took it to Turkey and the Middle East. By the eighteenth century tobacco smoking was introduced to Australia and nearby islands where it was used as payment for the cooperation and goodwill of the Indigenous people, thus supporting the early days of colonisation. As well as smoking, Native Americans chewed and sniffed tobacco, and it was Dutch traders who encouraged the European upper classes to use snuff. Throughout the world tobacco was marketed as a medicine, a cure for a wide variety of ailments, and something that calmed the mind, clarified thinking and promoted happy thoughts.

In 1603 James became King of Scotland, England and Ireland. He organised the first public debate on tobacco, where he displayed the black brains and tissues taken from the bodies of smokers. He taxed tobacco and it became an important stream of

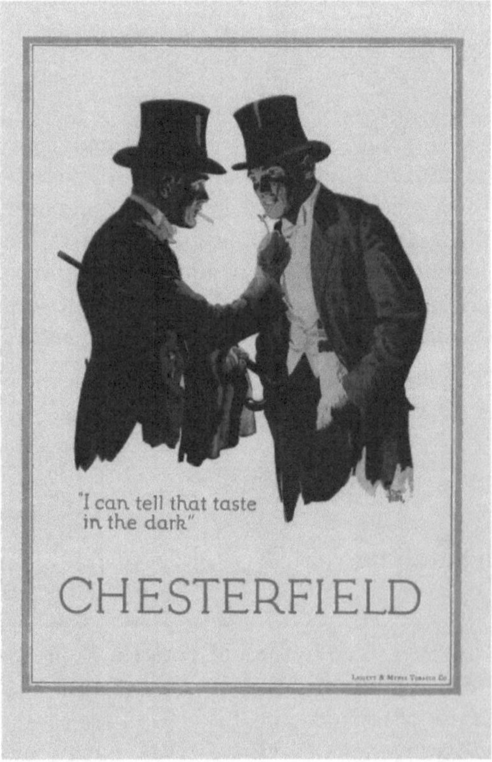

Figure 9.1 Advertisement for Chesterfield cigarettes, 1929
Source: Chesterfield cigarettes, Cosmopolitan magazine, 1929 https://commons.wikimedia.org/wiki/File:ChesterfieldCigarettes_02.jpg

revenue to the monarchy. In 1761, the English Dr John Hill reported the 'frightful symptoms of cancer' in the nasal passages due to snuff. He described breathing being obstructed by sore black swellings and an offensive discharge. Meanwhile, the Italian anatomist Giovanni Morgagni described lung cancer from his post-mortems but did not know the cause. Cancers of the lips, mouth and larynx became increasingly common.

'Segars', tobacco rolled and contained within a thin paper, were invented in Spain and Portugal. British soldiers fighting Napoleon in the Peninsula War brought these 'cigars' home. The Crimean War and the American Civil War encouraged the spread of smoking and chewing tobacco. In 1884 James Bonsack of Virginia perfected a cigarette rolling machine, and by 1890 Duke's American Tobacco Company was producing 90% of American cigarettes. Doctors noted that tobacco inflamed the mucous membranes of the mouth, throat and airways, it caused coughs and breathlessness, and affected blood circulation. They noted that cancer of the lip often occurred in the exact place that a pipe or a cigar was placed. Yet, most doctors continued to believe that tobacco was not particularly harmful.

The highly profitable tobacco companies multiplied into a tobacco industry. Cigarettes, endorsed by doctors, were included in the soldiers' rations during World War 1. Advertising promoted cigarettes as glamorous, fashionable and healthy. In the 1920s the tobacco companies increased their sales by deliberately targeting women, suggesting cigarettes projected female empowerment and could help with weight control. By the 1930s the world witnessed a marked increase in deaths from lung cancer, and researchers thought that tarmac, pollution from industry or coal, and car fumes were the most likely causes. In 1950, Richard Doll and Austin Bradford Hill studied patients with lung cancer in 20 London hospitals, and discovered that they all had tobacco smoking in common. Their study of doctors, published in 1954, led the British Government to advise the public that smoking and lung cancer were related.

Box 9.1 Doll and Hill's studies into smoking and lung cancer

<u>London patients' study</u>

Doll and Hill (1950) contacted 20 London hospitals and asked to be notified about any patients admitted with a range of cancers, including lung cancer. A sample of 1,732 patients with cancer, and under 75 years old, were interviewed using a standardised questionnaire. At four hospitals, interviews also took place with 743 patients who did not have cancer; these acted as a 'control' group. Patients were asked

a) if they had ever smoked
b) the ages at which they started and stopped smoking
c) the amount they smoked before the onset of the illness that brought them to hospital
d) the main changes in their smoking history and the maximum they had ever smoked
e) what proportion of their smoking was cigarettes or pipes
f) whether they inhaled when smoking

They concluded, "... smoking is a factor, and an important factor, in the production of carcinoma of the lung" (p.746).

British doctors' study

Doll and Hill (1954) sent a questionnaire to doctors which included asking them to classify themselves as

a) smoking at the moment
b) an ex-smoker who had now given up
c) someone who had never smoked regularly, e.g. one cigarette a day

40,564 questionnaires were completed and analysed. Twenty-nine months later the researchers noted those over 35 years old who had died, and analysed their causes of death. The research revealed,

> ... a significant and steadily rising mortality from deaths due to cancer of the lung as the amount of tobacco smoked increases. There is also a rise in the mortality from deaths attributed to coronary thrombosis as the amount smoked increases, but the gradient is much less steep ...
>
> (p.1455)

Tobacco wars

The tobacco industry moved to protect its vested interests, its highly profitable business. It already used its immense power to influence politics, the media, the law and policy, and now it aimed to shape and control scientific knowledge – to fight science with science. Under the guise of legitimate research and development, it aimed to

> ... undo what was now known: that cigarette smoking caused lethal disease. If science had historically been dedicated to the making of new facts, the industry campaign now sought to develop specific strategies to 'unmake' a scientific fact.
>
> (Brandt, 2012 p.64)

Brandt (2012) explains how the tobacco industry aimed to amplify doubts about smoking by building a public information campaign based on any statements by scientists and doctors who questioned whether smoking caused cancer. In 1954, they set up The Tobacco Industry Research Committee (TIRC). In an advert, disseminated to 400 newspapers, the industry explained that the Committee would aggressively pursue the science of tobacco to ensure the wellbeing of their consumers. For 40 years, their message remained that there was no clear evidence that smoking caused disease, millions of people derived pleasure from smoking and the TIRC would provide the scientific facts as soon as possible. They funded and disseminated cigarette research, promoting the perception that the science was inconclusive. Later, as independent medical research showing the harms of smoking grew, the industry argued that smoking was a personal, free choice. As a public relations campaign, it was a masterclass and the industry thrived.

Tobacco control means the combination of public health policy, research and practice that aims to prevent and reduce the use of tobacco. In the UK, the influence of the tobacco industry could be seen in the government's approach to preventing tobacco-related diseases. For decades, many public health interest groups, including Action on Smoking and Health, lobbied for a variety of tobacco control measures, including a ban on cigarette advertising, reducing smoking in public places, adding health warnings to cigarette packets and increasing cigarette tax. They met resistance from successive governments, who were mindful of the numbers employed by the industry and the billions of pounds they received from cigarette taxes. Governments entered into voluntary agreements with the tobacco industry and avoided legal measures. Between 1988 and 1990 Kenneth Clarke MP became UK Secretary of State for Health whilst holding a position within the tobacco company British American Tobacco. It wasn't until the 1990s that American lawyers found a way to successfully challenge tobacco companies (Table 9.1). Significant measures of tobacco control, such as legal bans on smoking in public places, were introduced across the Western world. In 2003, the World Health Organization took the lead with the WHO Framework Convention on Tobacco Control (WHO, 2003).

Today, the tobacco industry's largest companies are Philip Morris International, British American Tobacco, Imperial Tobacco, Altria Group and Japan Tobacco. As smoking has decreased due to health concerns in the West and some success with law suits, the tobacco industry focuses on new markets to entice new consumers, including children, to their products. They target low- and middle-income countries such as Africa where there are few aggressive tobacco control policies in place. They keep the prices of cigarettes low, threaten legal action as a first defence to any form of tobacco control and make high-value donations to charities to enhance their image. In what we might consider a conflict of interest, the chief executive of the state-owned China National Tobacco Corporation is responsible for both the sales of cigarettes and any tobacco control measures to limit their impact on health. Distrust of the industry continues because

> Thousands of internal tobacco industry documents released through litigation and whistleblowers reveal the most astonishing systematic corporate deceit of all time.
>
> (WHO, 2019b p.ii)

The tobacco industry

- does not accept smoking causes lung cancer
- maintains that nicotine is not physically and psychologically addictive in a similar way to heroin and cocaine
- maintains it is only interested in selling cigarettes to adults not children
- argues that advertising only encourages smokers to change brands, not that it increases cigarette consumption
- denies that advertising influences children to smoke

Table 9.1 Tobacco legal battles in the United States of America

Time line	*Reason for taking tobacco companies to court*	*Tobacco companies' response*
1950s law suits taken by individuals against tobacco companies	Tobacco industry failed to act with reasonable care when making and marketing cigarettes. Tobacco industry failed to warn consumers about the health risks of cigarettes. Fraud. Unfair and deceptive business practices.	Tobacco is not harmful to smokers. Cancer is caused by other factors. Smokers assume the risk of cancer when they choose to smoke. Tobacco companies won.
1980s law suits initiated by individuals against tobacco companies	Tobacco industry knew but did not warn consumers that cigarettes were addictive and caused lung cancer.	Consumers know the risks of cancer and other health problems when they choose to smoke. Tobacco companies won.
1990s law suits taken by US states against tobacco companies	Cigarettes cause health problems which incur significant costs to public healthcare systems.	Forty-six states and four of the largest tobacco companies settled out of court. The companies agreed to • refrain from certain advertising, including adverts aimed at children • pay billions of dollars to states to compensate for healthcare costs • create and fund an American public health education foundation
2006 a range of law suits		Florida Supreme Court found that tobacco companies had knowingly sold dangerous products and kept the health risks of smoking concealed. It paved the way for a further 8,000 smokers and families to sue tobacco companies.

Source: Michon (2019).

- does not accept, publicly, that low-tar cigarettes are just as harmful as other cigarettes
- continues to deny that second-hand smoke is a public health hazard
- continues to interfere with political and legal processes
- seeks to influence scientific and policy agendas
- makes unproven claims and discredits proven science
- exaggerates the importance of the industry to employment
- intimidates governments with litigation
- manipulates public opinion to gain the appearance of respectability

(WHO, 2019b p.ii; 2019c p.61)

The tobacco industry also seeks to maintain or increase its consumers by diversification into what it claims are less harmful products. In the 20th century it produced filtered then low-tar cigarettes. In the 21st century it, along with others, produced

Table 9.2 Tobacco and non-tobacco products

Tobacco			*Non-tobacco products*	
Smoking	*Vaping*	*Smokeless*	*Vaping*	*Other*
Inhalation of smoke from burning tobacco	Inhalation of vapour from heated tobacco	Tobacco is chewed or sniffed	Inhalation of vapour from e-liquid	Swallowed/ absorbed
Cigarettes Cigars Pipes Bidis and kreteks Waterpipes	Heated tobacco products	Chewing tobacco, e.g. gutka, tambaku paan, betel quid, zarda Sniffing tobacco, e.g. snuff, snus, toombak	E-cigarettes – electronic nicotine delivery systems (ENDS) E-cigarettes – electronic non-nicotine delivery systems (ENNDS)	Nicotine-replacement therapy, e.g. patches, gum, tablets

electronic cigarettes (e-cigarettes) which mimic the act of smoking but do not contain tobacco. In 2014, the tobacco industry launched its heated tobacco products. Sales are supported by industry-funded research and an aggressive marketing message that they are less dangerous than conventional cigarettes.

The powerful tobacco industry sells tobacco, a substance that causes disease and death across the world.

Smoking tobacco

Smoking tobacco products

Cigarettes

Cigarettes are paper tubes containing chopped tobacco leaf and fillers. The public health charity Action on Smoking and Health (ASH) (2018a) explain that fillers include other parts of the tobacco plant and a selection from hundreds of additives. Some of the additives extend the shelf life of cigarettes or make cigarette smoke more pleasant to inhale; others produce toxic chemicals when they are burned. Smoking produces mainstream smoke, that which the smoker inhales, and sidestream smoke, that which rises from the tip of a lit cigarette. Sidestream smoke contains higher concentrations of chemicals than mainstream partly because the more porous the paper around a cigarette, the more air is inhaled, thus diluting the inhaled smoke and the chemicals within it. Environmental smoke, or second-hand smoke, is made up of sidestream smoke and exhaled smoke. Smokers, including those who do not inhale, and bystanders, as passive smokers, are all inhaling poisons.

ASH (2018a) describe smoking as a process whereby the smoke carries the toxic chemicals into the smoker or into the air in the form of particulates, solids and gases.

Table 9.3 Some of the chemicals in tobacco smoke

Chemical	*Places, other than cigarettes, where these chemicals are often found*
Acetone	Nail-polish remover
Acetic acid	Hair dye
Ammonia	Household cleaner
Arsenic	Rat poison
Benzene	Rubber cement and petrol
Butane	Lighter fluid
Cadmium	Battery acid
Carbon monoxide	Car exhaust fumes
Formaldehyde	Embalming fluid
Hexamine	Barbecue-lighter fluid
Lead	Batteries
Naphthalene	Mothballs
Nicotine	Insecticide
Tar	Road paving
Toluene	Paint

Source: Adapted from American Lung Association (2019).

Particulates include tar and nicotine. Tar is the sticky brown substance that stains smokers' teeth and fingers. Tar is one of the chemicals that causes cancer. Nicotine is highly addictive and it is the craving for nicotine that often keeps people smoking. Lower-tar cigarettes are also lower in nicotine, but they are not safer or healthier because many smokers smoke more, or inhale more deeply, to get more nicotine, thus maintaining their overall tar inhalation.

When a cigarette is lit, nicotine contained in the moisture of the tobacco leaf evaporates and attaches to droplets in the smoke. On inhalation, it reaches the brain in 10 to 19 seconds, stimulating the nervous system and raising heart rate and blood pressure. The heart needs to works hard to get more oxygen. Filters, made of cellulose acetate, help to trap some of the nicotine, tar and other chemicals, and they cool the smoke, which makes it easier to inhale. Filtered cigarettes are no better for health than unfiltered ones because smokers who change to filtered cigarettes compensate by inhaling more deeply and smoking more cigarettes to meet the level of nicotine that they crave (Song *et al.*, 2017).

The gases in smoke include ammonia, hydrogen cyanide, acrolein and carbon monoxide. On inhalation, carbon monoxide binds with haemoglobin in the blood. Haemoglobin is the red molecule that transports both iron and oxygen through the body. When compromised by carbon monoxide, the haemoglobin cannot take enough oxygen to the tissues and organs. Smoking puts the whole body into a state of crisis as it struggles to get enough oxygen, a condition known as hypoxia. Nicotine cravings encourage repeat smoking, causing the accumulation of poisons in the body and increasingly damaging episodes of hypoxia.

Cigars

Cigars often contain whole-leaf tobacco, have no filters and often contain more nicotine and higher levels of cancer-causing chemicals than cigarettes. Most cigar smokers do not inhale, but this does not protect them, or bystanders, from inhaling poisons from sidestream smoke, nor does it protect smokers from direct damage to the mouth, tongue and throat (Viegas, 2009).

Pipes

Pipes comprise a small bowl, containing the burning tobacco, connected to a stem through which the smoke is drawn. Tobacco may be flavoured. Some smokers inhale, particularly if they were once a cigarette smoker, and some do not, which affects the location of health damage in the body (O'Connor, 2012).

Bidis and kreteks

Traditional Indian bidis are small amounts of tobacco flakes wrapped in a non-tobacco leaf and tied with string by hand. Traditional Indonesian kreteks are like manufactured cigarettes comprising tobacco, clove and other flavourings wrapped in paper. The health risks of both are very similar to cigarettes (O'Connor, 2012).

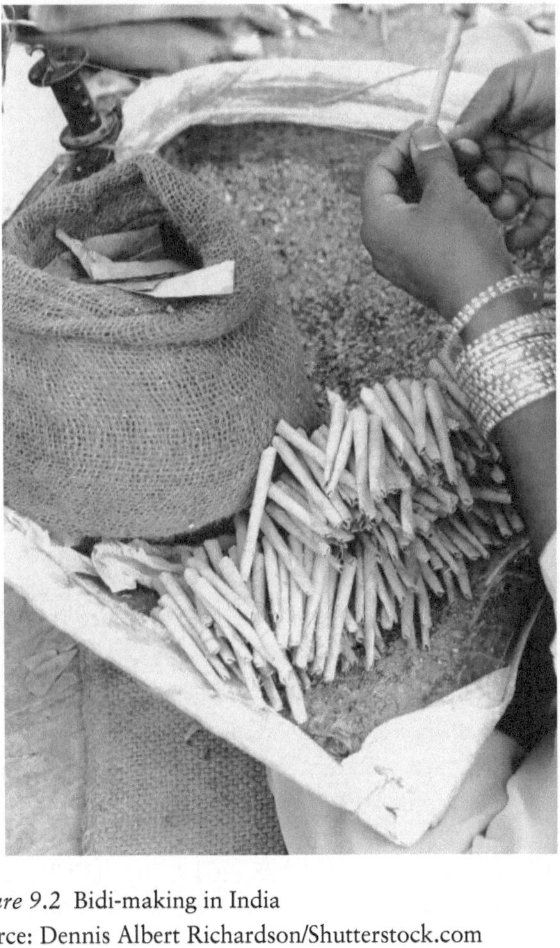

Figure 9.2 Bidi-making in India
Source: Dennis Albert Richardson/Shutterstock.com

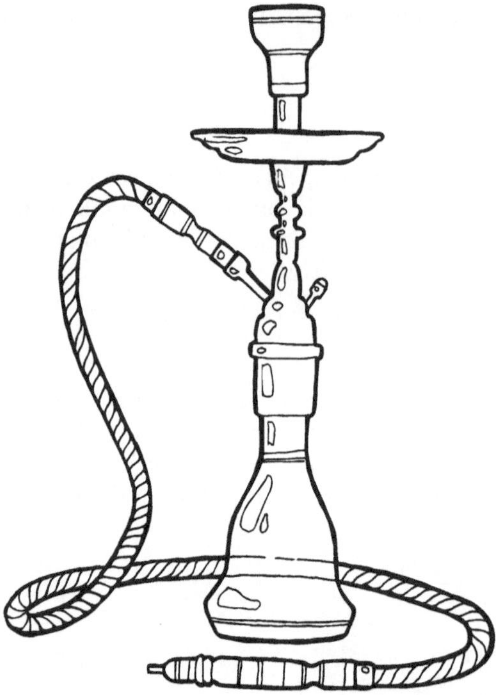

Figure 9.3 Shisha/hookah pipe
Source: Bukavik/Shutterstock.com

Waterpipes

Waterpipe tobacco smoking uses pipes, also called shisha, hookah, narghile or hubble bubble pipes. The apparatus includes a head containing tobacco separated from coal by foil. The coal heats the tobacco and the smoke passes downwards through a pipe into a bowl of water, which may be flavoured with mint, sugar or fruit. The smoker inhales through another pipe which runs down to just above water level. Despite the widespread belief that the water purifies the smoke, it does not. Smokers are susceptible to the same health risks from the tobacco as other types of tobacco smoking, and additional risks such as tuberculosis, herpes and hepatitis from the sharing of mouth pieces (Kadhum *et al.*, 2015). If an average shisha smoking session lasts an hour, this is equivalent to smoking more than 100 cigarettes (BHF, 2019).

Prevalence of smoking tobacco

The prevalence of smokers is rising in lower-income countries and falling in higher-income countries. China has the largest number of daily smokers. Smoking is rising among the young and females and in those countries that do not have tobacco control measures in place, such as in sub-Saharan Africa (ACS/VS, 2019). In the UK, there has been a significant decline in smoking since 2011, with the largest fall among the 18- to 24-year-olds (ONS, 2019).

Table 9.4 Prevalence of adult cigarette smokers in the UK, 2018

	Percentage of adults currently smoking
UK	14.7%
England	14.4%
Northern Ireland	15.5%
Scotland	16.3%
Wales	15.9%

Source: ONS (2019).

As smoking tobacco is a significant contributor to poor health, we can predict who is likely to suffer most smoking-related disease and early death in the future by noting who is smoking most now. In the UK

- the highest proportion of smokers are between 25 and 34 years old
- men (16.5%) smoke more than women (13%)
- people who work in jobs classified as routine and manual occupations (25.5%) smoke more than those who work in managerial and professional occupations (10.2%)
- smoking is notably high among adults with mental disorders and lesbian, gay and bisexual people
- about a tenth of women are smokers at the time of delivering their babies

(ONS, 2019)

Psychosocial reasons for smoking tobacco

Across Europe the most common age to start smoking is 15 to 16 years, but some start in their twenties and fewer start in their thirties (Marcon *et al.*, 2018). Delaney and colleagues (2018) interviewed smokers in Scotland about their reasons for starting and maintaining smoking. They found

- peer influence
- drinking alcohol

> ... going to clubs and having a drink ... you smoke more.
>
> (Louise, 22 years, p.5)

- transition to independent living, coupled with greater socialising, drinking, new social circles and control over their own finances

> ... there was nobody telling me that I couldn't ...
>
> (Rachel, 22 years p.5)

- transient employment in boring or stressful work environments

> It turned into more of a dependency when I was at work ... clock watching, waiting to get to my break.
>
> (Tom, 20 years, working in a call centre, p.4)

Table 9.5 Characteristics of smokers in the UK, 2018

Characteristic	*Highest prevalence of smoking (% smokers)*	*Lowest prevalence of smoking (% smokers)*
Housing tenure	Local authority renting (31%)	Owned property (8.3%)
Education	No qualifications (29.8%)	University degree (7.5%)
Economic activity	Unemployed people (29.2%)	Employed people (15%)
Country of birth	Poland (25.9%)	India (5.3%)
Relationship status	Single or cohabiting (21%)	Married or civil partnership (9.5%)
Religion (England only)	Muslim men (20.5%)	Sikh people (4.7%)
Ethnicity	Mixed ethnic group (20.4%)	Chinese (7.9%)

Source: ONS (2019).

People who live in poorer social and economic conditions may smoke because it is more acceptable within their social norms (Paul *et al.*, 2010). This includes friends who smoke, smoking as part of socialising, work environments that are conducive to smoking breaks or working outdoors. In contrast, people in higher socio-economic positions report smoking as unusual amongst their friends and smokers feeling embarrassed and judged.

People with mental, emotional or social problems smoke more than others. Among people who are depressed, smoking is linked to low mood and feelings of hopelessness (Clancy *et al.*, 2013):

> ... you sit down and cry half the day for no reason, well, all I do is smoke.
>
> (p.589)

> ... if you don't see a future ... there's no point in doing anything that's going to help you stay alive.
>
> (p.589)

Smoking provides a sense of control when someone feels they have no control over their life, a meaningful activity, a form of coping and it sometimes represents 'time out' (Clancy *et al.*, 2013):

> It's like a comfort thing ...
>
> (p.589)

People who experienced adverse childhood experiences such as abuse, neglect or household substance misuse are more likely to take up smoking, drink high levels of alcohol and have mental health problems, compared to those with happier more stable childhoods (Bellis *et al.*, 2015; CDC, 2020). Multiple adverse childhood experiences cause 'toxic stress', which leads to activities such as smoking as a way of coping with the past and consequent emotional difficulties (Ports *et al.*, 2019).

An additional reason why smoking is relatively high among people with mental disorders has been the reluctance of mental health staff to address smoking among service users. Their reluctance has been because of

- having low expectations of service users' ability to stop smoking
- lack of knowledge, seeing smoking as a choice rather than an addiction
- lack of knowledge about how smoking interacts with psychotic medications
- fear that addressing smoking would undermine the therapeutic relationship and an approach to care that aims to be respectful of service users' wishes

(Twyman *et al.*, 2019; ASH, 2019a)

In the UK, there is evidence that these attitudes are beginning to change, and practitioners are becoming more willing to learn how to address smoking cessation with service users (Simonavicius *et al.*, 2017).

Smoking tobacco and health

Smoking is more prevalent among some groups of people than others (Table 9.5) and, in turn, these differences track forward to those who develop smoking-related diseases and death. Smoking is a significant contributor to the inequalities in health discussed in Chapter 3.

Goldberg and colleagues (2014) carried out a large review of studies and concluded people are more likely to begin smoking if they are depressed or experiencing stressful events. The more cigarettes smoked per day, the lower was the person's quality of life. Compared to non-smokers, smokers report

- poorer physical health such as having a disability or problems with mobility and self-care
- poor social functioning which includes experiencing difficulties with social activities due to emotional or physical health problems
- poor vitality, feeling tired and worn out all the time
- problems with work or daily activities due to poor emotional health
- high levels of nervousness and depression

Smoking encourages chronic low-grade inflammation throughout the body. This inflammation is the mediator from which many other health conditions such as cancer and cardiovascular disease can follow. There is some evidence that having low-grade inflammation, which can be measured from a blood test, is associated with poor self-rated health (Warnoff *et al.*, 2016).

Hall and colleagues (2010) interviewed people who were living with severe chronic obstructive pulmonary disease (COPD) and concluded that living with COPD means

- living and seeing oneself decline

  I wasn't even able to eat. I was even more out of breath …

  (man with COPD, p.453)

- living and preparing to die

  [It] is like walking on a bomb. Each time I have a cold, I wonder whether this is the one that'll do it.

  (man with COPD, p.453, 454)

Table 9.6 Smoking tobacco and disease

The body	*Harms caused by smoking tobacco*	*Why smoking tobacco leads to illness and death*
Bones	Brittle bones	Bones will break easily (fractures). As older women often have lower bone density than men, smoking adds to their risk of developing osteoporosis.
Brain	Cerebrovascular accident (stroke) Smoking increases the risk of stroke by at least a half	Part of the brain dies due to a lack of blood and oxygen. If survived, it causes a range of problems depending on which part of the brain is damaged, e.g. inability to move one side of the body and problems with speech or expressing emotions.
Heart and circulation	Tachycardia (increased heart rate) Hypertension (high blood pressure) Myocardial infarction (heart attack) Atherosclerosis/ cardiovascular disease	A heart that pumps at a fast rate, trying to get blood and oxygen to the organs, will tire and eventually give up; a cardiac arrest causes death. Hypertension means that high-pressured blood enters organs, putting pressure on their structures and causing them to fail, e.g. the brain, heart and kidneys. The toxins in smoke harden blood vessels so that they cannot work, including those of the heart, encouraging splitting and death to part of the heart; a heart attack. The damage to blood vessels encourages atheroma, fatty plaques, which clog up the whole circulatory system.
Lungs	Coughs Asthma Pneumonia Emphysema Chronic obstructive pulmonary disease (COPD) Lung cancer In the UK, 84% of deaths from COPD and 83% of deaths from lung cancer are caused by smoking.	The airways and lungs are irritated by the smoke and toxins, causing them to narrow and produce mucous called phlegm or sputum. Breathing becomes difficult, the body cannot get enough oxygen and it tries to clear the phlegm by coughing. Together this encourages chest infections and death. Early signs of lung cancer include persistent coughing including coughing blood, recurrent chest infections, pain, tiredness, loss of appetite, weight loss, change in the appearance of fingers, wheezing and a hoarse voice. Tumours will continue to impede the functioning of the lungs, and the cancer can spread
Mouth and throat	Bad breath, stained teeth, gum disease, loss of taste Cancer of lips, tongue, larynx (voice box), throat and oesophagus In the UK, 93% cancers of the throat are caused by smoking.	Early signs of cancer include ulcers that do not heal, persistent white or red patches, lumps, unexplained loose teeth, difficulty with swallowing, persistent indigestion or acid reflux, loss of appetite, weight loss and pain. Speaking and swallowing becomes difficult, and there is a risk of food becoming lodged in the lungs, which can cause pneumonia. A tumour will continue to impede functioning and the cancer can spread.

Table 9.6 Cont.

The body	*Harms caused by smoking tobacco*	*Why smoking tobacco leads to illness and death*
Reproduction	Male impotence Harder to conceive Risks to baby's health Cervical cancer In the UK, 120,000 men in their 20s and 30s have smoking-related impotence. Smoking increases the risk of cot death by at least a quarter.	Sperm and eggs are harmed by the toxins in tobacco smoke. This makes conception harder and increases the chances of miscarriage, premature birth, death of foetuses and new-borns, low-birthweight babies and health problems in babies. For females who have contracted the HPV infection, which causes cervical cancer, smoking reduces the body's ability to get rid of the infection.
Skin	Premature ageing of the skin	The skin is starved of oxygen, causing it to become grey and dull, and toxins cause cellulite.
Stomach	Stomach ulcers Stomach cancer	Smoking weakens the sphincter that joins the lower oesophagus to the stomach, thus allowing stomach acid to reflux upwards (heartburn). Early signs of stomach cancer include nausea, frequent heartburn, pain, feeling full after eating only a small amount and tiredness. A tumour will continue to impede the functioning of the stomach, and the cancer can spread.

Sources: NHS.UK (2019a; 2019b).

- dying of COPD means suffocating

> … when the time comes I know for sure I'll be gasping for air.
>
> (woman with COPD, p.454)

COPD also has a significant impact on carers.

> My husband's illness fully dominates our daily routines. I get hardly any time of my own.
>
> (wife of a man with COPD, Lindqvist *et al.*, 2013, p.44)

> The goodnight kiss after he has coughed up a large amount of phlegm … is horrible, I do it, but I don't like it.
>
> (wife of a man with COPD, Lindqvist *et al.*, 2013 p.47)

A regular life-long smoker loses about 10 to 11 years of life compared to non-smokers (ACS/VS, 2019). In England, smoking is estimated to cause

- 54% of all deaths from types of cancer that can be caused by smoking
- 48% of deaths from types of respiratory disease that can be caused by smoking

Table 9.7 Deaths attributable to smoking tobacco in the UK, 2018

	Number of deaths per year
England	77,800
Northern Ireland	2,300*
Scotland	10,000*
Wales	5,500*

Source: ONS (2019) (*estimates).

- 45% of deaths from diseases of the digestive system that can be caused by smoking

(NHS Digital, 2019)

Smoking tobacco is strongly linked to disease and early death.

Vaping tobacco

Heated tobacco products (HTPs)

Tobacco companies produce heated tobacco products (HTPs), sometimes called 'heat-not-burn' products. HTPs are battery powered devices that heat tobacco or a tobacco stick, capsule, plug or pod. The vapour is sucked and inhaled. The aim of these products is to provide an alternative way of consuming tobacco without inhaling smoke from burning tobacco. These tobacco products normally comprise

- tobacco heated directly to produce a vapour
- tobacco which is heated in a vaporiser
- devices that produce a vapour from non-tobacco sources, but the vapour is passed over tobacco to provide flavour

Some products have been found to include the burning of tobacco (McNeil, 2018; Sohal *et al.*, 2019).

Prevalence of vaping heated tobacco products

In 2017, a large survey of adults in Great Britain found that 9% were aware of HTPs, and less than 2% had used them (Brose *et al.*, 2018). In 2018, a survey in Japan showed 2.7% used HTPs at least monthly; 1.7% daily. Two-thirds of HTP users were also smoking cigarettes and 1% had never smoked cigarettes (Sutanto *et al.*, 2019).

Vaping heated tobacco products and health

Vaping tobacco produces mainstream, sidestream and environmental/second-hand emissions. As HTPs have not been available for long, most of the research to date has been produced by the tobacco industry and is not bias-free. McNeill and colleagues

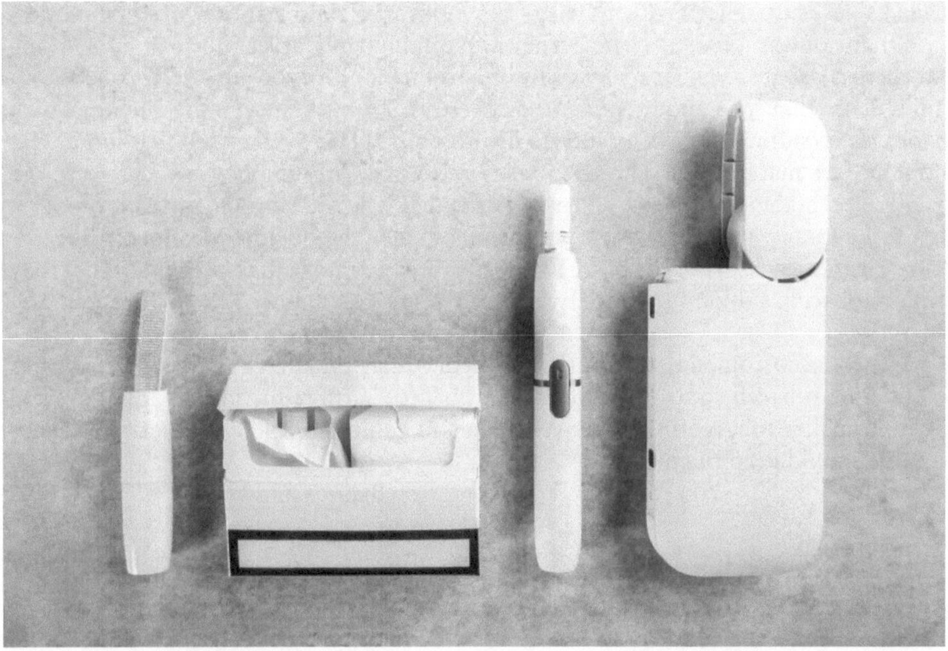

Figure 9.4 A heated tobacco device
Source: Anna Mente/Shutterstock.com

(2018) reviewed 20 studies, 12 of which were funded by the tobacco industry. Their key findings include

- there are a variety of HTPs, some of which heat tobacco and some also combust/burn it
- nicotine in the vapour reaches 70–84% of that in cigarette smoke
- HTPs deliver more nicotine in vapour than a cigalike e-cigarette and less nicotine than a tank-style e-cigarette
- when the consumer vapes the HTP freely, they absorb less nicotine into the body than cigarette users
- HTP users have a reduced urge to smoke tobacco
- cigarette smokers reported HTPs to be less rewarding than smoking a cigarette
- HTPs expose both users and bystanders to lower levels of potentially harmful chemicals than cigarette smoke
- HTP environmental emissions are probably more harmful compared to e-cigarettes

The World Health Organization (2019c) urges caution around the new HTPs.

- HTPs should be regulated like any other tobacco product
- HTPs produce toxic vapour, similar to the toxins found in cigarette smoke
- Users of HTPs are exposed to toxins in the mainstream vapour, and bystanders are exposed to toxins in second-hand vapour

The World Health Organization (2019c) warns that the tobacco industry's marketing of HTPs needs to be viewed with care. The industry claims that they are safer or less toxic than conventional cigarettes. They exploit any 'grey areas', for example noting that there is debate about *specific* forms of harm to confuse consumers. Tobacco companies claim that the vapour is *likely to cause less harm* than cigarette smoke, which is not clearly stating there is a reduced health risk. HTPs, such as IQOS, Ploom, Glo and PAX, are marketed as different to cigarettes, they are 'smoke-free' and therefore socially acceptable and environmentally friendly. They are promoted as a modern, high-tech, luxury product which complements a high-end lifestyle, much like the glossy cigarette adverts of the past. They sell a dream, rather than the reality that they contain tobacco, a toxic substance, whether it is smoked, eaten or vaped. In summary,

> The tobacco companies are using strategies that they have used for decades to fracture tobacco control and promote tobacco 'harm reduction' in an attempt to renormalize tobacco use ... Governments in countries where HTP are not available should keep them out.
>
> (Bialous and Glantz, 2018 p.s116)

Heated tobacco products are promoted as benign by the tobacco industry, but a public health danger by the World Health Organization.

Smokeless tobacco

Smokeless tobacco products

Tobacco products which are designed to be chewed or sniffed are often called smokeless tobacco. Chemicals such as nicotine are quickly absorbed into the blood stream through the mucous lining of the mouth or nasal passages. Chewing tobacco is normally made from tobacco leaves which are air cured and crushed, with added flavourings. Dipping is the process of holding the tobacco between the lip and the gum. Varieties include

- gutka – dried tobacco leaves, areca nut, slaked lime, catechu, flavourings and sweeteners
- mishri – burnt tobacco rubbed into gums, used for teeth cleaning
- nass/naswar/niswar – tobacco, ash, cotton or sesame oil and water, rolled into a ball
- snus – a Swedish form of snuff containing tobacco, moisturisers, sodium carbonate, salt, sweeteners and flavourings in small tea bags
- tambaku paan/betel quid – a combination of tobacco, areca nut and slaked lime folded into a betel leaf and chewed
- zarda – boiled and dried tobacco leaves with lime, spices, colourings, areca nut and flavourings

Varieties of sniffing tobacco include

- snuff – a mixture of finely ground tobacco that has been air or fire cured, with added flavourings and sometimes moistened with water

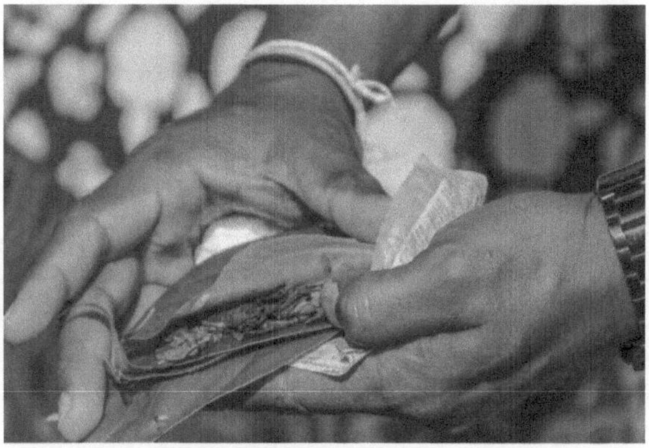

Figure 9.5 Betel quid
Source: D. Currin/Shutterstock.com

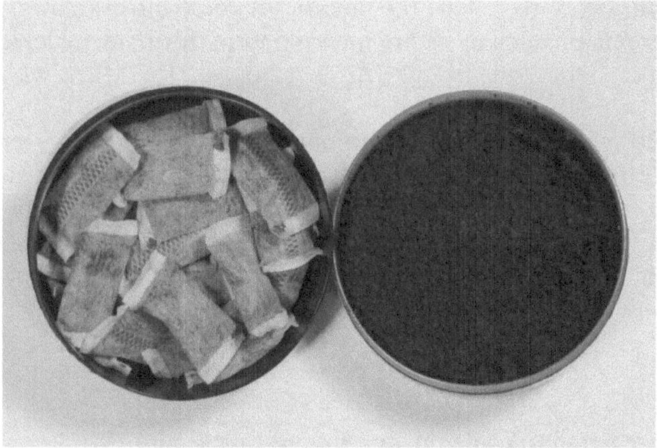

Figure 9.6 Swedish snus
Source: Adam Hoglund/Shutterstock.com

- creamy snuff – commercially produced paste of grounded tobacco, clove oil, glycerine, spearmint, menthol, camphor, salts and water
- snus – a powdered form of Swedish snuff
- toombak – a Sudanese form of snuff, which can also be eaten, contains tobacco, baking soda and water

Prevalence of using smokeless tobacco products

In 2016 there were 315,000 deaths across the world caused by smokeless tobacco, many of which were in South Asia (ACS/VS, 2019). In Great Britain, the most frequent consumers of smokeless tobacco products are ethnic minority groups, particularly people of South Asian origin.

Table 9.8 Ethnicity and use of smokeless tobacco in Great Britain, 2019

Use of smokeless tobacco	*White*	*Black/ African/ Caribbean*	*South Asian*				*Other/ mixed*
			All	*Indian*	*Bangladeshi*	*Pakistani*	
Ever tried	12%	19%	23%	16%	29%	21%	20%
Use at least monthly	1%	5%	7%	5%	12%	0%	3%
Never tried	86%	75%	64%	80%	68%	69%	75%

Source: Adapted from ASH (2019b p.4, 5).

Smokeless tobacco and health

Smokeless tobacco is consumed in a variety of forms with a range of additives. This lack of standardisation means that the health risks vary. Some of the most harmful compounds are the carcinogenic tobacco-specific nitrosamines. These can be 100 times higher in toombak than in plain chewing tobacco. Many tobacco products are now being processed in a way to reduce the amount of these nitrosamines, but other harmful components remain such as cadmium, polonium, formaldehyde, lead, polycyclic aromatic hydrocarbons and arsenic (Arain *et al.*, 2015; Mathews and Krishnan, 2019).

Fisher and colleagues (2019) compared the health of those who smoked cigarettes, consumers of smokeless tobacco and consumers of both. They found significantly higher risks of death from many causes including heart disease, cerebrovascular disease, cancer, respiratory disease, influenza and pneumonia, among the smokers and those who consumed both, compared to those who only used smokeless products. However, smokeless tobacco is associated with serious health risks for oral health. These include

- oral cancer
- leukoplakia, thick white patches inside the mouth, pre-cancerous
- erythroplakia, red area or red spots in the mouth, pre-cancerous
- oral submucous fibrosis (if tobacco is mixed with areca nut), progressive inflammation and fibrosing of the mouth which eventually leads to an inability to open the mouth, pre-cancerous
- staining of teeth
- increased dental caries and tooth loss (especially where tobacco has sweetening additives)
- recession of gums and inflammation

(Muthukrishnan and Warnakulasuriya, 2018)

Mishri is commonly used in India, where it has been linked to complications in pregnancy and raised numbers of still births (Pratinidhi *et al.*, 2010). Kakrani and colleagues (2015) carried out research, in a rural area of India, with 256 females aged 10 years and over who used mishri. A third had started using mishri before they reached 10 years old. Two-thirds used mishri to clean their teeth and rubbed it into their gums. They used it to get energy (16.8%), to relieve tension (12.9%), for time to pass (19.5%) and to get a kick (5.5%). Almost half (43.7%) had no awareness that the product was harmful to health.

> *Smokeless tobacco causes serious health problems, including oral cancer.*

Thinking point:

> How much should governments impose restrictions on the consumption of tobacco? Is it right that they restrict adults' freedom to make choices about their own health?

Non-tobacco products

In Great Britain, the prevalence of tobacco smokers has been falling for four decades while the numbers of people who have quit smoking has been steadily rising over the same period (ONS, 2019). This can be attributed to much greater awareness of the harmful effects of tobacco, legislation to ban smoking in pubic places, the introduction of widespread smoking cessation services, the use of nicotine-replacement therapy and the rise of vaping with electronic cigarettes which do not contain tobacco.

Nicotine-replacement therapy

Addiction to nicotine is often the reason that people keep smoking, sniffing or chewing tobacco. Nicotine-replacement therapy provides nicotine without the other harmful chemicals in tobacco. Products contain much lower levels of nicotine than tobacco and are normally provided as a course for up to 12 weeks because this is the time that it takes for the brain to adjust. Nicotine withdrawal symptoms include restlessness, irritability, frustration, tiredness, headaches, difficulty in sleeping and poor concentration. Nicotine cravings are usually at their worst during the first couple of weeks, but thereafter they become less frequent. Nicotine-replacement products, licensed in the UK as medicines, include

- gums
- inhalators
- lozenges
- microtabs, very small tablets which dissolve under the tongue
- nasal sprays
- patches
- tablets such a varenicline or bupropion

Electronic nicotine delivery systems (ENDS), e-cigarettes, are licensed in the UK as consumer products. It is illegal to sell these to under-18s or on behalf of under-18s, and advertising is limited. Products containing more than 20 mg per ml of nicotine cannot be sold without a medicinal licence.

Nicotine is much less harmful than tobacco, but it is not harmless. Short-term use of nicotine does little harm, aside from addiction (McNeill *et al.*, 2018). Longer-term use is associated with some cancers and damage to all the systems of the body, including cardiovascular, gastrointestinal, respiratory, immunological, renal and reproductive systems (Mishra *et al.*, 2015). Nicotine-replacement therapy alongside the face-to-face support and the expertise of smoking cessation services is the most effective way of transitioning from tobacco to low levels of nicotine to nothing (PHE, 2019).

Vaping non-tobacco products: e-cigarettes

Devices produced to replace cigarettes initially looked like cigarettes and were called electronic cigarettes, e-cigarettes. These battery-powered devices heat liquid to produce a vapour that can be inhaled. There are broadly two types

- electronic nicotine delivery systems (ENDS) – the liquid contains nicotine
- electronic non-nicotine delivery systems (ENNDS) – the liquid does not contain nicotine

Both may contain other toxic chemicals in the e-liquid.

Common battery-powered devices include

- one-time disposable products, sometimes called cigalikes
- reusable, rechargeable kits containing replaceable pods or cartridges
- reusable, rechargeable kits that allow the user to refill the liquid, sometimes called tanks or refillable pods
- reusable, rechargeable kits that enable the user to regulate the battery power

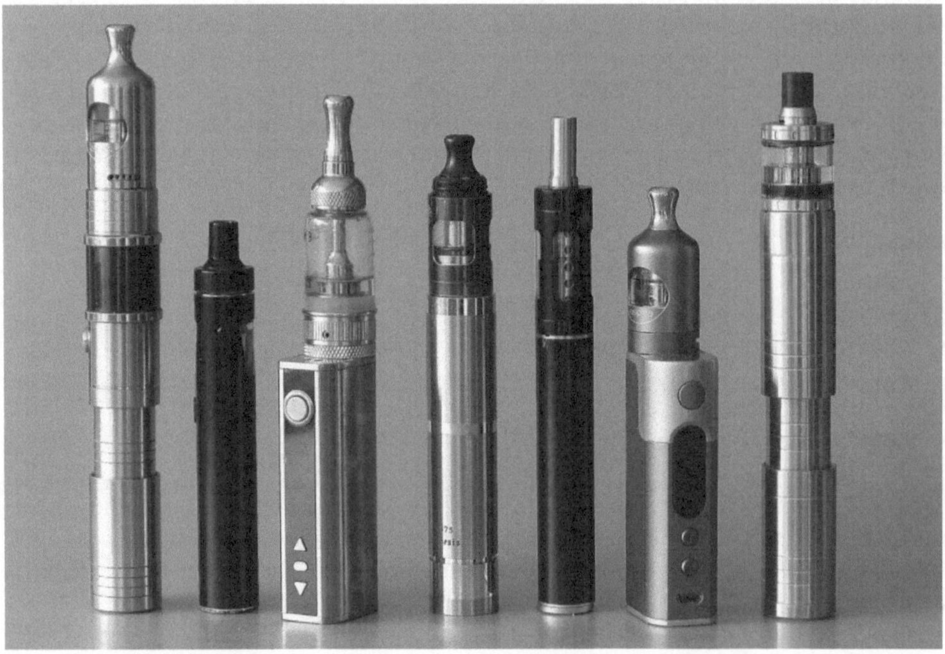

Figure 9.7 E-cigarettes
Source: Mano Kors/Shutterstock.com

Table 9.9 Reasons for vaping e-cigarettes in Great Britain, 2019 (n = 854)

Reasons for vaping	*Agree*	*Don't know*	*Disagree*
Health is my number one reason for taking up e-cigarettes	60%	26%	14%
I get a great deal of pleasure from vaping	51%	36%	12%
E-cigarettes have improved my quality of life	51%	37%	12%
Vaping is not a magic solution for stopping smoking	50%	24%	26%
Vaping is a medicine that I use in order to address my smoking addiction	50%	31%	20%
Lowering the levels of nicotine I consume through vaping is a priority for me	44%	34%	22%

Source: Adapted from ASH (2019c p.6).

Their design may resemble a memory-stick, pebble or pen, and other designs within box mods (modified vaporisers containing relatively larger batteries).

Prevalence of vaping e-cigarettes

The Office of National Statistics (2019) reported 6.3% of the British population, between 2.8 and 3.6 million people, were vaping with e-cigarettes in 2018. This was a significant increase compared to 2014. Men vaped more than women and the highest proportion of vapers were between 35 and 49 years old.

Reasons for vaping e-cigarettes

Many people vape e-cigarettes to help them to stop tobacco smoking, to cut down on smoking, to save money and because they enjoy it (ASH, 2019c) (Table 9.9).

Non-tobacco-products and health

Electronic nicotine delivery systems (ENDS)

Vaping with electronic nicotine delivery systems (ENDS) is encouraged as a form of short-term nicotine-replacement therapy, with a view to it being safer than tobacco for both the user and bystanders, and a step towards giving up nicotine completely. In addition to nicotine, e-liquid contains propylene glycol and glycerine, which, if overheated, can produce poisonous aldehydes. The flavourings appear to be safe and the small quantities of metal in the vapour are deemed too low to present a health risk.

Concerns about ENDS include

- perceptions that ENDS are as harmful as tobacco smoking, which they are not
- an increasing number of people who have never smoked tobacco are taking up ENDS, thus making them vulnerable to harms from nicotine
- over 80% of vapers in England use ENDS as opposed to healthier ENNDS
- many people use ENDS while continuing to smoke tobacco

(McNeill *et al.*, 2019; ASH, 2018b; 2019c; Robertson *et al.*, 2019)

Electronic non-nicotine delivery systems (ENNDS)

Vaping with e-liquid that does not contain nicotine is the healthiest choice, provided it is not overheated or ingested. There have been occasional accidents such as fire caused by the electrical elements of e-cigarettes, and users should not leave e-cigarettes charging overnight (ASH, 2018b).

> *Nicotine is a harmful, addictive substance, but does not contain the toxic chemicals found in tobacco. A product containing neither tobacco nor nicotine presents few health concerns.*

Benefits of quitting tobacco

Within the body, the benefits of quitting smoking tobacco begin after

- 20 minutes – the body begins to recover; the heart rate and blood pressure return to normal
- 8 hours – no nicotine in the body and cravings begin, which is where nicotine replacement is helpful. Coughing is the lungs trying to expel mucous.
- 24 hours – no carbon monoxide in the body, anxiety/stress levels are at their peak as a result of withdrawal, nicotine replacement is helpful
- 72 hours – breathing improves, airways relax, energy levels increase, food starts to smell and taste better
- One week – the worst withdrawal symptoms are over, but coughing may persist
- Two weeks – blood circulation, especially to teeth and gums, returns to normal and gum disease starts to heal
- One month – improved skin and hair, any residual anxiety goes
- Two months – lungs are working better, breathlessness is reduced
- Three months – cough is much improved
- Three to nine months – coughing, wheezing and breathing continue to improve as lungs heal and begin to work better
- One year – risk of heart attack falls to half of what it was as a smoker
- Five years – risk of type 2 diabetes is the same as a non-smoker
- Five to 10 years – circulation is much improved and the risk of having a stroke is the same as a non-smoker
- 10 years – risk of lung cancer falls to half of what it was as a smoker, and the risks of other cancers have reduced significantly
- 15 years – risk of heart attack is the same as someone who has never smoked

(NHS Lothian, 2014; ASH Wales, undated)

Those who quit smokeless tobacco will experience

- the symptoms of nicotine withdrawal for up to three days (anger, anxiety, stress, insomnia, headaches etc.)
- mouth sores will heal
- reduction in stained teeth

- breath smells better
- reduced risk of all smokeless tobacco-related diseases

(NCI, 2018; Mutukrishnan and Warnakulasuriya, 2018)

Some people gain weight because nicotine speeds up metabolism, food tastes better and food replaces one oral habit for another. Smokers who transfer to nicotine-replacement products have been shown to gain less weight (Wawryk-Gawda *et al.*, 2019), and one study suggested that the best combinations for both success at quitting smoking and the least weight gain were the nicotine patch 14 mg plus fluoxetine 40 mg, nicotine patch 14 mg plus fluoxetine 20 mg, or topiramate 200 mg (Hseih *et al.*, 2019).

Additional benefits of stopping tobacco smoking include reducing the chances of impotence, miscarriage, difficulties with getting pregnant, having premature babies or babies of low birth weight as well as reducing the risks to others from second-hand smoke (WHO, 2019d). Former smokers in Brazil (Zampier *et al.*, 2017) summed up their feelings:

> That terrible smell in my mouth and in my hair ... Now I am different.
>
> (p.4)

> I feel as if I have another body, my strength has changed.
>
> (p.3,4)

> Cash in my pocket improved a lot ... cigarettes cost money.
>
> (p.5)

> My life has changed one hundred percent, really!
>
> (p.6)

Summary

This chapter has

- described the rise and influence of the tobacco industry and its products
- explained who consumes tobacco, why and how
- shown how tobacco causes diseases that contribute to inequalities in health and early death
- discussed nicotine replacement as a short-term aid to quitting tobacco
- compared two types of e-cigarettes and their pros and cons for health
- presented the health benefits of quitting tobacco

Further reading

Milov, S. (2019) *The cigarette: a political history*. Cambridge, MA: Harvard University Press

Pickworth, W.B. (ed) (2020) *Smokeless tobacco products: characteristics, usage, health effects and regulatory implications*. London: Elsevier

World Health Organization (2019) *WHO report on the global tobacco epidemic, 2019*. Geneva: World Health Organization

Useful websites

Action on Smoking and Health. Available at: https://ash.org.uk
American Cancer Society/Vital Strategies *The Tobacco Atlas*. Available at: https://tobaccoatlas.org
World Health Organization *Tobacco*. Available at: www.who.int/health-topics/tobacco

References

Action on Smoking and Health (2018a) What's in a cigarette? Available at: https://ash.org.uk/information-and-resources/fact-sheets/whats-in-a-cigarette (Accessed 7th January 2020)

Action on Smoking and Health (2018b) Briefing: electronic cigarettes. Available at: https://ash.org.uk/wp-content/uploads/2019/04/E-Cigarettes-Briefing_PDF_v1.pdf (Accessed 7th January 2020)

Action on Smoking and Health (2019a) Smoking and mental health. Available at: https://ash.org.uk/wp-content/uploads/2019/08/ASH-Factsheet_Mental-Health_v3-2019-27-August-1.pdf (Accessed 7th January 2020)

Action on Smoking and Health (2019b) Tobacco and ethnic minorities. Available at: https://ash.org.uk/wp-content/uploads/2019/08/ASH-Factsheet_Ethnic-Minorities-Final-Final.pdf (Accessed 7th January 2020)

Action on Smoking and Health (2019c) Use of e-cigarettes (vaporisers) among adults in Great Britain. Available at: https://ash.org.uk/wp-content/uploads/2019/09/Use-of-e-cigarettes-among-adults-2019.pdf (Accessed 7th January 2020)

Action on Smoking and Health Wales (undated) Quitting smoking timeline. Available at: https://ash.wales/what-happens-hours-days-years-after-you-quit-smoking/ (Accessed 7th January 2020)

American Cancer Society/Vital Strategies (2019) The tobacco atlas. Available at: https://tobaccoatlas.org/ (Accessed 7th January 2020)

American Lung Association (2019) What's in a cigarette? Available at www.lung.org/stop-smoking/smoking-facts/whats-in-a-cigarette.html (Accessed 7th January 2020)

Arain, S.S., Kazi, T.G., Afridi, H.I., Talpur, F.N., Kazi, A.G., Brahman, K.D., Naeemullah, K., Panhwar, A., and Kamboh, M. (2015) 'Correlation of arsenic levels in smokeless tobacco products and biological samples of oral cancer patients and control consumers', *Biological Trace Element Research*, 168(2), pp.287–295

Bellis, M., Ashton, K., Hughes, K., Ford, K., Bishop, J., and Paranjothy, S. (2015) *Adverse childhood experiences and their impact on health-harming behaviours in the Welsh adult population*. Cardiff: Public Health Wales

Bialous, S.A., and Glantz, S.A. (2018) 'Heated tobacco products: another tobacco industry global strategy to slow progress on tobacco control', *Tobacco Control*, 27 doi:10.1136/tobaccocontrol-2018–054340

Brandt, A.M. (2012) 'Inventing conflicts of interest: a history of tobacco industry tactics', *American Journal of Public Health*, 102(1), pp.63–71

British Heart Foundation (2020) Shisha. Available at: www.bhf.org.uk/informationsupport/risk-factors/smoking/shisha (Accessed 7th January 2020)

Brose, L.S., Simonavicus, E., and Cheeseman, H. (2018) 'Awareness of "heat-not-burn" tobacco products in Great Britain', *Tobacco Regulatory Science*, 4(2) doi.org/10.18001/TRS.4.2.4

Centres for Disease Control and Prevention (2020) *Adverse childhood experiences (ACEs)*. Available at: www.cdc.gov/violenceprevention/acestudy/index.html (Accessed 5th September 2020)

Clancy, N., Zwar, N., and Richmond, R. (2013) 'Depression, smoking and smoking cessation: a qualitative study', *Family Practice*, 30(5), pp.587–592

Delaney, H., MacGregor, A., and Amos, A. (2018) '"Tell them you smoke, you'll get more breaks": a qualitative study of occupational and social context of young adult smoking in Scotland', *BMJ Open*, 8(12) doi:10.1136/bmjopen-2018–023951

Doll, R., and Hill, A. (1950) 'Smoking and carcinoma of the lung', *British Medical Journal*, 2(4682), pp.739–748

Doll, R., and Hill, A. (1954) 'The mortality of doctors in relation to their smoking habits', *British Medical Journal*, 1(4877), pp.1451–1455

Fisher, M.T., Tan-Torres, S.M., Gaworski, C.L., Black, R.A., and Sarkar, M.A. (2019) 'Smokeless tobacco mortality risks: an analysis of two contemporary nationally representative longitudinal mortality studies', *Harm Reduction Journal*, 16(27) doi:10.1186/s12954-019-0294-6

Goldenberg, M., Danovitch, I., and IsHak, W.W. (2014) 'Quality of life and smoking', *The American Journal of Addictions*, 23(6), pp.540–562

Hall, S., Legault, A., and Côté, J. (2010) 'Dying means suffocating: perceptions of people living with severe COPD facing the end of life', *International Journal of Palliative Nursing*, 16 (9), pp.451–457

Hsieh, M.T., Tseng, P.T., Wu, Y.C., Tu, Y.K., Wu, H.C., Hsu, C.W., Lei, W.T., Stubbs, B., Carvalho, A.F., Liang, C.S., Yeh, T.C., Chen, T.Y., Chu, C.S., Li, J.C., Yu, C.L., Chen, Y.W., and Li, D.J. (2019) 'Effects of different pharmacologic smoking cessation treatments on body weight changes and success rates in patients with nicotine dependence. A network meta-analysis', *Obesity Review*, 20(6), pp.895–905

Kadhum, M., Sweidan, A., Jaffery, A., Al-Saadi, A., and Madden, B. (2015) 'A review of the health effects smoking shisha', *Clinical Medicine*, 15(3), pp.263–266

Kakrani, V.A., Kulkarni, P.Y, Khedkar, D.T., and Bhawalkar, J.S. (2015) 'Perceptions and practices of smokeless tobacco use in the form of mishri among rural women above 10 years of age in Pune, Maharashtra, India', *International Journal of Medicine and Public Health*, 5(2), pp.173–178

Lindqvist, G., Albin, B., Heikkilä, K., and Hjelm, K. (2013) 'Conceptions of daily life in women living with a man suffering from chronic obstructive pulmonary disease', *Primary Health Care Research & Development*, 14(2), pp.40–51

Marcon, A., Pesce, G., Calciano, L., Bellisario, V., Dharmage, S.C., Garcia-Aymerich, J., Gislasson, T., Heinrich, J., Holm, M., Janson, C., Jarvis, D., Leynaert, B., Matheson, M.C., Pirina, P., Svanes, C., Villani, S., Zuberbier, T., Minelli, C., and Accordini, S. (2018) 'Trends in smoking initiation in Europe over 40 years: a retrospective cohort study', *Plos One*, 3(8) doi.org/101371/journal.pone.0201881

Mathews, L.M., and Krishnan, M. (2019) 'Oral cancer and smokeless tobacco – a review', *Drug Intervention Today*, 12(6), pp.1239–1243

McNeill, A., Brose, L.S., Calder, R., Bauld, L., and Robson, D. (2018) *Evidence review of e-cigarettes and heated tobacco products 2018*. London: Public Health England

McNeill, A., Brose, L.S., Calder, R., Bauld, L., and Robson, D. (2019) *Vaping in England: an evidence update February 2019*. London: Public Health England

Michon, K. (2019) Tobacco litigation: history and recent developments. Available at: www.nolo.com/legal-encyclopedia/tobacco-litigation-history-and-development-32202.html (Accessed 7th January 2020)

Mishra, A., Chaturvedi, P., Datta, S., Sinukumar, S., Poonam, J., and Garg, A. (2015) 'Harmful effects of nicotine', *Indian Journal of Medical and Paediatric Oncology*, 36(1) pp.24–31

Muthukrishnan, A., and Warnakulasuriya, S. (2018) 'Oral health consequences of smokeless tobacco use', *Indian Journal of Medical Research*, 148(1), pp.35–40

National Cancer Institute (2018) Smokeless tobacco and health risks. Available at: www.oncolink.org/risk-and-prevention/smoking-tobacco-and-cancer/smokeless-tobacco-and-health-risks (Accessed 3rd January 2020)

NHS Digital (2019) Statistics on Smoking England: 2019. Available at: https://digital.nhs.uk/data-and-information/publications/statistical/statistics-on-smoking/statistics-on-smoking-england-2019 (Accessed 7th January 2020)

NHS Lothian (2014) Your path to a smokefree life. Available at: www.nhslothian.scot.nhs.uk/HealthInformation/HealthAwareness/Smoking/Documents/SmokeFreeLife.pdf (Accessed 7th January 2020)

NHS.UK (2019a) Smokefree. How smoking affects your body. Available at: www.nhs.uk/smokefree/why-quit/smoking-health-problems (Accessed 7th January 2020)

NHS.UK (2019b) *Health A to Z*. Available at: www.nhs.uk/conditions (Accessed 7th January 2020)

O'Connor, R. (2012) 'Non-cigarette tobacco products: what have we learned and where are we headed', *Tobacco Control*, 21(2), pp.181–190

Office for National Statistics (2019) Adult smoking habits in the UK: 2018. Available at: www.ons.gov.uk/peoplepopulationandcommunity/healthandsocialcare/healthandlifeexpectancies/bulletins/adultsmokinghabitsingreatbritain/2018 (Accessed 7th January 2020)

Paul, C.L., Ross, S., Bryant, J., Hill, W., Bonevski, B., and Keevy, N. (2010) 'The social context of smoking: a qualitative study comparing smokers of high versus low socioeconomic position', *BMC Public Health*, 10(1) doi:10.1186/1471-2458-10-211

Ports, K.A., Holman, D.M., Guinn, A.S., Pampati, S., Dyer, K.E., Merrick, M.T., Buchanan Lunsford, N., and Metzler, M. (2018) 'Adverse childhood experiences and the presence of cancer risk factors in adulthood: a scoping review of the literature from 2005 to 2015', *Journal of Pediatric Nursing*, 44(2019), pp.81–96

Pratinidhi, A., Gandham, S., Shrotri, A., Patil, A., and Pardeshi, S. (2010) 'Use of "mishri" a smokeless form of tobacco during pregnancy and its perinatal outcome', *Indian Journal of Community Medicine*, 35(1) doi: 10.4103/0970-0218.62547

Public Health England (2019) *Health matters: stopping smoking – what works?* Available at: www.gov.uk/government/publications/health-matters-stopping-smoking-what-works/health-matters-stopping-smoking-what-works (Accessed 7th January 2020)

Ravenholt. R.T. (1990) 'Tobacco's global death march', *Population and Developmental Review*, 16(2), pp.213–240

Robertson, L., Hoek, J. Blank, M.L., Richards, R., Ling, P., and Popova, L. (2019) 'Dual use of electronic nicotine delivery systems (ENDS) and smoked tobacco: a qualitative analysis', *Tobacco Control*, 28(1), pp.13–19

Simonavicius, E., Robson, D., McEwen, A., and Brose, L.S. (2017) 'Cessation support for smokers with mental health problems: a survey of resources and training needs', *Journal of Substance Abuse Treatment*, 80 doi:10.1016/j.jsat.2017.06.008

Sohal, S.S., Eapen, M.S., Naidu, V.G.M., and Sharma, P. (2019) 'IQOS exposure impairs human airway cell homeostasis: direct comparison with traditional cigarette and e-cigarette', *ERJ Open Research*, 5(1) doi:10.1183/23120541.00159-2018

Song, M., Benowitz, N.L., Berman, M., Brasky, T.M., Cummings, K.M., Hatsukami, D.K., Marian, C., O'Connor, R., Rees, V.W., Woroszylo, C., and Shields, P.G. (2017) 'Cigarette filter ventilation and its relationship to increasing rates of lung adenocarcinoma', *Journal of the National Cancer Institute*, 109(12) doi:10.1093/jnci/djx075

Sutanto, E., Miller C., Smith, D.M., O'Connor, R.J., Quah, A.C.K., Cummings, K.M., Xu, S., Fong, G.T., Hyland, A., Ouimet, J., Itsuro, Y., Mochizuki, Y., Tabuchi, T., and Goniewicz, M.L. (2019) 'Prevalence, use behaviors, and preferences among users of heated tobacco products: findings from the 2018 ITC Japan survey', *International Journal of Environmental Research and Public Health*, 16(4630) doi:103390/ijerph16234630

Twyman, L, Cowles, C., Walsberger, S.C., Baker, A.L., Bonevski, B., and the Tackling Tobacco Mental Health Advisory Group (2019) '"They're going to smoke anyway": a qualitative study of community mental health staff and consumer perspectives on the role of social and living environments in tobacco use and cessation', *Frontiers in Psychiatry*, 10(503) doi:10.3389/fpsyt2019.00503

Viegas C.A. (2009) 'Noncigarette forms of tobacco use', *Jornal Brasileiro de Pneumologia: publicaçāo official de Sociedade Brasleira de Phneumologia e Tisilogia*, 34(12), pp.1069–1073

Warnoff, C., Lekander, M., Hemmingsson, T., Sorgonen, K., Melin, B., and Andreasson, A. (2016) 'Is poor self-rated health associated with low-grade inflammation in 43,100 late adolescent men? A cross-sectional study', *BMJ Open*, 6 doi:10.1136/bmjopen-2015–009440

Wawryk-Gawda, E., Zarobkiewicz, M.K., Chylińska-Wrzos, P., and Jodłowska-Jędrych, B. (2019) 'Lower weight gain after vaping cessation than after smoking quitting', *Annals of the National Institute of Hygiene*, 70(3), pp.253–258

World Health Organization (2003) *WHO framework convention on tobacco control*. Geneva: World Health Organization

World Health Organization (2019a) Tobacco. Available at: www.who.int/news-room/fact-sheets/detail/tobacco (Accessed 7th January 2020)

World Health Organization (2019b) Tobacco explained. The truth about the tobacco industry ... in its own words. Available at: www.who.int/tobacco/media/en/TobaccoExplained.pdf (Accessed 7th January 2020)

World Health Organization (2019c) *WHO Report on the global tobacco epidemic, 2019*. Geneva: World Health Organization

World Health Organization (2019d) Fact sheet about health benefits of smoking cessation. Available at: www.who.int/tobacco/quitting/benefits/en/ (Accessed 7th January 2020)

Zampier, V.S.B., Silva, M.H., Jesus, R.R., Oliveira, P.P., Jesus, M.C.P., and Merighi, M.A.B. (2017) 'Maintenance of tobacco withdrawal by former smokers: a phenomenological study', *Revista Gaúcha de Enfermagem*, 38(4) doi:10.1590/1983-1447.2017.04.2017-0027

10 Alcohol and health

Joanne Cairns and Sally Robinson

Key points

- Introduction
- Alcohol
- History of alcohol use
- Alcohol and health
- Measuring and defining alcohol use
- Trends and inequalities in alcohol consumption
- Reasons why people use and misuse alcohol
- Benefits of abstinence or drinking within recommended guidelines
- Summary

Introduction

This chapter explains how alcohol, and concerns about alcohol, have a long history. We describe how alcohol affects physical, mental, emotional, sexual, social and societal health. We will define the terminology that is used to describe alcohol use and alcohol misuse, and we will explain the criteria used to assess whether someone's drinking has become problematic. The trends and patterns of alcohol consumption in the UK will be presented. We end the chapter by considering the reasons why people use and misuse alcohol, including the role of the alcohol industry, and the benefits of reducing or giving up alcohol.

Alcohol

Alcohol, also called ethanol, is formed when yeast ferments sugars, such as those found in grapes for wine or apples for cider. The Office for National Statistics (2018a) reports beer (£27.6 billion) and wine (£17.8 billion) as the highest-selling alcoholic drinks in Europe. The UK is the second largest producer of beer (£3.7 billion) and the highest producer of whisky (£3.4 billion). While sales of beer have been falling, sales of gin grew 267% between 2009 and 2017, and the UK now produces three-quarters of all gin sales across Europe.

Alcoholic drinks are produced, marketed and sold by the alcohol industry who

- present alcohol as an important, desirable, valuable and legitimate product that is a normal part of modern life

- present the alcohol industry as trustworthy and benign; any regulation is unnecessary because alcohol is associated with health and wellbeing, and alcohol-related problems are caused by a minority of irresponsible drinkers
- work to embed alcohol into everyday life such as festivals, pubs, concerts, dining and through sponsorship of popular events such as sport

(Pettigrew *et al.*, 2018)

Alcohol is a psychoactive drug, meaning that it affects the brain and nervous system, and changes a person's mental state. Alcohol is a toxic substance, it kills cells, which is why it is used to sterilise and preserve food. The harm caused by alcohol, to the individual and to others, depends on the volume, frequency and quality of alcohol consumed. It is harmful because it

- directly poisons the body
- causes poor health and conditions that can be fatal
- contributes to accidents and injuries
- contributes to violent deaths and suicides
- harms other people
- causes wider social and economic problems

(PHE, 2016a)

History of alcohol use

The discovery of beer jugs from the Stone Age suggests that alcohol is likely to have been around a very long time (in 1967, the Flintstones cartoon characters were used to promote a brand of beer). According to one American professor, the cultivation of cereals during the Neolithic Revolution of around 10,000 BC may have been initially used for producing beer rather than flour (Braidwood *et al.*, 1953). Public health concerns about alcohol also have a long history. In the eighteenth century, the English painter and engraver William Hogarth depicted 'Beer Street' (Figure 10.1) as a place of economic prosperity and virtue. 'Gin Lane' (Figure 10.2) portrayed social disorder, vice and moral iniquity, reflecting the growing concerns about the Gin Craze at the time. Reverend James Townley, a friend and collaborator of Hogarth, wrote a poem to highlight some of the personal and societal consequences of gin consumption (Box 10.1).

Box 10.1 Gin Lane

Gin cursed Friend, with Fury fraught,
Makes human race a Prey;
It enters by a deadly Draught,
And steals our Life away.
Virtue and Truth, driv'n to Despair,
It's Rage compells to fly,
But cherishes, with hellish Care,
Theft, Murder, Perjury.
Damn'd Cup! that on the vitals preys,

That liquid Fire contains
Which madness to the Heart Conveys
And rolls it thro' the Veins.
(Source: James Townley, 1751 https://en.wikisource.org/wiki/Gin_Lane made available under a CC BY-SA 3.0 licence)

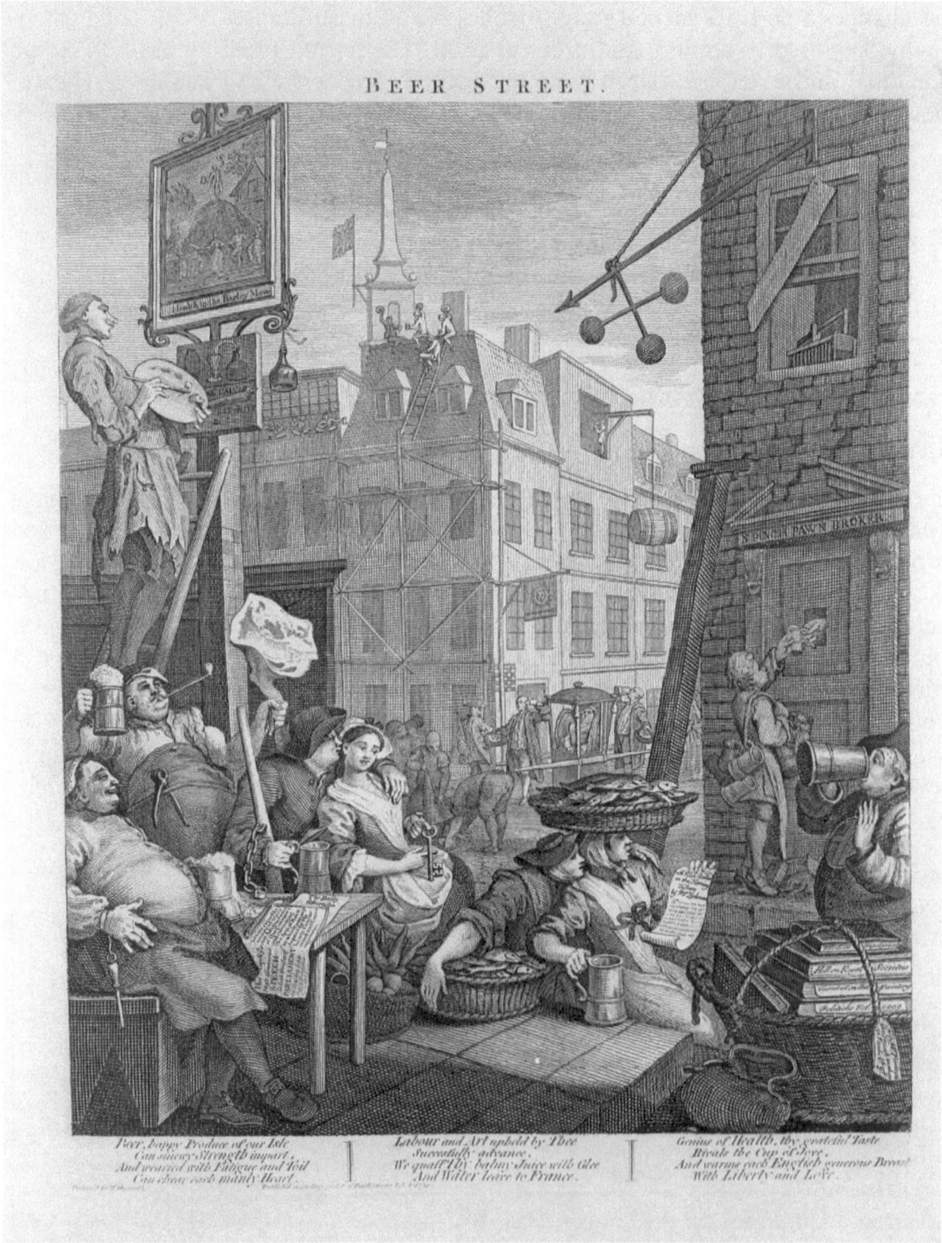

Figure 10.1 Beer Street by William Hogarth, 1751

Source: Wellcome Collection made available under a CC BY 4.0 licence https://creativecommons.org/licenses/by/4.0/

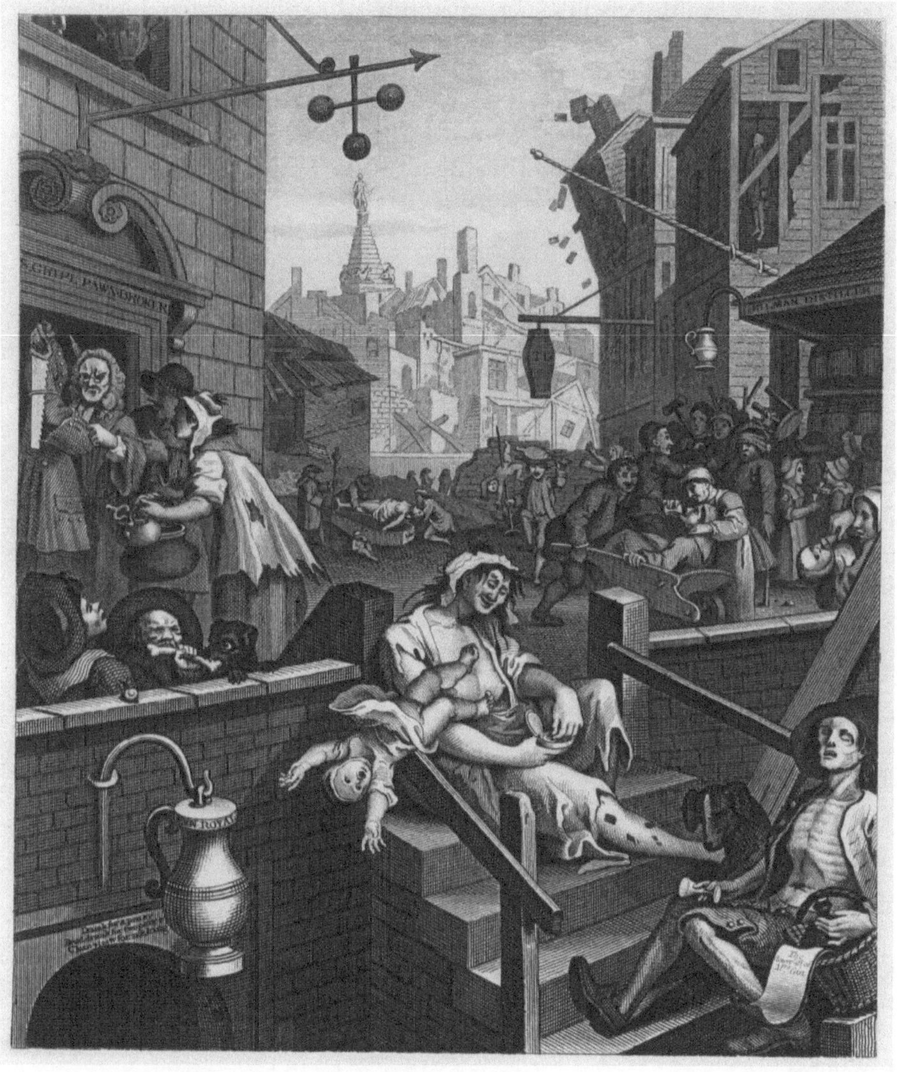

Figure 10.2 Gin Lane by William Hogarth, 1751

Source: Samuel Davenport, a re-engraving of William Hogarth's original, completed in 1806 to 1809, https://commons.wikimedia.org/wiki/File:William_Hogarth_-_Gin_Lane.jpg made available under a CC BY-SA 3.0 licence https://creativecommons.org/licenses/by-sa/3.0/

> *Throughout history, alcohol has been portrayed as a public asset and a public harm.*

Alcohol and health

Mortality and morbidity

Although individual research studies suggest that alcohol can be beneficial to people's health, reviewers of the whole body of evidence conclude that the harms from alcohol far outweigh any small gains (WHO, 2018; PHE, 2016a). The only exception seems to be women over the age of around 55 years, who may, on balance, gain some health benefits such as improved cardiovascular functioning, from light alcohol intakes of about five units per week (Sun *et al.*, 2011; Holmes *et al.*, 2016). The World Health Organization (2018) reported three million alcohol-related deaths across the world during 2016. This was 5.3% of all deaths, and a tenth of deaths in Europe. A quarter of these deaths were due to injuries and a fifth were due to cardiovascular and digestive diseases. In England, 358,000 hospital admissions were attributed to alcohol during 2018–2019 (NHS Digital, 2020). To summarise,

> Alcohol is a colossal global health issue and small reductions in health-related harms at low levels of alcohol intake are outweighed by the increased risk of other health-related harms, including cancer.
>
> (Burton and Sheron, 2018 p.987)

Alcohol and physical health

An individual's reaction to alcohol differs according to their age, sex, ethnicity, the proportion of fat to muscle in their body, the state of their liver, whether there is food in their stomach, how quickly it is drunk and how often the person drinks alcohol.

Alcohol and the body

Alcohol affects all parts of the body. Here is a summary of the immediate effects and the long-term effects from heavier or chronic alcohol consumption (AACNZ, 2012).

BRAIN AND NERVOUS SYSTEM

Immediate

- alcohol is a depressant which slows down the central nervous system
- impairs judgement
- loss of inhibitions and concentration
- drowsiness
- interferes with the process of laying down memories

Long term

- brain damage because alcohol is associated with the poor absorption of thiamine (vitamin B1). Thiamine deficiency causes a form of encephalopathy, which includes abnormal or paralysed eye movements and memory problems, and can be fatal
- cerebellum damage leads to problems with balance and walking
- increased risk of a cerebrovascular accidents (strokes) caused by bleeding in the brain
- peripheral nerve damage means that legs, toes, arms and hands become numb and insensitive

- if alcohol is used to treat insomnia, individuals are likely to become tolerant to it, leading to greater use of alcohol

MUSCLES AND BONES

Immediate

- impairs thinking and coordination, leading to clumsiness and injuries such as bruises, cuts and broken bones

Long term

- poor absorption of calcium, affecting bone strength, and leading to osteoporosis (brittle bones)
- osteonecrosis (bone death)
- gout (type of arthritis)
- muscle wasting and weakness

IMMUNE SYSTEM

Long term

- suppression of immune system, which is important for fighting infections

BLOOD

Immediate

The amount of alcohol in someone's blood, their blood alcohol concentration, will affect the types of symptoms they experience.

Table 10.1 The impact of blood alcohol concentration on a person

Blood alcohol concentration	*Individual signs and symptoms*
Less than 50 mg/dl	Talkative, relaxed, some impairment of physical coordination and thinking
50–150 mg/dl	Altered mood, e.g. well-being, unhappiness, shyness, argumentativeness, friendliness Impaired judgement and concentration Sexual disinhibition
150–250 mg/dl	Mood, personality and behaviour changes which may be sudden, angry and antisocial Slurred speech, drowsiness, unsteady walking Nausea, double vision, increased heart rate
300 mg/dl	Extremely drowsy, unresponsive Incoherent speech, confusion, memory loss Heavy breathing, vomiting
More than 400 mg/dl	Breathing shallow, slowed or stopped Coma or death

Source: Adapted from AACNZ (2012 p.6).

Long term

- blood abnormalities which lead to anaemia (shortness of breath, fatigue, dizziness) and low platelets, which are necessary for blood clotting

HEART AND BLOOD PRESSURE

Long term

- increased risks of coronary artery disease, irregular heartbeats, and cardiomyopathy (disease of the heart muscle), which leads to heart failure which is ultimately fatal
- high blood pressure

MOUTH AND THROAT

Immediate

- affects speech in accordance with mood changes

Long term

- increase risks of cancer of the mouth, throat, pharynx (upper throat) and larynx (voice box)

LUNGS

Immediate

- drowsiness and relaxation of the mouth and throat suppresses gagging and cough reflexes. Vomit and saliva become hard to clear and enter lungs, causing inflammation and infection which can lead to pneumonia

Long term

- pneumonia
- tuberculosis
- acute respiratory distress syndrome

OESOPHAGUS AND STOMACH

Immediate

- nausea, vomiting and diarrhoea leads to dehydration and chemical imbalance
- vomiting increases risks of heartburn (acid reflux from stomach), tearing the oesophagus, inhalation leading to lung infections and blockage of the airway causing breathing to stop
- heartburn (acid reflux from stomach into oesophagus) and gastritis (inflammation of stomach lining)

Long term

- cancer of the oesophagus (food pipe)
- oesophageal varices, where veins swell and burst, causing life-threatening bleeding

LIVER

Long term

- damage to the liver, whose function is to detoxify poisons such as alcohol
- fatty liver is where fat builds up in the liver; it may be reversible if drinking is reduced
- alcoholic hepatitis includes fatigue, jaundice (yellow skin), stomach swelling and enlarged, tender liver. Can cause death
- fibrosis is scar tissue caused by the liver attempting to repair itself
- cirrhosis is permanent damage, where most of the liver is replaced by scar tissue. It cannot function and can cause death
- liver cancer

PANCREAS AND GLUCOSE REGULATION

Immediate

- heavy consumption can lead to hypoglycaemia (low blood sugar), causing dizziness, shaking, sweating and, if severe, brain damage

Long term

- acute pancreatitis (inflammation and damage to the pancreas) causing abdominal and back pain, nausea and fever. It can be life-threatening
- chronic pancreatitis where the inflammation does not heal and symptoms worsen, including weight loss, type 2 diabetes, malnutrition and oily stools as fats in the diet are not digested and absorbed

INTESTINES

Long term

- cancer of the large bowel and rectum

WEIGHT

Long term

- high calories encourage weight gain, especially in those who are already overweight, those eating a high-fat diet and in men
- appetite stimulant, which encourages eating
- where alcohol is replacing food, malnutrition results

KIDNEYS AND FLUID BALANCE

Immediate

- as a diuretic, alcohol encourages the body to lose water via the kidneys and dehydrate, causing the need to urinate and thirst
- minerals are lost along with the water, exacerbated by alcohol-induced vomiting, which can lead to seizures and heart problems

BREAST (WOMEN)

Long term

- increased risk of breast cancer

HANGOVER

Immediate

- dehydration, which causes thirst, headache, dizziness and weakness
- irritation to the liver and stomach, causing nausea, vomiting and stomach pain
- low blood sugar causes fatigue and weakness
- disturbance of sleep can feel like 'jet lag'

ALCOHOL POISONING/ACUTE INTOXICATION

Immediate

- all the common symptoms of being drunk, such as slurred speech, poor coordination, change in mood or behaviour, are the result of alcohol poisoning
- lethal doses of alcohol, an 'overdose', leads to loss of consciousness, slowed breathing and death

PREGNANCY AND FOETAL ALCOHOL SPECTRUM DISORDER (FASD)

Immediate

Alcohol passes through the placenta to the foetus increasing risks of

- miscarriage
- premature birth
- stillbirth

Long term

Alcohol-related birth defects, collectively called foetal alcohol spectrum disorder, include

- restricted growth
- brain damage
- developmental delay
- behavioural challenges such as aggression
- low IQ
- poor social skills
- poor attention span

BREASTFEEDING

Alcohol passes into the breast milk and to the baby, which can affect the baby's development.

LOW-GRADE INFLAMMATION

Alcohol, particularly heavy drinking, causes chronic low-grade inflammation throughout the body, particularly in the intestines, which in turn contributes to conditions such as cancer, cardiovascular disease and type 2 diabetes (Imhof *et al.*, 2001; Bishehsari *et al.*, 2017).

Mental and emotional health

Alcohol travels in the blood to the brain's nerve cells, neurons, which changes how people think, feel and behave.

Positive feelings and behaviour

Alcohol encourages the production of endorphins, the chemicals that promote relaxation, reduce inhibitions and promote feelings of wellbeing. We feel more confident, less socially anxious and we may talk more (Mental Health Foundation, 2006).

Table 10.2 Positive reasons for drinking alcohol

	Percentage of responses (n = 1000)
Makes me feel relaxed	77%
Makes me feel happy	63%
Makes me feel more confident	41%
Helps me to fit in socially	44%
Makes me feel less anxious	40%
Makes me feel less depressed	26%
Makes me feel less inhibited	51%
Helps me to make friends more easily	31%

Source: Adapted from Mental Health Foundation (2006 p.8).

Negative feelings and behaviour

Drinking more than a little alcohol leads to exaggerated states of emotion such as anger, aggression, withdrawal and depression. Feeling anxious is the way in which the body warns us that a situation is potentially sensitive or unsafe. Alcohol takes away this warning system as well as interfering with thinking processes. These two factors mean that people who are normally adept at avoiding confrontation find themselves in negative verbal and physical confrontations.

Causes for concern include

- using alcohol to help with sleep
- drinking alcohol to cope with shyness, fear or anxiety
- avoiding social situations where there is no alcohol
- using alcohol to cope with stress, such as job stress

and there are

- significant associations between heavy alcohol use, depressive symptoms and anxiety
- concerns that alcohol problems are a high-risk factor for suicide, especially among males
- concerns that alcohol is a cause of other mental health problems

(Mental Health Foundation, 2006)

Using alcohol as a coping mechanism to deal with emotions is sometimes called self-medicating with alcohol. The Mental Health Foundation (2006) explain that, in the same way that the brain can induce anxiety, the brain can also reduce anxiety. If a person is using alcohol to relax and 'numb' their feelings of anxiety, increasing amounts of alcohol start to be required to have the same numbing effect. Alcohol also reduces serotonin in the brain, which leads to low/depressed feelings, so using alcohol to cope with low mood only adds to the problem. The underlying reasons for anxiety or low mood are not addressed. For example,

> Anger and depression and so on ... I had it all my life but I disguised it with alcohol ... I think deep down that I never wanted to be [gay] and I think that was half the problem ... I masked it with drinking, I medicated myself with drink.
>
> (gay male, 62, Maycock *et al.*, 2016 p.84)

Alcohol problems among those with mental disorders are common. Those with this 'dual diagnosis' self-medicate with alcohol to cope with the negative feelings of the disorder. Risks to their physical and mental health are compounded when alcohol is combined with prescription and other drugs (Shuckit, 2006; Turner *et al.*, 2018). Norström and Rossow (2016) reviewed a range of international studies and concluded that between 15% and 56% of people who attempted or completed suicide were misusing alcohol. The authors suggest that alcohol misuse is strongly associated with sadness, despair, hopelessness, depression, mental disorders, severe physical illness, aggression, loneliness, low self-esteem and social isolation. These predispositions to self-harm and suicide are likely to be worsened by alcohol.

Alcohol increases the risk of accidents and injuries because it slows down a person's reactions, their thinking processes, their co-ordination, vigilance, vision and hearing (Institute of Alcohol Studies, 2018). Unintentional and intentional injuries include road traffic injuries, drowning, burns, falls, suicide and interpersonal violence. In England, there were 77,728 hospital admissions for alcohol-related unintentional injuries in 2017 to 2018 (PHE, 2018).

Sexual health

Alcohol is associated with increased sexual arousal but decreased sexual performance. With greater consumption, men and women are more likely to

- report having multiple sexual partners
- have unprotected sex, especially men
- acquire more sexually transmitted infections

(RCP, 2011; PHE, 2016a)

The Royal College of Physicians (2011) explain how alcohol intoxication is often a frequent factor in sexual assault. Where the perpetrator has been drinking alcohol, the abuse and injuries are often greater. Alcohol is also associated with stranger rape and date rape.

Social and societal health

Alcohol affects people's relationships, adds to crime rates and, although the alcohol industry would argue that it adds to the economy, it also costs the economy.

Relationships

Alcohol can help and harm relationships. Endorphins play an important role in the process of forming human relationships, and so alcohol becomes associated with positive social bonding. It is about enjoying seeing friends, having a laugh, putting the

Table 10.3 Prevalence of harm caused by other people's alcohol consumption in England and Wales, 2015 to 2016

Examples of harms	*Estimated proportion of England's population*	*Estimated proportion of Wales's population*
Being kept awake due to noise or disruption	8%	29%
Felt uncomfortable or anxious at a social occasion (e.g. party)	6.8%	29.2%
Had a serious argument (no physical violence)	5.7%	20.3%
Felt physically threatened because of someone else's drinking	3.4%	17.7%
Stopped seeing or being in contact with someone because of their drinking	2.5%	15.5%
Felt forced or pressured into sex or something sexual	0.7%	1.8%

Sources: Adapted from Benyon *et al.* (2019) p.4; Quigg *et al.* (2016 p.3).

world to rights, getting out, being in a nice atmosphere and relaxation (McQueen *et al.*, 2017). However, researchers estimate that about a fifth of people in England and half of the people in Wales experience harm from someone else's alcohol consumption each year (Benyon *et al.*, 2019; Quigg *et al.*, 2016). Relationships where one or both partners engage in severe problematic drinking are more likely to break down than relationships of lower or no drinking (PHE, 2016a). There is strong association between alcohol consumption and intimate partner violence/domestic violence. Alcohol intoxication can cause the violence, and it can be a way of coping with the consequences of violence (PHE, 2016a).

Crime

Alcohol-related crime takes many forms, including driving after consuming more than the legal limit of alcohol, assault, robbery and homicide (Table 10.4). Data are likely to under-represent the true scale of crimes, as only the ones reported to the police are recorded. In Scotland, in 2017/2018, 39% of prisoners reported being under the influence of alcohol when they were arrested (Giles and Robinson, 2019). Wider costs of alcohol-related crime to society include

- fear of crime
- emergency services and healthcare
- street cleaning
- noise and light pollution
- increased insurance payments

(PHE, 2016a)

Economic impact of alcohol

The main financial costs of alcohol, paid for by the public, relate to healthcare, social care, reduced employment and productivity, crime and public order, environmental health, alcohol education and other prevention measures. Estimates suggest, each year, alcohol costs

- £7.2 billion to Scotland (3.4% of gross domestic product)
- £21 billion to England and Wales (1.7% of gross domestic product)

Table 10.4 Incidents where the victim(s) believed the offender(s) to be under the influence of alcohol

Percentage of incidents known to police			
England and Wales 2016/2017		*Scotland 2017/2018*	
Theft	12.4%		
Criminal damage	20.6%		
Hate crime	21.5%		
Violent incidents	46.2%	Violent incidents	46%
Victims of sexual assault in own home	32.6%	Homicide	81%
Victims of sexual assault in offender's home	35.9%		
Victims of sexual assault in pub/club/street	57.1%		

Sources: ONS (2018b); Giles and Robinson (2019).

- £679.8 million to Northern Ireland (2.2% of gross domestic product)
- £1.2 to £1.4 billion to the UK due to people working under the influence of alcohol or working with hangovers

(IAS, 2016; Bhattacharya, 2016; 2019)

Alcohol contributes to significant physical, mental, emotional, sexual, social and societal harms to the public's health and wellbeing.

Measuring and defining alcohol use

Units of alcohol and guidelines

Counting alcohol units was first introduced in the UK in 1987 to help the public to keep track of their drinking (HCSTC, 2012). A unit of alcohol is 8 grams or 10 ml of ethanol. This takes the body around an hour to process but this

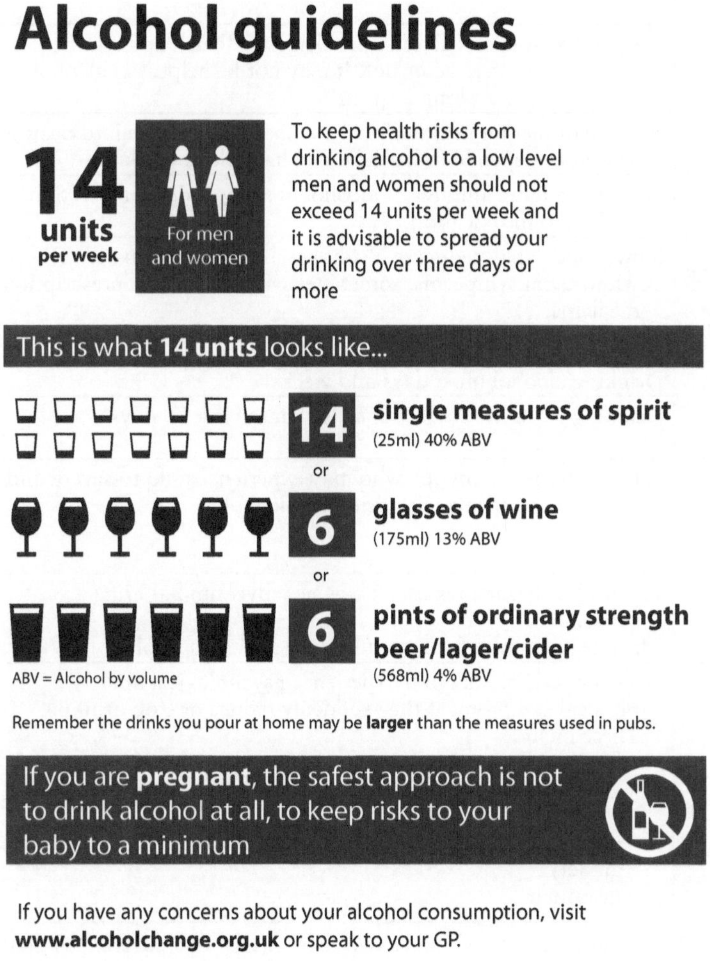

Figure 10.3 UK low risk drinking guidelines

Source: Alcohol Change UK, 2020a. Reproduced with permission from Alcohol Change UK.

Table 10.5 Alcohol terminology

Terms	*Definition*	
Dependent drinking Alcohol dependence Severe alcohol use disorder Alcohol addiction	A strong desire to drink alcohol and difficulties in controlling its use. Persistent drinking despite harmful consequences. Giving alcohol a higher priority than other activities.	Alcohol misuse
Harmful drinking High-risk drinking	Drinking 35 units a week or more for women and 50 units a week or more for men. Alcohol consumption is causing mental or physical harm.	
Hazardous drinking Heavy drinking Increasing risk drinking	Drinking between 14 and 35 units a week for women and between 14 and 50 units for men. Drinking that increases a person's risk of harm, physically, mentally or socially.	
Moderate drinking Lower risk drinking	Drinking up to 14 units per week	
Alcoholism	A term that suggests alcohol problems are 'black and white', like having a disease or not. It may not be helpful as alcohol problems occur along a spectrum.	
Alcohol-use disorders	A range of mental health disorders that include acute intoxication as well as dependent, harmful and hazardous drinking.	
Binge drinking	Drinking a large amount of alcohol in a single drinking session leading to intoxication.	
Detoxification	Slowly and safely reducing alcohol consumption to avoid withdrawal symptoms, sometimes with the help of prescription medicine.	
Excessive drinking	Either harmful or hazardous drinking	
Frequent drinking	Drinking alcohol most days and weeks	
Heavy episodic drinking	Drinking 7.5 units at least once within the last 30 days.	
Problem drinkers Problematic drinking Alcohol problems	A broad term for anyone who may experience mild to severe and/or changing problems with drinking alcohol.	
Substance misuse Substance abuse	Harmful or hazardous use of psychoactive/mind-altering substances. The most common form of substance misuse is alcohol.	
Withdrawal	Dependent drinkers often experience psychological and physical symptoms if they suddenly reduce or stop drinking. These include • hand tremors • sweating • visual hallucinations • depression • anxiety • insomnia	

Sources: Berridge *et al.* (2009); NICE (2010); DH (2016); Alcohol Change UK (2020b); NHS (2020); WHO (2018).

varies according to the sex, age, weight and health of the individual. All alcohol is harmful; only abstinence is risk-free. People who choose to drink alcohol can minimise harms to their health by drinking within the UK Chief Medical Officers' Low Risk Drinking Guidelines (DH, 2016). These are based on studying the average risks of alcohol to populations, not an individual's personal risk, which may be higher if they have certain mental or physical health problems, low weight or are taking medications.

The Guidelines recommend that men and women should consume a maximum of 14 units per week spread over three days or more. Heavy drinking should be avoided, even over a small number of days. When five to seven units of alcohol are consumed within a period of three to six hours, the risks of injury increase by a factor of between two and five. The Guidelines do not state limits for 'single occasion drinking episodes' in units because individuals' risks of harm vary. Instead, they recommend that levels of consumption on a single occasion are kept to a minimum. Pregnant women should abstain from alcohol as it could harm the unborn baby.

Chapter 11 includes a discussion about the meanings associated with using different terminology (Table 10.5) and the World Health Organization's classification of substance use and addictive behaviour, which includes alcohol (p.308–313).

Assessment of alcohol use

The World Health Organization developed the Alcohol Use Disorders Identification Test (AUDIT) (Table 10.6) to assess alcohol consumption and identify any potential alcohol problems (Babor *et al.*, 2001).

> *Alcohol use and misuse occur along a scale which can be measured in units or using the AUDIT screening tool.*

Trends and inequalities in alcohol consumption

The World Health Organization (2018) reports that alcohol is consumed by more than half the population of the Americas, Europe and Western Pacific, with the highest drinking occurring among 15- to 19-year-olds in Europe. Across the world, the prevalence of heavy episodic drinking has decreased from 22.6% in 2000 to 18.2% in 2016, but remains high in some sub-Saharan African countries and in parts of Eastern Europe.

Trends and inequalities in UK alcohol consumption

In the UK, alcohol consumption generally declined following the era of Hogarth's 'Gin Lane', with two notable dips during the two World Wars. Historians suggest that consumption started to rise in the 1960s due to

- popularity of stronger drinks such as wine, spirits and strong white cider
- alcohol becoming more affordable due to rising incomes and alcohol tax not rising in line with inflation

Table 10.6 Alcohol Use Disorders Identification Test (AUDIT)

Questions	*Scoring system*				
	0	*1*	*2*	*3*	*4*
How often do you have a drink containing alcohol?	Never	Monthly or less	2–4 times per month	2–3 times per week	4 or more times per week
How many units of alcohol do you drink on a typical day when you are drinking?	0–2	3–4	5–6	7–9	10 or more
How often have you had 6 or more units if female, or 8 or more if male, on a single occasion in the last year?	Never	Less than monthly	Monthly	Weekly	Daily or almost daily
How often during the last year have you found that you were not able to stop drinking once you had started?	Never	Less than monthly	Monthly	Weekly	Daily or almost daily
How often during the last year have you failed to do what was normally expected from you because of your drinking?	Never	Less than monthly	Monthly	Weekly	Daily or almost daily
How often during the last year have you needed an alcoholic drink in the morning to get yourself going after a heavy drinking session?	Never	Less than monthly	Monthly	Weekly	Daily or almost daily
How often during the last year have you had a feeling of guilt or remorse after drinking?	Never	Less than monthly	Monthly	Weekly	Daily or almost daily
How often during the last year have you been unable to remember what happened the night before you had been drinking?	Never	Less than monthly	Monthly	Weekly	Daily or almost daily
Have you or somebody else been injured as a result of your drinking?	No		Yes		Yes, during the last year
Has a relative or friend, doctor or other health worker been concerned about your drinking or suggested that you cut down?	No		Yes		Yes, during the last year

AUDIT Scoring

- 0–7 indicates low risk
- 8–15 indicates increasing risk
- 16–19 indicates higher risk
- 20 or more indicates possible dependence

Source: PHE (2017). Reproduced under the terms of the Open Government Licence v.3.0.

- aggressive promotion of alcohol by retailers
- liberal regimes for off-licence sales
- increased alcohol consumption by women and young people

(HCHC, 2009)

Total consumption

A large survey across Great Britain asked 7,100 people about their alcohol consumption during the previous week (ONS, 2018c). It showed

- people were drinking slightly less than they were in 2005
- 29.2 million people drank alcohol; this represented 57.5% of respondents in England, 53.5% of the respondents in Scotland and half the respondents in Wales
- 61.9% of men drank alcohol compared to 52.4% of women
- people aged 45–64 were the highest drinkers and 16- to 24-year-olds were the lowest, continuing the downward trend among the younger age group

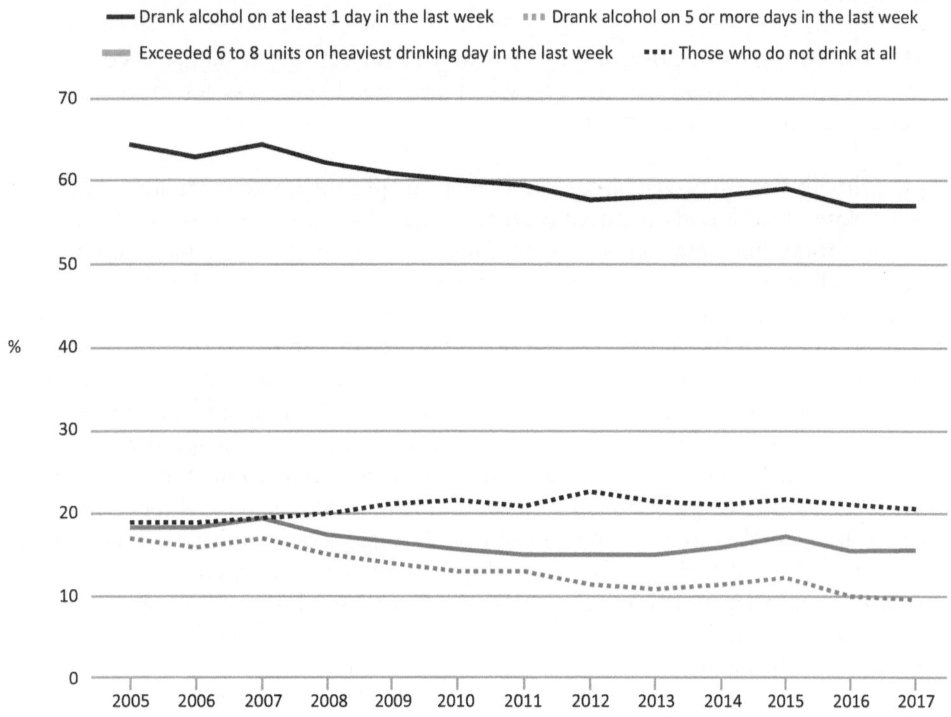

Figure 10.4 Self-reported drinking habits in Great Britain, 2005 to 2017 (n = 7,100)
Source: ONS, 2018c. Reproduced under the terms of the Open Government Licence v.3.0

Teetotalism

The British survey examined alcohol abstention and found

- 20.4% did not drink alcohol at all
- teetotalism had increased among the 16- to 24-year-olds and decreased among the over-65s since 2005
- 27.9% of women over 65 years were teetotal, which is a fall of 10% since 2005
- London had the highest proportion of teetotallers

(ONS, 2018c)

Socio-economic circumstances and alcohol consumption

With higher socio-economic position, more alcohol was consumed. For example,

- people working in managerial and professional jobs drank more frequently than those in routine and manual jobs
- people with higher incomes drank more than those with lower incomes

(ONS, 2018c)

Thinking point:

> If those in higher socio-economic positions, and earning a higher income, are drinking more alcohol than others, which group is likely to suffer more alcohol-related diseases and early death?

People who live in deprived areas experience disproportionately greater negative alcohol-related health consequences than those who live in more affluent areas, even when their total consumption is similar. This is called the 'alcohol harm paradox'. Bellis and colleagues (2016) found that people who lived in areas of deprivation were more likely to binge drink, consume beer and spirits rather than wine, to smoke, eat a poorer diet, be less active and carry excess weight compared to those living in affluent communities. They concluded that although total alcohol consumption was not different to those living in affluent areas, their binge drinking adds, cumulatively, to the health risks from other behaviours, thus leading to greater hospital admissions and early death. However, Katikireddi and colleagues (2017) compared people in lower socio-economic positions to those in higher socio-economic positions, as measured by a combination of education, occupation, income and other risk factors such as smoking and weight. The researchers found that even after accounting for their different patterns of drinking, including bingeing, smoking and obesity, those in lower socio-economic positions still suffered greater alcohol-related harms. For now, the reasons for the alcohol harm paradox remains unclear.

Ethnicity and alcohol consumption

The British survey found that 61% of those who drank alcohol described themselves as White (ONS, 2018c). This chimes with another survey, carried out in England, which found that those identifying as 'White British' or 'White other' consumed alcohol to a hazardous, harmful or dependent level more than people of other ethnicities (Drummond *et al.*, 2016). The British survey found that the highest level of teetotalism, abstinence from alcohol, was in London (26.6%), the most ethnically diverse area in the UK. Many UK studies show that teetotalism is higher among the non-White population, especially South Asians from Pakistani, Bangladeshi and Muslim backgrounds (Hurcombe *et al.*, 2010). There are diverse reasons for drinking habits, such as:

> Sikh men positively associate drinking with work life, whereas Pakistani men express the opposite view.
>
> (Hurcombe *et al.*, 2010 p.38)

Lesbian, gay, bi and trans people and alcohol consumption

The charity Stonewall researched 5,000 lesbian gay, bi and trans (LGBT) people across Great Britain. It found that 16% drank alcohol almost every day, with more men (20%) doing so than women (11%) (Figure 10.5).

Problematic alcohol consumption

The British survey defined binge drinking as exceeding six units for females and eight units for males on their heaviest drinking day. It found

- binge drinking was the most common in Scotland (37.3%), then Wales (30.4%) and England (26.2%)
- 28.7% of men and 25.6% of women binged at least once that week
- the over 65s were the least likely to binge drink
- 16 to 24 year olds binged to the highest level, for example excess drinking on a Friday or Saturday night

(ONS, 2018c)

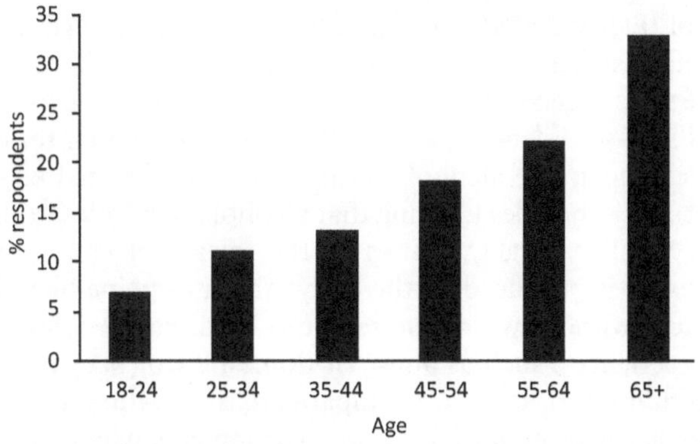

Figure 10.5 British lesbian, gay, bi and trans (LGBT) people's daily consumption of alcohol by age

Source: Bachmann and Gooch, 2018 p.17. Reproduced with permission from Stonewall.

Table 10.7 Patterns of alcohol consumption among over 16s in England, Scotland and Wales

	*England 2014 (%) (n = 7,500)**	*Scotland 2014/15 (%) (n = 5,000)**	*Wales 2016/17/18/19 (%) (n = 10,000)***
Dependent drinking	1.2%	1%	2%
Harmful drinking (higher risk)		2%	
Hazardous drinking (increasing risk)	16.6%	15%	16%
Moderate drinking (low risk)	57.5	82%	61%
Non-drinker (or very rarely drinks)	22.8%		21%

Notes: *based on AUDIT scores
**based on units of alcohol

Sources: Drummond *et al.* (2016); Gray and Leyland (2016); StatsWales (2020).

An analysis of the numbers of people who present to their family doctors (general practitioners) in the UK showed alcohol dependence was more common in males than females, in deprived areas and in Northern Ireland and Scotland (Thompson *et al.*, 2017). In England, it is estimated that 10.8 million adults are drinking at a level that is putting their health at risk, and about 1.6 million have some level of alcohol dependence (PHE, 2016b).

Alcohol consumption in the UK is concerning, especially among White, 45- to 65-year-olds. Levels of alcohol misuse, heavy drinking and binge drinking are too high.

Reasons why people use and misuse alcohol

The misuse of alcohol may be perceived as a moral failure, for which the individual is held responsible and judged, or it may be understood as a disease, an addiction, beyond an individual's control (Pickard *et al.*, 2015). Here we present a third, more holistic, view. Alcohol use and misuse is thought to be approximately 40% to 60% genetically inherited; there are several genes that scientists think combine to encourage a propensity towards alcohol misuse (Edenberg *et al.*, 2019). The remaining reasons are due to environments which encourage alcohol consumption as a learned behaviour from others (PHE, 2016a). This includes learning that alcohol is a way to produce feelings of relaxation and sociability, largely thanks to the release of endorphins. Endorphin means 'endogenous', it is produced by the body, and 'morphine-like'. For some, alcohol becomes a crutch, without which life feels too hard. People who have suffered adverse childhood experiences, such as abuse or domestic violence, are four times more likely to be a harmful/high-risk drinker compared to those who grew up in more stable, happier households (Bellis *et al.*, 2015). In environments where alcohol consumption is the norm, perhaps socially expected, the use of alcohol can become a destructive relationship. This combination of the biological, psychological and social/

environmental reflects the biopsychosocial model described by Engel in 1977, and it is this model that informs a holistic approach to understanding alcohol use today. For example,

- biological factors include genetics and functioning of the body
- psychological factors include learning from others to buy a round of drinks and to use alcohol to cope with negative feelings
- social/environmental factors include the selling and consuming of alcohol as part of everyday, 'normal', living

Thinking point:

> Consider your own alcohol consumption/teetotalism. What factors have influenced your own decisions and behaviour?

Alcohol and family upbringing

Adults' use of alcohol influences their children and their future relationship with alcohol as adults. Across the UK, 300,000 children under 16 are thought to live with someone who drinks at harmful levels, 3.4 million live with one binge-drinking parent and almost a million with two (Velleman and Templeton, 2016). In England, 200,000 children live with a parent or carer who is dependent on alcohol and in Scotland 51,000 children live with an adult who has alcohol problems (McGovern *et al.*, 2018; Scottish Government, 2012). Parents and carers instil certain attitudes and norms around alcohol. Some introduce children to alcohol believing that it equips them to make sensible choices about alcohol outside the home, increases children's resistance to peer influence and protects them from problematic drinking (PHE, 2016a). However, research studies clearly show that early initiation to alcohol by parents/carers is associated with increased alcohol consumption and alcohol-related harms in the next generation, and parents are advised to avoid glamorising alcohol and to promote a healthy relationship with it through authoritative parenting and clear behavioural expectations (PHE, 2016a; Rossow *et al.*, 2016a; 2016b; Foster *et al.*, 2017).

Alcohol and workplace

The types of working conditions that are associated with greater alcohol use include shift/night work, long hours, business travel and job stress (Nicholson and Mayho, 2016). Among service personnel, such as police officers, alcohol is often used to cope with post-traumatic stress disorder (Green, 2008), and Browne and colleagues (2008) found that members of the UK Armed Forces scored more highly on the AUDIT than the general population. Alcohol can affect people's performance at work, not just in terms of taking time off work, absenteeism, but also being at work but not able to work effectively, a form of presenteeism. Thørrisen and colleagues (2019) reviewed a range of studies and found a relationship between higher levels of alcohol consumption and poorer work performance.

Alcohol consumption in later life

Retirement brings with it changes such as having more time and, for some, more disposable money, which means alcohol is more affordable. Some older people increase their drinking because they have fewer responsibilities and can attend more social occasions (Britton and Bell, 2015). In England, a large group of older people were studied over 10 years and the authors found that the frequency of their alcohol consumption changed as their health changed (Holdsworth *et al.*, 2016). Those who reported being in good health were often frequent drinkers, but the study could not say whether alcohol or alcohol-related socialising caused their good health.

One study showed that when people retired, many switched to home drinking as their main or only drinking location (Edgar *et al.*, 2016). This did not necessarily suggest hidden or problem drinking, although those concerns exist, but it was often due to fewer opportunities to socialise, costs and a preference for drinking at home perhaps before or during a meal. Men were more likely to drink in public spaces compared to women, who tended to drink in the home either alone, with family or with friends. It was noted that caring responsibilities, most often undertaken by women, were associated with social isolation and might encourage domestic rather than public drinking. One woman explained:

> It's so much easier just to have a glass of wine than making a cup of tea ... I just think it's the way we are nowadays ... it's become part of life really.
>
> (female; Edgar *et al.*, 2016 p.35)

Harmful alcohol consumption among older people may be triggered or exacerbated by age-related life changes and stressors, such as

- becoming a carer
- bereavement
- boredom
- fewer lifestyle constraints
- financial changes
- health problems and chronic illnesses
- loneliness
- loss of friends
- loss of independence
- loss of occupation
- loss of social status
- reduced self-esteem

(Phillips, 2014)

Alcohol-saturated culture

The alcohol industry promotes its products through mainstream and social media, product placement in films or television, sports and arts sponsorship and many other marketing opportunities. These strategies encourage individuals to develop positive beliefs about alcohol and increase the range of environments in which alcohol consumption becomes socially acceptable and normalised (Sudhinaraset *et al.*, 2016). They also encourage the onset of drinking, binge drinking, increased drinking and allegiance to certain brands (Tanski *et al.*, 2015). The industry targets the young to become drinkers, for example through its introduction of flavoured alcoholic drinks and alcopops in the 1980s and 1990s. The industry claims that its advertising only influences people's choices of brands and does not increase consumption of alcohol (Schmitt, 2012). It cites its alcohol industry-funded research and uses its wealth and power to influence policy-makers through its International Center for Alcohol Policies (Cambridge and Mailon, 2018). These are the same tactics long employed by the tobacco industry and they should be open to the same scepticism from the public.

Box 10.2 Celebrity-endorsed alcohol marketing

Diageo, a British alcohol company, produces Smirnoff vodka, Cîroc vodka, Johnnie Walker whiskey, Guinness beer and Baileys liqueur. Puff Daddy, also known as P. Diddy, is an American rapper, record producer and actor. Since 2007, the American marketing of Cîroc vodka has been handled by Puff Daddy, with the profits being split between himself and Diageo.

Cîroc vodka had been marketed with the message that it was the only vodka made from grapes, but this was not engaging consumers. Puff Daddy changed the message. He provided a story to connect the brand with a lifestyle. He intertwined the vodka with his music videos, his lyrics and VIP events.

In an interview he said, "There's no vodka out there that spoke my language ... I didn't think there was a vodka whose marketing spoke to my lifestyle, that made me feel like I wanted to feel. I've branded myself as the king of celebration, and that's what this alliance is about" (AdAge.com, 2007) (p.100).

(Source: Arpad Papp-Vary, 2016)

People use and misuse alcohol due to a combination of biological, psychological and social/environmental reasons.

Benefits of abstinence or drinking within recommended guidelines

Abstinence or drinking within the Low Risk Drinking Guidelines (DH, 2016) are the healthier options for individuals and for society. Participants who gave up alcohol for a month said:

> I felt more in control; not getting wasted all the time. If I was out with friends, I went home when I wanted to.
>
> (De Visser and Lockwood, 2018 p.17)

> Waking up and feeling completely alive without any signs of feeling dull around the edges.
>
> (De Visser and Lockwood, 2018, p.17)

Table 10.8 UK adults' views of the benefits of giving up alcohol for one month

Benefits at the end of the month	*Percentage of respondents (n = 1,715)*
I have a sense of achievement	93%
I have saved money	88%
I am thinking more deeply about my relationship with alcohol	82%
I feel more in control of my drinking	80%
I have reset my relationship with alcohol	78%
I have learnt more about when and why I drink	76%
The quality of my sleep has improved	71%
I have realised that I don't need to drink to relax or enjoy myself	71%
My general health has improved	70%
I have more energy	67%
My levels of concentration are better	57%
My skin looks better	54%
I have lost weight	57%
I have spent more time with friends and family	41%

Source: Adapted from De Visser and Lockwood, (2018 p.16).

Charlet and Heinz (2016) reviewed 63 international research studies which reported on the effects of alcohol reduction for individuals who had been hazardous, harmful or dependent drinkers. They found,

- reduced alcohol-associated injuries
- improved functioning of the heart muscle
- lowered blood pressure
- normalisation of blood chemistry
- reduction in body weight
- the progression of alcohol-induced liver fibrosis slowed down
- improvement in the health of liver cells, where cirrhosis was not present
- reduced withdrawal symptoms
- reduced mental-health-related hospital admissions
- improved in symptoms of anxiety and depression
- improved self confidence
- improved quality of life
- lowered stress
- better social functioning
- improved work productivity
- reduced healthcare costs

In Scotland, Tom, Sam and Steve were among 10 people who were interviewed about their experiences six months after reducing or ceasing drinking alcohol with professional support (McQueen *et al.*, 2017). Some discussed the loss of the social events which revolved around friends and alcohol. While some avoided them, the solution for Tom was to switch to non-alcoholic drinks. Others met their friends and were pleasantly surprised when they were congratulated and admired for giving up alcohol.

> ... they say, "Well done, I wish I could do that".
>
> (Sam; McQueen *et al.*, 2017 p.7)

Each interviewee had personal gains which acted as motivators to maintain changes. Steve, a diabetic, noticed how he felt better because he was able to manage his insulin regime.

> Well it's my health, really it's much better ...
>
> (Steve; McQueen *et al.*, 2017 p.6)

Sam felt proud of his willpower, was enjoying meals out and holidays. The most important benefit was

> ... for my wife ... she says she's got the man back she married. It's been really good and not just for me as well, for my wife and my daughter.
>
> (Sam; McQueen *et al.*, 2017 p.6)

Summary

This chapter has

- put alcohol use into a UK historical context
- described how alcohol harms health
- explained how alcohol use is defined and measured
- described UK trends and patterns of alcohol consumption
- offered explanations for why alcohol is used and misused
- identified the benefits of abstinence or drinking within recommended guidelines

Further reading

Barrie, K., and Scriven, A. (2014) *Alcohol misuse*. London: Churchill Livingstone/Elsevier

Useful websites

Alcohol Change UK. Available at: www.alcoholchange.org.uk
Institute of Alcohol Studies. Available at: www.ias.org.uk

References

Alcohol Advisory Council of New Zealand (2012) *Alcohol – the body and health effects*. Wellington: Alcohol Advisory Council of New Zealand

Alcohol Change UK (2020a) Check your drinking. Available at: https://alcoholchange.org.uk/alcohol-facts/interactive-tools/check-your-drinking (Accessed 23rd June 2020)

Alcohol Change UK (2020b) How do we talk about alcohol? Available at: https://alcoholchange.org.uk/policy/policy-insights/how-do-we-talk-about-alcohol (Accessed 30th January 2020)

Babor, T.F., Higgins-Biddle, J.C., Saunders, J.B., *et al.* (2001) *AUDIT: The alcohol use disorders identification test: guidelines for use in primary care*. 2nd edn. Geneva: World Health Organization

Bachmann, C.L., and Gooch, B. (2018) LGBT in Britain: health report. Available at: www.stonewall.org.uk/system/files/lgbt_in_britain_health.pdf (Accessed 6th February 2020)

Bellis, M., Ashton, K., Hughes, K., Ford, K., Bishop, J., and Paranjothy, S. (2015) *Adverse childhood experiences and their impact on health-harming behaviours in the Welsh adult population*. Cardiff: Public Health Wales

Bellis, M.A., Hughes, K., Nicholls, J., Sheron, N., Gilmore, I., and Jones, L. (2016) 'The alcohol harm paradox: using a national survey to explore how alcohol may disproportionately impact health in deprived individuals', *BMC Public Health*, 16(111) doi:10.1186/s12889-016-2766-x

Benyon, C., Bayliss, D., Mason, J., Sweeney, K., Perkins, C., and Henn, C. (2019) 'Alcohol-related harm to others in England: a cross-sectional analysis of national survey data', *BMJ Open*, 9(5) doi:10.1136/bmjopen-2017–021046

Berridge, V., Herring, R., and Thom, B. (2009) 'Binge drinking: a confused concept and its contemporary history', *Social History of Medicine*, 22(3), pp.597–607

Bhattacharya, A. (2016) Dereliction of duty: are UK alcohol taxes too low? Institute of Alcohol Studies. Available at: www.ias.org.uk/uploads/pdf/Derelictionofduty.pdf (Accessed 7th February 2020)

Bhattacharya, A. (2019) Financial headache. Institute of Alcohol Studies. Available at: www.ias.org.uk/uploads/pdf/IAS%20reports/rp35062019.pdf (Accessed 7th February 2020)

Bishehsari, F., Magno, E., Swanson, G., Desai, V., Voigt, R.M., Forsyth, C.B., and Keshavarzian, M.D. (2017) 'Alcohol and gut-derived inflammation', *Alcohol Research*, 38(2), pp.163–171

Braidwood, R. J., Sauer, J.D., Helbaek, H., Mangelsdorf, P.C., Cutler, H.C., Coon, C.S., Linton, R., Steward, J., and Oppenheim, A.L. (1953) 'Did man once live by beer alone?', *American Journal of Anthropology*, 55(4), pp.515–526

Britton, A., and Bell, S. (2015) 'Reasons why people change their alcohol consumption in later life: findings from the Whitehall II cohort study', *PLoS One*, 10(3), doi:10.1371/journal.pone.0119421

Browne,T., Iversen, A., Hull, L., Workman, L., Barker, C., Horn, O., Jones, M., Murphy, D., Greenberg, N., Rona, R., Hotopf, M., Wessely, S., and Fear, N.T. (2008) 'How do experiences in Iraq affect alcohol use among male UK armed forces personnel?', *Occupational Environmental Medicine*, 65(9), pp.628–633

Burton, R., and Sheron, N. (2018) 'No level of alcohol consumption improves health', *The Lancet*, 392(10152), pp.987–988

Cambridge, J., and Mialon, M. (2018) 'Alcohol industry involvement in science: a systematic review of the perspectives of the alcohol research community', *Drug and Alcohol Review*, 37(5), pp.565–579

Charlet, K., and Heinz, A. (2016) 'Harm reduction – a systematic review on effects of alcohol reduction on physical and mental symptoms', *Addiction Biology*, 22(5), pp.1119–1159

Department of Health (2016) UK chief medical officers' low risk drinking guidelines. Available at: https://assets.publishing.service.gov.uk/government/uploads/system/uploads/attachment_data/file/545937/UK_CMOs__report.pdf (Accessed 7th February 2020)

De Visser, R., and Lockwood, N. (2018) Dry January. Evaluation of Dry January 2018. University of Sussex. Available at: https://s3.eu-west-2.amazonaws.com/files.alcoholchange.org.uk/documents/R.-de-Visser-Dry-January-evaluation-2018.pdf?mtime=20191221120711 (Accessed 5th February 2020)

Drummond, C., McBride, O., Fear, N., and Fuller, E. (2016) 'Chapter 10: Alcohol dependence', in McManus, S., Bebbington, P., Jenkins, R., and Brugha, T. (eds) *Mental health and wellbeing in England: adult psychiatric morbidity survey 2014*. Leeds: NHS Digital, pp.238–264

Edenberg, H.J., Gelernter, J., and Agrawal, A. (2019) 'Genetics of alcoholism', *Current Psychiatry Reports*, 21(4) doi:10.1007/s11920-019-1008-1

Edgar, F., Nicholson, D., Duffy, T., Seaman, P., Bell, K. and Gilhooly, M. (2016) Alcohol use across retirement: a qualitative study into drinking in later life. Glasgow Centre for Population Health. Available at: www.gcph.co.uk/assets/0000/5529/Alcohol_use_across_retirement_-_March_2016_-_Final.pdf (Accessed 22nd December 2019)

Engel, G. (1977) 'The need for a new medical model: a challenge for biomedicine', *Science*, 196(4286), pp.129–136

Foster, J., Bryant, L., and Brown, K. (2017) "Like sugar for adults": The effect of non-dependent parental drinking on children and families. Institute of Alcohol Studies/Alcohol Focus Scotland/ Alcohol and Families Alliance. Available at: www.ias.org.uk/uploads/pdf/IAS%20reports/rp28102017.pdf (Accessed 7th February 2020)

Giles, L., and Robinson, M. (2019) *Monitoring and evaluating Scotland's alcohol strategy: monitoring report*. Edinburgh: NHS Scotland

Gray, L., and Leyland, A.H. (2016) 'Chapter 4 alcohol', in Campbell-Jack, D., Hinchliffe, S., and Rutherford, L. (eds) *The Scottish health survey*. Edinburgh: Scottish Government, pp.82–113

Green, B. (2008) 'Post-traumatic stress disorder in UK police officers', *Current Medical Research and Opinion*, 20(1), pp.101–105

Holdsworth, C., Mendonça, M., Pikhart, H., Frisher, M., de Oliveira, C., and Shelton, N. (2016) 'Is regular drinking in later life an indicator of good health? Evidence from the English longitudinal study of ageing', *Journal of Epidemiology and Community Health*, 70(8), pp.764–770

Holmes, J., Angus, C., Buykx, P., Ally, A., Stone, T., Meier, P., and Brennan, A. (2016) Mortality and morbidity risks from alcohol consumption in the UK. University of Sheffield. Available at: www.sheffield.ac.uk/polopoly_fs/1.538671!/file/Drinking_Guidelines_Final_Report_Published.pdf (Accessed 7th February 2020)

House of Commons Health Committee (2009) *Alcohol. First report of session 2009–10. Volume 1*. London: The Stationery Office

House of Commons Science and Technology Committee (2012) *Alcohol guidelines. Eleventh report of session 2010–12*. London: The Stationery Office

Hurcombe, R., Bayley, M., and Goodman, A. (2010) Ethnicity and alcohol: a review of the UK literature. Joseph Rowntree Foundation. Available at: www.jrf.org.uk/sites/default/files/jrf/migrated/files/ethnicity-alcohol-literature-review-summary.pdf (Accessed 7th February 2020)

Imhof, A., Froehlich, M., Brenner, H., Boeing, H., Pepys, M.B., and Koenig, W. (2001) 'Effect of alcohol consumption on systematic markers of inflammation', *Lancet*, 357(9258), pp.763–767

Institute of Alcohol Studies (2016) The economic impacts of alcohol. Available at: www.ias.org.uk/uploads/pdf/Factsheets/FS%20economic%20impacts%20042016%20webres.pdf (Accessed 7th February 2020)

Institute of Alcohol Studies (2018) Accidents and injuries. Available at: www.ias.org.uk/Alcohol-knowledge-centre/Health-impacts/Factsheets/Accidents-and-injuries.aspx (Accessed 7th February 2020)

Katikireddi, S.V., Whitley, E., Lewsey, J., Gray, L., and Leyland, A. (2017) 'Socioeconomic status as an effect modifier of alcohol consumption and harm: analysis of linked cohort data', *Lancet Public Health*, 2(6) doi:10.1016/S2468-2667(17)30078-6

Mayock, P., Bryan, A., Carr, N., and Kitching, K. (2009) Supporting LGBT lives: a study of the mental health and wellbeing of lesbian, gay, bisexual and transgender people. Gay and lesbian equality network. Available at: www.hse.ie/eng/services/publications/mentalhealth/suporting-lgbt-lives.pdf (Accessed 23rd December 2019)

McGovern, R., Gilvarry, E., Addison, M., Alderson, H., Carr, L, Geijer-Simpson, E., Hrisos, N., Lingam, R., Minos, D., Smart, D., and Kaner, E. (2018) *Addressing the impact of non-dependent parental substance misuse upon children*. London: Public Health England

McQueen, J.M, Ballinger, C., and Howe, T.E. (2017) 'Factors associated with alcohol reduction in harmful and hazardous drinkers following alcohol brief intervention in Scotland: a qualitative enquiry', *BMC Health Services Research*, 17(1) doi:10.1186/s12913-017-2093-7

Mental Health Foundation (2006) Cheers report: understanding the relationship between alcohol and mental health. Available at: www.drugsandalcohol.ie/15771/1/cheers_report%5B1%5D.pdf (Accessed 26th April 2020)

National Institute for Health and Care Excellence (2010) Alcohol-use disorders: prevention. Public health guideline [PH24]. *Available at:* www.nice.org.uk/guidance/ph24/chapter/8-Glossary (Accessed 30th January 2020)

National Health Service Digital (2020) Statistics on alcohol, England 2020. Available at: https://digital.nhs.uk/data-and-information/publications/statistical/statistics-on-alcohol/2020/part-1 (Accessed 11th February 2020)

National Health Service (2020) Overview. Alcohol misuse. Available at: www.nhs.uk/conditions/alcohol-misuse/ (Accessed 30th January 2020)

Nicholson, P.J., and Mayho, G. (2016) 'Alcohol, drugs, and the workplace: an update for primary care specialists', *British Journal of General Practice*, 66(652), pp.556–557

Norström, T., and Rossow, I. (2016) 'Alcohol consumption as a risk factor for suicidal behaviour: a systematic review of associations at the individual and population level', *Archives of Suicide Research*, 20(4), pp.489–506

Office for National Statistics (2018a) UK manufacturers' sales: a focus on the beverages industry. Available at: www.ons.gov.uk/businessindustryandtrade/manufacturingandpro ductionindustry/articles/ukmanufacturerssalesafocusonthebeveragesindustry/2018-11-27 (Accessed 3rd February 2020)

Office for National Statistics (2018b) Data on alcohol related incidents, years ending March 2011 to March 2017, Crime Survey for England and Wales. Available at: www.ons.gov.uk/peoplepopulationandcommunity/crimeandjustice/adhocs/009372dataonalcoholrelatedi ncidentsyearsendingmarch2011tomarch2017crimesurveyforenglandandwales (Accessed 1st February 2020)

Office for National Statistics (2018c) Adult drinking habits in Great Britain: 2017. Available at: www.ons.gov.uk/peoplepopulationandcommunity/healthandsocialcare/drugusealcoholandsmoking/bulletins/opinionsandlifestylesurveyadultdrinkinghabitsingreat britain/2017 (Accessed 3rd February 2020)

Papp-Vary, A. (2016) 'Product placement in music videos – the Lady Gaga phenomenon', in Milkovic, M., Kozina, G., and Primorac, D. (eds) *Economic and Social Development 12th International Scientific Conference on Economic and Social Development*. Bangkok, 18–20th February, pp.94–105

Pettigrew, S., Hafekost, C., Jongenelis, M., Pierce, H., Chikritzhs, T., and Stafford, J. (2018) 'Behind closed doors: the priorities of the alcohol industry as communicated in a trade magazine', *Frontiers in Public Health*, 6(217) doi:10.3389/fphbh.2018.00217

Phillips, A. (2014) 'One too many: alcohol consumption and the health risks', *Nursing and Residential Care*, 16(4), pp. 206–209

Pickard, H., Ahmed, S.H., and Foddy, B. (2015) 'Alternative models of addiction', *Frontiers in Psychiatry,* 6(20) doi: 10.3389/fpsyt.2015.00020

Public Health England (2016a) The public health burden of alcohol and the effectiveness and cost-effectiveness of alcohol control policies. Available at: https://assets.publishing.service.gov.uk/government/uploads/system/uploads/attachment_data/file/733108/alcohol_public_health_burden_evidence_review_update_2018.pdf (Accessed 5th February 2020)

Public Health England (2016b) Health matters: harmful drinking and alcohol dependence. Available at: www.gov.uk/government/publications/health-matters-harmful-drinking-and-alcohol-dependence (Accessed 3rd February 2020)

Public Health England (2017) Alcohol use screening tests. Available at: www.gov.uk/government/publications/alcohol-use-screening-tests (Accessed 22nd December 2019)

Public Health England (2018) Public health profiles. Available at: https://fingertips.phe.org.uk/search/injuries#page/3/gid/1/pat/6/par/E12000004/ati/102/are/E06000015/iid/91417/age/1/sex/4 (Accessed 24th July 2019)

Quigg, Z., Bellis, M.A., Grey, H., Ashton, K., Hughes, K., and Webster, J. (2016) *Alcohol's harms to others: the harms from other people's alcohol consumption in Wales*. Liverpool: Public Health Institute, Liverpool John Moores University

Rossow, I., Felix, L., Keating, P., and McCambridge, J. (2016a). 'Parental drinking and adverse outcomes in children: A scoping review of cohort studies', *Drug and Alcohol Review*, 35(4), pp.397–405

Rossow, I., Keating, P., Felix, L., and McCambridge, J. (2016b). 'Does parental drinking influence children's drinking? A systematic review of prospective cohort studies', *Addiction*, 111(2), pp.204–217

Royal College of Physicians (2011) *Alcohol and sex: a cocktail for poor sexual health. Report of the alcohol and sexual health working party*. London: Royal College of Physicians

Schmitt, P. (2012) 'Alcohol advertising affects brand choice but not consumption', *The Drinks Business*, 27*th* April. Available at: www.thedrinksbusiness.com/2012/04/alcohol-advertising-affects-brand-choice-but-not-consumption/ (Accessed 3rd February 2020)

Scottish Government (2012) *Final business and regulatory impact assessment for minimum price per unit of alcohol as contained in alcohol (minimum pricing) (Scotland) Bill*. Edinburgh: Scottish Government

Shuckit, M. (2006) 'Comorbidity between substance use disorders and psychiatric conditions', *Addiction*, 101(1), pp. 76–88

StatsWales (2020) National survey for Wales. Adult lifestyles. Available at: https://statswales.gov.wales/Catalogue/National-Survey-for-Wales/Population-Health/Adult-Lifestyles (Accessed 3rd February 2020)

Sudhinaraset, M., Wigglesworth, C., and Takeuchi, D.T. (2016) 'Social and cultural contexts of alcohol use. Influences in a social-ecological framework', *Alcohol Research*, 38(1), pp.35–45

Sun, Q., Townsend, M.K., Okereke, O.I., Rimm, E.B., Hu, F.B., Stampfer, M.J., and Grodstein, F. (2011) 'Alcohol consumption at midlife and successful ageing in women: a prospective cohort analysis in the nurses' health study', *Plos Medicine*, 337(24), pp.1705–1714

Tanski, S.E., McClure, A.C., Li, Z., Jackson, K., Morgenstern, M., Zhongze, L., and Sargent, J.D. (2015) 'Cued recall of alcohol advertising on television and underage drinking behaviour', *Journal of the American Medical Association Pediatrics*, 169(3), pp.264–271

Thompson, A., Wright, A.K., Ashcroft, D.M., van Staa, T.P., and Pirmohamed, M. (2017) 'Epidemiology of alcohol dependence in UK primary care: results from a large observational study using the Clinical Practice Research Datalink', *PLoS One*, 12(3) doi:10.1371/journal.pone.-174818

Thørrisen, M., Bonsaksen, T., Hashemi, N., Kjeken, I., van Mechelen, W., and Aas, R.G. (2019) 'Association between alcohol consumption and impaired work performance (presenteeism): a systematic review', *BMJ Open*, 9(7) doi:10.1136/bmjopen-2019–029184

Turner, S., Mota, N., Bolton, J., and Sareen, J. (2018) 'Self-medication with alcohol or drugs for mood and anxiety disorders: a narrative review of the epidemiological literature', *Depression and Anxiety*, 35(9), pp.851–860

Velleman, R., and Templeton, L. (2016) 'Impact of parents' substance misuse on children: an update', *BJPsych Advances*, 22(2), pp.108–117

World Health Organization (2018) *Global status report on alcohol and health.* Geneva: World Health Organization

11 Drugs and health

Sally Robinson

Key points

- Introduction
- Definitions and classifications of drugs
- Natural and synthetic drugs
- Drugs: medicinal/recreational
- Controlled drugs
- Drugs and health
- Criminal justice versus public health
- Benefits of recovery
- Summary

Introduction

This chapter will define a drug and suggest three ways of classifying drugs. Drugs include alcohol and tobacco, but as these are discussed in previous chapters they are not included. It will describe the seven types of drugs, how they affect health and how their use is 'controlled' by UK laws. The chapter explains some of the reasons why people take drugs outside of medical supervision, and how disorders and dependency may develop. The health risks associated with drug use are explained; some of them lead to 'deaths of despair'. The chapter illuminates why drug use is a public health issue.

Definitions and classifications of drugs

The word 'drug' has different meanings

- in medicine, it is a substance which has the potential to prevent or cure a disease or enhance health and wellbeing
- in pharmacology, it is a chemical agent that alters the biochemical and physiological processes of the body
- in everyday language, the term often refers to psychoactive drugs or illicit drugs where there may, or may not, be medical reasons for their use

(WHO, 1994)

Drugs can be classified in different ways, according to

- natural or synthetic origins
- medicinal or recreational use
- levels of legal control

There are many overlaps no matter how we classify drugs. For example, cannabis can be either natural or synthetic and it can be used for medical or recreational purposes. The group of drugs called opioids are both natural, from opium poppies (opiates), and synthetically made. Opioids are in common painkillers available over the counter with low levels of legal control as well as in diamorphine used in medicine and heroin for recreational use, both of which are subject to high levels of legal control.

Natural and synthetic drugs

Natural and synthetic medicinal drugs

Approximately 30% to 50% of medicinal drugs used in Western medicine are plant-based and the rest are synthetic (Anand *et al.*, 2019). Historically all medicines were derived from plants as herbal medicines. They remain the mainstay of traditional medicine including Chinese, Ayurveda, Kampo, traditional Korean medicine and Unani (Yuan *et al.*, 2016). There continues to be much interest in learning from plants.

Phytochemicals

A plant's phytochemicals help it to thrive and fight disease. Some plants seem to have immunity-enhancing properties which may be useful for the development of vaccines and, as microorganisms are unable to develop resistance to phytochemicals, they are of interest to a world worried about antibiotic resistance (Anand *et al.*, 2019).

Table 11.1 Drugs developed from plants and used in Western medicine

Plant species	*Medicine*	*Therapeutic purpose*
Filipendula ulmaria (L.) Maxim	Aspirin	Painkiller, anti-inflammatory
Papaver somniferum L.	Codeine, morphine	Painkiller
Digitalis purpurea	Digoxin	Atrial fibrillation, helps heart to beat stronger and in regular rhythm
Cannabis sativa L.	Cannabidiol (CBD)/ cannabis oil	Anxiety, chronic pain, epileptic seizures
Garlic (*Allium sativum* L.)	Allicin	Anti-fungal
Taxus brevifolia Nutt.	Paclitaxel (Taxol)	Chemotherapy drug for breast cancer
Atropa belladonna L.	Apomorphine hydrochloride (Apokyn)	Restores balance of dopamine in the brain, used in Parkinson's disease

Source: Adapted from Anand *et al.* (2019 p.6).

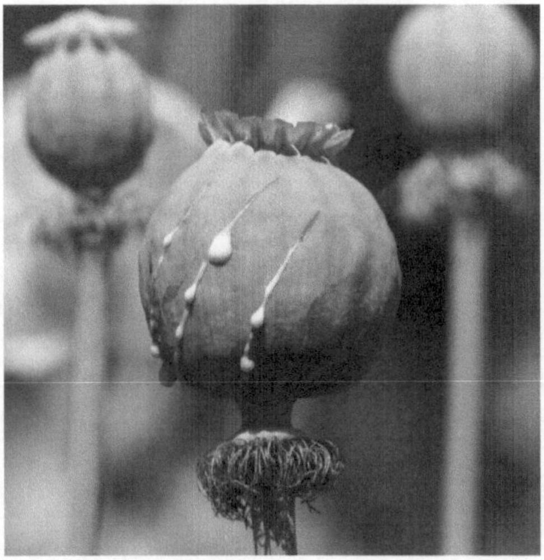

Figure 11.1 Opium resin in the unripe seed pod of an opium poppy (*Papaver somniferum* L.)
Source: Daniel Prudek/Shutterstock.com

Synergistic compounds

The pharmaceutical industry often focuses on developing 'one drug for one target to deal with one disease'. Plant-based medicines are combinations of compounds with synergistic effects, meaning each compound enhances the other. Current drug research is turning towards a 'multi-compound and multi-target' approach, believing that it may be more effective for tackling complex diseases such as cancer and cardiovascular disease (Yuan *et al.*, 2016; Luo *et al.*, 2019).

Genetics

The genes from plants and other natural microorganisms have evolved through natural selection, and advances in gene mining and manipulation are beginning to open up new possibilities for drug development (Wright, 2018).

Natural and synthetic recreational drugs

Recreational drugs are substances taken for pleasure or leisure, perhaps as part of someone's lifestyle, without medical supervision. They come from

- raw plants, e.g. cannabis, magic mushrooms
- refined plants, e.g. heroin from opium poppies, cocaine from coca plants
- synthetic, e.g. amphetamine-type stimulants, new psychoactive substances

Drugs may be made of natural or synthetic compounds, sometimes both. Natural plant compounds continue to provide information for the development of new drugs.

Drugs: medicinal/recreational

There are seven types of drugs: depressants, stimulants, opioids, cannabinoids, hallucinogens, nitrites, and performance- and image-enhancing. All drugs can be used for medicinal or recreational reasons.

Psychoactive drugs

Psychoactive drugs, also known as psychotropic substances, affect the central nervous system, including the brain, and cause changes in thinking, feelings, perceptions, behaviour and consciousness. They may be prescribed for a therapeutic purpose or be used for recreational reasons. They often create rewarding sensations such as relaxation or heightened alertness, which is one reason why some people may take these drugs to the point of dependency.

Medicines

Medicines are used for therapeutic purposes, normally under medical supervision or guidance. They help to prevent, diagnose and treat disease. They are often classified according to their therapeutic effects, for example

- analgesics for pain relief
- antibiotics to prevent or treat infection from microorganisms
- anticonvulsants to prevent and treat epileptic seizures
- antifungals to prevent or treat fungal infections such as athlete's foot
- anti-inflammatory medicines to reduce inflammation or swelling
- antiseptics for preventing multiplication of microorganisms around wounds or burns
- antitoxins are made by an organism and used to prevent or treat diseases caused by biological toxins such as tetanus
- antivirals prevent the growth of viruses or kill existing ones
- bronchodilators for widening the bronchi and relaxing the chest muscles to improve breathing.
- chemoprevention drugs prevent some cancers
- oral contraceptives to prevent conception
- statins help to lower blood cholesterol
- vaccines protect against infectious diseases and some cancers by providing active acquired immunity

Seven types of drugs and their health effects

Depressants

- Alcohol, sedatives, tranquillisers, sedative hypnotics, GHB (gamma hydroxybutyrate), GBL (gamma butyrolactone), benzodiazepines, e.g. diazepam, non-benzodiazepines, barbiturates, pregabalin, gabapentin, volatile substances such as nitrous oxide (laughing gas), glue, petrol and paint. Opioids in high doses act as depressants

- 'Downers', 'relaxants'
- Psychoactive
- Slow down the central nervous system, slowing down messages between the brain and the body. This is not the same as a 'depressed mood'
- Therapeutic aims are to promote relaxation, sedation, relief from muscle spasms or nerve pain and decrease anxiety
- Long-term effects include slurred speech, poor concentration, memory loss, confusion, headache, dizziness, dry mouth, slowed breathing, low blood pressure and dependency
- Misuse/overdose can cause breathing to stop, loss of consciousness, long-term brain damage through lack of oxygen, coma or death

(NIDA, 2018a; MIND, 2020)

Stimulants

- Caffeine, nicotine, amphetamines, cocaine, crack, khat, 3,4-methylene dioxymethamphetamine (MDMA) (ecstasy), methylphenidate (Ritalin); synthetic cathinones, e.g. α-pyrrolidinopentiophenone
- 'Uppers', 'speed', 'crystal meth', 'charlie', 'coke', 'dust', 'white', 'base', 'rock', 'E', 'yaba', 'crank', 'Tina', 'ice', 'bath salts', 'flakka' ('zombie drug'), 'bliss', 'cloud nine', 'vanilla sky', 'lunar wave'
- Psychoactive
- Speed up the central nervous system making people feel more alert. Increase all body processes including heart rate, blood pressure, breathing and hunger. Later tiredness, hunger and depression
- Therapeutic aims are to help with attention deficit disorder (ADHD), narcolepsy (sleeping sickness) and rarely depression
- Long-term effects include restlessness, tremors, rapid breathing, confusion, aggression, hallucinations, panic attacks and dependence

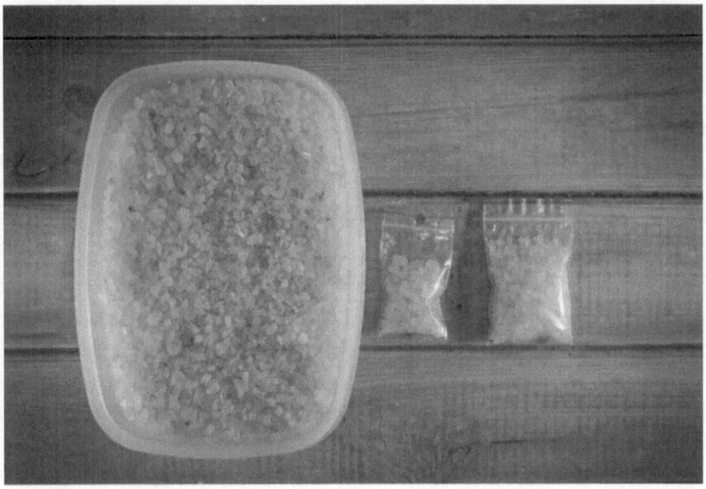

Figure 11.2 Synthetic cathinone: 'flakka' or 'bath salts'
Source: Anastasika Yar/Shutterstock.com

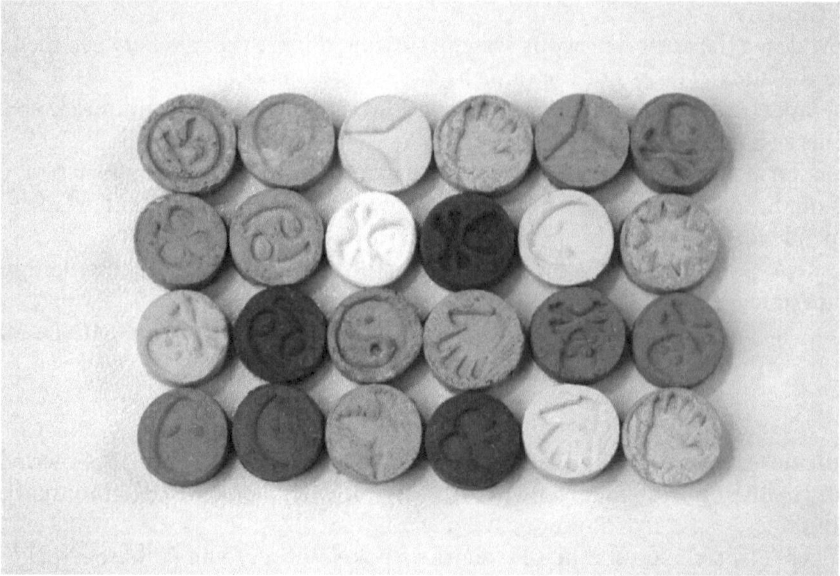

Figure 11.3 MDMA/ecstasy
Source: Couperfield/Shutterstock.com

- Synthetic cathinones also cause paranoia, hallucinations, increased friendliness and sex drive, panic attacks, extreme agitation and violent behaviour
- Misuse/overdose can lead to heart problems leading to a heart attack and nerve problems can lead to seizures, coma and death

(NIDA, 2018b; 2018c; Drugwise, 2016a)

Opioids

- Codeine, dihydrocodeine (DF118), oxymorphone, tramadol, buprenorphine, fentanyl, oxycodone, opium, morphine, diamorphine, pethidine, methadone, temgesic, physeptone
- 'Heroin', 'boy', 'brown', 'china white', 'gear', 'dragon', 'H', 'junk', 'skag', 'smack'
- Psychoactive
- They mimic endorphins, the body's natural painkillers, and produce feelings of wellbeing
- Therapeutic aims are to relieve pain and promote relaxed, pleasant feelings. Can induce confusion, drowsiness, nausea, constipation, euphoria and slowed breathing
- Long-term use can lead to tolerance, meaning that more is needed to get the same effect, leading to dependence. In high doses, opioids act like depressants, slowing the central nervous system
- Misuse /overdose can lead to breathing slowing and stopping, reduced oxygen to the brain leading to brain damage, coma and death

(NIDA, 2020; Drugwise, 2017a)

Cannabinoids

Cannabis plant

- 'Marijuana', 'weed', 'pot', 'grass', 'dope', 'ganja', 'herb', 'pot', 'broccoli', 'skunk', 'Mary Jane', 'boom', 'ashes', 'peng', 'zoot', 'teahead'
- Psychoactive
- The cannabis plant contains cannabinoids, including THC (tetrahydrocannabinol), which gets someone 'high', and CBN (cannabinol), which is calming. The 'high and the calming' go together
- Cannabis encourages 'high', happy, spacey, euphoric, relaxed feelings. It can alter senses, change mood, alter sense of time, impair memory and affect body movement
- Long-term use can lead to dependence and high doses cause breathing problems and lung illness if smoked, heart problems, a range of developmental problems in children if used during and after pregnancy, intense vomiting, temporary paranoia, hallucinations and suicidal thoughts

Synthetic cannabinoids, cannabinoid receptor agonists (SCRAs)

- 'Spice', 'K2', 'black mamba', 'annihilation', 'exodus damnation', 'happy joker', 'fake weed', 'synthetic marijuana'
- Psychoactive
- Can be up to 800 times more potent than cannabis. They induce the 'high' but not so much the 'calming'. They are much more likely than plant cannabis to cause altered perceptions/hallucinations, psychosis, e.g. extreme anxiety, confusion, paranoia, hallucinations. Also, twitchy unusual movements, violent behaviour and suicidal thoughts, alongside a racing heart, raised blood pressure, chest pain, vomiting, kidney damage, overheating, seizures and death

Medicinal cannabis

- Cesamet and canemes contain nabilone; marinol and syndros contain dronabinol; sativex contains nabiximols; epidiolex contains cannabidiol
- Subject to stringent clinical and marketing regulations
- Psychoactive effects are very low
- Contain either synthetic THC, plant-based CBD, or plant-based THC and CBD
- Therapeutic aims are to help with chronic pain, cancer pain, nausea caused by chemotherapy, anxiety disorders, depression, sleep disturbances, spasms caused by multiple sclerosis and epileptic seizures
- Can cause dizziness, disorientation, dry mouth, euphoria, nausea, confusion and drowsiness
- There is little research into the long-term use of medicinal cannabis

(NIDA, 2018d; 2019a; Drugwise, 2017b; EMCDDA, 2018)

Hallucinogens

Classic hallucinogens

- LSD (D-lysergic acid diethylamide); psilocybin (4-phosphoryloxy-*N*,*N*-dimethyltryptamine); peyote (mescaline); DMT (*N*,*N*-dimethyltryptamine); 251-NBOMe
- 'acid', 'blotter acid', 'cheer', 'flash', 'Lucy', 'dots', 'drop', 'rainbows', 'stars', 'tripper', 'mellow yellow'; 'magic mushrooms', 'little smoke', 'shrooms'; 'button', 'cactus', 'mesc.'; 'N Bomb', '251'
- Psychoactive
- Hallucinogens alter sensory perceptions, thoughts, feelings and awareness of surroundings. They cause hallucinations, images or sensations that seem real, but are not
- Interfere with serotonin in the brain, which regulates mood, hunger, sleep, sensory perception, body temperature, sexual behaviour and intestinal muscle control
- Not used therapeutically, but mental health-related research is ongoing
- Can cause increased heart rate and nausea
- Long-term use and misuse can cause persistent psychosis which includes paranoia, mood changes and disturbances in thinking and vision

Dissociative hallucinogens

- PCP (phencyclidine); ketamine; dextromethorphan (DXM); salvia (*Salvia divinorum*)
- 'Angel dust', 'hog', 'love boat', 'peace pill'; 'special K', 'cat valium'; 'robo'; 'diviner's sage', 'maria pastora', 'sally-d', 'magic mint'
- Psychoactive
- Encourage sensations of being disconnected from the body and the environment, and feelings of being out of control
- Interfere with glutamate in the brain, which regulates learning and memory, emotion, perception of pain and responses to the environment
- Not used therapeutically, but mental health-related research is ongoing
- Can cause numbness, disorientation, loss of coordination, increased heart rate and blood pressure, raised body temperature. In high doses can cause memory loss, panic, seizures, inability to move, psychotic symptoms and problems with breathing. Risk of dependency depends on the drug
- Long-term use and misuse are associated with speech problems, memory loss, anxiety, depression and suicidal thoughts

(NIDA, 2019b)

Nitrites

- Butyl nitrite, isobutyl nitrite
- 'poppers', 'hardware', 'liquid gold', 'locker room', 'ram', 'rush', 'TNT'
- Psychoactive, though they do not 'directly' stimulate or depress the central nervous system

- Enhance sexual pleasure
- Can cause blood rush to the head, quickened heart rate, headache, dizziness, light-headedness, slowed-down sense of time and loss of consciousness if the individual is very active. Also, high blood pressure, heart attack if there is an existing heart condition and eye damage if there is an existing glaucoma
- Long-term use and misuse are associated with skin problems and, if swallowed, they can be fatal

(Drugwise, 2016b)

Performance- and image-enhancing drugs

- Anabolic steroids, peptides, growth hormones, selective androgen receptor modules (SARMs), insulin-like growth factors (IGF-1), mechano growth factor (MGG), xanthines, thyroid hormones
- Non-psychoactive

Anabolic steroids

- Anabolic steroids are synthetic versions of testosterone and testosterone-like substances. Their function is to grow skeletal muscle and male sexual characteristics
- Therapeutic uses are to treat delayed puberty, low levels of testosterone in men and concerns related to male mood and sexual performance
- Can cause increased muscularity, aggression and violence, and females may develop male features
- Long-term use or misuse is associated with high blood pressure, liver abnormalities, stunted growth in young people, low sperm count, initially raised sex drive but then lowered, over-development of male breast tissue, sleep disorders, depression, psychological dependence and paranoia

Peptides

- Synthetic peptides promote increases in human growth hormone, which develops muscle and bone
- Can cause water retention, numbness and tiredness

(Drugwise, 2017c; NIDA, 2018e)

New psychoactive substances (NPS)

For decades, the only type of synthetic recreational drugs were amphetamine-type stimulants such as ecstasy. Peacock (2019) explains how, in the early to mid-2000s, many diverse synthetic psychoactive substances emerged and rapidly proliferated across the world, often using on-line trade and outwitting existing legal and scientific controls. These new psychoactive substances may be sold to unwary customers under the name of a traditional drug such as LSD or ecstasy. Although they are often used as part of illicit drug use, they are also used within medicines, adulterated medicines and counterfeit medicines.

Table 11.2 Categories of traditional and synthetic psychoactive drugs according to effects on central nervous system

Effects of drug on central nervous system	*Example of traditional drug*	*Example of synthetic new psychoactive substances*
Depressants	Diazepam	Etizolam, conazolam
Stimulants	Cocaine, methamphetamine	4-Fluoroamphetamine, dimethylcathinone
Opioids	Morphine	Furanyl, fentanyl, ocfentanil
Cannabinoids	Cannabis	AB-PINACA, ADB-FUBINACA
Hallucinogens - classic dissociatives	LSD, 2C-B phencyclidine	1p-LSD, 2C-1 3-methoxyphencyclidine, deschloroketamine

Source: Adapted from UNODC (2018 p.6).

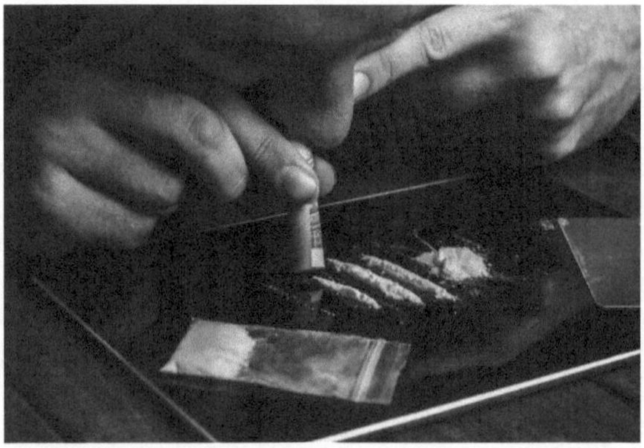

Figure 11.4 Snorting cocaine
Source: DedMityay/Shutterstock.com

International reports suggest:

> ... users are unaware of the content and the dosage of the psychoactive substances .... This potentially exposes users of NPS to additional serious health risks. Little or no scientific information is available to determine the effects that these products may have and how best to counteract them.
>
> (UNODC, 2017 p.8)

There are seven types of drugs which are used for medicinal and recreational purposes.

Controlled drugs

The selling and use of alcohol, tobacco and solvents are limited by UK drug laws, but in this section we focus on controlled drugs. Controlled drugs are those that are 'controlled' under the Misuse of Drugs Regulations 2001, the Misuse of Drugs Act 1971 and the Psychoactive Substances Act 2016. Drug activity that occurs outside of these drug laws is illegal/illicit.

Misuse of Drugs Regulations 2001

The Misuse of Drugs Regulations clarify who is authorised to supply and possess controlled drugs in their professional capacity as doctors, pharmacists, midwives, nurses and others who are independent prescribers. The purpose is to prevent controlled drugs being illegally obtained and causing harm. Drugs are categorised into five schedules which relate to imports, exports, production, supply, possession, prescribing and record keeping.

Box 11.1 The Five Schedules for controlled drugs in the Misuse of Drugs Regulations 2001

Schedule 1, e.g. cannabis resin/oil, LSD, ecstasy (MDMA)
These drugs are highly addictive and have no therapeutic value. To acquire them, someone, normally a researcher, requires a Home Office licence. A register must be kept.

Schedule 2, e.g. morphine, diamorphine (heroin), pethidine, cocaine, codeine, amphetamine, alfentanil, fentanyl, ketamine, cannabis-based medicinal products
These drugs have therapeutic value and are highly addictive. They must be stored in a locked container. A register must be kept. Prescription only.

Schedule 3, e.g. midazolam, temazepam, phentermine, tramadol
These drugs have therapeutic value. Do not need to be locked away but they do have special prescription requirements.

Schedule 4, e.g. benzodiazepines such as diazepam (valium) and lorazepam; anabolic and androgenic steroids such as testosterone and nandrolone; cannabis oral spray (Sativex)
These drugs have therapeutic value. Prescription only.

Schedule 5, e.g. low-concentrate codeine such as dihydrocodeine, low-concentrate morphine

Some controlled drugs are exempt from full control when they are present as part of a medicine in low strength because the risks of misuse are reduced. Most are available 'over the counter'.

(Source: Dangerous drugs: the misuse of drugs regulations, 2001; Home Office, 2019a; Barber, 2019)

Over the counter medicines

In the UK, there are three categories of 'over the counter' medicine.

- 'Prescription only' medicines must be prescribed by an authorised professional and dispensed from a pharmacy or another place with a specific licence. These are normally for conditions that need to be diagnosed and managed by a health professional and include antibiotics and medicines for treating high blood pressure. Many controlled drugs fall within this category.
- 'Pharmacy medicines' can be bought from pharmacies. These are normally for treating short-term conditions, and need to be used more carefully, possibly with additional advice from a pharmacist. They include larger packs of paracetamol, medicines containing codeine and emergency contraception. Many controlled drugs fall within this category.
- 'General sales list' medicines can be bought from retailers such as supermarkets. These are for common, easy to recognise, health concerns. The risks of harm are relatively low if they are inappropriately used. They include antihistamines for allergies and small packs of paracetamol. Some controlled drugs fall within this category.

(Gov.UK, 2019)

Misuse of Drugs Act 1971

The Misuse of Drugs Act classifies drugs as Class A, Class B or Class C. There is a temporary classification for new drugs, which means they can be banned until they are researched and classified. People can be fined or imprisoned for

- possessing drugs, e.g. taking or carrying
- supplying drugs, e.g. selling, dealing, sharing
- producing drugs, e.g. making, growing

The penalty depends on the type of drug, the amount and whether the person is dealing or producing the drug.

Psychoactive Substances Act 2016

The 2016 Act was a response to the rise in new psychoactive substances. People can be fined or imprisoned for

- carrying a psychoactive substance with the intention to supply to another
- supplying a psychoactive substance, e.g. selling, dealing, sharing
- producing a psychoactive substance

Food, nicotine, alcohol, caffeine, nitrites and medicines are not included.

Table 11.3 Penalties relating to controlled drugs according to UK law

Class	*Examples of drug*	*Penalty for possession*	*Penalty for supply and production*
A	Crack cocaine, MDMA (ecstasy), heroin, LSD, magic mushrooms, methadone, methamphetamine (crystal meth)	Maximum 7 years in prison and/or unlimited fine.	Maximum of life in prison and/or unlimited fine.
B	Amphetamines, barbiturates, cannabis, codeine, ketamine, methylphenidate (Ritalin), synthetic cannabinoids, synthetic cathinones (e.g. mephedrone, methoxetamine)	Maximum 5 years in prison and/or unlimited fine.	Maximum of 14 years in prison and/or unlimited fine.
C	Anabolic steroids, benzodiazepines (diazepam), gamma-hydroxybutyrate (GHB), piperazines (BZP), khat	Maximum 2 years in prison and/or unlimited fine. (Except anabolic steroids, where it is not an offence to possess them for personal use.)	Maximum of 14 years in prison and/or unlimited fine or both.
Temporary class drugs	Some methylphenidate substances (ethylphenidate, 3,4-dichloromethylphenidate (3,4-DCMP), methylnaphthidate (HDMP-28), isopropylphenidate (IPP or IPPD), 4-methylmethylphenidate, ethylnaphthidate, propylphenidate) and their simple derivatives	None, but police can take away a suspected temporary class drug.	Maximum of 14 years in prison and/or unlimited fine.
Psychoactive substances		None, unless the person is in prison.	Maximum of 7 years in prison and/or unlimited fine.

Source: Adapted from Gov.UK (2020).

The Crime Survey for England and Wales collects data on drug use (Home Office, 2019b). During the year 2018/19, 2.4% of 16- to 59-year-olds described themselves as frequent users of drugs, that is more than once a month. The figure rose to 4.9% among the 16- to 24-year-olds. More men than women took drugs across all age groups. Cannabis was the most popular drug, with 9.2% of 16- to 59-year-olds taking it once or twice a week.

Table 11.4 Use of controlled drugs during 2018 to 2019 in England and Wales

Class of drug		*Percentage of 16- to 59-year-olds*	*Percentage of 16- to 24-year-olds*
	Any drug	9.4% (3.2 million people)	20.3% (1.3 million people)
Class A	Any Class A drug	3.7%	8.7%
	Cocaine powder	2.9%	6.2%
	Crack cocaine	0.1%	0%
	Ecstasy	1.6%	4.7%
	LSD	0.4%	1.3%
	Magic mushrooms	0.5%	1.6%
	Heroin	0.1%	0%
	Methadone	0.1%	0%
Class A/B	Amphetamines	0.6%	1.0%
	Methamphetamines	0%	0%
Class B	Cannabis	7.6%	17.3%
	Ketamine	0.8%	2.9%
	Mephedrone	0%	0%
Class B/C	Tranquillisers	0.4%	0.6%
Class C	Anabolic steroids	0.2%	0.3%
New psychoactive substances	Nitrous oxide	2.3%	8.7%

Source: Adapted from Home Office (2019b p.11).

Controlled drugs are those 'controlled' by three specific UK legal regulations.

Thinking point:

Consider the pros and cons of these drugs being controlled by UK law.

Drugs and health

Drugs are xenobiotics. These are chemical compounds which are foreign/unexpected to an organism and include natural substances which are ingested in very high concentrations, industrial pollutants, toxins in tobacco and many household and gardening chemicals/products. In today's world we cannot avoid xenobiotics and sometimes, when used carefully, the benefits to health outweigh the harms. However, xenobiotics promote chronic low-grade inflammation throughout the body which, in turn, can lead to several conditions such as cancer, cardiovascular disease, autoimmune diseases and type 2 diabetes (Furman *et al.*, 2019).

Drugs can potentially harm people's health by the choice of drug, the way it is taken, how much is taken, how frequently it is taken, the individual's own characteristics and the environment in which the drug is taken. This is called the 'drug, set and setting' model. Drug-related harm results from the interaction of the

- drug – its pharmacological properties, e.g. potency, purity, how it is used
- set – the characteristics of the person, e.g. physical, psychological ('mind set'), personal reasons
- setting – the physical and social environment, e.g. noisy, stressful, supportive, culture

(Zinberg, 1986)

Self-medication

Self-medication is the use of drugs to treat self-recognised symptoms. Rodrigues (2020) explains that self-medication has always been the subject of debate between medical professionals who cite health risks and others who cite convenience, consumer choice and the economic benefits of self-management, especially for minor conditions. Medicines are tied into social, political and economic concerns relating to the power of the medical profession, the pharmaceutical industry, national and international laws and cultural understandings. Self-medication includes those in the UK called the 'general sales medicines' available in supermarkets as well as medicines which, in the UK, would require a medical consultation and prescription. Online information has increased consumer demand and further blurred the boundaries between drugs for medicinal or recreational use. Online selling has hidden the market-place, enhanced its links with crime, promoted like-minded communities, produced cheaper products, allowed anonymous purchase and provided convenience (Mounteney *et al.*, 2015).

Additional concerns about self-medication include

- it is fuelling the world antibiotic-resistance crisis
- using medications to deal with symptoms rather than underlying problems, such as the causes of anxiety or pain
- unwanted side effects
- non-optimal treatment
- increased drug use
- access by vulnerable people who may need special advice
- poisoning

(Mahmood *et al.*, 2019; Perrot *et al.*, 2019; Torres *et al.*, 2019; Rodrigues, 2020)

Box 11.2 UK government warns students about self-medication

Press release

26th September 2017

The Medicines and Healthcare products Regulatory Agency warns students about the risk of self-prescribing and self-medicating with medicines bought online.

Freshers warned against self-prescribing: you're not doctors yet

Another academic year begins, freshers and university students are being warned of the possible dangers to their health from self-prescribing and self-medicating with powerful prescription medicines.

The purchasing of prescription-only medicines such as anti-anxiety medicines and benzodiazepines outside the regulatory supply chain remains prevalent despite repeated warnings about self-medication.

When buying medicines outside the regulated supply chain you risk ending up with potentially dangerous or useless unlicensed medicines sold by illegal online suppliers. It also increases the risk of being ripped off through credit-card fraud or having your identity stolen.

There is no assurance of quality and standards. Medicines purchased this way could have the wrong active ingredient, no active ingredient or indeed the incorrect dosage.

Prescription medicines are, by their very nature, potent.

Self-diagnosis and self-medication can be dangerous.

Visit https://fakemeds.campaign.gov.uk/ for tips on buying medicines safely online.

(Source: Gov.UK, 2017 reproduced under the Open Government Licence v3.0)

Routes of administration and health risks

Table 11.5 shows the health risks associated with how drugs are administered.

Thinking point:

Why do you think people start taking recreational drugs and then continue to do so?

Patterns of drug use and health

Heather (2018) explains how historical perceptions of the word 'addiction' took two forms: the moral approach where an addict is someone who has free choice and is fully responsible for their addictive behaviours, or a medical approach where a person has a disease and their addictive behaviour is involuntary, the result of compulsion. These two views continue to be consistently challenged as we develop more interdisciplinary

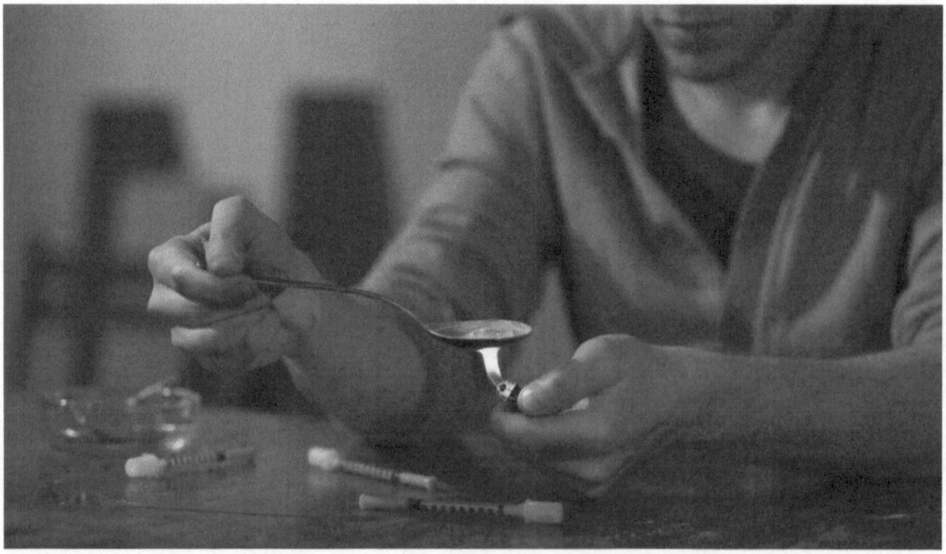

Figure 11.5 Heating heroin ready for injecting
Source: Mortortion Films/Shutterstock.com

Table 11.5 Routes of administration for drugs and their health risks

Medical terminology	*Routes of administration*	*Examples of recreational drugs*	*Recreational terminology*	*Health risks related to the route of administration*
Oral	By mouth	Alcohol, cannabis, heroin, ecstasy, amphetamines, LSD, magic mushrooms	Popping pills, bombing, kissing (exchanging drugs mouth to mouth)	Safer way to take drugs as they are slowly absorbed, but also unpredictably absorbed. Periodontitis, tooth decay, burns and infections in the mouth.
Sublingual	Under the tongue	Buprenorphine		
Buccal	Between gum and cheek	Tobacco, cannabis		
Intravenous	Injection into a vein	Pethidine, morphine, ketamine, heroin, amphetamines, cocaine	Shooting, slamming, smashing, pinning, banging, jacking-up	Most dangerous route as it bypasses body defences. Risks of HIV, hepatitis and other viral, bacterial and fungal infections due to contaminated/ shared needles. Scarring, inflammation and collapse of veins. Damage at injection site e.g. inflammation, sepsis, haemorrhaging, gangrene, thrombosis. Can cause sudden death.
Intramuscular	Injection into a muscle			
Intrathecal	Injection into the space around the spinal cord			
Subcutaneous	Just under the skin	Cocaine, anabolic steroids, heroin, barbiturates	Skin popping	Skin abscesses and infection, risk of hepatitis and other infections due to contaminated/shared needles.
Rectal	Into the anus/rectum	Cocaine, ecstasy, methamphetamine, cannabis, heroin, LSD	Plugging, boofing	Damage, burn, perforation or death of rectal or colon membrane. Can cause sudden death.
Vaginal	Into the vagina	Cocaine, ecstasy, heroin, cannabis, amphetamines, LSD		Damage, burn or perforation of vaginal walls. Can cause sudden death.

(*Continued*)

Table 11.5 Cont.

Medical terminology	*Routes of administration*	*Examples of recreational drugs*	*Recreational terminology*	*Health risks related to the route of administration*
Ocular	Liquid into the eye	Heroin, cocaine, crack cocaine, topical anaesthetics methamphetamine, bath salts		Damage to conjunctiva and pupil, may cause cornea to become anaesthetised leading to injuries and ulcers.
Otic	Into the ear	Oxymorphone	Crushed into ear	Hearing loss
Nasal	Powder or liquid into the nose	Snuff, cocaine, ecstasy, heroin, amphetamines	Snorting, sniffing, tooting	Damage to nasal cavity, destruction of septum, nosebleeds, ulceration. Sharing of equipment (straws, pens, bank notes) can spread infections such as hepatitis C and HIV.
Nasal/oral inhalation	Gas, smoke, vapour via the nose and mouth into lungs	Tobacco, cannabis, heroin, crack cocaine, nitrites, volatile substances	Smoking, huffing, glue sniffing, dusting, bagging, chroming	Mouth, nose, throat irritation, impaired breathing, respiratory disease
Nebulisation of liquid and inhalation of vapour	Via the nose into lungs	Heroin	Chasing	
Cutaneous	Applied to skin for a topical (local) or systemic (whole body) effect			Hard to gauge correct dosage, hence development of skin patches
Transdermal	Patch applied to skin for systemic effect	Fentanyl, nicotine, testosterone		Adverse skin reactions such as burns

Sources: DH (2011); Peragallo *et al.* (2013); Shekarchizadeh *et al.* (2013); MacDonald *et al.* (2015); Pastore *et al.* (2015); Allen and Bridge (2017); Alcohol rehab (2020).

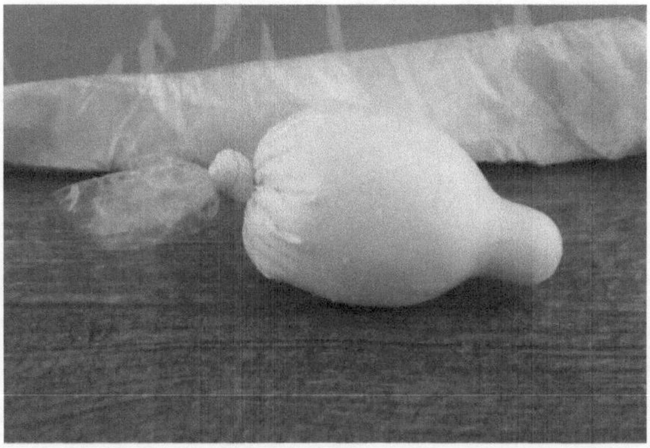

Figure 11.6 Heroin in condom for vaginal or rectal smuggling
Source: gaikova/Shutterstock.com

and holistic understandings of people and their behaviours. Heather focuses less on the person, and more on addictive behaviours:

> A person is addicted to a specific behaviour if they have demonstrated repeated and continuing failures to refrain from or radically reduce the behaviour despite resolutions to do so.
>
> (Heather, 2018 p.24)

Others prefer to use the word 'dependence' rather than addiction. Their reasons include that addiction implies a disease from which 'addicts' will never recover or change; or 'addiction' suggests 'all or nothing' which does not reflect the graded experience of much drug use; and perhaps mostly because the word 'addiction' has dehumanising and negative connotations which are neither deserved nor helpful (Drugwise, 2017d; Alcohol Change UK, 2020).

Between abstinence and dependency are phrases such as use, misuse and disorders. 'Use' implies no judgement, whereas

> Abuse and misuse imply that the use is harmful or done in the wrong way ... is dependent or part of ... problematic or harmful behaviour. Those who believe drug taking is wrong ... will tend to use the term misuse ... The Government, for example still uses the term ...
>
> (Drugwise, 2017e)

The World Health Organization (2019) brings the health effects of drugs (substances), which includes alcohol and tobacco, under its umbrella of mental disorders within their International Statistical Classification of Diseases, Injuries and Causes of Death (ICD-11). This brings together psychological and physical signs and symptoms caused by repetitive substance use and those caused by repetitive/addictive behaviours such as gambling because the two have much in common.

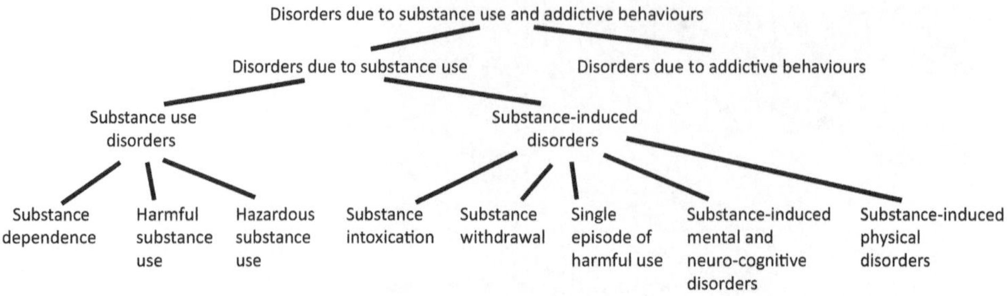

Figure 11.7 Disorders due to substance use and addictive behaviours
Source: World Health Organization, 2019

Substance use disorders, the disorders of use

- Substance dependence

Dependence is an inability to regulate the use of substances. It feels like a primitive, internal drive to use the substance and continue using it. It relates to the mesolimbic part of the brain, the 'reward pathway', where the brain 'remembers the pleasure' of previous exposure to the substance. The person has

- impaired control over the substance – its use may be inappropriate, it may be excessive and it is difficult to stop
- salience – it is prioritised over other necessary activities, even when it is causing significant harm
- physiological tolerance to the substance – needing more to get the same effect and repeating use to prevent or cope with withdrawal symptoms

A person needs to be exhibiting two of these characteristics repeatedly over 12 months or continuously over one month.

- Harmful substance use

Harmful substance use is characterised by a repetitive pattern of use, but not yet dependency. There is also the presence of significant harm to the person's mental or physical health, or behavioural problems that are adversely affecting others.

- Hazardous substance use

Hazardous use is a condition characterised by a repetitive pattern of substance use, but no harm has yet occurred. It is known that continuing this pattern of use will have harmful consequences.

Substance-induced disorders, the consequences of substance use

- Substance intoxication

Intoxication means the immediate, acute, time-limited, consequences of substance use, which will differ according to the substance.

- Substance withdrawal

Withdrawal means the consequences of substance dependence or a pattern of taking high doses. It lasts between a few days and a few months.

- Single episode of harmful use

A person has experienced harm related to taking a substance, but there is insufficient information for another diagnosis to be made.

- Substance-induced mental and neurocognitive disorders

Mental and neurocognitive disorders can be caused or exacerbated by a substance, for example, substance-induced anxiety disorder, substance-induced psychotic disorder, substance-induced obsessive compulsive disorder and many more. Some will diminish after the substance use stops but others, such as amphetamine-induced psychosis, may take several months.

- Substance-induced physical disorders

The physical conditions known to be associated with substance use include alcoholic cirrhosis, cancer and lung disease.

Disorders due to addictive behaviours

These disorders include gaming disorder and gambling disorder. Like substance dependence, both manifest impaired control, salience and physiological tolerance.

The route to disorders and dependency

The United Nations Office on Drugs and Crime and the World Health Organization (2017) report about 10% of people who start to use drugs go on to develop a drug disorder. Some are genetically programmed to be at greater risk of dependence. Risk can be modified by protective or detrimental early life experiences. For example, trauma, deprivation and chronic stress increase vulnerability.

When a vulnerable person is exposed to drugs, it interferes with the brain's reward pathway. Evolution designed the reward pathway to reinforce our important behaviours such as eating, drinking, paternal behaviours and social interaction, now it has learnt to reward a drug with a 'high'. Environments become strongly associated with the new learnt behaviour, and they trigger the desire for drug-seeking behaviour. Stress can also become a trigger. While the impulse to use a drug is easily triggered, the ability to control the desire is weakened. As the brain is not functioning normally, decision-making is poor and people find themselves engaging in illegal, unethical, immoral behaviours to obtain drugs, and do so increasingly under the influence of drugs.

Box 11.3 Trauma, self-medication and drug use

Adverse childhood experiences include experiencing or witnessing violence or abuse; having a family member die or attempt suicide; growing up in a household where there is drug-taking and having a parent with a mental health problem. Children from poorer backgrounds who have experienced adverse childhood experiences are much more likely than others to take drugs to self-medicate their emotional pain for the rest of their lives, and many develop a drug disorder. Trauma in adulthood, such as bereavement, being a victim of violence or in a violent relationship, being in a combat zone and homelessness are also associated with drug use and disorders.

(Source: Anda *et al.*, 2008; Gadd *et al.*, 2019; HCSAC, 2019)

Drug dependence is the result of cumulative biological and environmental disadvantages such as

- child neglect and abuse
- poor parenting and family support
- dysfunctional household
- poor emotional support
- social isolation and exclusion
- unemployment
- excess workload, poor working conditions
- poverty, poor neighbourhoods, homelessness, hunger
- exploitation, violence

(UNODC/WHO, 2017; HCSAC, 2019)

For example:

> The area that I was living in was being pulled down. It was an area of urban deprivation. There was high unemployment and crime. It seemed that nobody was working … I grew up during the miners' strike, you know. It was probably a sense of hopelessness throughout the area. There was no investment in the area. There was no community centre as such. For me looking back, it was a sense of no hope and no sense of purpose … Just that: feeling heartbreak, feeling 'what's the point?' and I coped with that by using substances.
>
> (Colin; HCSAC, 2019, p.9. Reproduced under Open Parliament Licence v3.0)

Substance-linked sex

Chemsex is a term used to describe the use of drugs, usually methamphetamine, mephedrone and GBH/GBL by men who have sex with men, to facilitate and enhance the sexual experience. Lawn and colleagues (2019) carried out an international survey with 22,289 respondents across the UK, Australia, Canada and those European countries that have adopted the Euro currency. Their average age was 31.4 years. The researchers coined the term substance-linked sex (SLS) as a broader term to encompass the use of any drug-related sex by anyone. It is:

> The act of engaging in sexual activity while under the influence of $\geq$ 1 [one or more than one] drugs applicable across a range of licit and illicit substances as well as across different sexes and sexual orientations, in various scenarios.
>
> (Lawn *et al.*, 2019 p.2)

The researchers asked about experiences over the previous 12 months.

- SLS was most strongly associated with being younger, having higher income and being from the UK
- At least a fifth used drugs to enhance their sexual experience, rising to 45% among homosexual men
- Men had SLS more than women. SLS was more common among homosexual and bisexual men than heterosexual men. Bisexual women had SLS more than heterosexual women
- More than half had taken alcohol, a third cannabis and just under one-sixth MDMA as part of SLS. The fourth choice for most was cocaine, but for homosexual men it was poppers.
- Heterosexual men took cannabis for SLS more than other men. Homosexual and bisexual men took MDMA, GHB/GBL, methamphetamine, mephedrone, poppers, ketamine and Viagra more than heterosexual men
- All groups rated GHB/GBL then MDMA as the best for sexual enjoyment, but thereafter there were differences in perceptions of other drugs

SLS presents concerns because it is associated with increased health risks, including sexually transmitted infections, unplanned pregnancies, loss of consciousness during sex and for some it has led to wider negative impacts on their lives (Paquette *et al.*, 2017; Glynn *et al.*, 2018).

Pregnancy

Taking drugs in pregnancy, without medical supervision, presents many potential health risks.

- Alcohol – miscarriage, still birth, heart abnormalities, foetal alcohol spectrum disorders, long-term developmental concerns
- Cannabis – associated with premature labour, low birth weight, poor foetal brain growth and later academic and behavioural concerns
- Cocaine – placental abruption (detachment), premature birth, impact on cognitive development
- Methamphetamine – miscarriage, still birth, maternal high blood pressure, low birth weight, developmental problems
- Opioids – bleeding in pregnancy, low birth weight, respiratory problems, risk of neonatal abstinence syndrome (baby has withdrawal symptoms), poor growth

- Smoking – miscarriage, increased risk of ectopic pregnancy, premature birth, low birth weight
- Drug use may affect early maternal-infant bonding

(Forray, 2016)

Co-occurring mental health and substance use conditions

Mental health problems can be a cause and a consequence of drug, including alcohol, use. These co-occurring conditions are a concern because Public Health England (2017) report

- about 70% of drug users have mental health problems
- about half of those receiving support from mental health services have a problem with substance use
- half of suicides are thought to be related to a history of substance use
- co-occurring conditions are the 'norm' rather than the exception among those in prison
- women are increasingly using substances to cope with psychological and physical harm from violence
- people with co-occurring mental health and substance use conditions are more likely to smoke and suffer from smoking-related illnesses and premature death

In Scotland, researchers interviewed 123 people over 35 years old who had a 'drug use problem'. Ninety-five percent reported having depression, 89% had anxiety and 53% had chronic pain (Matheson *et al.*, 2017).

Adulterants

Counterfeit and illegal drugs, especially those in pill or powder form, can be dangerous because the dose of the active substance is unknown. They can include potentially poisonous adulterants such as lead (metal), strychnine (pesticide), clenbuterol (decongestant), local anaesthetics, levamisole (worm treatment), aluminium and glass (DH, 2011). One woman said:

> I'm seeing more diversity in drugs and quality of drugs due to the darknet markets ... we're injecting drugs that we don't know exactly what they are or the strength any more. So called 'liquid Xanax' for example – it's clearly not etizolam when it has floaties in it.
>
> (Australian woman, quoted in Peacock *et al.*, 2019 p.1679)

Poly-drug use

Examples of risks associated with mixing two drugs include

- cocaine + alcohol = increased intoxication and increased risks to cardiovascular system
- cannabis + alcohol = poor driving performance

- opioids + benzodiazepines = increases the depression (slowing) of the central nervous system
- nitrites + Viagra = abnormally low blood pressure

(DH, 2011)

Deaths of despair

Drug-related deaths

> ... are often referred to as 'deaths of despair' because most relate to people who have little hope for the future due [to] their experience of poverty [and] inequality of opportunity.
>
> (HCSAC, 2019 p.9. Reproduced under Open Parliament Licence v3.0)

Defining a drug-related death is complex. In the UK, the Office of National Statistics includes a drug-related death as one recorded within the World Health Organization's ICD-11 category 'mental and behavioural disorders due to psychoactive substance use', and the death relates to opioids, cannabinoids, sedatives or hypnotics, cocaine, other stimulants including caffeine, hallucinogens, multiple drug use or use of other psychoactive substances. In addition, drug-related deaths include those where a substance listed within the Misuse of Drugs Act was in the body at the time of death. Some of the exceptions to recording a death as drug-related include some painkillers and cold remedies.

Drug-related deaths rose significantly in 2018 across the UK. There were 4,359 drug-related deaths in England and Wales, representing a 16% increase on the previous year (ONS, 2019). There were 189 deaths in Northern Ireland, representing a rise of 39% since the previous year (NISRA, 2020). In Scotland, there were 1,187 deaths, the highest ever recorded (Figure 11.8). At 161 deaths per million of the population, this was three times the death rate of the whole UK, which was 54 per million (NRS, 2019). Of these, 72% were male and two-thirds were aged between 35 and 54 years old.

Table 11.6 Percentage of UK drug-related deaths due to specific drugs, 2018

Drug detected	*Scotland*	*Northern Ireland*	*England and Wales*
Opioids/opiates	79.1%	60.8%	51%
Heroin and/or morphine	41.3%	21.2%	
Methadone	42.9%	7.9%	
Amphetamines	3.5%	7.9%	3.6%
Ecstasy-type drugs	2.7%	5.8%	1.5%
Cocaine	21.1%	14.8%	11.1%
Pregabalin	16.4%	28.6%	
Gabapentin	15.2%	2.6%	
Psychoactive substances	575 deaths	5.3%	125 deaths

Note: Based on ONS definition.

Sources: NRS (2019); NISRA, 2020; ONS (2019).

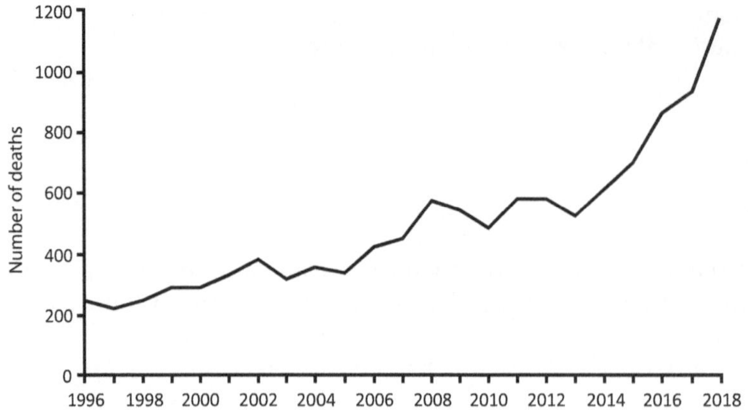

Figure 11.8 Drug-related deaths in Scotland, 1996 to 2018
Source: HCSAF, 2019 reproduced under the terms of the Open Parliament Licence v3.0

An inquiry into Scotland's drug crisis found that drug-related deaths have risen because of

- poly-drug use
- increased strength and toxicity, e.g. benzodiazepines were 10 times as strong as the diazepam people used to take
- an ageing cohort. The cohort who began taking drugs in the 1980s are now middle-aged and have a range of health conditions such as respiratory or circulatory disease, which increases their risk of death
- a rise in blood-borne viruses. In 2015, Glasgow had a major HIV outbreak which has been perpetuated by the sharing of syringes. Deaths from HIV-related infections and hepatitis C have been high. A third of Scotland's drug-related deaths in 2018 were in Greater Glasgow and Clyde.

(HCSAC, 2019)

Stigma

International reports show that although developing a substance use/induced disorder can have lethal consequences, less than one in six people, across the world, receive the treatment that they need (UNODC/WHO, 2017). Their reasons could include cost, delays, personal denial of a problem and lack of knowledge, but often help is not sought because of stigma. People with substance use problems are frequently judged, isolated, marginalised, ostracised and the victims of discrimination. Very many live alone with little social interaction (Matheson *et al.*, 2017). In Scotland, the language used in the media has been described as horrendous and dehumanising, reinforcing drug use as a moral failing rather than a complex health issue (HCSAC, 2019). Social stigma can be internalised into a powerful self-stigma so that the individual judges themselves in the same way, they become their own harshest critic, and they believe that they are not worthy of help and are overwhelmed by feelings of shame (Hammarlund *et al.*, 2018). For example,

> I don't trust nobody ... I keep myself to myself unless they ask anything but part from that I feel isolated. Put [this way], if I was deid, nobody would miss me.
>
> (Woman, 39 years; Matheson *et al.*, 2017 p.i)

Taking drugs outside of medical supervision carries serious health risks. Those who are poor and vulnerable are more likely to develop disorders and dependency. Social stigma is a major barrier to early intervention and obtaining help.

Criminal justice versus public health

The UK's drug laws are influenced by the United Nations' Conventions on psychoactive drugs signed in 1961 and 1971. The Global Commission on Drug Policy (2019) explains how these conventions were based on securing controlled drugs for medicinal use while preventing their diversion into recreational use. Today tobacco and alcohol remain legal and enable their respective industries to make huge profits, while the illegal drug market thrives and organised crime benefits. The cost has been in terms of public health, security, prison overcrowding, discrimination, violence, corruption and poor access to essential medicines. The Commission argues that the distinction between what is legal and illegal is the result of historic culture, power and politics. It is

> ... too often influenced by ideology, prejudice and discrimination of marginalized populations, not to mention the financial interests of the pharmaceutical industry. Science is rarely part of the decision process ...
>
> (Global Commission on Drugs Policy, 2019 p.3)

The Commission is calling for a review of the current classification of drugs across the world and using the World Health Organization and other interdisciplinary scientific research groups to guide an evidence-based approach.

A similar debate is ongoing within the UK where the UK government primarily treats drug use as a matter for the criminal justice system and the Scottish government believes it needs to be treated as a public health issue (HCSAC, 2019). The inquiry into concerns about drug use in Scotland prompted criticisms of a criminal justice approach, arguing it

- reinforces social stigma/discrimination and marginalises/demonises those who take drugs, so some don't come forward for treatment when they need it
- increases health risks because it pushes drug markets 'underground' where quality and safety cannot be monitored, and dealers are forced into 'dark alleys' for fear of arrest
- prison sentences encourage loss of home, family, jobs and networks, which makes recovery harder
- drugs in prisons are prevalent, it is where some develop a drug use, others get into increased difficulties

The arguments for a public health approach included that it

- can reduce harm to the most vulnerable by reducing stigma
- would reduce harm and costs to communities
- would include the expertise of multiple agencies, including criminal justice

The call from Scotland is:

> The Government must revise its strategy for addressing problem drug use in line with a public health approach ... to transfer lead responsibility for drugs policy from the Home Office to the Department for Health and Social Care.
>
> (HCSAC, 2019 p.24)

Benefits of recovery

The benefits of stopping the use or misuse of drugs partly depends on the types of drugs and how they are administered. Timpson and colleagues (2016) interviewed 32 people from across the UK who were participating in various types of recovery communities, each offering different types of support. For some, recovery meant abstinence and for others it was about recognising a need to change; each was on their own individual journey towards becoming someone different to who they had been. Many spoke of having a purpose, re-connecting with family and friends, with employment or education, and developing a sense of control over themselves, their lives and their relationships with others.

Summary

This chapter has

- defined drugs and some of the ways they can be classified
- explained the seven types of drugs and how they affect health
- described UK drug laws and how they define and apply to controlled drugs
- examined some of the reasons behind drug use and why dependency may develop
- described patterns of drug use and health
- outlined the health risks associated with drug use
- presented some arguments for rethinking drug policy away from criminal justice towards public health

Further reading

Nutt, D. (2020) *Drugs without the hot air*. Cambridge: UIT Cambridge Ltd.
Pycroft, A. (2015) *Key concepts in substance misuse*. London: Sage

Useful websites

Drugwise. Available at: www.drugwise.org.uk
FRANK. Available at: www.talktofrank.com
European Monitoring Centre for Drugs and Drug Addiction. Available at: www.emcdda.europa.eu

References

Alcohol Change UK (2020) How do we talk about alcohol? Available at: https://alcoholchange.org.uk/policy/policy-insights/how-do-we-talk-about-alcohol (Accessed 30th January 2020)

Alcohol rehab (2020) Ways of taking drugs. Available at: https://alcoholrehab.com/drug-addiction/routes-of-drug-administration (Accessed 17th February 2020)

Allen, J.R., and Bridge, W. (2017) 'Strange routes of administration for substances of abuse', *The American Journal of Psychiatry Residents' Journal*, 12(12) doi:10.1176/appi.ajp-rj.2017.121203

Anand, U., Jacobo-Herrera, N., Altermimi, A., and Lakhssassi, N. (2019) 'A comprehensive review of medicinal plants as antimicrobial therapeutics: potential avenues of biocompatible drug discovery', *Metabolites*, 9(258) doi:10.3390/metabo9110258

Anda, R.F., Brown, D.W., Felitti, V.J., Dube, S.R., and Giles, W.H. (2008) 'Adverse childhood experiences and prescription drug use in a cohort study of adult HMO patients', *BMC Public Health*, 8(1) doi:10.1186/1471-2458-8-198

Barber, S. (2019) Medical use of cannabis. Briefing paper No.8355. Available at: https://researchbriefings.files.parliament.uk/documents/CBP-8355/CBP-8355.pdf (Accessed 3rd March 2020)

Dangerous drugs: the misuse of drugs regulations (2001) (SI 2001/3998). Available at: www.legislation.gov.uk/uksi/2001/3998/pdfs/uksi_20013998_en.pdf (Accessed 1st March 2020)

Department of Health (2011) *A summary of the health harms of drugs*. London: Department of Health

Drugwise (2016a) Stimulants. Available at: www.drugwise.org.uk/stimulants/ (Accessed 12th February 2020)

Drugwise (2016b) Nitrites. Available at: www.drugwise.org.uk/nitrites/ (Accessed 17th February 2020)

Drugwise (2017a) Opioid analgesics. Available at: www.drugwise.org.uk/analgesic/ (Accessed 12th February 2020)

Drugwise (2017b) Spice. Synthetic cannabinoids (SCRAs). Available at: www.drugwise.org.uk/wp-content/uploads/Spice-info-sheetv1.3-Interactive-national.pdf (Accessed 12th February 2020)

Drugwise (2017c) Performance and image enhancing drugs. Available at: www.drugwise.org.uk/performance-and-image-enhancing-drugs-pieds/ (Accessed 16th February 2020)

Drugwise (2017d) What is addiction? Available at: www.drugwise.org.uk/what-is-addiction/ (Accessed 18th February 2020)

Drugwise (2017e) Drug misuse. Available at: www.drugwise.org.uk/drug-misuse/ (Accessed 18th February 2020)

European Monitoring Centre for Drugs and Drug Addiction (2018) *Medical use of cannabis and cannabinoids*. Luxembourg: Office of the European Union

Forray, A. (2016) 'Substance use during pregnancy, *F1000 Research*, 5(887) doi:10.12688/f1000research.7645.1

Furman, D., Campisi, J., Verdin, E., Carrera-Bastos, P., Targ, S., Franceschi, C., Ferrucci, L., Gilroy, D.W., Fasano, A., Miller, G.W., Miller, A.H., Mantovani, A, Weyand, C.M., Barzilae, N., Goronzy, J.J., Rando, T.A., Effros, R.B., Lucia, A., Kleinstreuer, N., and Slavich, G.M. (2019) 'Chronic inflammation in the etiology of disease across the life span', *Nature Medicine*, 25(12), pp.1822–1832

Gadd, D., Henderson, J., Radcliffe, P., Stephens-Lewis, D., Johnson, A., and Gilchrist, G. (2019) 'The dynamics of domestic abuse and drug alcohol dependency', *The British Journal of Criminology*, 60(1) doi:10.1093/bjc/azz063

Global Commission on Drugs Policy (2019) Classification of psychoactive substances. When science was left behind. Available at: www.drugsandalcohol.ie/30714/1/2019Report_EN_web.pdf (Accessed 16th February 2020)

Glynn, R.W., Byrne, N., O'Dea, S., Shanley, A., Codd, M., Keenan, E., Ward, M., Igoe, D., and Clarke, S. (2018) 'Chemsex, risk behaviours and sexually transmitted infections among men who have sex with men in Dublin, Ireland', *International Journal of Drug Policy*, 52, pp.9–15

Gov.UK (2017) Press release. Freshers warned against self-prescribing: you're not doctors yet. Available at: www.gov.uk/government/news/freshers-warned-against-self-prescribing-youre-not-doctors-yet (Accessed 3rd March 2020)

Gov.UK (2019) Medicines: reclassify your product. Available at: www.gov.uk/guidance/medicines-reclassify-your-product (Accessed: 11th February 2020)

Gov.UK (2020) *Drugs penalties.* Available at: www.gov.uk/penalties-drug-possession-dealing (Accessed 11th February 2020)

Hammarlund, R., Crapanzano, K.A., Luce, L., Mulligan, L., and Ward, K.M. (2018) 'Review of the effects of self-stigma and perceived social stigma on the treatment-seeking decisions of individuals with drug-and alcohol-use disorders', *Substance Abuse and Rehabilitation*, 9, pp.115–136

Heather, N. (2018) 'Rethinking addiction', *The Psychologist*, 31(1), pp.24–29

Home Office (2019a) List of the most commonly encountered drugs currently controlled under the misuse of drugs legislation. Available at: www.gov.uk/government/publications/controlled-drugs-list--2/list-of-most-commonly-encountered-drugs-currently-controlled-under-the-misuse-of-drugs-legislation (Accessed: 11th February 2020)

Home Office (2019b) Drug misuse: findings from the 2018 to 2019 crime survey for England and Wales. Available at: www.gov.uk/government/statistics/drug-misuse-findings-from-the-2018-to-2019-csew (Accessed 20th February 2020)

House of Commons Scottish Affairs Committee (2019) Problem drug use in Scotland. First Report of Session 2019. Available at: https://publications.parliament.uk/pa/cm201919/cmselect/cmscotaf/44/44.pdf (Accessed 25th February 2020)

Lawn, W., Aldridge, A., Xia, R., and Winstock, A.R. (2019) 'Substance-linked sex in heterosexual, homosexual, and bisexual men and women: an online, cross-sectional "Global Drug Survey" report', *The Journal of Sexual Medicine*, 16(5) doi:10.1016/j.jsxm.2019.02.018

Luo, M., Jiao, J., and Wang, R. (2019) 'Screening drug target combinations in disease-related molecular networks', *BMC Bioinformatics*, 20(198) doi:10.1186/s12859-019-2730-8

MacDonald, L.E., Onsrud, J.E., and Mullins-Hodgin, R. (2015) 'Acute sensorineural hearing loss after abuse of an inhaled, crushed oxymorphone extended-release tablet', *Pharmacotherapy*, 35(7) doi:10.1002/phar.1605

Mahmood, K., Rezaee-Momtaz, M., Tavousi, M., Montazeri, A., and Araban, M. (2019) 'Risk factors associated with self-medication among women in Iran', *BMC Public Health*, 19(1033) doi: 10.1186/s12889-019-7302-3

Matheson, C., Liddell, D., Hamilton, E., and Wallace, J. (2017) Older people with drug problems in Scotland: a mixed methods study exploring health and social support needs. Scottish Drugs Forum. Available at: www.sdf.org.uk/wp-content/uploads/2017/06/OPDP-mixed-methods-research-report-PDF.pdf (Accessed 20th February 2020)

MIND (2020) Recreational drugs and alcohol. Available at: www.mind.org.uk/information-support/types-of-mental-health-problems/drugs-recreational-drugs-alcohol/recreational-drugs-a-z/ (Accessed 12th February 2020)

Mounteney, J., Bo, A., Klempova, D., Oteo, A. and Vandam, L (2015) The internet and drug markets. European Monitoring Centre for Drugs and Drug Addiction. Available at: www.emcdda.europa.eu/attachements.cfm/att_234684_EN_Internet%20and%20drug%20markets%20study.pdf (Accessed 19th February 2020)

National Institute on Drug Abuse (2018a) Prescription CNS depressants. Available at: www.drugabuse.gov/publications/drugfacts/prescription-cns-depressants (Accessed 12th February 2020)

National Institute on Drug Abuse (2018b) Prescription stimulants. Available at: www.drugabuse.gov/publications/drugfacts/prescription-stimulants (Accessed 12th February 2020)

National Institute on Drug Abuse (2018c) Synthetic cathinones ('bath salts'). Available at: www.drugabuse.gov/publications/drugfacts/synthetic-cathinones-bath-salts (Accessed 14th February 2020)

National Institute on Drug Abuse (2018d) Synthetic cannabinoids (K2/Spice). Available at: www.drugabuse.gov/publications/drugfacts/synthetic-cannabinoids-k2spice (Accessed 12th February 2020)

National Institute on Drug Abuse (2018e) Steroids and other appearance and performance enhancing drugs (APEDs). Available at: www.drugabuse.gov/publications/research-reports/steroids-other-appearance-performance-enhancing-drugs-apeds/what-are-different-types-apeds (Accessed 16th February 2020)

National Institute on Drug Abuse (2019a) Marijuana. Available at: www.drugabuse.gov/publications/drugfacts/marijuana (Accessed 12th February 2020)

National Institute on Drug Abuse (2019b) Hallucinogens. Available at: www.drugabuse.gov/publications/drugfacts/hallucinogens (Accessed 14th February 2020)

National Institute on Drug Abuse (2020) Opioids. Available at: www.drugabuse.gov/drugs-abuse/opioids (Accessed 12th February 2020)

Office for National Statistics (2019) Deaths related to drug poisoning in England and Wales: 2018 registrations. Available at: www.ons.gov.uk/peoplepopulationandcommunity/birthsdeathsandmarriages/deaths/bulletins/deathsrelatedtodrugpoisoninginenglandandwales/2018registrations (Accessed 21st February 2020)

National Records of Scotland (2019) Drug-related deaths in Scotland in 2018. Available at: www.nrscotland.gov.uk/files//statistics/drug-related-deaths/2018/drug-related-deaths-18-pub.pdf (Accessed 21st February 2020)

Northern Ireland Statistics and Research Agency (2020) Drug-related and drug-misuse deaths 2008–2018. Available at: www.nisra.gov.uk/publications/drug-related-and-drug-misuse-deaths-2008–2018 (Accessed 21st February 2020)

Pastore, M.N., Yogeshvar, K.N., Horstmann, M., and Roberts, M.S. (2015) 'Transdermal patches: history, development and pharmacology', *British Journal of Pharmacology*, 172(9), pp.2179–2209

Paquette, R., Tanton, C., Burns, F., Prah, P., Shahmanesh, M., Field, N., Macdowall, W., Gravningen, K., Sonnenberg, P., and Mercer, C.H. (2017) 'Illicit drug use and its association with key sexual risk behaviours and outcomes: findings from Britain's third national survey of sexual attitudes and lifestyles lNatsal-3)', *PloS One*, 12(5) doi:10.1371/journal.pone.0177922

Peacock, A., Bruno, R., Gisev, N., Degenhardt, L., Hall, W., Sedefov, R., White, J., Thomas, K.V., Farrell, M., and Griffiths, P. (2019) 'New psychoactive substances: challenges for drug surveillance, control and public health responses', *The Lancet*, 394(10209), pp.1668–1884

Peragallo, J., Biousse, V., and Newman, N.J. (2013) 'Ocular manifestations of drug and alcohol abuse', *Current opinion in ophthalmology*, 24(6), pp.566–573

Perrot, S., Citée, J., Louis, P., Quentin, B., Robert, C., Milon, J.Y., Bismut, H., and Baumelou, A. (2019) 'Self-medication in pain management: the state of the art of pharmacists' role for over-the-counter analgesic use', *European Journal of Pain*, 13(10), pp.1747–1762

Public Health England (2017) Better care for people with co-occurring mental health and alcohol/drug use conditions. Available at: https://bit.ly/2JyYRAl (Accessed 23rd February 2020)

Rodrigues, C.F. (2020) 'Self-medication with antibiotics in Maputo, Mozambique: practices, rationales and relationships', *Palgrave Communications*, 6(6) doi:10.1057/s41599-019-0385-8

Shekarchizadeh, H., Khami, M.R., Mohebbi, S.Z., Ekhtiari, H., and Virtanen, J.I. (2013) 'Oral health of drug abusers: a review of health effects and care', *Iranian Journal of Public Health*, 42(9), pp.929–940

Timpson, H., Eckley, L., Sumnall, H., Pendlebury, M., and Hay, G. (2016) '"Once you've been there, you're always recovering": exploring experiences, outcomes, and benefits of substance misuse recovery', *Drugs and Alcohol Today*, 16(1), pp.29–38

Torres, N.F., Chibi, B., Middleton, L.E., Solomon, V.P., and Mashamba-Thompson, T.P. (2019) 'Evidence of factors influencing self-medication with antibiotics in low and middle income countries: a systematic scoping review', *Public Health*, 168, pp.92–101
United Nations Office on Drugs and Crime (2017) *Global synthetic drugs assessment.* Vienna: United Nations
United Nations Office on Drugs and Crime/World Health Organization (2017) International standards for the treatment of drug use disorders. Available at: www.who.int/substance_abuse/activities/msb_treatment_standards.pdf (Accessed 18th February 2020)
United Nations Office on Drugs and Crime (2018) Understanding the synthetic drug market: the NPS factor. Global Smart Update Volume 19. Available at: www.unodc.org/documents/scientific/Global_Smart_Update_2018_Vol.19.pdf (Accessed 12th February 2020)
Wright, G. (2018) 'Unlocking the potential of natural products in drug discovery', *Microbial Biotechnology*, 12(1), pp.55–57
World Health Organization (1994) Lexicon of alcohol and drug terms published by the World Health Organization. Available at: www.who.int/substance_abuse/terminology/who_lexicon/en/ (Accessed: 11th February 2020)
World Health Organization (2019) Model list of essential medicines. 21st list. Geneva: World Health Organization
World Health Organization (2019) International statistical classification of diseases and related health problems 11th revision (ICD-11). Available at https://icd.who.int/browse11/l-m/en (Accessed 18th February 2020)
Yuan, H., Ma, Q., Ye, L., and Piao, G. (2016) 'The traditional medicine and modern medicine from natural products', *Molecules*, 21(5) doi:10.3390/molecules21050559
Zinberg, N. (1986) *Drug, set and setting: basis for controlled intoxicant use.* London: Yale University Press

12 Weight and health

Sally Robinson

Key points

- Introduction
- Weight statistics
- Measuring weight and shape
- Body fat and health
- The experience of weight
- Influences on weight
- A healthy weight
- Summary

Introduction

This chapter will present information about adult weight across the world, including illustrations from the UK. It will explain how we measure weight and shape and the ways in which being overweight or underweight are associated with quality of life, illness and early death. It will examine how excess body fat leads to disease, and the impact of undernutrition on people's health. The chapter discusses how people experience weight, including weight stigma and eating disorders. It concludes with an overview of the influences on people's weight and provides a description of a healthy weight.

Weight statistics

Overweight data

Across the world, more than 1.9 billion adults are overweight and 650 million are obese (BMI over 30) (WHO, 2018). This represents a tripling of obesity across the world between 1975 and 2016 (Table 12.1). In the UK, there was a rapid rise in overweight and obesity during the 1990s, but since 2000 the rate of increase has slowed (Table 12.2).

In England, 31% of men and 45% of women with learning disabilities are obese, which compares to 24% of men and 27% of women in the general population (Gov. UK, 2016). Adults of Chinese heritage are less overweight or obese compared to other ethnicities (Figure 12.1).

Table 12.1 Comparison of adult overweight and obesity (BMI ≥25) (age-standardised estimate) in some regions of the world between 1975 and 2016

	Percentage overweight or obese		
	Population	*Male*	*Female*
1975			
World	21.5%	20.4%	22.7%
Europe	39.2%	39.1%	38.8%
Africa	11.6%	7.9%	15.0%
Americas	36.6%	37.0%	36.1%
South-East Asia	21.9%	19.7%	24.1%
2016			
World	38.9%	38.5%	39.2%
Europe	58.7%	63.1%	54.3%
Africa	31.1%	22.8%	38.8%
Americas	62.5%	64.1%	60.9%
South-East Asia	5.8%	4.7%	7.0%

Source: Adapted from WHO (2017a).

Table 12.2 Adult overweight and obesity across the UK as a percentage of population

	Overweight and obese (BMI ≥ 25)	*Obese (BMI ≥30)*	*Obese men (BMI ≥ 30)*	*Obese women (BMI ≥ 30)*
England (2017)	64%	29%	27%	30%
Northern Ireland (2017/2018)	64%	27%	26%	27%
Scotland (16–64 years) (2017)	65%	29%	27%	30%
Wales (2016/2017)	60%	24%	24%	22%

Sources: NHS Digital (2019); Public Health Wales NHS Trust (2019); Scottish Government (2018); Department of Health (2018).

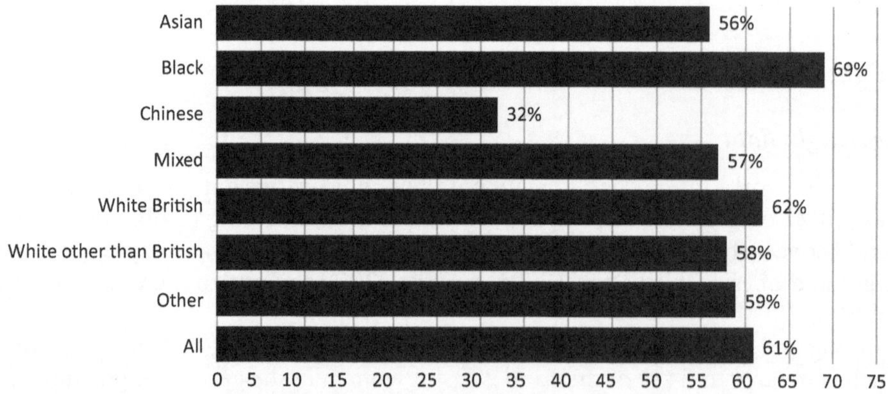

Figure 12.1 Percentage of overweight or obese adults in England by ethnicity, 2016 to 2017
Source: adapted from Gov.UK, 2018. Reproduced under the terms of the Open Government Licence v3.0

Table 12.3 Comparison of adult underweight (BMI <18) (age standardised estimate) in some regions of the world between 1975 and 2016

	Percentage underweight		
	Population	*Male*	*Female*
1975			
World	14.3%	13.8%	14.8%
Europe	3.4%	2.6%	4.2%
Africa	18.7%	19.7%	17.8%
Americas	5.3%	4.6%	5.9%
South-East Asia	33.2%	32.5%	34.0%
2016			
World	9.0%	8.6%	9.4%
Europe	1.6%	0.8%	2.3%
Africa	10.7%	12.1%	9.5%
Americas	1.8%	1.2%	2.3%
South-East Asia	20.5%	20.2%	20.9%

Source: Adapted from WHO (2017b).

Underweight data

Nine per cent of the world's adult population are underweight (BMI less than 18). This represents a reduction since 1975 (WHO, 2017b) (Table 12.5). In the UK, 1% of the adult population are underweight, which is half of what it was in 1975 (WHO, 2017b).

The world has seen the prevalence of overweight and obesity rising and underweight falling over the last 40 years.

Measuring weight and shape

Body mass index (BMI)

Nuttall (2015) explains how American life insurance data, published in 1901, contained information about people's heights and weights. The data suggested a relationship between the ratio of weight to height, their 'body build', and people's life expectancy. Tables of weight/height were developed and used to classify people as overweight, underweight or 'ideal' weight. The cut-off points were related to the reference population, those who had applied for insurance. For example, if a person's weight:height ratio was 20% higher than the average of others at that height, they were overweight. Insurers were interested in limiting the financial risks of insuring people who were not 'ideal' weight, but others were interested in understanding the health risks.

The calculations were refined with the aim to define someone's fat mass as a proportion of their total mass, regardless of their height or the size of their skeleton. The research community agreed that the mathematical formula Quetelet's Index, weight divided by height squared, would be the most accurate though it was recognised that it did not accurately represent a person's percentage of body fat. In 1972, Ancel Keys and colleagues used this to calculate indices of relative weight and obesity and used the term body mass index.

Body mass index (BMI) is a calculation of a person's weight in kilograms divided by the square of their height in metres.

$$\frac{\text{Weight (kg)}}{\text{Height (m)}^2}$$

Table 12.4 International classification of adult underweight, overweight and obesity according to BMI

Classification	*Body mass index (BMI) (kg/m²)*
Underweight	Less than 18.5
Severe thinness	Less than 16
Moderate thinness	16–16.99
Mild thinness	17–18.49
Normal range	18.50–24.99
Overweight	More than 25
Pre-obese	25–29.99
Obese	More than 30
Obese I	30 to 34.99
Obese II	35–39.99
Obese III	More than 40

Source: Adapted from World Health Organization (2019).

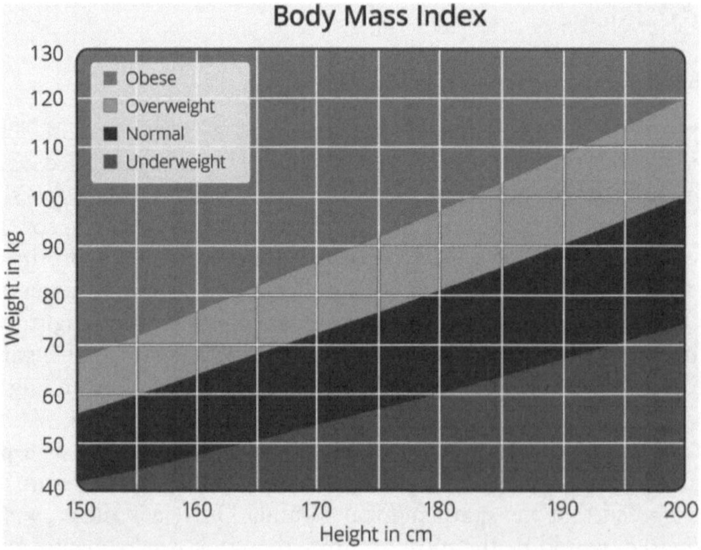

Figure 12.2 Classification of body mass index
Source: Zerbor/Shutterstock.com

The World Health Organization established the four categories underweight, normal, overweight and obese that are used today (Table 12.4). The 'cut off points' for the classifications emerged from studying a large reference population of Europeans and obesity-related disease (WHO, 1998). In 1997 the International Obesity Task Force modified 'overweight' to 'pre-obesity' and categorised obesity into three classes.

Criticisms of body mass index (BMI)

Nuttall (2015) draws on a wide range of evidence to argue why using BMI, alone, to understand disease and death is limited.

- The introduction of the term 'pre-obese', rather than 'overweight', with its connotation that people are moving towards obesity, means that people within this category are sometimes included alongside the other obese categories. Together this exaggerates the perceptions of the scale of obesity, even though they are well within the expected normal distribution of BMI within the reference population
- BMI does not differentiate between lean body mass, such as muscle, and fat mass. People, such as well-muscled athletes, can have a high BMI, but low body fat mass. As a proxy measure of body fat, it fails
- BMI does not capture the location of body fat
- BMI does not account for important variables such as sex, ethnicity, age and leg length. For example, women generally have a lower BMI than men, but they tend to have higher body fat
- BMI is designed to be used with large populations, not with individuals
- The relationship between BMI and disease or death does not consider factors such as family history, genetics, past and current health-related behaviours such as smoking, duration and history of weight gain, occupations or medication. This may explain the 'obesity paradox', where some people with lower and higher BMIs have longer life expectancy compared to those in the 'normal range'
- Several large studies show little association between BMIs and death rate, especially in the 24 to 28 BMI range

BMI, mortality and morbidity

In terms of preventing early death, a BMI of 23 seems to be ideal for under 70-year-olds, and a BMI of 25 or higher into the overweight range for those who are older (Flegal *et al.*, 2013; Nuttall, 2015; Bhaskaran *et al.*, 2018) (Table 12.5). Nyberg and colleagues (2018) found, with increasing BMI, the number of years Europeans who lived with disease increased *regardless* of being smokers, non-smokers, physically active or inactive, and across socio-economic groups (Table 12.6). These studies are not saying that a high BMI directly causes illness, rather that it is associated with more ill health and early death as we age, regardless of our lifestyles or socio-economic background.

Table 12.5 Expected age of death at 40 years among UK non-smokers

Body mass index (BMI)	*Men (years)*	*Women (years)*
Underweight (<18.5)	77.9	79.8
Normal range (18.5–24.9)	82.2	84.3
Overweight (25–29.9)	81.2	83.5
Obese I (30–34.9)	78.7	81.9
Obese II (35–39.9)	76.2	79.6
Obese III (>40)	73.1	76.6

Source: Adapted from Bhaskaran *et al.* (2018).

Table 12.6 Estimated additional number of years with disease according to BMI between 40 to 75 years

Body mass index (BMI)	*Additional years of disease compared to having a BMI in normal range (18.5–24.9)*	
	Men (years)	*Women (years)*
Underweight (<18.5)	1.8	0
Normal range (18.5–24.9)	-	-
Overweight (25–29.9)	1.1	1.1
Obese I (30–34.9)	3.9	2.7
Obese II & III (35+)	8.5	7.3

Source: Nyberg *et al.* (2018).

High BMI is a marker that signals a higher risk of developing illness and early death in populations.

Waist circumference

Storing visceral and sub-cutaneous fat in the abdomen/upper body, 'apple' shape, is more strongly associated with diabetes, high blood pressure and coronary heart disease than storing fat across the pelvis and thighs, 'pear' shape. With age, both sexes accumulate more fat in the trunk, increasing the health risks, even among those within a 'normal range' BMI. Although total body fat is important, many studies demonstrate that waist circumference and/or the ratio of waist to hip is a better predictor of disease, and better than BMI (Periera *et al.*, 2012; Sahakyan *et al.*, 2015; Tran *et al.*, 2018) (Figure 12.3).

Generally, a person's waist should be less than half their height. Weight loss is recommended for Europeans, regardless of BMI, if a man's waist is approximately 94 cm (37 inches) and a woman's is 80 cm (31.5 inches) (Table 12.7). A European adult may be classified as having abdominal obesity if their waist circumference is more than 102 cm for men and 88 cm for women. Bates and colleagues selected a sample of people with an ethnic mix that broadly represented the population of England and found waist circumference was greater among older adults (Bates *et al.*, 2019) (Table 12.8).

Figure 12.4 does not distinguish between type 1 and type 2 diabetes, but as type 2 is much more prevalent, we can assume that the majority of measurements came from those with type 2. It shows that 9% of women and 12% of men with very large waist circumferences had diabetes.

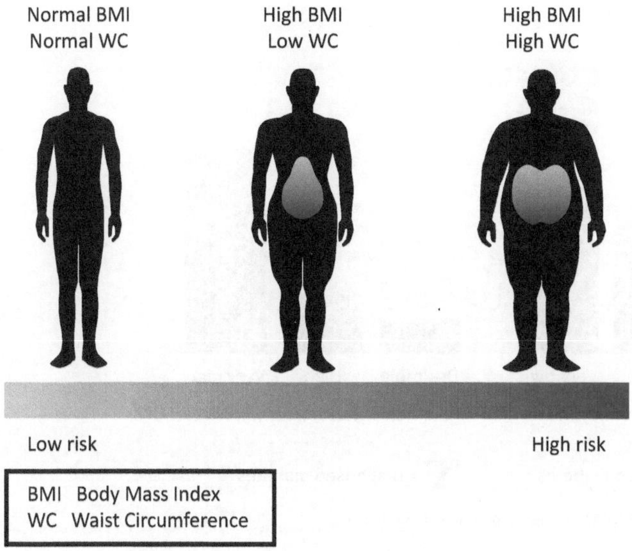

Figure 12.3 Mortality and morbidity risk from excess total fat and intra-abdominal fat
Source: adapted from Fu *et al.*, 2015 p.508

Table 12.7 Maximum waist circumference thresholds

	Europeans	*South Asians*	*Chinese*	*Japanese*	*Ethnic south and central Americans*	*Sub-Saharan Africans*
Men	94 cm	90 cm	90 cm	90 cm	Until better data are available, use south Asian recommendations	Until better data are available, use European recommendations
Women	80 cm	80 cm	80 cm	80 cm		

Source: Adapted from NICE (2013 p.52, 53).

Table 12.8 Waist circumference in England

	Weight loss recommended	*Abdominal obesity*	*Mean waist circumference of adults in England*	
			19–64 years	*65+ years*
Men	94 cm	102 cm	96 cm	103.2 cm
Women	80 cm	88 cm	86.6 cm	92.6 cm

Source: Bates *et al.* (2019).

A body shape index (ABSI)

A body shape index (ABSI) measures the risk of waist circumference relative to height and BMI (Krakauer and Krakauer, 2012). A high score indicates that a person's waist circumference is greater than expected, given their weight and height.

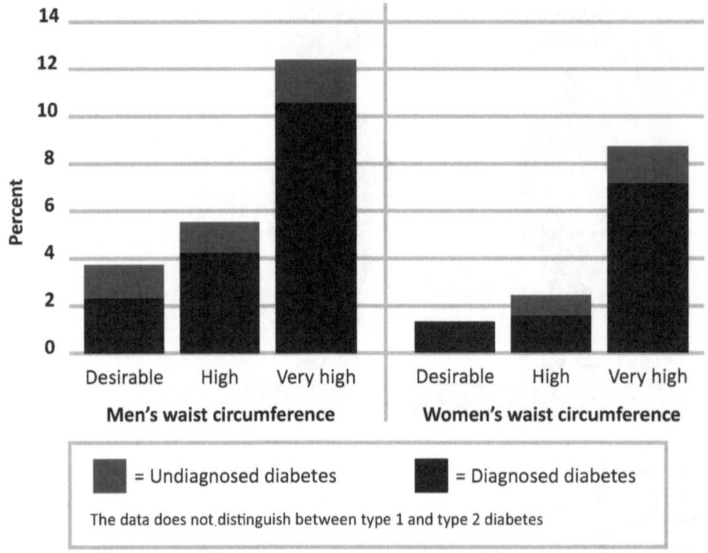

Figure 12.4 Relationship between diabetes and waist circumference in England, 2017 to 2018
Source: adapted from PHE, 2019a. Reproduced under the terms of the terms of the Open Government Licence v3.0

$$\text{ABSI} = \frac{\text{Waist Circumference (WC)}}{\text{BMI}^{2/3} \times \text{height}^{1/2}}$$

Studies show that an ABSI score predicts risks of early death, because it identifies high abdominal fat. It does so more accurately than BMI, waist circumference or waist/height ratio alone (Krakauer and Krakauer, 2014; Grant *et al.*, 2017; Bertoli *et al.*, 2017). ABSI calculators are available on-line.

Measuring disease and early death using body mass index has limitations, therefore other measures are used.

Body fat and health

Body fat

Body fat is essential to protect the organs of the body, to keep the body warm, to help the body to absorb fat-soluble vitamins, to store and provide energy, to support the growth of cells and to produce some hormones. Fat cells are stored in adipose tissue, a connective tissue found throughout the body. Sub-cutaneous fat sits beneath the skin. Visceral fat is in the abdomen, surrounding and infiltrating the major internal organs.

Excess body fat and health

Overweight and obesity are defined as having an excess of body fat to a degree that impairs health.

Atherosclerosis/cardiovascular disease

Too much fat in the body interferes with the lining of the arteries and encourages raised blood cholesterol, which forms atheroma, the fatty plaque that can clog the flow of the blood. This causes cardiovascular conditions such as high blood pressure, clots/thromboses, strokes and heart attacks.

Insulin resistance

Insulin, a hormone produced by the pancreas, removes glucose from the blood and helps it to enter the body's cells where it is used for energy. Insulin resistance means that this process is not working and excess glucose remains in the blood, a state called hyperglycaemia. The pancreas tries to rectify this by producing more insulin, leading to the condition hyperinsulinemia. Eventually the pancreas may not be able to keep up, and falters, leading to type 2 diabetes. Insulin resistance is associated with body fat, but it can exist in people who are not overweight.

Type 2 diabetes

Body fat and insulin resistance are strongly associated with developing type 2 diabetes. Unstable/high blood sugar damages blood vessels and encourages atheroma to stick to the sides. Together this exacerbates high blood pressure and cardiovascular disease.

Metabolic syndrome

High levels of visceral fat are associated with combinations of insulin resistance, diabetes, high blood pressure and high blood cholesterol. Together these are called metabolic syndrome, which is strongly associated cardiovascular disease and type 2 diabetes.

Non-alcoholic fatty liver disease

Non-alcoholic fatty liver disease occurs because of an accumulation of fat in the liver. Not only does this damage the liver, but it is linked to developing type 2 diabetes, high blood pressure and kidney disease.

Cancer

Body fat sends out instructions which affect the functions of the body, including metabolism and growth. Body fat leads to a greater production of hormones such as insulin and encourages chronic low-grade inflammation. All of these can encourage cells to divide more frequently, thus increasing the chance of some dividing uncontrollably and becoming cancer.

Being overweight or obese throughout adulthood increases the risk of cancer of the

- mouth
- oesophagus, stomach, pancreas, liver and bowel

- breast (postmenopausal)
- ovary and endometrium
- prostate
- kidney

  and gaining weight in adulthood increases the risk of postmenopausal breast cancer.

(WCRF/AICR, 2018)

COVID-19

High body fat is associated with severe illness and death from the COVID-19 coronavirus. Tan and colleagues (2020) explain that studies carried out in early 2020 suggest that critical illness from the virus increased by between 27% and 44% for those who were overweight and doubled for the obese. They suggest this may occur due to the adipose tissue being a 'target and viral reservoir' for the virus before it spreads to other organs; it may be because of greater body fat weakening the immune response; and it may be because fat reduces the ability of the lungs and airways to expand to full capacity and enable administered oxygen to move from the lungs into the blood stream and then around the body.

Low-grade inflammation

Cells secrete cytokines which affect how cells communicate with one another. Some of these are inflammatory. Fat cells are cells which store fat. As fat cells increase in size, more inflammatory cytokines, such as leptin, are produced. These activate a process which perpetuates chronic low-grade inflammation within the body. The body's inflammation response is a healthy defence to cope with injured cells, but chronic low-grade inflammation is harmful and associated with cancer, diabetes and cardiovascular disease.

Musculoskeletal conditions

Excess body fat places strain on the musculoskeletal system, causing pain, injury and long-term disability to the back, hips, knees, ankles, feet and to bones, joints and soft tissues. It is a major contributor to osteoarthritis, a condition where the cartilage at the ends of bones is worn down, causing painful joints.

Biomechanical and physiological limitations

Excess body fat affects how the body functions.

- Body movement is impaired; it is less mechanically efficient. This is associated with a greater reluctance to engage in physical activity
- The body's agility, flexibility and balance are reduced, resulting in poorer functioning during work and leisure activities
- The fat around the airways leads to sleep apnoea, a condition where breathing stops and starts
- The ability to tolerate heat is reduced

- In the event of a fall, fat around the hip bone may prevent a fracture, but the combination of poorer agility and balance, along with relative muscle weakness, increases the risk of falls
- Body fat can provide warmth in a cold climate, but it is less flexible than wearing additional clothing
- An obese person is more buoyant in water, but there is greater drag as the body emerges from the water
- Having excess body fat is only helpful during times of prolonged starvation

(Shephard, 2018a)

Psychosocial consequences of excess weight

Excess body fat has been linked to individuals experiencing psychological and social consequences, especially for those who are obese.

- An obese adult may carry the scars of having been an obese child, where studies show they may have experienced bullying, teasing, social isolation, a reluctance to participate in sports, poor self-image, low self-esteem, above average absenteeism from school, increased illness and poorer academic achievement
- Finding and buying clothes can be challenging and embarrassing
- Travelling may be impeded by the size of the vehicle/aeroplane, seats and seat belts
- Seating in public facilities such as cinemas, toilets or restaurants may be too small

Table 12.9 Self-reported overall happiness and general health according to weight

	Happy (n = 155,555)	*Unhappy (n = 7,511)*	*Good health (n = 118,609)*	*Poor health (n = 44,457)*
BMI				
Underweight (<18.5)	0.47%	0.89%	0.47%	0.54%
Normal weight (18.5–24.9)	33.7%	32.03%	37.09%	20.88%
Overweight (25–29.9)	42.57%	37.73%	43.83%	38.39%
Obese I (30–34.9)	17.49%	19.54%	14.54%	25.71%
Obese II (35–39.9)	4.93%	6.20%	24.54%	25.71%
Obese III (>40)	1.84%	3.59%	3.23%	9.66%
Waist circumference (men/women)				
Normal weight (<94 cm/<80 cm)	39.62%	37.86%	44.87%	25.32%
Overweight (94–101 cm/ 80–87 cm)	26.86%	23.92%	27.65%	24.26%
Obese (≥102 cm/≥88 cm)	33.52%	38.21%	27.48%	50.42%
Waist-hip-ratio (men/women)				
Normal weight (<0.90/0.80)	35.80%	33.10%	40.36%	23.15%
Overweight (0.90–0.99/ 0.80–0.84)	40.00%	39.17%	39.36%	41.55%
Obese (≥1/≥0.85)	24.21%	27.73%	20.27%	35.30%
Body fat percentage (men/women)				
Normal weight (≤25%/≤32%)	34.45%	36.07%	38.62%	23.57%
Obese (≤25%/≤32%)	65.55%	63.93%	61.38%	76.43%

Source: Adapted from Ul-Haq *et al.* (2014 p.23).

- Participation in sport, especially for women, is hampered by not being chosen to play and being asked to wear scanty clothing
- Negativity from others, such as those personal trainers or doctors who brand obese individuals as lazy, can deter individuals from participating in sports and healthcare
- Recruitment to employment, wages, continued employment and opportunities for promotion are negatively affected by obesity
- Excess body fat can reduce prospects of marriage, though this can vary across cultures
- These adverse psychosocial factors are associated with a reduced quality of life that is independent of any co-existing medical conditions, and may explain why obese individuals are prone to anxiety, depression and suicide

(Shephard, 2018b)

Academics from across the UK came together to study how 163,066 adults described their health and happiness (Ul-Haq *et al.*, 2014) (Table 12.9). They cross-checked the findings against the adults' weight, using measures of BMI, waist circumference, waist-hip ratio and body fat percentage. Those who were underweight, overweight or obese reported poorer health than those of 'normal' weight. They found,

- overweight and obese individuals were more likely to report poor health
- obese men were more likely to report poor health
- obese women were more likely to report unhappiness
- women reported feeling unhappy if they were obese I, II or III
- men only reported feeling unhappy if they were obese III
- underweight women only reported unhappiness if they also reported poor health
- being obese is associated with unhappiness, and this unhappiness seems to be related to experiencing poor health

Fit but fat

With regular physical activity, the lungs work better, we inhale and utilise more oxygen, and the heart muscle is strengthened and better able to pump highly oxygenated blood around the body. Having cardiorespiratory fitness may protect people from some of the negative physical and mental health consequences of carrying excess fat (Ortega *et al.*, 2018).

Maternal overweight and obesity

Excess weight at conception and during pregnancy is a concern because a third of UK women who die during pregnancy/childbirth are obese and a fifth are overweight (Knight *et al.*, 2018). Complications of being obese (BMI >30) during pregnancy affect both the mother and the baby.

An obese pregnant woman has an increased risk of

- miscarriage, loss of a pregnancy during the first 23 weeks
- diabetes during the pregnancy (gestational diabetes)

- pre-eclampsia, a condition of high blood pressure and protein in the urine which causes seizures and death
- thrombosis, blood clots
- needing labour to be medically induced
- caesarean, surgical, delivery and wound infection
- post-birth haemorrhage/bleeding
- anaesthetic complications such as epidural failure
- difficulties with starting breastfeeding
- postnatal depression

A foetus/baby with an obese mother has an increased risk of

- still birth, a death after 24 weeks of pregnancy
- prematurity
- being larger than average size
- neonatal death, in the first month of life
- congenital anomalies, being born with medical conditions
- injuries from birth
- need for intensive care

(Chodankar *et al.*, 2017)

Societal costs of obesity

Financial costs

Obesity has risen to the top of political agendas because of the potential impacts on wider society. These include costs of chronic healthcare and absenteeism from work, state benefits for people unable to work, and the costs of social care and early death. Public Health England (2017) report:

> The UK-wide NHS costs attributable to overweight and obesity are projected to reach £9.7 billion by 2050, with wider costs to society estimated to reach £49.9 billion per year.

That obesity is costly is not disputed; we need to ask who is providing the figure, for what purpose, and what evidence it is based upon. For example, in 2018 Simon Stevens, chief executive of NHS England, said:

> We are now spending more on obesity-related conditions in this country than we are on the police or the fire service.
>
> (BBC, 2018)

BBC journalists found that the claim was made based on research that double-counted the costs of obesity-related diabetes as well as diabetes not caused by obesity (BBC, 2018). They also found that it was based on the 'protection' budget for the police, fire services, law courts and prisons.

National security

The American writers Voss and colleagues (2019) cite people's physical fitness for military service and the costs of supporting members of the military with obesity-related chronic disease as two reasons why obesity threatens national security.

> *Having excessive body fat is associated with medical risks and subsequent costs to society.*

Underweight and health

Underweight is defined as having a BMI of under 18.5 but, as we have seen, BMI has limitations.

Underweight is a warning sign

Being underweight may be

- a symptom of conditions such as cancer, tuberculosis, diabetes or anorexia nervosa
- a sign that nutrients are not being properly digested or absorbed due to a problem with the gastrointestinal tract
- the result of not consuming enough calories in food and drink for the body's activities.
- the result of undertaking excessive physical activity without enough food and drink to provide enough calories

Undernutrition

People who are underweight are often undernourished, they are consuming too few nutrients for their body's needs and are very likely to have many nutritional deficiencies. In the UK, we often see the word malnutrition being used inaccurately as a synonym for undernutrition. Malnutrition means there is an imbalance of nutrition and comprises both overnutrition and undernutrition. Anyone, of any weight, can be malnourished if they are eating a poor diet.

When undernourished, the body will preserve and use what nutrients it can, but quickly becomes deficient and no longer has the raw material with which to grow, repair and function. Nutritional deficiencies will start to develop, such as

- anaemia, due to lack of iron, vitamin B12 or folate
- osteoporosis and fractures due to lack of vitamin D or calcium
- loss of muscle, hair, hunger and fatigue due to lack of protein

Protein-energy malnutrition means that the body is deficient in many nutrients, particularly in protein and energy (calories). Starvation means suffering or death due to lack of food. In these circumstances, the body normally turns to its stored glycogen and body fat to provide energy so that it can function. Once these are depleted, the body breaks down its own muscles and tissues to obtain energy to keep its organs, such as the heart, working. If starvation continues, muscles shrink, weight is lost; body temperature falls; concentration becomes difficult; weakness and fatigue set in; sleep deteriorates; skin becomes dry and may develop downy hair; fertility falls and immunity against infections lowers. Increasingly, chemicals such as sodium, potassium and magnesium become imbalanced and calcium is leeched out of bones, making them fragile. The major organs shrink, become strained and eventually fail, culminating in death.

Psychosocial consequences of starvation

No matter whether starvation is due to famine, war or an eating disorder, common features observed in both men and women include:

- difficulties in making decisions as the brain requires calories to function
- concentration is impaired, including having recurrent thoughts about food
- low mood and irritability
- inflexibility, obsessiveness, rigidity, an inability to be spontaneous
- inward-looking and self-focussed
- tendency to hoard
- social withdrawal, isolation
- loss of sense of humour
- neglect of personal hygiene

Maternal undernutrition

Maternal undernutrition is defined as having a BMI of under 18.5. During pregnancy, the mother will not improve her nutritional status due to the demands of the foetus. This increases the risks of

- maternal nutritional deficiencies such as anaemia
- maternal death
- a low-birth-weight baby, which is associated with illness and death in new-borns, and life-long physical and mental health consequences

(Ahmed *et al.*, 2012)

In the UK, underweight women are advised to gain about three stones (19 kg) during pregnancy (BDA, 2016).

Being underweight and undernourished is associated with serious medical risks.

The experience of weight

People who are unhappy about their weight often have

- a fear or dislike of body fat
- anxieties about food and/or physical activity
- distressing emotions

> I eat if I'm happy, I eat if I'm sad. I eat to celebrate ... it can be a self-esteem thing, it can be a social coping kind of thing, it can fill a void if you're anxious, if you have no friends ... It's still miserable ... a fight every day.
>
> (Lilia, who describes herself as obese, in Moola and Norman, 2017 p.271)

> I can more or less eat what I want but ... I think the worse, my worst thing would be [to be] overweight, that's what I worry about most.
>
> (Lee, a British man between 18 and 45 years old, in Janowski *et al.*, 2018 p.1351)

> I went into a cycle of dieting, I went off the diet, dieted often, and got fatter, and fatter, and fatter ... I had borderline eating problems ...
>
> (Carmen, lesbian, in Smith *et al.*, 2019 p.1183)

Jenny, with a 'normal range' BMI of 21, was asked how she would feel if she was unable to exercise for a week.

> You might as well say to me "stop eating", or "stop breathing" ... I should be really depressed, I should be suicidal ... by the end of it all, I just wouldn't be able to cope ... without exercising, the weight going on and the anxiety building up, I would get depressed.
>
> (Jenny, in Bamber *et al.*, 2000 p.427)

Some people have concerns about being too thin.

> I am a tall skinny man ... I hate my body. I would hate someone to laugh at me and I know girls don't like skinny men.
>
> (anonymous man, in Boynton, 2017)

Some want to be both thin and muscular.

> Being a male, in general you are expected to be a bigger and more athletic person to maintain that standard of masculinity ... you have to be ... kind of like processed masculine for the queer community ... we all want to be simultaneously slim and muscular at the same time.
>
> (22 year old gay male, in VanKim *et al.*, 2016 p.3680)

People's negative experiences of weight are the result of a combination of historical, cultural, social, familial influences, sometimes combined with biological and psychological traits that make a person particularly vulnerable.

British attitudes to overweight

In 2015, the British Social Attitudes Survey examined the attitudes of Britain towards overweight (Curtice, 2016).

Thinking point:

Participants were given the following scenario. How would you respond?

Table 12.10 British attitudes towards those who are very overweight

Statements	*n =1,841 weighted sample; 1,858 unweighted sample*		
	Agree	*Neither agree nor disagree*	*Disagree*
Most very overweight people are lazy	28%	29%	40%
Most very overweight people could lose weight if they tried	53%	20%	24%
People who are very overweight care just as much about their appearance as anyone else	57%	23%	16%
People who are very overweight should have the same right as anyone else to receive expensive NHS treatments	48%	25%	23%

Source: Adapted from Curtice (2016 p.19).

> Say two people who are equally well qualified apply for a job as an office manager. One person is very overweight and the other is not. Who do you think would be more likely to be offered the job – the very overweight person, the person who is not very overweight, or would they both have an equal chance of getting it?
>
> (Curtice, 2016 p.22. Reproduced with permission from Public Health England)

Three quarters of respondents said that the person who was not overweight would get the job, 22% thought both would have an equal chance, and 1% thought that it would go to the overweight person (Table 12.10). The survey's authors concluded that toleration of overweight, in themselves and others, was greater among men than women. People of a healthy weight were more likely to hold negative attitudes towards people who are obese than people who are overweight or obese themselves. Although respondents recognised social reasons for obesity, such as processed foods produced by the food industry, many held the view that losing weight was an individual and medical problem for which the solution was personal willpower.

Weight stigma

Williams and Annandale (2018) describe weight stigma in terms of blaming, shaming, discrimination and loss of status, casting the obese as the 'other', a burden to society. Weight stigma affects women more than men, and it is found in multiple sectors including healthcare settings and among doctors, nurses, medical students and dietitians (Tomiyama *et al.*, 2018; Henderson *et al.*, 2018). A person does not have to be overweight to experience feelings of weight stigma, the perception of being overweight is enough.

Weight stigma, among the overweight or obese, has been found to encourage poor health and weight gain because it

- is a stressor that increases the hormone cortisol, which encourages the storage of body fat

- is linked to physical risks such as high blood pressure and high blood cholesterol, as well as anxiety disorders and depression
- is internalised and self-loathing encourages behaviour that is detrimental to the individual's health
- decreases self-regulation, which encourages the rejection of dietary advice, binge eating and avoidance of exercise
- is associated with greater experience of physical pain because social and physical pain seem to be processed through the same biological pathways
- is associated with lowered functional mobility, perhaps because it attacks a person's self-concept as a fully functioning person
- attaches moral connotations to people's behaviour, which blur people's subjective and objective experiences of their bodies. For example, genuinely feeling heavier/fatter along with resulting lowered self-worth because of prior eating behaviour even when no weight has in fact been gained
  (Olson *et al.*, 2018; Tomiyama *et al.*, 2018; Williams and Annandale, 2018)

Researchers at University College London carried out a study of 5,056 older adults as part of the English Longitudinal Study of Ageing. They concluded that about 40% of the negative psychological effects associated with obesity can be attributed to feelings of weight discrimination (Jackson *et al.*, 2015).

Moola and Norman (2017) explain that women who have the slimmer bodies that are closer to what UK culture presents as ideal may suffer less discrimination from others, but they can nevertheless experience acute body shame. Burns and colleagues (2001) found that women's quality of life was negatively affected by their perception of their weight status and their history of weight loss, much more than men, regardless of their actual weight. Susie Orbach, author of the book *Fat is a Feminist Issue*, argues that women feel bad about their bodies because of the visual images which

> … reward not the human body as a place we dwell in but as an object to enhance the profits of the beauty, fashion, diet, cosmetic surgery and exercise industries, no matter one's age.
>
> (Orbach, 2018)

Eating disorders

Eating disorders are normally a symptom of experiencing very difficult emotions. They are characterised by excessive concerns about weight and shape, which drive harmful weight-control behaviours. The National Centre for Eating Disorders (Jade, 2019) define the most common eating disorders as follows.

Anorexia nervosa

Anorexia nervosa is a mental disorder whereby sufferers refuse to maintain a normal body weight and shape. They are motivated by an extreme fear of some, or all, food which they consider to be either fattening or impure. The more they lose weight, the fatter they 'feel', and they exhibit all the signs of starvation. Many include strenuous exercise, probably as a way of reducing anxiety and keeping warm. They may include episodes of binging and purging, such as vomiting or taking laxatives. They often hear an inner voice which encourages them to keep losing weight. It is a condition with an average lifespan of seven years, and it has the highest death rate of any mental health condition. About eight in ten people recover, though some will need to work hard to keep their weight up. In 2019, research suggested that anorexia might be partly caused by genes which affect a person's metabolism (Watson *et al.*, 2019).

Bulimia nervosa

Bulimia nervosa is characterised by binge eating and purging. They are 'normal' weight or overweight. Typically, they crave food which is 'fattening' and eat, and eat, until their anxiety is reduced. They feel bad, so they purge. It can cause damage to the point of being life-threatening.

Binge eating disorder and compulsive overeating

Binge eating disorder means that people are unable to prevent themselves from eating large amounts of food, often in a short time span. Eating feels out of control. Compulsive overeating is a milder form of binge eating. It could include recurrent trips to the cupboard looking for something to eat, constant nibbling or a lack of control around certain foods such as chocolate. Both include eating faster than normal, beyond feeling full; eating when not hungry; eating alone or in secret; feeling guilty or upset after eating; feeling 'taken over' and then trying to compensate for the overeating by dieting. Someone with these conditions is likely to be overweight.

Compulsive exercise

Compulsive or excessive exercise is when someone has a rigid exercise regime to manage their emotions. It is continued despite rain, snow, injury or illness because, without it, intense anxiety, distress, guilt and/or depression return. It can be used to give permission to eat. Compulsive exercise may lead to a loss of bone density, chronic bone and joint pain and persistent fatigue. Coupled with an eating disorder, it adds to loss of weight, and can be fatal.

Table 12.11 English hospital admissions due to eating disorders, 2017 to 2018

Age (years)	*Male*	*Female*
18	8	85
19	5	97
20	9	77
21	5	70
22	5	66
23	1	62
24	5	45

Source: Adapted from Public Health England (2019b).

People's experiences of their weight are influenced by widespread weight stigma. At worst, it can fuel negative body images, serious psychological problems and eating disorders.

Influences on weight

The UK Government's Foresight Programme published its world-leading analysis of obesity in 2007, with the obesity system map demonstrating how obesity is a complex multi-dimensional problem requiring cross-society support (Government Office for Science, 2007). It placed energy balance in the centre, representing 'calories in, calories out', and grouped the key influences as biology, individual activity, activity environment, food consumption, food production, individual psychology and societal influences. These influences are related to one another through numerous pathways, chains of events, that ultimately feed into the centre and determine weight gain or loss.

Biology

Foresight explained that individuals who seem to be naturally slim may have finely tuned appetite-control systems which match their energy/calorie intake to their energy/calorie needs. Other individuals' systems may be less attuned, making them more vulnerable to weight gain unless they exert conscious control. In times of food shortages this difference was less apparent, but in the context of food abundance it has become visible. While hunger is a powerful drive to seek out food, feelings of fullness/satiety are relatively weak and can be easily overridden, such as 'giving in' to the appearance of a tasty dessert or snack. The basic functioning of the body, the physiology, of a slim person is no different to that of a fatter person, but there may be genetic differences which encourage different responses to the same environment. In 2019, Cambridge

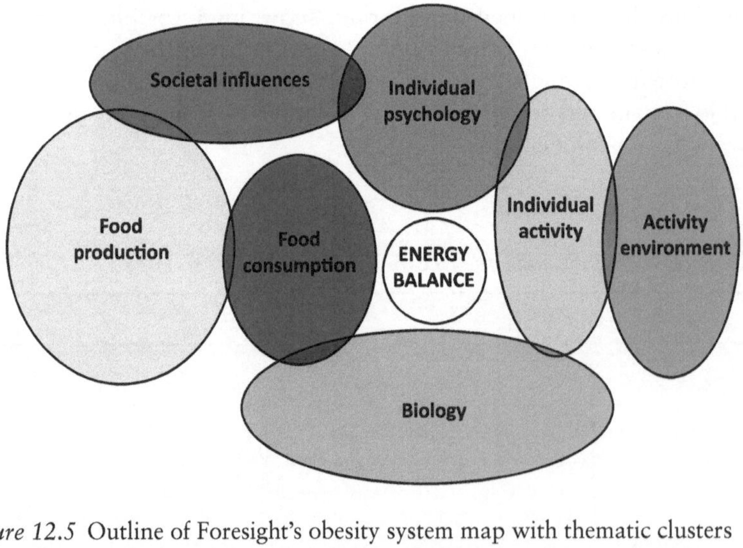

Figure 12.5 Outline of Foresight's obesity system map with thematic clusters

Source: Government Office for Science, 2007 p.121. Reproduced with permission from Government Office for Science.

University announced the results of a large study that showed persistently thin people have fewer of the tiny variations within genes that are known to encourage weight gain compared to people who experience severe early-onset obesity (Riveros-McKay *et al.*, 2019).

Individual food consumption and physical activity

Foresight argue that there are subtle shifts in both physical activity and diet that influence weight, and one is not more important than the other. People's decisions and behaviours may be influenced by what they want, such as sweet food or peer approval, and their desire to be healthy and/or a certain weight. Add to these mixed feelings habits which have become automatic, beliefs about the positive and negative outcomes of a behaviour, the ability to translate good intentions into actions and perceptions about what is morally right or wrong, and it becomes clear that weight-related behaviour is not simple.

Physical and social environment

In the UK, the physical and social environment simultaneously encourages weight gain through the obesogenic environment, and encourages slim, muscular body ideals and weight loss (Figure 12.6 and Table 12.12). The tensions between the two feed into weight discrimination and stigma, body image concerns, eating distress, eating disorders, questionable surgery, and a range of physical and mental health problems.

An obesogenic environment comprises

> The sum of the influences that the surroundings, opportunities or conditions of life have on promoting obesity in individuals and populations.
>
> (Swinburn *et al.*, 1999 p.564)

Food insecurity means not being able to obtain the quantity and quality of food that enables people to stay healthy and well. It includes worrying about food and going without food, and it leads to food poverty. This is discussed in Chapter 4.

Alongside environments which encourage and discourage weight, we must also add culture and the ever-changing aesthetic tastes related to the body and how it is clothed. These reflect the contemporary social beliefs, concerns and aspirations of their time. Consider the current emphasis on sustainable clothing. The journalist Sarah Vine observes:

> The Victorians kept female sexuality in check through tight corseting. In the Twenties, an androgynous shape was considered all the rage, while an hourglass was preferable in the bountiful Fifties ... now the world seems awash with the kind of lean, sculpted physiques more characteristic of a twentysomething athlete.
>
> (Vine, 2019 p.42)

Thinking point:

> To what degree is the current 'obesity epidemic' a medical problem, a behavioural problem or a social problem? Where do we focus our efforts?

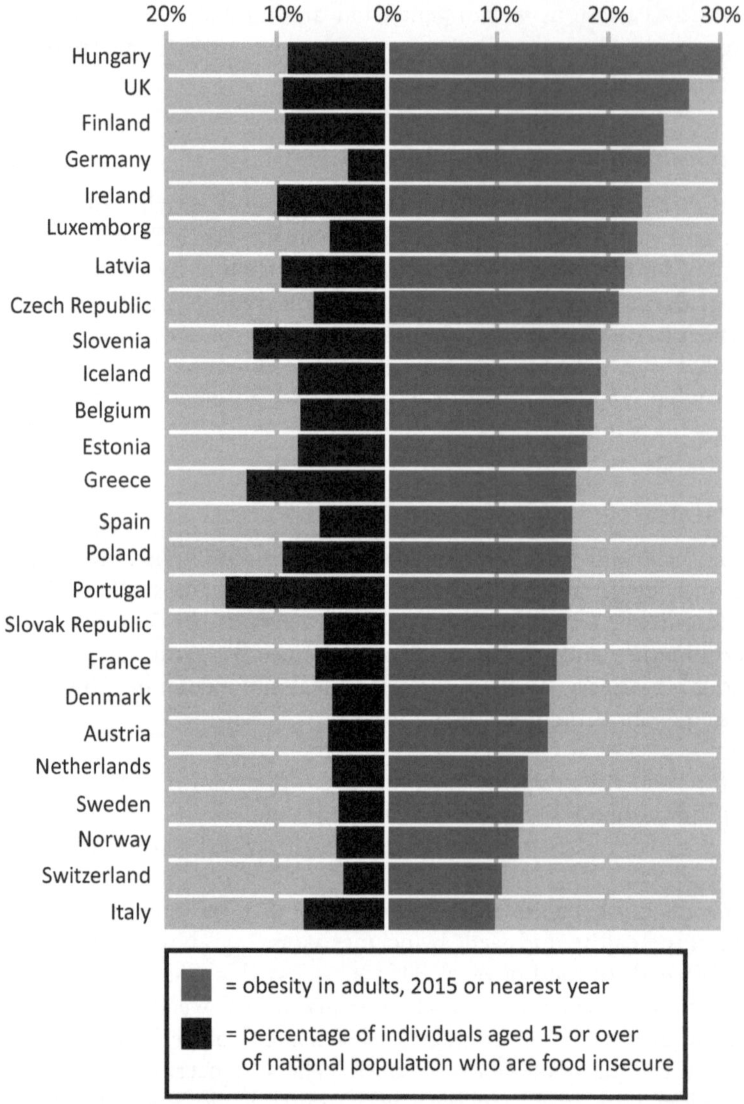

Figure 12.6 Adult obesity and food insecurity
Source: adapted from The Food Foundation, 2017 p.4

A healthy weight

Encouraging individuals to try to keep to a healthy weight makes sense based on medical and epidemiological research. The risks of early death and disease are decreased if people are a healthy weight. We know that measuring weight, alone, is too simplistic and people's body shapes provide a better measure of potential risks of ill health. These measures are imprecise and we wait for the development of personalised medicine, that is understanding each person as a unique combination of our genes, lifestyles and environment, to be able to identify the healthy weight for each individual.

Table 12.12 Environmental influences on weight gain and weight loss

Obesogenic environment	*Environments that encourage underweight*
Widely available cheap high-calorie food	Food insecurity/food poverty
Many take-away/fast-food outlets	Fashion industry
Sugar-sweetened drinks	Dieting industry
Large portion sizes	Exercise industry
Food promotions	Social media promoting eating-disordered behaviour or fat-shaming
Sedentary lifestyles, screen time	Social acceptance of weight stigma
Environments and cultures which promote long periods of sitting	Cultures where thinness is associated with success
Neighbourhoods which are not 'walkable' nor promote active travel such as cycling	Portrayal of idealised/slim bodies in mass media, such as television and advertising, or social media
No nearby physical activity facilities	Portrayal of idealised/slim bodies in visual arts
No nearby green spaces, parks, gardens, community gardens or allotments	

A healthy weight is not 'merely the absence of disease'. How we feel matters too. A healthy weight to someone suffering weight stigma is not a number, be that in kilograms or a clothes size, it is about having a positive body image and, in turn, a healthy self-image. Generally, if we see ourselves as fitting within societal norms, we feel more at ease. A healthy weight is about the body functioning well; having good levels of physical and mental energy; being able to think, rest and sleep; feeling good about our bodies and feeling accepted within society. The responsibility for enabling people to live well at their own healthy weight lies with individuals and everyone who helps to create the society in which we live.

Summary

This chapter has

- noted the rise of overweight and obesity across the world
- described measures of weight and shape, and how they indicate risk of disease and early death
- shown how having excess body fat or being undernourished have physical, psychological costs for individuals and wider costs to society
- explored the negative impact of weight stigma on people's experience of their weight and their health
- explained how eating disorders are harmful weight-control behaviours
- outlined how weight is influenced by biology, individual behaviour and the physical and social environment
- proposed a holistic definition of a healthy weight

Further reading

Brownell, K.D., and Walsh, B.T. (2017) *Eating disorders and obesity. A comprehensive handbook*. 3rd edn. New York: The Guildford Press

Lake, A.A., Townshend, T.G., and Alvanides, S. (eds) (2011) *Obesogenic environments. Complexities, perceptions and objective measures.* Chichester: Blackwell/John Wiley

Useful websites

Association for the Study of Obesity. Available at: www.aso.org.uk
National Centre for Eating Disorders. Available at: https://eating-disorders.org.uk

References

Ahmed, T., Hossain, M., and Sanin, K.I. (2012) 'Global burden of maternal and child undernutrition and micronutrient deficiencies', *Annals of Nutrition and Metabolism*, 61(s1), pp.8–17

Bamber, D., Cockerill, I.M., Rodgers, S., and Carroll, D. (2000) '"It's exercise or nothing": a qualitative analysis of exercise dependence', *British Journal of Sports Medicine*, 34(6), pp.423–430

Bates, B., Collins, D., Cox, L., Nicholson, S., Page, P., Roberts, C., Steer, T., and Swan, G. (2019) *National diet and nutrition survey. Years 1 to 9 of the rolling programme (2008/2009–2016/2017): time trend and income analyses.* London: Public Health England

BBC (2018) News. Reality check: does obesity cost more than police and fire service? Available at: www.bbc.co.uk/news/health-43897286 (Accessed 24th July 2019)

Bhaskaran, K., dos-Santos-Silva, I., Leon, D.A., Douglas, I.J., and Smeeth, L. (2018) 'Association of BMI with overall and cause-specific mortality: a population-based cohort study of 3.6 million adults in the UK', *The Lancet*, 6(12), pp.944–953

Bertoli, S., Leone, A., Krakauer, N.Y., Bedogni, G., Vanzulli, A, Radaelli, V.I., De Amicis, R., Vignati, L., Krakauer, J.C., and Battezzati, A. (2017) 'Association of Body Shape Index (ABSI) with cardiometabolic risk factors: a cross sectional study of 6081 caucasian adults', *Plos One*, 12(9) e0185013 doi.org/10.1371/journal.pone.0185013

Boynton, P. (2017) 'I'm a skinny man and scared to let women see me naked', *The Telegraph*, 30th April. Available at: www.telegraph.co.uk/women/life/skinny-man-scared-let-women-see-naked (Accessed 27th July 2019)

British Dietetic Association (2016) *Food fact sheet. Pregnancy.* Available at: www.bda.uk.com/foodfacts/Pregnancy.pdf (Accessed 5th September 2019)

Burns, C.M., Tijhuis, M.A.R., and Seidell, J.C. (2001) 'The relationship between quality of life and perceived body weight and dieting history in Dutch men and women', *International Journal of Obesity*, 25(9), pp.1386–1392

Chodankar, R., Middleton, G., Lim, C., and Mahmood, T. (2017) 'Obesity in pregnancy', *Obstetrics, Gynaecology and Reproductive Medicine*, 28(2), pp.53–56

Curtice, J. (2016) British social attitudes. Attitudes to obesity, Public Health England. Available at: www.bsa.natcen.ac.uk/media/39132/attitudes-to-obesity.pdf (Accessed 24th July 2019)

Department of Health (2018) *Health survey (NI) first results 2017/18.* Available at: www.health-ni.gov.uk/publications/health-survey-northern-ireland-first-results-201718 (Accessed 15th July 2019)

Flegal, K.M., Kit, B.K., Orpana, H., and Graubard, B.I. (2013) 'Association of all-cause mortality with overweight and obesity using standard body mass index categories: a systematic review and meta-analysis', *Journal of the American Medical Association*, 309(1), pp.71–82

Fu, J., Hofker, M., and Wijemenga, C. (2015) 'Apple or pear: size and shape matter', *Cell Metabolism*, 21(4) doi:10.1016/j.cmet.2015.03.016

Gov.UK (2016) Guidance. Obesity, weight management and people with learning disabilities. Available at: www.gov.uk/government/publications/obesity-weight-management-and-people-with-learning-disabilities (Accessed 27th July 2019)

Gov.UK (2018) Overweight adults. Available at: www.ethnicity-facts-figures.service.gov.uk/health/diet-and-exercise/overweight-adults/2.1 (Accessed 26th April 2020)

Government Office for Science (2007) *Foresight. Tackling obesities: future choices – project report*. London: Department for Innovation, Universities and Skills

Grant, J., Chittleborough, C.R., Shi, Z., and Taylor, A.W. (2017) 'The association between A Body Shape Index and mortality: results from an Australian cohort', *Plos One*, 12 (7) e0181244 doi.org/10.1371/journal.pone.0181244

Henderson, E., Norrenberg, A., Cairns, J., and Gadsby, E. (2018) 'How can primary care help to reduce weight stigma?' *British Journal of General Practice* (BJGP), 68(1) doi.org/10.3399/bjgp18X696665

Jackson, S.E., Beeken, R.J., and Wardle, J. (2015) 'Obesity, perceived weight discrimination, and psychological well-being in older adults in England', *Obesity*, 23(5), pp.1105–1111

Jade, D. (2019) National Centre for Eating Disorders. Information. Available at: https://eating-disorders.org.uk/information/ (Accessed 28th July 2019)

Jankowski, G.S., Gough, B., Fawkner, H., Halliwell, E., and Diedrichs, P.C. (2018) 'Young men's minimisation of their body dissatisfaction', *Psychology and Health*, 33(11), pp.1343–1363

Knight, M., Bunch, K., Tuffnell, D., Jayakody, H., Shakespeare, J., Kotnis, R., Kenyon, S., and Kurinczuk, J.J. (eds) on behalf of MBRRACE-UK (2018) *Saving lives, improving mothers' care. Lessons learned to inform maternity care from the UK and Ireland confidential enquiries into maternal deaths and morbidity 2014–16*. Oxford: National Perinatal Epidemiology Unit, University of Oxford

Krakauer, N.Y., and Krakauer, J.E. (2012) 'A new body shape index predicts mortality hazard independently of body mass index', *Plos One*, 7(7) doi:10.1371/journal.pone.0039504

Krakauer, N.Y., and Krakauer, J.E. (2014) 'Dynamic association of mortality hazard with body shape', *Plos One*, 9(2) doi:10.1371/journal.pone.0088793

Moola, F.J., and Norman, M.E. (2017) 'On judgement day: anorexic and obese women's phenomenological experience of the body, food and eating', *Feminism and Psychology*, 27(3), pp.259–279

National Institute for Health and Care Excellence (2013) BMI: preventing ill health and premature death in black, Asian and other minority ethnic groups. Available at: www.nice.org.uk/guidance/ph46/resources/bmi-preventing-ill-health-and-premature-death-in-black-asian-and-other-minority-ethnic-groups-pdf-1996361299141 (Accessed 27th April 2020)

NHS Digital (2019) Statistics on obesity, physical activity and diet. England: 2019. Available at: https://digital.nhs.uk/data-and-information/publications/statistical/statistics-on-obesity-physical-activity-and-diet/statistics-on-obesity-physical-activity-and-diet-england-2019 (Accessed 15th July 2019)

Nuttall, F.Q. (2015) 'Body Mass Index. Obesity, BMI and health: a critical review', *Nutrition Research*, 50(3), pp.117–128

Nyberg., S.T., Batty, G.D., Pentti, J., *et al.* (2018) 'Obesity and loss of disease-free years owing to major non-communicable diseases: a multicohort study', *Lancet Public Health*, 18 e490-97 doi.org/10.1016/S2468-2667(18)30139-7

Olson, K.L., Landers, J.D., Thaxton, T.T., and Emery, C.F. (2018) 'The pain of weight-related stigma among women with overweight or obesity', *Stigma and Health*, 4(3), pp.243–246

Orbach, S. (2018) 'Forty years since Fat Is A Feminist Issue', *The Guardian*, 24th June. Available at: www.theguardian.com/society/2018/jun/24/forty-years-since-fat-is-a-feminist-issue (Accessed 27th July 2019)

Ortega, F.B., Ruiz, J.R., Labayen, I., Lavie, C.J., and Blair, S.N. (2018) 'The fat but fit paradox; what we know and don't know about it', *British Journal of Sports Medicine*, 52(3), pp.151–153

Pereira, P.F., Serrano, H.M., Carvalho, G.Q., Lamounier, J.A., Peluzio, M.doC.G., Franceschini, S.doC.C., and Priore, S.E. (2012) 'Body fat location and cardiovascular disease risk factors in overweight female adolescents and eutrophic female adolescents with high percentage body fat', *Cardiology in the Young*, 22(2), pp.162–169

Public Health England (2017) Guidance. Health matters: obesity and the food environment. Available at: www.gov.uk/government/publications/health-matters-obesity-and-the-food-environment/health-matters-obesity-and-the-food-environment--2 (Accessed 24th July 2019)

Public Health England (2019a) Statistics on obesity, physical activity and diet, England, 2019. NHS Digital. Available at: https://digital.nhs.uk/data-and-information/publications/statistical/statistics-on-obesity-physical-activity-and-diet/statistics-on-obesity-physical-activity-and-diet-england-2019/part-3-adult-obesity (Accessed 29th August 2019)

Public Health England (2019b) Hospital admissions as a result of eating disorders for young people: summary and data. Available at: www.gov.uk/government/publications/eating-disorders-in-young-people (Accessed 29th August 2019)

Public Health Wales NHS Trust (2019) Obesity in Wales. Available at: www.publichealthwalesobservatory.wales.nhs.uk/obesityinwales (Accessed 29th August 2019)

Riveros-McKay, F., Mistry, V., Bounds, R., Hendricks, A., Keogh, J.M., Thomas, H., Henning, E., Corbin, L.J., Understanding Society Scientific Group, O'Rahilly, S., Zeggini, E., Wheeler, E., Barroso, I., and Farooqi, I.S. (2019) 'Genetic architecture of human thinness compared to severe obesity', *PLoS Genetics*, 15(1) doi:10.1371/journal.pgen.1007603

Sahakyan, K.R., Somers, V.K., Rodriguez-Escudero, J.P., Hodge, D.O., Carter, R.E., Sochor, O., Coutinho, T., Jensen, M.D., Roger, V.L., Singh, P., and Lopez-Jimenez, F. (2015) 'Normal weight central obesity: implications for total cardiovascular mortality', *Annals of Internal Medicine*, 163(11), pp.827–835

Scottish Government (2018) Obesity indicators. Progress report October 2018. Available at: www.gov.scot/binaries/content/documents/govscot/publications/statistics/2018/10/obesity-indicators/documents/00542529-pdf/00542529-pdf/govscot%3Adocument/00542529.pdf (Accessed 29th August 2019)

Shephard, R. (2018a) 'Does it matter if I am overweight? 1. Some biomechanical, physiological and performance-related consequences', *Health and Fitness Journal of Canada*, 11(2), pp.15–52

Shephard, R. (2018b) 'Does it matter if I am overweight? 2. Some psycho-social consequences', *Health and Fitness Journal of Canada*, 11(2), pp.22–66

Smith, M.L., Telford, E., and Tree, J.J. (2019) 'Body image and sexual orientation: the experiences of lesbian and bisexual women', *Journal of Health Psychology*, 24(9), pp.1178–1190

Swinburn, B., Egger, G., and Raza, F. (1999) 'Dissecting obesogenic environments: the development and application of a framework for identifying and prioritizing environmental interventions for obesity', *Preventive Medicine*, 29(6 Pt 1), pp.563–570

Tan, M., He, F.J., and MacGregor, G.A. (2020) 'Obesity and COVID-19: the role of the food industry', *BMJ*, 369 doi.org/10.1136/bmj.m2237

The Food Foundation (2017) UK and global malnutrition: the new normal. International learning series/1. Available at: https://foodfoundation.org.uk/wp-content/uploads/2017/09/1-Briefing-Malnutrition_vF2.pdf (accessed 29th August 2019)

Tomiyama, A.J., Carr, D., Granberg, E.M., Major, B., Robinson, E., Sutin, A.R., and Brewis, A. (2018) 'How and why weight stigma drives the obesity "epidemic" and harms health', *BMC Medicine*, 16(123) doi:10.1186/s12916-018-1116-5

Tran, N.T.T., Blizzard, C.L, Luong, K.N., van Truong, N.L., Tran, B.Q., Otahal, P., Nelson, M., Magnussen, C., Gall, S., Bui, T.V., Srikanth, V., Au, T.B., Ha, S.T., Phung, H.N., Tran, M.H., and Callisaya, M. (2018) 'The importance of waist circumference and body mass index in cross-sectional relationships with risk of cardiovascular disease in Vietnam', *Plos One*, 13(5) doi.org/10.1371/journal.pone.0198202

Ul-Haq, Z., Mackay, D.F., Martin, D., Smith, D.J., Gill, J.M.R., Nicholl, B.I., Cullen, B., Evans, J., Roberts, B., Deary, I.J., Gllacher, J., Hotopf, M., Craddock, N., and Pell, J.P. (2014) 'Heaviness, health and happiness: a cross-sectional study of 163 066 UK Biobank participants', *Journal of Epidemiology and Community Health*, 68(4), pp. 340–348

VanKim, N., Porta, C.M., Eisenberg, M.E., Neumark-Sztainer, D., and Laska M.N. (2016) 'Lesbian, gay and bisexual college student perspectives on disparities in weight-related behaviours and body image: a qualitative analysis', *Journal of Clinical Nursing*, 25(23/24), pp.3676–3686

Vine, S. (2019) 'Spare me the forty-something celebrities with the bodies of twenty-year-old athletes ... they are turning every beach into a body shaming battleground', *Daily Mail*, Saturday 13th July, pp.42

Voss, J.D., Pavela, G., and Stanford, F.C. (2019) 'Obesity as a threat to national security: the need for precision engagement', *International Journal of Obesity*, 43(3), pp.437–439

Waton, J.J., Yilmaz, Z., Thornton, L.M., *et al.* (2019) 'Genome-wide association study identifies eight risk loci and implicates metabo-psychiatric origins for anorexia nervosa', *Nature Genetics*, 51(8) doi:10.1038/s41588-019-0439-2

Williams, O., and Annandale, E. (2018) 'Obesity, stigma and reflexive embodiment: feeling the "weight" of expectation', *Health: An Interdisciplinary Journal for the Social Study of Health, Illness and Medicine*, 14 doi:10.1177/1363459318812007

World Cancer Research Fund/American Institute for Cancer Research (2018) *Body fatness and weight gain and the risk of cancer*. London: World Cancer Research Fund International

World Health Organization (1998) *Obesity: preventing and managing the global epidemic. WHO technical report series 894*. Geneva: World Health Organization

World Health Organization (2017a) Global health data repository. Prevalence of overweight among adults, BMI >25, age standardised. Estimates by WHO Region. Available at: http://apps.who.int/gho/data/view.main.GLOBAL2461A?lang=en (Accessed 10th July 2019)

World Health Organization (2017b) *Prevalence of underweight among adult, BMI <18, crude estimates by WHO region*. Available at: http://apps.who.int/gho/data/view.main.NCDBMILT18CREGv (Accessed 19th July 2019)

World Health Organization (2018) Obesity and overweight. Key facts. Available at: www.who.int/news-room/fact-sheets/detail/obesity-and-overweight (Accessed 15th July 2019)

World Health Organization (2019) BMI classification. Available at: http://apps.who.int/bmi/index.jsp?introPage=intro_3.html (Accessed 30th August 2019)

Part III

Non-communicable diseases

13 Cardiovascular disease

Sally Robinson

Key points

- Introduction
- The heart and the circulatory system
- Cardiovascular disease
- Causes of cardiovascular disease
- Primary prevention of cardiovascular disease
- Secondary prevention of cardiovascular disease
- Tertiary prevention of cardiovascular disease
- Summary

Introduction

Cardiovascular disease is the second highest cause of death in the UK. This chapter outlines the function of the heart and the circulatory system before describing some of the more common cardiovascular conditions and the extent to which they cause poor health and death in the UK. We examine atherosclerosis in depth, focusing on the causes of atheroma and damage to blood vessels and blood flow. These include health-related behaviours, the socio-economic and physical environment and non-modifiable risk factors. The chapter concludes with the priorities for the primary, secondary and tertiary prevention of cardiovascular disease.

Box 13.1 The number one cause of death across the world

Cardiovascular disease causes more death across the world than any other disease. This amounts to 31% of all deaths, of which 85% are due to a heart attack or stroke. More than three-quarters of deaths occur in low- and middle-income countries.

(Source: WHO, 2020)

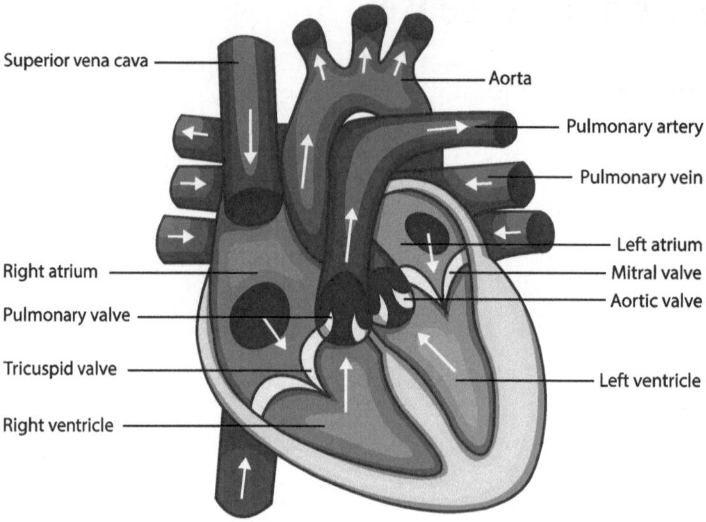

Figure 13.1 The heart
Source: Mari-Leaf/Shutterstock.com

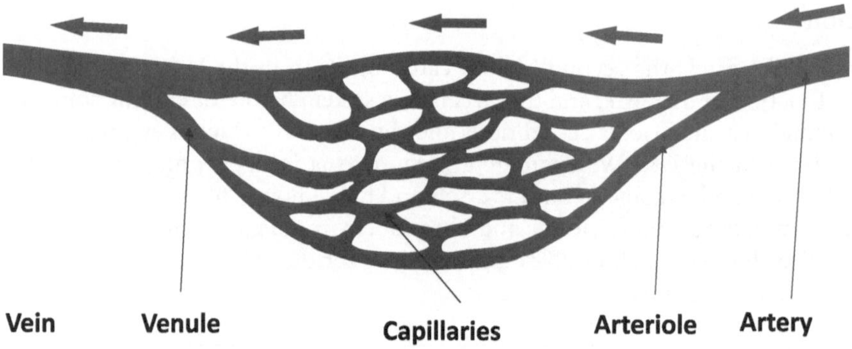

Figure 13.2 Blood circulation from arteries into veins
Source: NelaR/Shutterstock.com

The heart and the circulatory system

The heart is a muscular organ that acts as a pump. It has small nodes which produce electrical impulses causing the heart to contract and push the blood around the circulatory system of the body. The rate of the pumping action is the heartbeat and the waves are felt throughout the arteries of the body. We feel these as pulses. The arteries carry blood containing nutrients and the oxygen which it has picked up via the lungs to every cell of the body. Anything that impedes this process, such as damage to the heart or to the blood vessels, means that cells, tissues and organs of the body will start to fail.

Box 13.2 The function of the heart

The heart is a muscular cavity containing four chambers. Blood which has circulated around the body, and is very low in oxygen, arrives back at the heart via the veins. It enters the right atrium, goes through the tricuspid valve, and into the right ventricle where it is pumped via the pulmonary artery into the circulatory system of the lungs. The oxygen we breathe into the lungs is transferred into the blood stream. This oxygenated blood leaves the lungs and travels inside the pulmonary vein into the left atrium of the heart. It passes through the mitral valve into the left ventricle. As the ventricle contracts, the blood is pumped up through the aorta. The aorta, a large artery, travels down the centre of the body and has many arteries branching from it. The blood travels down these arteries into the branching arterioles to reach the capillaries in the periphery of the body, such as the hands and feet. As the blood circulates, the oxygen and nutrients are transferred across the blood vessel wall into the tissues, enabling all organs and body parts to function. The deoxygenated blood enters the tiny venules which become larger veins. The lack of oxygen darkens the colour of the blood. Eventually the blood reaches the large vein, the superior vena cava. It enters the right atrium of the heart and the cycle repeats.

Cardiovascular disease

Cardiovascular disease is a collective term for many conditions which affect the heart and the circulatory system. The international classification of diseases (ICD-11) uses the term 'diseases of the circulatory system' (WHO, 2019). Some of the more common conditions include

- endocarditis – inflammation/swelling of the inner lining of the heart often due to infection
- myocarditis – inflammation/swelling of the middle/muscular layer of the heart often due to infection
- pericarditis – inflammation/swelling of the outer lining of the heart often due to infection
- cardiomyopathies/diseases of the myocardium, the muscular layer of the heart
- heart valve diseases – one or more of the heart's four valves does not open/shut properly
- cardiac arrhythmia – irregular heartbeat
- atrial fibrillation – a common cause of irregular heartbeat, caused by a problem with the electrical impulses of the heart causing the right atrium to twitch. It increases the risk of having a cerebrovascular accident
- heart failure – the heart does not pump the blood properly
- diseases of coronary arteries, the vessels that supply blood to the heart
- coronary heart disease/ischaemic heart disease – the blood supply in one or more coronary arteries is impeded

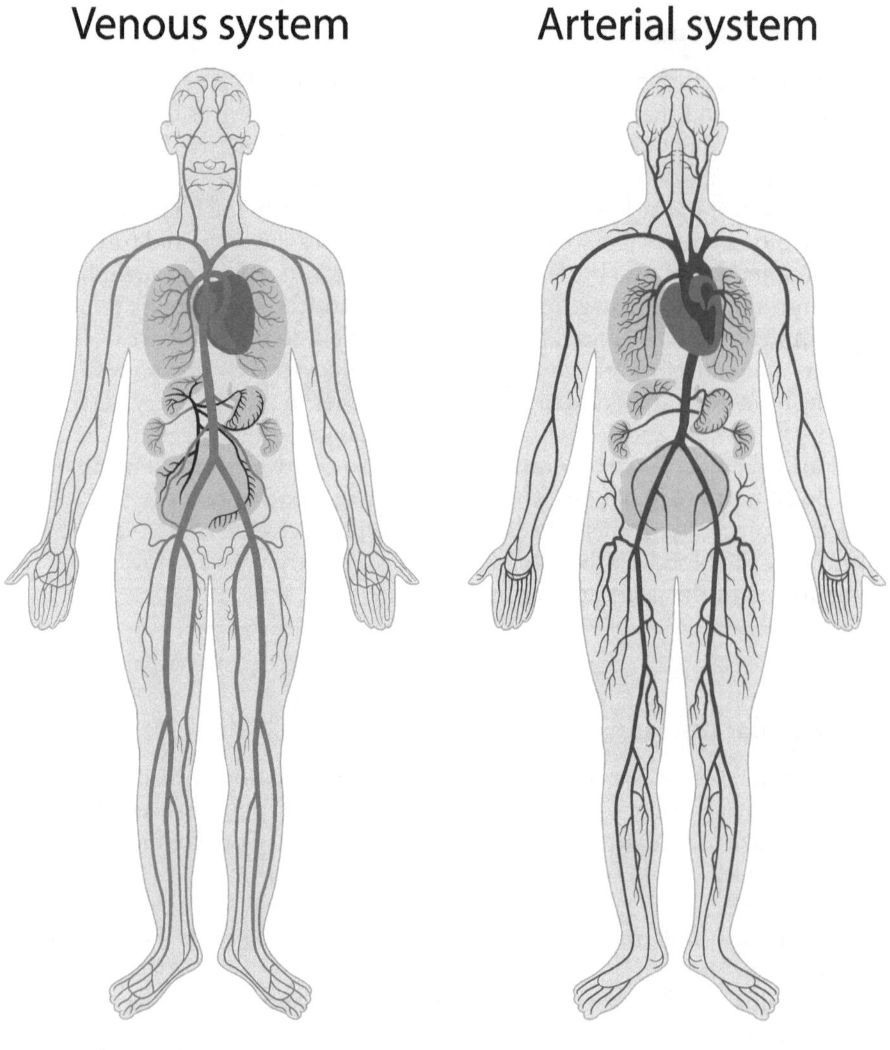

Figure 13.3 The circulatory system
Source: Olga Bolbot/Shutterstock.com

- myocardial infarction – a heart attack, the death of an area of heart muscle due to the blood supply being cut off
- peripheral arterial disease – the arteries, arterioles and capillaries taking blood to the peripheries of the body become blocked and tissue begins to die
- hypertensive diseases – diseases that cause high blood pressure
- hypotension – low blood pressure
- cerebrovascular accident – a stroke caused by a burst blood vessel, or a blood clot that has blocked a blood vessel, in the brain. Both stop the blood supply and some brain tissue dies
- trans ischaemic attack – 'mini-stroke', the blood supply in the brain is blocked partially/temporarily

- vascular dementia – reduced blood supply to cells in the brain
- pulmonary heart disease – high blood pressure in the lungs causes part of the heart to fail

Atherosclerosis

Many cardiovascular conditions are caused and/or aggravated by atherosclerosis. Atherosclerosis is the accumulation of fatty material, called atheroma or plaque, on the inner surface of the arteries. This causes them to narrow, making it hard for the blood to circulate. Without a good supply of oxygen and nutrients, the tissues struggle to survive (ischaemia). The atheroma may rupture, causing the blood around it to clot. The blood clot (thrombus) can lead to a complete blockage of the artery. The clot may travel and cause a blockage somewhere else (embolism). A blockage in circulation will cause the surrounding tissue to die (infarct); in the heart it causes a heart attack, in the brain it causes a stroke and in the feet it causes gangrene.

The burden of cardiovascular disease in the UK

The British Heart Foundation (2020a; 2020b) reports 7.4 million people in the UK have cardiovascular disease, which costs the UK economy about £19 billion each year. This is twice as many people as those living with Alzheimer's disease and cancer combined. It causes 460 deaths every day and makes up 27% of all UK deaths. Of the 167,116 people who died in 2018, 44,262 were under the age of 75 years. Death

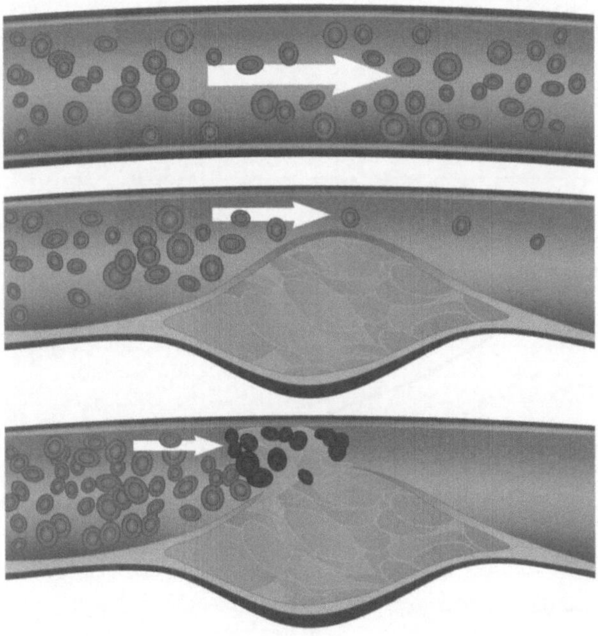

Figure 13.4 Atherosclerosis: development of atheroma followed by rupturing and blood clot formation

Source: Diamond_Images/Shutterstock.com

Box 13.3 Medical terminology

- aneurysm – bulge in blood vessel
- arterio ... – artery or arteriole
- athero ... – gruel-like/soft/pasty
- cardio ... /cardiac – heart
- cerebro ... – brain
- ecto ... – out/outside
- embolus – particles, often part of a blood clot, that travel and may block a capillary
- endo ... – in/within
- haem ... – blood
- infarct/infarction – localised death caused by the obstruction of blood supply to tissues or part of an organ
- ischaemia – shortage of oxygen to tissues or part of an organ due to restricted blood supply
- ...itis – inflammation
- myo ... – muscle
- ... oma – a mass
- ... pathy – disease/suffering
- peri ... – surrounding
- ... sclerosis – hardening
- ... thelium – layer of body tissue
- thrombus/thrombosis – blood clot
- vascular/vaso ... – blood vessels
- venous – vein

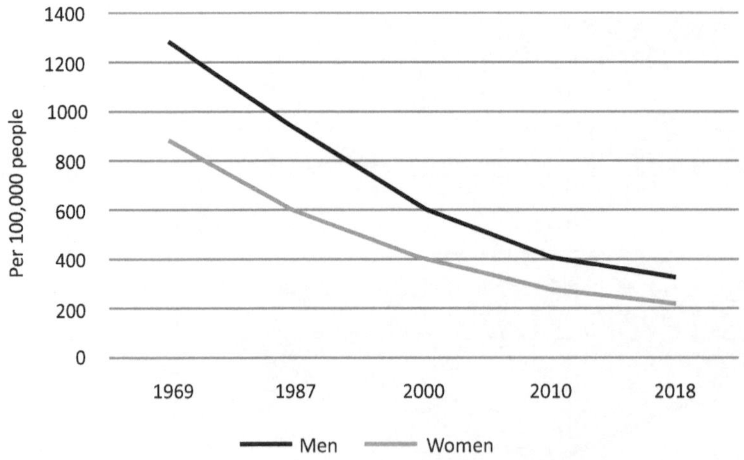

Figure 13.5 Age-standardised death rates from cardiovascular disease, UK 1969–2018
Source: British Heart Foundation, 2020b

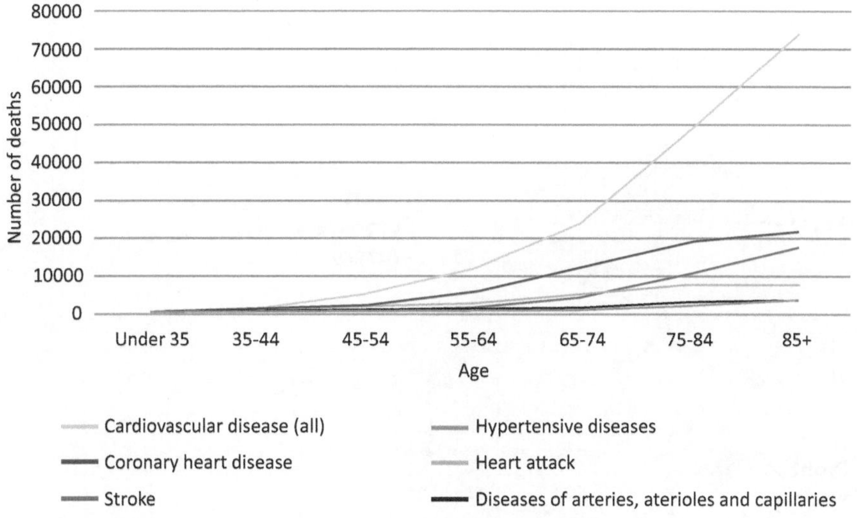

Figure 13.6 UK deaths from cardiovascular disease by age, 2018
Source: British Heart Foundation, 2020b

rates are higher in men than women, and they rise with age. Scotland, South Wales, the North of England and areas of higher deprivation see more premature deaths from cardiovascular disease than the rest of the country. Compared to 1969, when half of all deaths were caused by cardiovascular disease, we have made some progress (Figure 13.5), but cardiovascular disease remains the second highest cause of death in the UK, only surpassed by dementia.

Coronary heart disease

Coronary heart disease, also called ischaemic heart disease, means that the coronary arteries which supply blood to the heart have become narrowed, usually by atherosclerosis, so that the blood supply is impeded. As insufficient oxygen and nutrients reach the heart muscle, the individual feels chest tightening/pain and/or a choking sensation on exertion, but this goes away once they are at rest. This is angina. Without treatment, it can be a precursor to having a heart attack. Descriptions of angina include:

> ... a feeling of tightness in the middle of the chest ... particularly um when walking and I need to stop and rest and that helps ... I had the feeling of er sort of breathlessness.
>
> (male, 87 years; Jones *et al.*, 2010 p.738)

and

> I never had a chest pain ... I had this discomfort.
>
> (female, 77 years; Jones *et al.*, 2010 p.738)

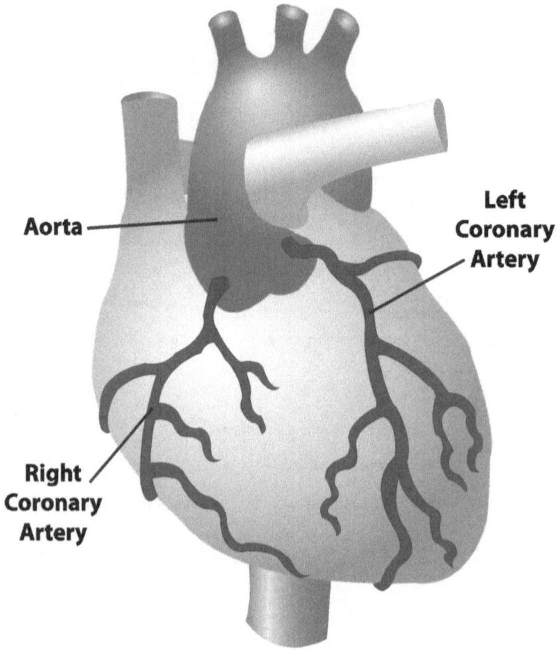

Figure 13.7 Coronary arteries supply oxygen to the heart muscle
Source: OSweetNature/Shutterstock.com

Table 13.1 Prevalence of UK coronary heart disease, 2018 to 2019

	Number of people living with coronary heart disease seeing their General Practitioner	*Percentage of population*
England	1,855,339	3.1%
Scotland	225,000	3.9%
Wales	117,733	3.6%
Northern Ireland	74,154	3.7%
UK	2,272,226	3.2%

Source: Adapted from British Heart Foundation (2020b).

The British Heart Foundation (2020b) report almost 2.3 million people living with coronary heart disease in the UK. It is the leading cause of death across the world and causes about 64,000 deaths in the UK each year. This is about 180 per day or one every eight minutes. One in seven men and one in 12 women die from coronary heart disease. It is the leading cause of male deaths in the UK (ONS, 2020) and it kills twice as many women as breast cancer (British Heart Foundation, 2020a).

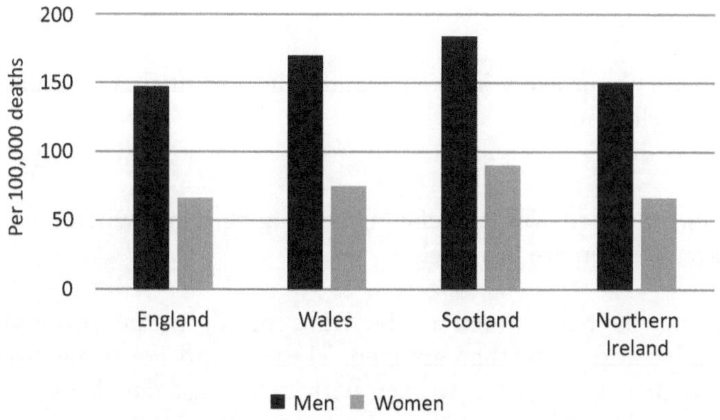

Figure 13.8 Age-standardised UK deaths from coronary heart disease, by sex 2016 to 2018
Source: British Heart Foundation, 2020b

Heart attack

A heart attack, also called a myocardial infarction, occurs because the blood supply to the heart muscle, travelling in the coronary arteries, has been cut off, causing some heart tissue to die. The symptoms of a heart attack are

- discomfort or pain in the chest that does not go away
- mild to severe pain that spreads to the arms, neck, jaw, stomach or back
- nausea, sweating, feeling short of breath and light-headed
- none or only some of the above

The individual should

- call an ambulance as this is a medical emergency
- stay calm and sit down
- take 300 mg of aspirin immediately

(British Heart Foundation, 2020c)

The long-term impact of a heart attack depends on how much damage has been done to the heart and how quickly medical treatment is obtained.

Coronary heart disease and heart attacks have been traditionally associated with men, supported by research carried out with men, to the disadvantage of women. The stereotypical heart attack involves a man clutching his chest with crushing pain. Some women describe chest pain that radiates down the arm, but others describe more vague, intermittent and non-specific symptoms such as feeling generally unwell. Leslie Davis (2017) interviewed women who said:

> It didn't hurt as bad as I thought a heart attack would hurt.
>
> (p.492)

> It didn't occur to me that it could be my heart.
>
> (p.493)

> I don't like to complain about every little ache and pain. I want to make sure it's "something" before I tell him.
>
> (p.493)

The male stereotype contributes to women delaying seeking help and when they do, they often get worse care. Women are less likely

> ... to receive aspirin, be resuscitated or be transported to the hospital in ambulances using lights and sirens than are men. These factors contribute to the disproportionately higher mortality in women with cardiovascular disease than men. A major shift in thinking is required ... about who gets and dies from heart disease.
>
> (editorial, *The Lancet*, 2019 p.959)

Box 13.4 Young men's thoughts about having a heart attack

Christopher Merritt and colleagues interviewed 10 men of mixed ethnicities who had experienced a heart attack. They were between 30 and 44 years old and receiving healthcare in London. Some of the themes which emerged from their discussions were described as follows.

- Denial of having the heart attack, the symptoms don't match, I am too young
- It's not my fault, it's someone/something else's fault, I am confused, I should have, they should have
- I'm less of a man, I'm physically weak, I can't do that anymore, I've lost my independence and need support, I can't be a provider

  "I used to have this thing about, if I saw someone picking on someone in the street I'd step in, but now ... I can't ... you are not as male or as macho male as you were before ..."

  (Rajesh p. 596)
- Life's short, when will it happen again? What will happen to my children? I need to change jobs, reassessing what is important
- Life loses its colour, I'm bored, medicine is a life sentence, ... but risk factors are fun

  "... I don't go to pubs no more because I'd be tempted."

  (Ahmed, p.600)

- Rehabilitation takes time, I need to rebuild, I have no choice, I've decided to change, what can I do?
- It's not all bad, I'm becoming an expert, change can be good, helping others is good

(Source: Merritt *et al.*, 2017)

The British Heart Foundation (2020a) report 100,000 people are admitted to a UK hospital having suffered a heart attack each year (Figure 13.9). This is 280 per day or one every five minutes. About 70% of people survive a heart attack each year and about 23,000 people under the age of 75 years die. People who have had a heart attack are twice as likely to have a stroke compared those who have not and across the world it is the most common cause of heart failure (Cahill and Kharbanda, 2017).

Heart failure

Heart failure means that the heart has difficulty pumping the blood, often due to strain or damage. For example, this might be caused by atherosclerosis, high blood pressure, a heart attack or damage to the heart valves. As the blood is not circulating properly, tissue fluid builds up in the body rather than being absorbed into the blood stream (oedema). Gravity encourages the fluid to sit in the lower legs, ankles, feet, lower abdomen or lower back. Symptoms of heart failure include

- shortness of breath, even at rest
- tiredness and/or feeling weak
- swelling in the legs, ankles, feet, lower abdomen or lower back

(British Heart Foundation, 2020c)

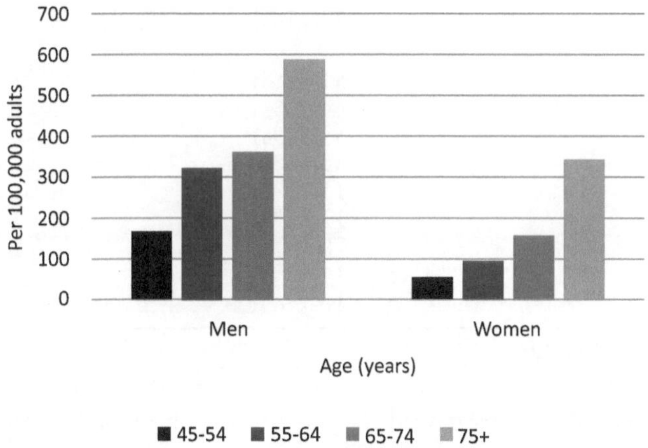

Figure 13.9 Incidence rates (new cases) of heart attacks by sex and age, UK 2017
Source: British Heart Foundation, 2020b

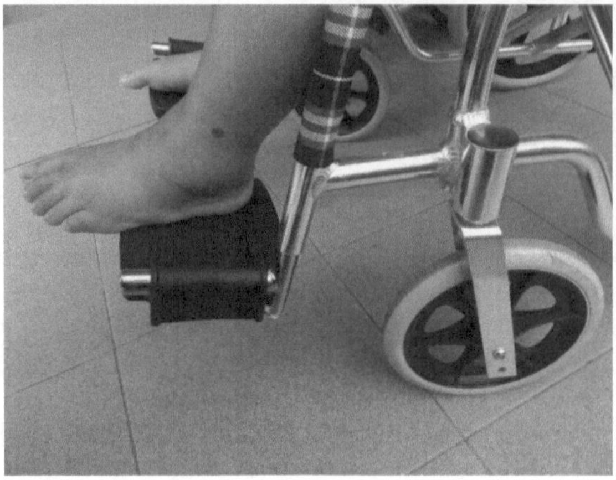

Figure 13.10 Swollen ankles due to oedema
Source: AppleDK/Shutterstock.com

Table 13.2 Symptoms described by people with heart failure

	Number of patients (%) (n = 63)
Symptoms	
Shortness of breath	50(79%)
Tiredness	54(86%
Swelling in legs, ankles, feet	42(67%)
Pain (general)	20(5%)
Chest pain	27(43%)
Numbness	18(29%)
Irregular heartbeat	24(38%)
Dry mouth	18(29%)
Cough	13(21%)
Impact of heart failure	
Limitations to physical activity	51(81%)
Physical mobility difficulties	44(70%)
Emotional impacts	53(84%)
Impacts to daily living activities	35(56%)
Sleep disturbance	15(24%)
Cognition/thinking	17(27%)
Self-care	7(11%)
Social interaction	14(22%)
Weight gain	1(2%)

Source: Adapted from Gwaltney *et al.* (2012).

Gwaltney and colleagues (2012) interviewed 63 patients with heart failure in the United States of America. They heard people describe:

> I can start walking down the hall and literally have to lean up against the wall … gasping for breath.

> I can't sweep, mop or run the vacuum cleaner. I get totally exhausted.

Table 13.3 Prevalence of UK heart failure, 2018 to 2019

	Number of people living with heart failure seeing their general practitioner	*Percentage of population*
England	558,168	0.9%
Scotland	48,000	0.8%
Wales	34,453	1.1%
Northern Ireland	18,323	0.9%
UK	658,944	0.9%

Source: Adapted from British Heart Foundation (2020b).

> ... my hands will tingle like they are asleep, but then they hurt and burn.
>
> (p. 3)

The authors collated the symptoms to show that tiredness and shortness of breath were mentioned by the most people (Table 13.2).

The British Heart Foundation (2020a; 2020b) estimate there are 920,000 people in the UK living with heart failure and 658,944 are seeing their general practitioner for treatment (Table 13.3). People who have heart failure are two to three times more likely to have a stroke compared to those without.

Peripheral arterial disease

Peripheral arterial disease, sometimes called peripheral vascular disease, means that the blood circulation to the peripheries of the body, such as the hands and feet, is blocked, usually due to atherosclerosis. The individual feels pain as the tissues fail to receive the oxygen they need (ischaemia). The damage can lead to ulcers and eventually to gangrene, which necessitates an amputation.

Box 13.5 Swedish patients' experiences of leg/foot amputations due to peripheral arterial disease

Some patients have been in pain for a while and know that it may end in an amputation, while for others it is a complete shock because they assume the doctor will be able to fix it. There is no choice; if they want to survive, they need an amputation. It happens very quickly and patients would have liked time for more discussion about the future before the operation. Perhaps the healthcare professionals put off the decision until the last minute because of their own discomfort. It is about nine days between the operation and leaving the hospital to start rehabilitation. It is a 'vacuum phase' in which some realise that once the operation is done the surgeons no longer visit, they are of no interest to surgeons any more. The nine days are a period marked by overwhelming loss, waking up to realise they have one leg and the contours of the sheets show the absence of a foot. Patients long to become 'normal' again and wait anxiously to get their prosthetic limb. On the plus side, the pain has gone and meeting the prosthetic technician gives them hope for the future, though they don't know what it will look like. The waiting and not knowing is the hardest journey and being able to share these feelings with another is helpful. Some experience delays as they wait for their wound to heal. Using a wheelchair is an obstacle because friends and family get nervous, they avoid them or speak to them in a loud voice as if the amputation happened in their heads. Some friends don't understand why the patients 'let' the doctors cut off their leg, as if it could have been avoided. Later, for most, their quality of life gradually improves, they feel happier, people say they look younger and they begin to think about learning to drive and being independent again. The prosthesis is a symbol of normality, they are 'just like everyone else'.

(Source: Torbjörnsson *et al.*, 2017)

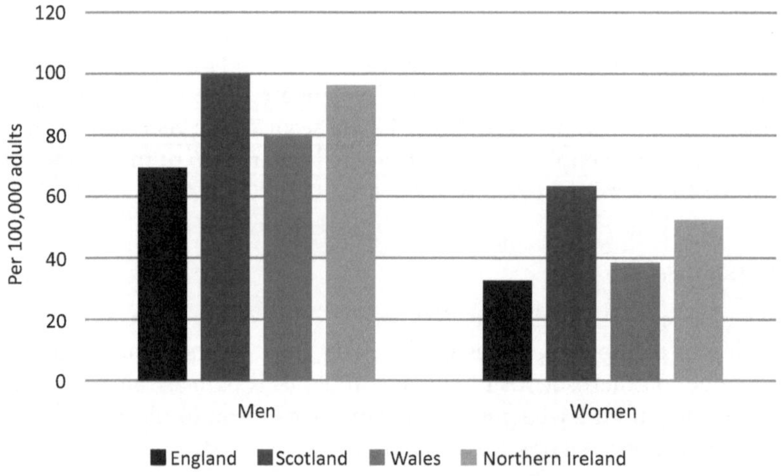

Figure 13.11 Incidence rates (new cases) of peripheral arterial disease, UK 2017
Source: British Heart Foundation, 2020b

Thinking point:

> Consider the experiences of the Swedish patients (Box 13.5). What do they suggest about personal and social perceptions of physical disability?

In 2018 to 2019 there were 361,833 people in England and 48,000 people in Scotland seeing their general practitioner for peripheral arterial disease (British Heart Foundation, 2020b).

Cerebrovascular disease

Cerebrovascular disease refers to several conditions that affect the blood vessels in the brain. A cerebrovascular accident (CVA), or a stroke, means that the blood

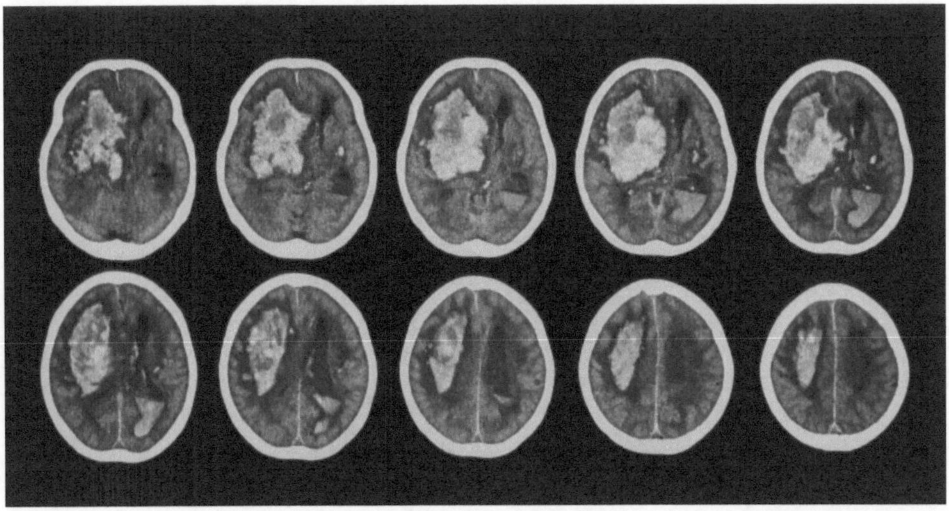

Figure 13.12 Computed tomography (CT) scan of the brain showing a haemorrhagic stroke
Source: Suttha Burawonk/Shutterstock.com

supply to part of the brain has been interrupted. Most strokes are ischaemic, meaning they are caused because of a blood clot, often due to atherosclerosis. Some are the result of a haemorrhage, meaning a blood vessel burst. The symptoms of a stroke include

- the face may drop on one side, the individual may be unable to smile
- an inability to lift both arms and keep them there
- slurred or garbled speech

(NHS, 2019a)

A transient ischaemic attack, often called a TIA, means that the blood supply to part of the brain has been temporarily disrupted. This may cause a temporary loss of speech, but individuals feel completely well again quite quickly.

Symptoms of a CVA/TIA are a medical emergency because treatment needs to be given within four and a half hours for long-term damage to be prevented. Stroke is the most common cause of severe disability in the UK. Its effects depend upon where the damage occurs in the brain, as each part of the brain contains neurons that control different functions in the body (Figure 13.13). There are sensory neurons (senses), motor neurons (movement) and interneurons that connect neurons together into a circuit.

The effects of a stroke can include many or some of the following symptoms.

Physical effects such as

- difficulties with movement such as weakness in one side of the body or one limb
- balance problems because balance is a combination of all the senses working with muscles and joints

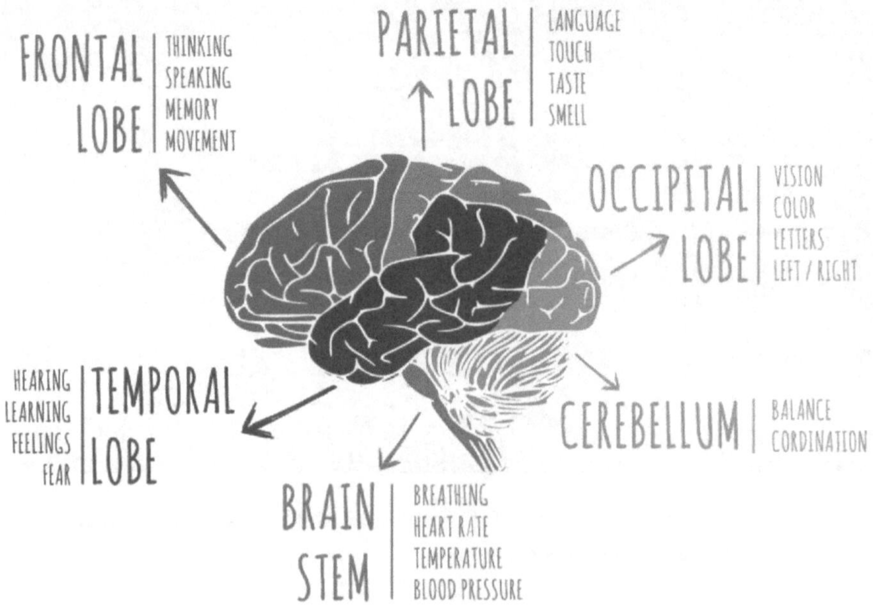

Figure 13.13 Areas of the brain and some key functions
Source: Noiel/Shutterstock.com

Table 13.4 Prevalence of UK strokes or transient ischaemic attacks (TIA), 2018 to 2019

	Number of people who have had a stroke or a TIA	*Percentage of population*
England	1,063,319	1.8%
Scotland	130,000	2.3%
Wales	68,870	2.1%
Northern Ireland	38,234	1.9%
UK	1,300,423	1.8%

Source: Adapted from British Heart Foundation (2020b).

- continence problems, an inability to control the bladder and/or bowels
- headaches due to fluid accumulating in the brain after a haemorrhage, or side effects of medicines
- seizures or epilepsy due to a disturbance in the electrical signals passing along the nerves of the brain to the body
- pain caused by muscle contractions and spasms
- swallowing problems because of an inability to control mouth and throat muscles
- sensory problems such as loss of smell or taste

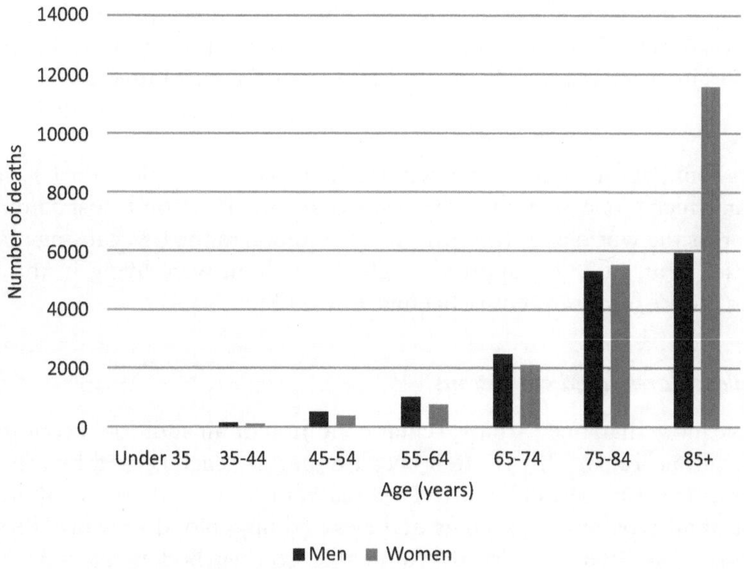

Figure 13.14 UK deaths from a stroke by sex, 2018
Source: British Heart Foundation, 2020b

- vision problems such as loss of some sight or eye movement, as well as the processing of visual images

Communication problems such as being unable to

- speak
- speak clearly because of an inability to control muscles in the mouth, throat and face
- understand others
- read
- write

Fatigue because

- the brain is healing, especially in the early phases
- the recovery process takes a lot of energy
- anxiety and depression can add to tiredness

(Stroke Association, 2020)

Many early symptoms will improve with support and motivation as the neurons in the brain 're-wire', and some people recover completely. For others, the symptoms of a stroke, the recovery/rehabilitation process and the long-term impact can be life-changing with significant personal, social and financial consequences. One person explained:

> My life is turned upside-down, and I have to ask for help ... and it feels very weird not to be able to do things myself ... I used to be a very social person, and now I am afraid to go out. I have to think and do things differently than I did before, and this makes me very sad ... I do not feel free – not the way I used to be.
>
> (case 9; Pedersten *et al.*, 2019 p.6)

The British Heart Foundation (2020a) reports more than 100,000 people in the UK have a stroke each year, which is one every five minutes. Strokes are the second most common cause of death across the world and the fourth most common in the UK, causing about 36,000 deaths each year. In 2018, approximately 1.3 million were living in the UK having survived a stroke or a transient ischaemic attack (Table 13.4).

Multiple cardiovascular-related conditions

Many people have more than one cardiovascular condition or an additional condition at the same time (Table 13.5). This is often because they are each caused by atherosclerosis, such as a stroke or peripheral arterial disease, or because they contribute to the development of atherosclerosis, such as diabetes and high blood pressure. People with cardiovascular conditions are already vulnerable, so their bodies easily develop serious complications that increase their risk of dying when faced with additional challenges, such as the COVID-19 coronavirus (British Heart Foundation, 2020a).

> *Cardiovascular disease is a collective term for conditions which affect the heart and circulatory system. It is the highest cause of death in the world and second highest in the UK.*

Causes of cardiovascular disease

Many of the more common cardiovascular conditions are caused and/or aggravated by atherosclerosis. Atherosclerosis is the result of two elements:

- the accumulation of fatty atheroma in the blood
- damage to the blood vessel walls and blood flow

Table 13.5 Percentage of people with coronary heart disease who have additional conditions, UK 2018

	Heart failure	*Stroke or transient ischaemic attack*	*Peripheral arterial disease*	*High blood pressure*	*Diabetes*
England	13.3%	12.8%	5.7%	55.8%	28.1%
Wales	14.3%	13.6%	5.6%	56.6%	29.4%
Scotland	13.0%	14.2%	7.3%	51.4%	25.3%
Northern Ireland	13.5%	13.7%	8.2&	55.8%	28.3%
UK	13.4%	12.9%	5.9%	55.5%	27.9%
UK over-75-year-olds who are obese (BMI >30)	19.1%	18.1%	7.1%	71.2%	39.2%

Source: Adapted from British Heart Foundation (2020d).

Table 13.6 Risk factors for atherosclerosis

Modifiable risk factors	
Atheroma High blood cholesterol Poor diet	Damage to blood vessels and blood flow High blood pressure High blood glucose Tobacco/e-cigarettes Physical inactivity and sedentary behaviour Alcohol Chronic stress Adverse childhood experiences Air pollution
Excess body fat/abdominal fat	
Socio-economic and physical environment	
Non-modifiable risk factors	
Middle/older age South Asian, African, African Caribbean Family history/genetics Sex	

If both are present, the atheroma sticks to the inside wall of the blood vessel causing narrowing. The atheroma may rupture, causing a blockage. Atherosclerosis is often described as a chronic inflammatory disease because the whole process is driven by chronic low-grade inflammation in the body, a process where free-radical molecules cause oxidative stress which damages cells and triggers disease (Singh *et al.*, 2015; Ruparelia and Choudhury, 2020). Low-grade inflammation is encouraged by age, poor diet, tobacco, excess body fat and stress (Pahwa *et al.*, 2020).

Atheroma

Atheroma is a fatty plaque made up of cell debris, calcium, fibrin and cholesterol carried in the blood. Raised levels of blood cholesterol leads to the creation and accumulation of atheroma. High blood cholesterol is encouraged by diet and excess body fat.

High blood cholesterol

All fatty substances carried in the blood are called lipids. When we eat fat in the diet, it is digested to become triglycerides (smaller fat molecules) and glycerol. These travel in the bloodstream from the intestine to the liver. Blood cholesterol is a lipid. It is mostly made in the liver. It is vital for certain body functions. The liver converts the triglycerides and cholesterol into packages called lipoproteins. There are two kinds of lipoproteins, both of which make up the total amount of cholesterol in the body.

- Low-density lipoproteins (LDL) deliver cholesterol around the body to tissues for the vital functions of membrane and hormone synthesis

then the

- High-density lipoproteins (HDL) take some of the cholesterol back to the liver where it is used to make bile acids, which are vital for digestion

LDLs are associated with creating more atherosclerosis. HDLs are protective because evidence shows that *low* levels of HDL in the blood are associated with more atherosclerosis.

Dietary cholesterol is present in foods of animal origin. An individual's liver compensates for how much cholesterol is eaten. If an individual eats a lot, their liver will make less; if an individual eats a little, their liver will make more. The cholesterol eaten in food does not normally affect blood cholesterol levels, and so foods high in cholesterol such as eggs are not a risk for atherosclerosis.

Poor diet

A diet high in saturated fats, trans fat and salt and low in dietary fibre, omega 3 fats, fruit and vegetables is strongly associated with the development of atherosclerosis and cardiovascular disease. In the UK a third of deaths from cardiovascular disease are associated with a poor diet (British Heart Foundation, 2020b).

- Saturated fats

Saturated fats increase blood cholesterol, and they raise the LDLs. Most people in the UK need to eat less of these.

- Polyunsaturated fats (omega 6)

Omega 6 fats lower blood cholesterol by lowering the LDLs and the HDLs. Eating more of these is not helpful, but it is helpful to replace saturated fat with polyunsaturated fats.

Table 13.7 Foods which encourage atherosclerosis

Foods high in saturated fat	*Foods high in trans fats*	*Foods high in salt*
Butter Ghee Margarine Suet Full-fat milk Cream Meat Poultry Cheese Processed meats, e.g. sausages, burgers, bacon Cakes Biscuits Ice-cream	'Hydrogenated oils'/ `hydrogenated fat' in margarine, spreads and processed food manufactured outside the UK, e.g. biscuits, cakes Takeaways, e.g. kebabs, and where vegetable oils are heated to very high temperatures or reheated Natural trans fats in beef lamb milk milk products	Many processed foods, e.g. biscuits breakfast cereal canned food crisps gravy products green pesto ketchup meat spread salted nuts savoury rice smoked fish some breads soups

Source: PHE/FSA (2015).

- Polyunsaturated fats (omega 3)

Omega 3 fats lower the risk of blood clots (thrombosis). Most people in the UK need to eat more of these in addition to replacing saturated fats.

- Monounsaturated fats

Monounsaturated fats lower LDLs, but not the 'protective' HDLs. Eating more of these is not helpful, but it is helpful to replace saturated fat with monounsaturated fats.

- Trans fats

Trans fats increase LDLs. People who regularly eat processed or takeaway foods may be eating too many of these.

- Dietary fibre

Diets low in dietary fibre including cereals and wholegrains are associated with higher levels of cardiovascular disease. Most people eat too little of this.

- Fruit and vegetables

Diets low in fruit and vegetables are associated with higher levels of cardiovascular disease. They are high in dietary fibre, protect against stiffening blood vessels and high blood pressure, and contain antioxidants which may be protective. Most people in the UK eat too little of these foods.

- Salt

Too much salt is associated with raised blood pressure. People who regularly eat processed foods may be eating too much salt.

- Plant sterols and stanols

Plant stanols and sterols, sometimes added to foods, help to reduce LDLs.

(Macready *et al.*, 2014; NICE, 2014; British Dietetic Association, 2017; SACN, 2019)

> *Saturated fats and trans fats increase blood cholesterol, including harmful LDLs, which encourage atheroma in the blood stream.*

Damage to blood vessel walls and blood flow

Blood vessel walls can be damaged by high blood pressure, high blood glucose and chemicals associated with tobacco/e-cigarettes, physical inactivity and sedentary behaviour, alcohol, stress, air pollution and excess body fat/abdominal fat. Most damage affects arteries as they need to be able to dilate and constrict to move the blood along, but some damage affects the veins as well.

High blood pressure (hypertension)

Blood pressure is the pressure inside the arteries. It rises (systolic pressure) when the heart contracts and falls (diastolic pressure) when the heart relaxes. Hypertension means the pressure is too high. The heart is needing to work hard to move the blood, and the pressure in the arteries causes them to bulge (aneurysm), which damages

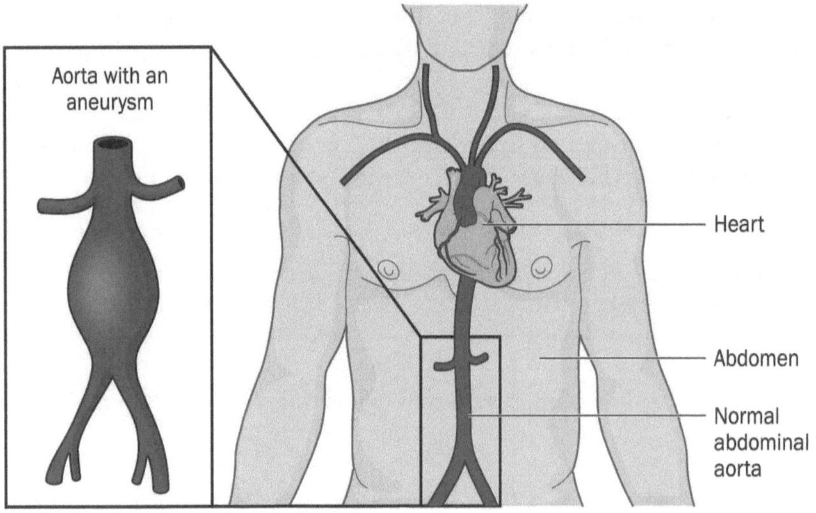

Figure 13.15 Aortic aneurysm
Source: Blamb/Shutterstock.com

Table 13.8 Symptoms and risk factors for high blood pressure

Symptoms of high blood pressure	*Factors which encourage high blood pressure*
Headaches	Over 65 years old
Dizziness	African, Caribbean, Indian, Irish heritage
Blurred vision	Chinese or Pakistani women
Nosebleeds	Genetics/a relative with high blood pressure
Shortness of breath	Overweight/excess body fat
Chest pain	Diet with too much salt and too few fruit and vegetables
No symptoms	Inactivity/sedentary behaviour
	Alcohol
	Excess caffeine-based drinks
	Smoking tobacco
	Stress
	Disturbed/inadequate sleep
	Low socio-economic status
	Noise pollution
	Air pollution

Sources: British Heart Foundation (2020d); NHS (2019b); PHE (2014); Műnzel and Sørensen (2017); Sanidas *et al.* (2017); Basner *et al.* (2020).

the artery walls. This is more likely to happen if the arteries are already narrowed by atherosclerosis. It is a vicious circle. At some point an artery may burst/haemorrhage. High blood pressure tires the heart and encourages poor blood flow which leads to tissue and organ damage. The causes, symptoms and prevalence of high blood pressure are summarised in Tables 13.8 and 13.9.

High blood glucose

High blood glucose means the amount of glucose in someone's blood rises too high because the body is not producing enough insulin or because the body's cells are unable to absorb the glucose from the blood. It occurs in diabetes, but also in prediabetes and some other medical conditions. The 'sugary blood' irritates the lining of the blood vessels, which encourages atherosclerosis. Adults with diabetes are two to three times more likely to develop cardiovascular disease compared to others and one-third of adults with diabetes die from cardiovascular disease (British Heart Foundation, 2020a). The causes and symptoms of type 2 diabetes are summarised in Table 13.10.

Tobacco/e-cigarettes

Tobacco contains many harmful chemicals which damage the artery walls.

- Nicotine is an addictive stimulant that increases the heart rate and blood pressure. It is found in all tobacco products (smoking, heated, smokeless) and e-cigarettes (electronic nicotine delivery systems).
- Carbon monoxide is produced when tobacco is burnt in smoking and heated tobacco products. When a person inhales the tobacco smoke, the carbon

Table 13.9 Prevalence of UK hypertension, 2018 to 2019

	Number of people living with high blood pressure seeing their general practitioner	*Percentage of population*
England	8,353,678	14%
Scotland	790,000	13.7%
Wales	512,542	15.8%
Northern Ireland	273,895	13.8%
UK	9,930,115	14.0%

Source: Adapted from British Heart Foundation (2020b).

Table 13.10 Symptoms and risk factors for diabetes

Symptoms of high blood glucose/diabetes	*Factors which encourage type 2 diabetes (type 1 is not preventable)*
Thirst	Over 25 years old and Asian, sub-Saharan African or Caribbean descent
Frequent urination	
Tiredness	Over 40 years old and White
Unexpected weight loss	Genetics/a close relative with diabetes
Blurred vision	Smoking tobacco/vaping e-cigarettes
Genital itching	Alcohol
Slow healing wounds	Excess body fat/abdominal fat
	Inactivity/sedentary behaviour
	Diet high in refined grains, sugar and sugary drinks; low in wholegrains, fruit and vegetables
	Obesogenic environments
	Environments with higher levels of traffic, noise and air pollution

Sources: Diabetes UK (2020); Kolb and Martin (2017); Basner *et al.* (2020).

Table 13.11 Estimated percentage of UK cardiovascular disease-related deaths attributable to high LDL blood cholesterol, high blood pressure, high blood glucose and smoking tobacco, 2017

	Percentage of deaths from cardiovascular disease	*Percentage of deaths from coronary heart disease*	*Percentage of deaths from stroke*
High LDL blood cholesterol	24.9%	44.5%	11.3%
High blood pressure	45.4%	49.9%	45.6%
High blood glucose	23.5%	32.9%	26.1%
Tobacco smoking (active and passive)	11.4%	15.3%	9.0%

Source: British Heart Foundation (2020b).

monoxide decreases the amount of oxygen in the blood, which puts a strain on all organs, especially the brain and heart, and damages artery walls which encourages atherosclerosis.

Only e-cigarettes which are electronic *non*-nicotine delivery systems are relatively safe. About 20,000 people die each year in the UK due to cardiovascular disease related to smoking tobacco (British Heart Foundation, 2020a).

Physical inactivity and sedentary behaviour

Physical inactivity and sedentary behaviour are treated as separate risk factors for cardiovascular disease, as each has a specific meaning. Physical inactivity means an individual is not engaging in enough physical activity to meet the guidelines for good health (Tremblay *et al.*, 2017). In the UK, for 19- to 64-year-olds, these are 150 minutes of moderate-intensity activity per week or 75 minutes of vigorous activity along with muscle-strengthening activities on two days per week (DHSC, 2019). Physical inactivity is associated with atherosclerosis because it has been linked to

- impaired blood glucose regulation, which increases the risk of high blood glucose
- impaired blood flow
- stiffening of the artery walls

(Lavie *et al.*, 2019)

High levels of sedentary behaviour, such as sitting and watching television, are also associated with increased atherosclerosis. In one study, people who watched television for more than 21 hours per week increased their chances of developing atherosclerosis by 80% (Lazaros *et al.*, 2019). In another review of several studies, Pandie and colleagues (2016) found more atherosclerosis, coronary heart disease, heart attacks, strokes and cardiovascular-related deaths among those people who had been sedentary for more than 10 hours per day. Sedentary behaviour encourages cardiovascular disease by

- reducing the enzyme lipoprotein lipase, an enzyme which breaks down LDLs thus reducing their damage

- lowering the rate of blood flow and damaging the inner lining of blood vessels. Together these encourage vasoconstriction and raised blood pressure
- lowering levels of heart and respiratory fitness, which means the body's ability to deliver oxygen around the body is reduced, adding strain on the heart

(Carter *et al.*, 2017; Lavie *et al.*, 2019)

There is not a straightforward linear relationship between degrees of sedentary behaviour and degrees of cardiovascular disease (Pandie *et al.*, 2016). Sedentary behaviour seems to be most harmful to people who also have very low levels of physical activity (Lavie *et al.*, 2019; Walker *et al.*, 2019).

Alcohol

Regular alcohol consumption, even at moderate levels, is associated with high blood pressure. It is thought that alcohol acts on the inner lining of the arteries, preventing them from dilating properly, possibly in response to low-grade inflammation (Husain *et al.*, 2014). Blood pressure is at its highest about 10 hours after consumption (McFadden *et al.*, 2005). The damage accumulates over time, and excess alcohol has been linked to damage to the heart muscle and abnormal heart rhythm. It also contributes to increased body fat/weight gain. The only people for whom a little alcohol, up to five units per week, has cardiovascular benefits are women over 55 years (Holmes *et al.*, 2016).

Chronic stress

When we are stressed, the body's instinct to survive kicks in, and we are primed to 'fight', 'flight' or 'freeze'. The hormone cortisol triggers the release of glucose into the bloodstream. It also increases chronic low-grade inflammation throughout the body, which encourages the blood vessel walls to become scarred and constricted, so blood pressure rises. At the same time, adrenaline increases the heart rate, quickens the blood flow to the brain and muscles, and also increases blood pressure. We are in high alert. After the stress has passed, the parasympathetic nervous system returns the body to rest. However, for people experiencing high levels of chronic stress, their bodies remain in a state of readiness with the high blood glucose, rapid heart rate and high blood pressure damaging their heart and the artery walls. How we deal with stress, such as drinking alcohol, smoking tobacco, eating 'comforting' high fat/sugar foods or being sedentary, can also contribute to atherosclerosis.

Song and colleagues (2019) researched 136,637 patients with diagnosed stress disorders, such as post-traumatic stress disorder and acute stress reaction, from 1987 to 2013, to see who subsequently developed cardiovascular disease. The sample was compared to their siblings, who did not have a stress disorder. The authors found a stress-related disorder increased heart failure, cerebrovascular disease, heart conduction disorders and cardiac arrest within the first year of the diagnoses of the stress-related disorders. The patients were four times more likely to have a cardiac arrest, where the heart stops beating, within six months of the stress diagnosis compared to their sibling. The British Heart foundation explain:

> A cardiac arrest usually happens without warning. If someone is in cardiac arrest, they collapse suddenly. [They] will be unconscious ... unresponsive and won't be breathing or breathing normally ... making gasping noises. Without immediate treatment ..., the person will die.
>
> (British Heart Foundation, 2019)

Adverse childhood experiences

We have known since the 1990s that adverse childhood experiences (ACEs) are associated with a range of adult physical and mental health conditions. Barr (2017) explains how ACEs, especially when severe and prolonged, are so stressful that children experience 'toxic stress'. Toxic stress affects the developing brain and damages bodies. It causes children's cortisol to rise and damages/thickens blood vessel walls. These atherosclerotic changes continue to worsen and are clinically recognised as a predictor of later cardiovascular disease in adulthood. As in adults, the stress in children related to ACEs seems to be associated with other risks for cardiovascular disease such as increased weight (body mass index) and waist circumference (Pretty *et al.*, 2013). We also know that combinations of childhood ACEs are associated with adult tobacco smoking, heavy alcohol consumption, physical inactivity and type 2 diabetes (high blood glucose) (Hughes *et al.*, 2017). In summary,

> ACEs are consistently an avoidable risk factor for some of the largest threats to public health and costs to health services across Europe and north America ...

Table 13.12 Multiple adverse childhood experiences and adult disease

Adverse childhood experiences (ACE)	*Strength of evidence that multiple ACEs are associated with adult disease*	*Adult health-related behaviour/disease*
Emotional abuse Physical abuse Sexual abuse	Very strong	Drug misuse Interpersonal violence Self-directed violence
Emotional neglect Physical neglect Mother treated violently	Strong	Sexual risk-taking Mental health problems
Substance misuse in household Mental illness in household Separation/divorce Imprisonment of member of household	Moderate	Cardiovascular disease Cancer Respiratory disease Smoking Heavy alcohol consumption Poor self-rated health
	Weak/modest	Physical inactivity Overweight/obesity Type 2 diabetes

Source: Hughes *et al.* (2017).

> [The financial] costs of cardiovascular disease attributable to ACEs were substantially higher than for most other causes of ill health.
>
> (Bellis *et al.*, 2019 p.e517, 518)

Air pollution

Air pollution is the fifth most common cause of cardiovascular disease across the world. Air pollution caused by fossil fuel emissions from cars and industry, such as ozone, nitrogen dioxide, carbon monoxide and sulphur dioxide, and particulates such as soot and dust, is clearly associated with heart attacks, strokes, heart failure, irregular heart rates and sudden death (Estol, 2020). Pollution accelerates atherosclerosis by

- damaging the inside walls of the arteries
- causing arteries to become rigid, which increases blood pressure and puts added strain on the heart
- encouraging blood clotting (thrombosis)
- encouraging insulin resistance, so blood glucose remains high
- interfering with the electrical impulses of the heart, causing irregular heart beats
- damaging the structure of the heart, encouraging heart failure

(British Heart Foundation, 2020e; Estol, 2020)

Damage to blood vessel walls and impeded blood flow encourage atheroma to stick and create high blood pressure – which itself damages blood vessel walls.

Excess body fat/abdominal fat

The combination of a high-calorie diet and high levels of sedentary behaviour is associated with weight gain. In 2017, in the UK, 14.7% of deaths from cardiovascular disease occurred where individuals were obese (BMI >30) (British Heart Foundation, 2020b). Some people may have relatively high body fat without being overweight; this is sometimes called 'skinny fat'. Excess body fat encourages atheroma and damages the blood vessels and blood flow.

Body fat releases inflammatory cytokines from fat cells that encourage low-grade inflammation throughout the body. This raises blood cholesterol, including the LDLs, which encourage atheroma. Body fat also leads to insulin resistance, which means the body's cells become less able to absorb glucose from the blood stream, resulting in high blood glucose/type 2 diabetes which irritates the lining of the arteries.

These problems are compounded if much of the body's fat sits around the organs in the abdomen, creating an 'apple shape' and making it hard for the organs to function. This visceral fat makes it difficult for the heart and arteries to pump the blood around the body, which leads to high blood pressure. Older people who are not overweight but have a relatively large waist measurement suffer more atherosclerosis and cardiovascular disease than those who are not 'apple shaped' (Chen *et al.*, 2019; Fan *et al.*, 2016).

Box 13.6 Metabolic syndrome

Metabolic syndrome is a combination of high blood pressure, high blood glucose and excess abdominal body fat. All contribute to atherosclerosis. If someone has three or more of these symptoms, they are diagnosed with metabolic syndrome, which puts them at very high risk of developing cardiovascular disease and/or type 2 diabetes.

- large waist circumference

80 cm or more in European and South Asian women; 94 cm or more in European men; 90 cm or more in South Asian men

- low levels of HDL blood cholesterol
- high blood pressure
- high triglyceride levels in the blood
- high blood glucose/inability to control blood glucose
- increased risk of blood clots
- swelling/irritation of body tissue

(Source: NHS, 2019c)

Body fat contributes to both atheroma and damage to blood vessels and blood flow.

Socio-economic and physical environment

In the UK, we see more deaths from cardiovascular disease (Table 13.13) and more multiple conditions in areas of deprivation compared to more affluent ones (Figure 13.16).

Table 13.13 Age-standardised death rates among under 75s from cardiovascular disease by deprivation, UK 2016 to 2018

	Local authority/ Unitary authority/ District council	*Level of deprivation (1 is most deprived and 317 is least deprived/most affluent)*	*Deaths under 75 years per 100,000 people*
Highest premature death rate			
Scotland	Glasgow City	4	138.0
Greater Manchester, England	Manchester	2	124.6
Lancashire, England	Blackpool	1	122.7
North Yorkshire, England	Middlesbrough	16	118.6
Gwent, Wales	Blaenau Gwent	1	116.4
Lowest premature death rate			
Surrey, England	Waverley	313	42.2
East Midlands, England	Rutland	303	41.8
Worcestershire, England	Malvern Hills	187	41.3
Essex, England	Rochford	286	40.8
Surrey, England	Mole Valley	294	40.0
Hampshire, England	Hart	317	39.1

Source: British Heart Foundation (2020b).

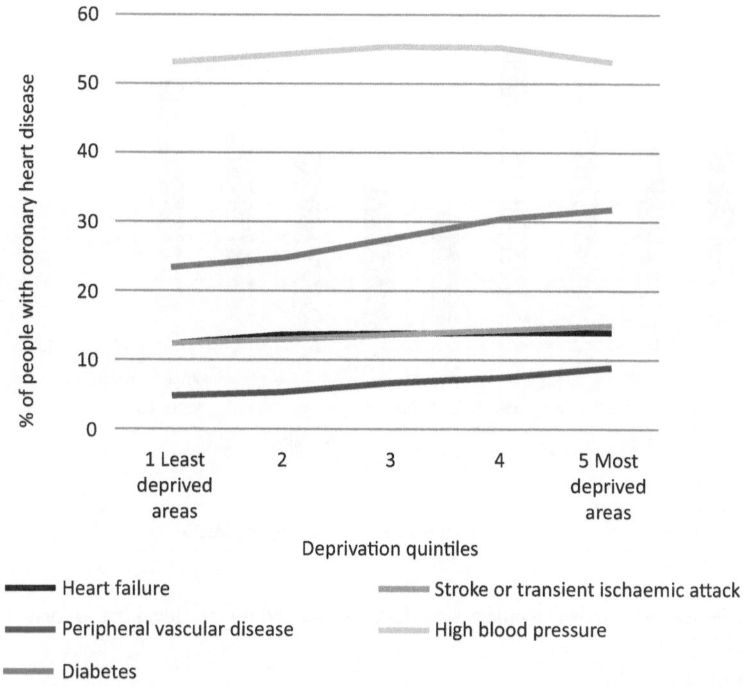

Figure 13.16 Percentage of people with coronary heart disease who have additional conditions, by deprivation, UK 2018

Source: British Heart Foundation, 2020b

Excessive body fat and health-related behaviours, such as inactivity, poor diet and smoking, are more common in areas of deprivation, while heavy alcohol consumption is more variable (McLean and Dean, 2020; Scholes, 2018) (Figure 13.17).

Health-related behaviours are shaped by the social, economic and physical environment in which people live and work. Ramsey and colleagues (2015) carried out a study of 24 British towns and concluded that neighbourhood-level deprivation is more strongly associated with early death from cardiovascular disease than people's occupation or health-related behaviours, particularly neighbourhoods with average low educational achievement and average low income (Ramsey *et al.*, 2015). Malambo and colleagues (2016) carried out a review of many research studies from across the world and concluded that cardiovascular risks, such as poor diet, inactivity, weight gain and high blood pressure, were greater in environments with

- high residential density
- high-density traffic and poor safety from traffic
- low street connectivity
- few walkable areas
- few recreational facilities
- high density of fast-food restaurants
- low density of supermarkets/grocers

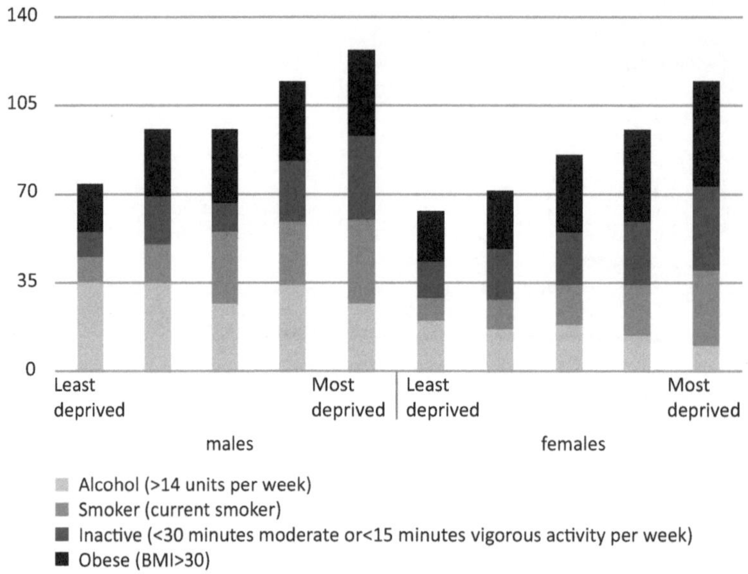

Figure 13.17 Prevalence of cardiovascular risk factors according to level of deprivation, Scotland 2018

Source: McLean and Dean, 2020

They found the most diagnosed cardiovascular conditions in areas of

- high-density traffic
- proximity to roads
- high density of fast-food restaurants

Thinking point:

How might the environment shape each of the factors associated with increasing atherosclerosis in the body outlined in Table 13.6 on p.373?

Atherosclerosis, and therefore cardiovascular disease, is encouraged by a range of health-related behaviours and factors in the socio-economic and physical environments in which people live.

Non-modifiable risk factors for cardiovascular disease

There are four non-modifiable risk factors associated with the development of atherosclerosis and cardiovascular disease.

- Age

The risks increase with age. For males, this is linear, for females, risks increase post-menopause

- Ethnicity

People with a South Asian, African or African Caribbean heritage are at higher risk because they develop type 2 diabetes more than the rest of the UK population. People with African or African Caribbean heritage are more likely to develop high blood pressure and to have a stroke compared to other ethnic groups. People with a South Asian heritage are at greater risk of developing coronary heart disease compared to Europeans

- Family history/genetics

An individual is at higher risk of developing cardiovascular disease if it is present in the family. This may be due to several genes which in combination encourage high blood pressure or high blood cholesterol. Familial hypercholesterolaemia, which means very high LDL blood cholesterol, is an example of an inherited condition caused by at least one parent passing on a mutated gene

- Sex

There are differences between male and female experiences of cardiovascular disease which are not accounted for by health-related behaviours alone and are not fully understood. Differences may be genetic, causing differing heart responses to stress, or related to sex hormones; for example, oestrogen, which is high in premenopausal women, seems to be protective. Females increase their risks of developing atherosclerosis/cardiovascular disease in the short and/or long term if they experience

- polycystic ovary syndrome
- early menopause
- pregnancy-induced high blood pressure/preeclampsia
- gestational diabetes
- pre-term birth

(Gao *et al.*, 2019; British Heart Foundation, 2020f)

Age, ethnicity, family history/genetics and sex can increase or decrease people's risks of developing atherosclerosis and cardiovascular disease

Primary prevention of cardiovascular disease

The primary prevention of cardiovascular disease focuses on promoting healthy cardiovascular circulation for the whole population.

Reduce the build-up of atheroma in the blood stream

The aim is to reduce blood cholesterol, reduce LDLs, protect HDLs, reduce risks of blood clots and discourage excess body fat.

Keep the blood vessel walls healthy and flexible

The aim is to avoid irritants and toxins which directly damage artery walls and make arteries narrow and inflexible. These include avoiding

- the causes of excess glucose in the blood (e.g. excess body fat or frequent high-sugar drinks)
- tobacco
- alcohol
- air pollution

Keep a healthy heart, heartbeat and blood flow

We protect the heart and blood flow by avoiding

- atheroma and damage to artery walls
- all causes of high blood pressure
- excess salt
- alcohol
- nicotine
- carbon monoxide in tobacco smoke
- air pollution
- physical inactivity and sedentary behaviour
- chronic stress
- toxic stress in childhood
- excess body fat

and encouraging

- physical activity
- good mental health

Table 13.14 Foods which help to protect against developing cardiovascular disease

Eat foods rich in omega 3 fats	*Replace saturated fats with monounsaturated fats*	*Replace saturated fats with polyunsaturated fats*	*Eat wholegrain (insoluble) dietary fibre*	*Eat soluble dietary fibre*	*Eat foods fortified with plant sterols and stanols*
Oily fish, e.g. sardines, mackerel, trout, tuna, salmon, herrings, pilchards Green leafy vegetables Walnuts, linseeds Foods fortified with omega 3 fats	Olive oil Rapeseed oil Avocados Walnuts Almonds Pecan nuts	Sunflower oil Corn oil Rapeseed oil Spreads made from these oils Nuts Seeds	Wholegrain bread, pasta, rice, breakfast cereal e.g. Shredded Wheat, Weetabix, low-sugar granola Fruit Vegetables	Oats Fruit Vegetables Pulses, e.g. baked beans, kidney beans, soya beans, lentils, chickpeas, lentils	Usually in milks, yoghurts, fat spreads

Source: British Dietetic Association (2017).

- weight management
- fresh, not processed, foods

Address the underlying causes of atherosclerosis

The aim is to create a health promoting environment which makes healthier living accessible and affordable. This includes opportunities for

- physical activity
- healthy eating
- alternatives to recreation associated with alcohol and tobacco

as well as

- clean fresh air for all
- improving communities with high socio-economic deprivation
- creating places with high walkability and low quantities of traffic
- replacing fast-food outlets with local supermarkets/grocers
- raising awareness that adverse childhood experiences are associated with adult disease, including cardiovascular disease

The World Health Organization's (2020) key recommendations to countries to prevent cardiovascular disease include

- comprehensive tobacco-control policies
- taxation of foods high in fat, sugar and salt
- more walking and cycle paths
- strategies to reduce harmful alcohol use
- healthy school meals

Secondary prevention of cardiovascular disease

Secondary prevention is normally carried out by healthcare professionals in primary care settings, and is aimed at people who are known to be at higher risk of developing cardiovascular disease such as those

- in middle and older age
- of South Asian, African, African Caribbean heritage
- with a family history or specific genetic risks
- with certain medical conditions such as atrial fibrillation, chronic kidney disease and severe mental disorders

The aim is to treat early signs quickly and prevent disease from taking hold. Along with encouraging healthy behaviours, the main tasks include monitoring, treating and reducing

- high blood pressure
- high blood cholesterol

- high blood glucose levels
- blood clotting risks

and checking for medical conditions which increase any of these.

(NICE, 2018)

There is an urgent, need for healthcare professionals to integrate asking about stress and adverse childhood experiences into secondary screening (Su *et al.*, 2015; Bellis *et al.*, 2019).

Box 13.7 Blood cholesterol test

An individual might be asked not to eat anything for up to 12 hours before the blood sample is taken. The sample is analysed in a laboratory. Generally, healthy results are

total cholesterol ... 5 mmol/l or below
HDL ... 1 or above mmol/l
LDL ... 3 or below mmol/l
non-HDL means total cholesterol minus HDL 4 mmol/l or below
triglycerides ... 2.3 mmol/l or below

(Source: NHS, 2019d)

> *More than half of all cardiovascular disease in the UK is avoidable if we put into practice all that is understood about the primary and secondary prevention of the disease.*
>
> (ONS, 2019)

Tertiary prevention of cardiovascular disease

People who may be referred to a cardiac rehabilitation service include those who have angina or heart failure, a heart attack or heart surgery. Cardiac rehabilitation has been shown to reduce cardiovascular-related deaths and hospital admissions, and to improve the functioning of the body and people's perceptions of their quality of life (BACPR 2017).

Cardiac rehabilitation means:

> The coordinated sum of activities required to influence favourably the underlying cause of cardiovascular disease, as well as to provide the best possible physical, mental and social conditions, so that the patients may, by their own efforts, preserve or resume optimal functioning in their community and through improved health behaviour, slow or reverse progression of disease.
>
> (BACPR, 2017 p.1)

The British Association for Cardiovascular Prevention and Rehabilitation outlines six core components of cardiac rehabilitation which need to be delivered by a multi-disciplinary team.

- Health-related behaviour change and education
  e.g. goal-setting, regular assessment, tobacco cessation, healthy eating, occupational factors, sexual relations, weight management
- Lifestyle risk-factor management
  e.g. tailored physical activity and exercise plan, personalised dietary assessment and advice, individual support with smoking cessation
- Psychosocial health
  e.g. assessment of psychological stressors and quality of life, support with sexual concerns or alcohol/drug misuse
- Management of medical risks
  e.g. assessment of blood pressure, blood cholesterol and heart rate, examining beliefs about taking prescribed medicines
- Long-term strategies
  e.g. signposting to local heart/activity/weight management groups and communication with healthcare services to ensure appropriate ongoing support
- Evaluation/audit
  e.g. evaluate cardiac rehabilitation services to assess programmes and outcomes against national standards

(BACPR, 2017)

Summary

This chapter has

- outlined the heart and circulatory system
- described common types of cardiovascular disease
- explained the burden of cardiovascular disease for people's health
- examined the causes of atherosclerosis
- outlined the priorities for primary, secondary and tertiary prevention of cardiovascular disease

Further reading

Jones, J., Buckley, J., Furze, G., and Sheppard, G. (eds) (2020) *Cardiovascular prevention and rehabilitation in practice.* 2nd edn. London: Wiley/Blackwell

Useful websites

British Heart Foundation. Available at: www.bhf.org.uk
Stroke Association. Available at: www.stroke.org.uk

References

Barr, D.A. (2017) 'The childhood roots of cardiovascular disease disparities', *Mayo Clinic Proceedings*, 92(9), pp.1415–1421

Basner, M., Riggs, D.W., and Conklin, D.J. (2020) 'Environmental determinants of hypertension and diabetes mellitus: sounding off about the effects of noise', *Journal of the American Heart Association*, 9(6) doi:10.1161/JAHA.120.016048

Bellis, M.A., Hughes, K., Ford, K., Rodriguez, G.R., Sethi, D., and Passmore, J. (2019) 'Lifecourse health consequences and associated annual costs of adverse childhood experiences across Europe and North America: a systematic review and meta-analysis', *Lancet Public Health*, 4(10) doi:10.10.1016S2468-2667(19)30145–8

British Association for Cardiovascular Prevention and Rehabilitation (2017) The BACPR standards and core components for cardiovascular disease prevention and rehabilitation 2017. Available at: www.bacpr.com/resources/BACPR_Standards_and_Core_Components_2017.pdf (Accessed 12th August 2020)

British Dietetic Association (2017) Heart health. Available at: www.bda.uk.com/uploads/assets/5693cba0-4d26-463d-8f4e27d4e6ab6ba4/Heart-Health-food-fact-sheet.pdf (Accessed 7th August 2020)

British Heart Foundation (2019) Cardiac arrest. Available at: www.bhf.org.uk/informationsupport/conditions/cardiac-arrest (Accessed 10th August 2020)

British Heart Foundation (2020a) BHF statistics factsheet – UK. Available at: https://bit.ly/39FPsBz (Accessed 3rd August 2020)

British Heart Foundation (2020b) Heart and circulatory disease statistics 2020. British Heart Foundation/University of Birmingham. Available at: www.bhf.org.uk/what-we-do/our-research/heart-statistics/heart-statistics-publications/cardiovascular-disease-statistics-2020 (Accessed 3rd August 2020)

British Heart Foundation (2020c) Conditions. Available at: www.bhf.org.uk/informationsupport/conditions (Accessed 4th August 2020)

British Heart Foundation (2020d) High blood pressure – symptoms and treatment. Available at: www.bhf.org.uk/informationsupport/risk-factors/high-blood-pressure/symptoms-and-treatment (Accessed 6th August 2020d)

British Heart Foundation (2020e) What is air pollution? Available at: www.bhf.org.uk/informationsupport/risk-factors/air-pollution#:~:text=Air%20pollution%20can%20be%20harmful,the%20strain%20on%20your%20heart (Accessed 10th August 2020)

British Heart Foundation (2020f) Risk factors. Available at: www.bhf.org.uk/informationsupport/risk-factors (Accessed 10th August 2020)

Cahill, T., and Kharbanda, R.K. (2017) 'Heart failure after myocardial infarction in the era of primary percutaneous coronary intervention: mechanisms, incidence and identification of patients at risk', *World Journal of Cardiology*, 9(5), pp.407–415

Carter, S., Hartman, Y., Holder, S., Thijssen, D.H., and Hopkins, N. (2017) 'Sedentary behaviour and cardiovascular disease risk: mediating mechanics', *Exercise, Sport Sciences Review*, 45(2), pp.80–86

Chen, G., Arthur, R., Iyengar, N.M., Kamensky, V., Xue, X., Wassertheil-Smoller, S., Allison, M.A., Shadyab, A.H., Wild, R.A., Sun, Y., Banack, H.R., Chai, J.C., Wactawski-Wende, J., Manson, J.E., Stefanick, M.L., Dannenberg, A.J., Rohan, T.E., and Qi, Q. (2019) 'Association between regional body fat and cardiovascular disease risk among postmenopausal women with normal body mass index', *European Heart Journal*, 40(34), pp.2849–2855

Davies, L.L. (2017) 'A qualitative study of symptom experiences of women with acute coronary syndrome', *Journal of Cardiovascular Nursing*, 32(5), pp.488–495

Department of Health and Social Care (2019) UK chief medical officers' physical activity guidelines. Department of Health and Social Care/Welsh Government/Department of Health/Scottish Government. Available at: https://assets.publishing.service.gov.uk/government/uploads/system/uploads/attachment_data/file/832868/uk-chief-medical-officers-physical-activity-guidelines.pdf (Accessed 10th August 2020)

Diabetes UK (2020) Diabetes risk factors. Available at: www.diabetes.org.uk/preventing-type-2-diabetes/diabetes-risk-factors (Accessed 6th August 2020)

Editorial (2019) 'Cardiology's problem women', *The Lancet*, 393(10175), pp.959

Estol, C.J. (2020) 'Air pollution and cardiovascular disease: a proven causality', in Al-Dalaimy, W., Ramanathan, V., and Sánchez Sorondo, M. (eds) *Health of people, health of planet and our responsibility*. New York: Springer, pp.193–204

Fan, H., Li, X., Zheng, L., Chen, X., Ian, Q., Wu, H., Ding, X., Qian, D., Shen, Y., Yu, Z., Fan., L., Chen, M., Tomlinson, B., Chan, P., Zhang, Y., and Liu, Z. (2016) 'Abdominal obesity is strongly associated with cardiovascular disease and its risk factors in elderly and very elderly community-dwelling Chinese', *Scientific Reports*, 6 doi:10.1038/srep21521

Gao, A., Chen, Z., Sun, A., and Deng, X. (2019) 'Gender differences in cardiovascular disease', *Medicine in Novel Technology and Devices*, 4 doi:10.1016/j.medntd.2019.100025

Gwaltney, C.J., Slagle, A.F., Martin, M., Ariely, R., and Brede, Y. (2012) 'Hearing the voice of the heart failure patient: key experiences identified in qualitative interviews', *The British Journal of Cardiology*, 19(25) doi:10.5837/bjc.2012.004

Holmes, J., Angus, C., Buykx, P., Ally, A., Stone, T., Meier, P., and Brennan, A. (2016) Mortality and morbidity risks from alcohol consumption in the UK. University of Sheffield. Available at: www.sheffield.ac.uk/polopoly_fs/1.538671!/file/Drinking_Guidelines_Final_Report_Published.pdf (Accessed 12th August 2020)

Hughes, K., Bellis, M.A., Hardcastle, K.A., Sethi, D., Butchart, A., Mikton, C., Jones, L., and Dunne, M.P. (2017) 'The effect of multiple childhood experiences on health: a systematic review and meta-analysis', *Lancet Public Health*, 2, e356-366 doi:10.1016/S2468-2667(17)30118-4

Husain K., Ansari, R.A., and Ferder, L. (2014) 'Alcohol-induced hypertension: mechanism and prevention', *World Journal of Cardiology*, 6(5), pp.245–252

Jones, M.M., Somerville, C., Feder, G., and Foster, G. (2010) 'Patients' descriptions of angina symptoms: a qualitative study of primary care patients', *British Journal of General Practice*, 60(579), pp.735–741

Kolb, H., and Martin, S. (2017) 'Environmental/lifestyle factors in the pathogenesis and prevention of type 2 diabetes', *BMC Medicine*, 15(131) doi:10.1186/s12916-017-0901-x

Lavie, C.J., Ozemek, C., Carbone, S., Ktzmarzyk, P.T., and Blair, S.N. (2019) 'Sedentary behaviour, exercise, and cardiovascular health', *Circulation Research*, 124(5), pp.799–815

Lazaros, G., Oikonomou, E., Vogiatzi, G., Chjristoforatou, E., Tsalamandris, S., Goliopoulou, A., Tousouli, M., Mystakidou, V., Chasikidis, C., and Tousoulis, D. (2019) 'The impact of sedentary behaviour patterns on carotid atherosclerotic burden: implications from the Corinthia epidemiological study', *Atherosclerosis*, 282, pp.154–161

Macready, A.L., George, T.W., Chong, M.F., Alimbetov, D.S., Jin, Y., Vidal, A., Spencer, J.P.E., Kennedy, O.B., Tuohy, K.M., Minihane, A., Gordeon, M.H., Lovegrove, J.A., FLAVURS Study Group (2014) 'Flavonoid-rich fruit and vegetables improve microvascular reactivity and inflammatory status in men at risk of cardiovascular disease – FLAVURS: a randomized controlled trial', *American Journal of Clinical Nutrition*, 99(3), pp.479–489

Malambo, P., Kengne, A.P., de Villiers, A., Lambert, E.V., and Puoane, T. (2016) 'Built environment, selected risk factors and major cardiovascular disease outcomes: a systematic review', *PLoS ONE*, 11(11) doi:10.1371/journal.pone.0166846

McFadden, C.B., Brensinger, C.M., Berlin, J.A., and Townsend, R.R. (2005) 'Systematic review of the effect of daily alcohol intake on blood pressure', *American Journal of Hypertension*, 18(2), pp.276–286

McLean, J., and Dean, L (eds) (2020) *The Scottish health survey. 2018 edition: amended in February 2020. Volume 1*. Scottish Government. Available at: www.gov.scot/publications/scottish-health-survey-2018-volume-1-main-report/ (Accessed 11th August 2020)

Merritt, C.J., de Zoysa, N., and Hutton, J. (2017) 'A qualitative study of younger men's experience of heart attack (myocardial infarction)', *British Journal of Health Psychology*, 22(3), pp.589–608

Műnzel, T., and Sørensen, M. (2017) 'Noise pollution and arterial hypertension', *European Cardiology Review*, 12(1), pp.26–29

National Health Service (2019a) Overview. Stroke. Available at: www.nhs.uk/conditions/stroke/ (Accessed 4th August 2020)

National Health Service (2019b) Overview. High blood pressure (hypertension). Available at: www.nhs.uk/conditions/high-blood-pressure-hypertension/ (Accessed 6th August 2020)

National Health Service (2019c) Metabolic syndrome. Available at: www.nhs.uk/conditions/metabolic-syndrome/ (Accessed 11th August 2020)

National Health Service (2019d) Getting tested. High cholesterol. Available at: www.nhs.uk/conditions/high-cholesterol/getting-tested/ (Accessed 7th August 2020)

National Institute for Health and Care Excellence (2014) *Prevention of cardiovascular disease. Evidence update January 2014*. London: NICE

National Institute for Health and Care Excellence (2018) NICE impact cardiovascular disease prevention. Available at: www.nice.org.uk/media/default/about/what-we-do/into-practice/measuring-uptake/nice-impact-cardiovascular-disease-prevention.pdf (Accessed 12th August 2020)

Office for National Statistics (2019) Avoidable mortality in the UK: 2017. Available at: https://bit.ly/2IaIDg1 (Accessed 12th August 2020)

Office for National Statistics (2020) Leading causes of death, UK: 2001 to 2018. Available at: www.ons.gov.uk/peoplepopulationandcommunity/healthandsocialcare/causesofdeath/articles/leadingcausesofdeathuk/2001to2018 (Accessed 4th August 2020)

Pahwa, R., Goyal, A., Bansai, P., and Jialal, I. (2020) 'Chronic inflammation', in *StatPearls. Treasure Island (FL)*. Available at: www.ncbi.nlm.nih.gov/books/NBK493173/ (Accessed 2nd September 2020)

Pandie, A., Salahuddin, U., Garg, S., Ayers, C., Kulinski, J., Anand, V., Mayo, H., Kumbhani, D.J., de Lemos, J., and Berry, J.D. (2016) 'Continuous dose-response association between sedentary time and risk for cardiovascular disease', *JAMA Cardiology*, 1(5), pp.575–583

Pedersen, S.G., Anke, A., Aadal, L., Pallesen, H., Moe, S., and Arntzen, C. (2019) 'Experiences of quality of life the first year after stroke in Denmark and Norway. A qualitative analysis', *International Journal of Qualitative Studies on Health and Well-being*, 14(1) doi:10.1080/17482631.2019.1659540

Pretty, C., O'Leary, D.D., Cairney, J., and Wade, T.J. (2013) 'Adverse childhood experiences and the cardiovascular health of children: a cross-sectional study', *BMC Pediatrics*, 13 (208) doi:10.1186/1471-2431-13-208

Public Health England (2014) Tackling high blood pressure. From evidence to action. Available at: https://assets.publishing.service.gov.uk/government/uploads/system/uploads/attachment_data/file/527916/Tackling_high_blood_pressure.pdf (Accessed 6th August 2020)

Public Health England/Food Standards Agency (2015) *McCance and Widdowson's the composition of foods*. 7th edn. London: Royal Society of Chemistry

Ramsey, S.E., Morris, R.W., Whincup, P.H., Subramanian, S.V., Papacosta, A.O., Lennon, L.T., and Wannamethee, S.G. (2015) 'The influence of neighbourhood-level socioeconomic deprivation on cardiovascular disease mortality in older age: longitudinal multilevel analyses from a cohort study of older British men', *Journal of Epidemiology and Community Health*, 69(12),pp.1224–1231

Ruparelia, N., and Choudhury, R. (2020) 'Inflammation and atherosclerosis: what is on the horizon? *Heart (British Cardiac Society)*, 106, pp.80–85

Sanidas, E., Papadopoulos, D.P., Grassos, H., Velliou, M., Tsioufis, K., Barbetseas, J., and Papademetriou, V. (2017) 'Air pollution and arterial hypertension. A new risk factor is in the air', *Journal of the American Society of Hypertension*, 11(11), pp.709–715

Scholes, A. (2018) Health survey for England 2017. Multiple risk factors. NHS Digital. Available at: http://healthsurvey.hscic.gov.uk/media/78655/HSE17-MRF-rep.pdf (Accessed 11th August 2020)

Scientific Advisory Committee on Nutrition (2019) Saturated fats and health. London. Available at: www.gov.uk/government/publications/saturated-fats-and-health-sacn-report (Accessed 9th August 2020)

Singh, R., Devi, S., and Gollen, R. (2015) 'Role of free radical in atherosclerosis, diabetes and dyslipidaemia: larger-than-life', *Diabetes/Metabolism Research and Reviews*, 31(2), pp.113–126

Song, H., Fang, F., Arnberg, F.K., Mataix-Cols, D., Fernández de la Cruz, L., Almqvist, C., Fall, K., Lichtenstein, P., Thorgeirsson, G., and Valdimarsdóttir, U.A. (2019) 'Stress related disorders and risk of cardiovascular disease: population based, sibling controlled cohort study', *BMJ*, 365 doi:10.1136/bmj.11255

Stroke Association (2020) Effects of stroke. Available at: www.stroke.org.uk/effects-of-stroke (Accessed 5th August 2020)

Su, S., Jimenez, M.P., Roberts, C.T.F., and Loucks, E.B. (2015) 'The role of adverse childhood experiences in cardiovascular disease risk: a review with emphasis on plausible mechanisms', *Current Cardiology Reports*, 17(10), 88 doi:10.1007/s11886-015-0645-1

Torbjörnsson, E., Ottosson, C., Blomgren, L., Boströn, L., and Fagerdahl, A. (2017) 'The patient's experience of amputation due to peripheral arterial disease', *Journal of Vascular Nursing*, 35(2), pp.57–63

Tremblay, M.S., Aubert, S., Barnes, J.D., Saunders, T.J., Carson, V., Latimer-Cheung, A.E., Chastin, S.F.M., Altenburg, T.M., Chinapaw, M.J.M., and SBRN terminology consensus project participants (2017) 'Sedentary Behavior Research Network (SRBN) – terminology consensus project process and outcome', *International Journal of Behavioral Nutrition and Physical Activity*, 14(1) doi:10.1186/s12966-017-0525-8

Walker, T.J., Heredia, N.I., Lee, M., Laing, M., Laing, S.T., Fisher-Hoch, S.P., McCormick, J.B., and Reininger, B.M. (2019) 'The combined effect of physical activity and sedentary behaviour on subclinical atherosclerosis: a cross-sectional study among Mexican Americans', *BMC Public Health*, 19(161) doi:10.1186/s12889-019-6439-4

World Health Organization (2019) International statistical classification of diseases and related health problems 11th revision (ICD-11). Available at: https://icd.who.int/browse11/l-m/en#/ (Accessed 29th July 2020)

World Health Organization (2020) Cardiovascular diseases. Available at: www.who.int/newsroom/fact-sheets/detail/cardiovascular-diseases-(cvds) (Accessed 12th August 2020)

14 Cancer

Sally Robinson

Key points

- Introduction
- Cancer
- Cancer sites in the body
- The burden of cancer
- Causes of cancer
- Primary prevention of cancer
- Secondary prevention of cancer
- Tertiary prevention of cancer
- Summary

Introduction

In the UK, a new cancer is diagnosed every two minutes. This chapter explains how cancer starts, grows and spreads. It describes types of cancer cells, stages of cancer and the most common sites in the body where malignant tumours are found, with their symptoms. The burden of cancer is described through an overview of current epidemiological data. The non-modifiable and modifiable causes of cancer are explained with recommendations for how to prevent 40% of cancers. The chapter ends with an outline of the secondary and tertiary prevention of cancer.

Cancer

The human body is made up of nearly two trillion cells. These cells are constantly replaced with fresh new ones to keep the body healthy and well. The whole body is replaced about every seven years. Each cell divides itself into two identical new cells, a process called mitosis. Both cells have the same chromosomes containing many genes, each with their DNA. Sometimes there is a problem with mitosis. When cells multiply into a mass, they create a tumour, or a neoplasm. As the tumour grows, it may be possible to see it with medical imaging, such as X-rays, or to feel the lump under the skin. Tumours made up of normal cells are called benign tumours. They stay in the same place, grow slowly and do not invade other tissues. They are not cancer.

In cancer, a single cell mutates into an abnormal cell. The abnormal cells, sometimes called cancer cells, multiply into a malignant tumour which may be detected as a lump. The body supplies these cells with blood and oxygen, enabling them to spread. Some cells

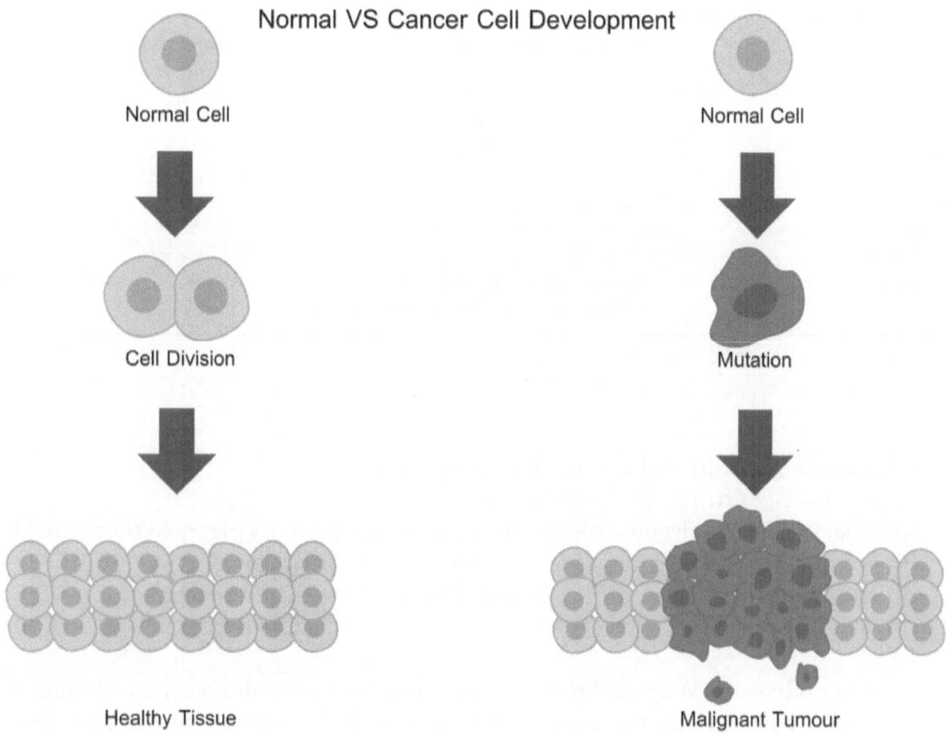

Figure 14.1 The development of normal cells versus cancer cells
Source: 1168group/Shutterstock.com

may break away from the primary tumour and travel in the blood stream, or through the lymphatic system, to another part of the body. This process is called metastasis. On arrival the cells start to multiply, and another tumour grows; these are 'secondary' tumours.

Both benign and malignant tumours can damage the part of the body where they are growing, interfere with the body's normal functioning and cause unpleasant symptoms. However, because malignant tumours spread further and faster, and disperse their cancer cells, they cause extensive damage which leads to disability and death. Some cells are defined as pre-cancerous when they are currently benign but show abnormalities which suggest they could become malignant.

Cancer cells

The genes inside a cell oversee the process of mitosis. At the point a cell divides, a gene may mutate, for example it may be lost or damaged. This interferes with the creation of the new cell, which starts to grow abnormally and reproduces itself at high speed. A mutated gene may be inherited or a gene may mutate due to external factors coming into the body: the modifiable causes of cancer. Unlike healthy cells, cancer cells

- are often abnormally shaped
- do not stop growing and dividing

Table 14.1 Types of cancer cells

Types of cancer cells	*Site of the primary tumour*	*Percentage of all UK cancers*
Carcinomas	Skin or tissue that cover internal organs	85%
Brain and spinal cord cancers	Central nervous system	3%
Leukaemia	Bone marrow	3%
Lymphomas	Lymphatic system	5%
Myelomas	Plasma cells	1%
Sarcomas	Connective tissues found in bones, cartilage, fat, muscle or blood vessels	1%

Source: Cancer Research UK (2017b).

- form a tumour, a lump that continues to grow
- ignore messages from other cells telling them to stop growing
- lose their surface molecules which normally keep a cell in its place, so they spread
- do not mature; they are immature and do not work properly
- do not repair themselves, no matter the damage, they keep on going

(Cancer Research UK, 2017a)

The human body is made up of different types of cells such as blood cells and muscle cells. Cancer is defined by the type of cells within which the abnormal cells first appear, where the cancer starts. For example, if someone's primary tumour begins in a muscle, and comprises abnormal muscle cells, it is called a sarcoma. If some cells break away from this tumour, travel through the blood stream and settle in the lung, the secondary tumour is also a sarcoma.

Carcinomas

Carcinomas are malignant cells which emerge in the sheets of epithelial tissue that cover all the surfaces of the body, including all organs. Epithelial tissue is made up of cells that include squamous cells, adenomatous cells and transitional cells.

- Squamous cell carcinoma starts in areas such as the skin or the lining of the oesophagus
- Adenocarcinoma starts in glands
- Transitional cell carcinoma starts in tissues that can stretch, such as the lining of the bladder
- Basal cell carcinoma starts in the cells that make up the deepest layer of skin

Brain and spinal cord cancers

The brain and spinal cord make up the central nervous system. The brain controls the electrical messages that are sent down the nerve fibres through the spinal cord and out to the wider parts of the body. The brain comprises nerve cells called neurons and connective tissue made up of glial cells.

- Glioma starts in the brain
- Mixed neuronal-glial tumours start in the brain or spinal cord

Leukaemia

Bone marrow produces red blood cells, platelets and white blood cells. Blood cells begin life as immature stem cells inside the marrow. Lymphoid stem cells develop into white blood cells called lymphocytes. Myeloid stem cells develop into white blood cells (monocytes and granulocytes), red blood cells and platelets. A mutation in the stem cells will cause the production of abnormal blood cells. These do not form tumours but accumulate in the blood stream. Leukaemia is cancer of white blood cells. Acute forms develop very quickly, and chronic forms develop slowly.

- Acute myeloid leukaemia starts with immature, abnormal myeloid blood cells in the bone marrow (Figure 14.2)
- Acute lymphoblastic leukaemia starts with immature, abnormal lymphocytes in the bone marrow
- Chronic lymphocytic leukaemia starts with almost mature, abnormal lymphocytes
- Chronic myeloid leukaemia starts with almost mature, abnormal granulocytes

Lymphomas

The lymphatic system is a drainage system that circulates around the body. It collects excess extracellular fluid, called lymph, from tissues and directs it back into the bloodstream via lymphatic capillaries and larger vessels. Lymph contains infection-fighting lymphocytes. At intervals, the lymphatic system has lymph nodes, small masses of lymph tissue.

- Lymphomas start with abnormal lymphocytes in the lymph

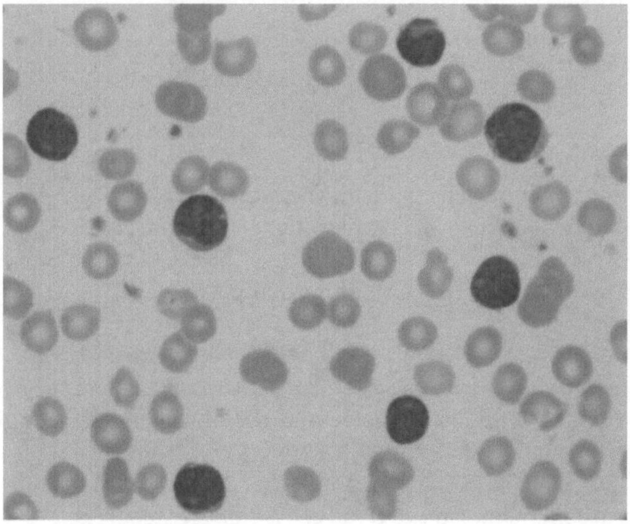

Figure 14.2 High number of immature, abnormal myeloid blood cells pick up dark stain in bone marrow

Source: Schira/Shutterstock.com

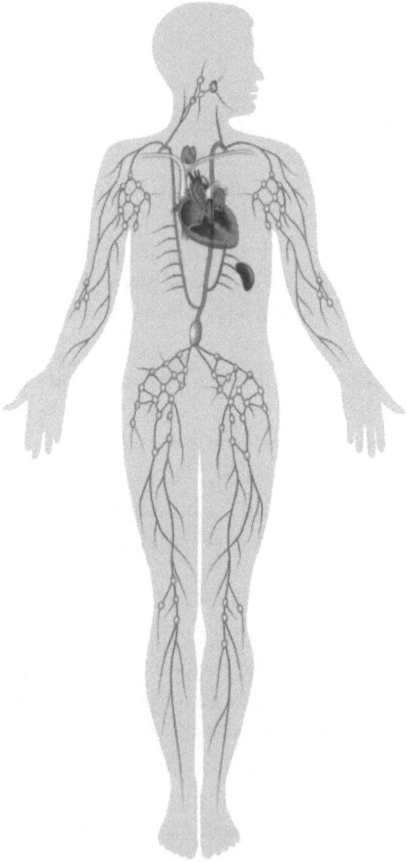

Figure 14.3 The lymphatic system
Source: Alila Medical Media/Shutterstock.com

Myelomas

Plasma cells are a type of white blood cells made in the bone marrow. They produce antibodies (immunoglobulins) which help the body to fight infections.

- Myeloma, or multiple myelomas, starts with abnormal plasma cells

Sarcomas

Connective tissues include bones, tendons, cartilage and the fibrous tissue that gives support to organs.

- Bone sarcomas (osteosarcoma) start in the bone cells, called osteocytes
- Soft tissue sarcomas start in cartilage or muscle cells

Table 14.2 Stages of cancer

Stage	*Description of cancer*
Stage 0	There is a group of abnormal cells which may be pre-cancerous, but there is no tumour. This is sometimes called a 'carcinoma in situ'.
Stage I	The tumour is relatively small and contained within the organ where it started.
Stage II	The tumour is larger than Stage I but has not spread into neighbouring tissues. It might have spread into lymph nodes.
Stage III	The tumour is larger than Stage II, it has spread into neighbouring tissues, cancer cells are in the lymph nodes.
Stage IV	Cells from the primary tumour have travelled (metastasised) and entered another part of the body, creating a secondary tumour(s).

Source: Cancer Research UK (2017c).

Stages of cancer

In the UK, healthcare professionals may describe the stage of someone's cancer using a number system. The larger the tumour and the more it has spread, the more damage is occurring in the body, and the harder it is to treat. In Scotland, the most common stages at which breast cancer was diagnosed in 2018 was Stage I (41%) and Stage II (38%), in contrast to 46% of lung cancer and 21% of bowel cancer diagnoses which had reached Stage IV (PHS, 2020).

> *Cancer is the process of a cell mutating into an abnormal cell and then replicating into a tumour.*

Cancer sites in the body

A tumour will affect the normal functioning of the area of the body in which it sits, regardless of whether it is the primary tumour or a secondary tumour. Symptoms of cancer may also be symptoms of other conditions; it is vital to seek medical advice quickly.

Lung cancer

Lung cancer may imply cancer in the lungs, but the term can also refer to cancer in the respiratory system.

Common symptoms of lung cancer include

- a persistent cough
- a cough which may be different from normal, e.g. painful, coughing phlegm or blood
- breathlessness
- pain in chest or shoulder
- recurrent chest infections
- loss of appetite
- weight loss
- fatigue

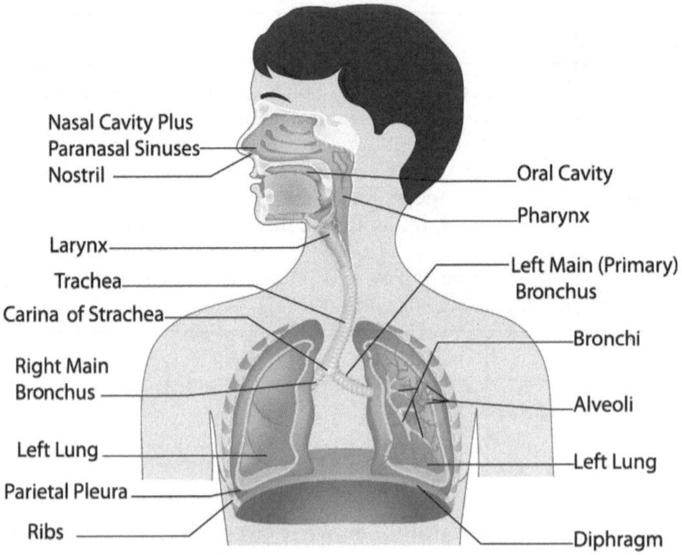

Figure 14.4 The respiratory system
Source: snapgalleria/Shutterstock.com

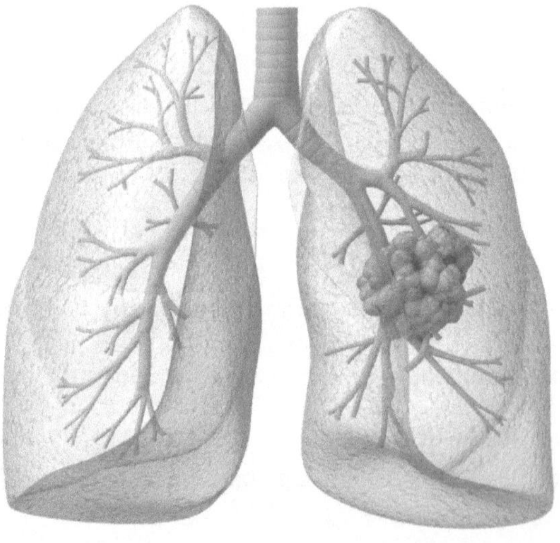

Figure 14.5 Lung cancer
Source: SceiPro/Shutterstock.com

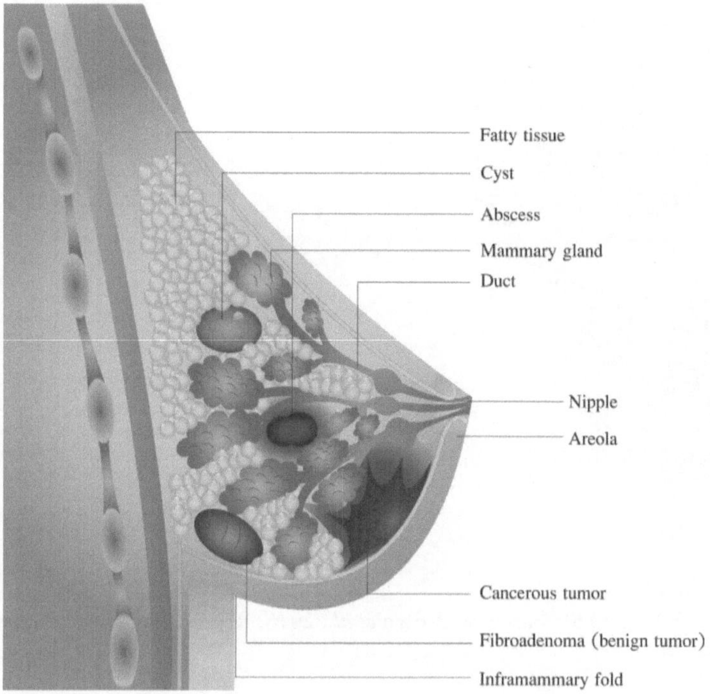

Figure 14.6 Breast cancer
Source: Tefi/Shutterstock.com

Breast cancer

Breast cancer refers to cancer in the breast tissue. This can occur in men and women, but it is far more common in women.

Common symptoms of breast cancer include

- a lump in the breast or armpit
- a change in shape, size or feel of the breast
- skin changes such as dimpling, redness or a rash
- a change in the position of the nipple
- fluid leaking from the nipple in the absence of pregnancy or breastfeeding

Prostate cancer

Prostate cancer is cancer occurring in the prostate, a gland at the base of the bladder. Its normal function is to produce a fluid which becomes part of semen.

Common symptoms of prostate cancer include

- needing to urinate frequently and urgently, including during the night
- difficulty in passing urine
- blood or semen in the urine

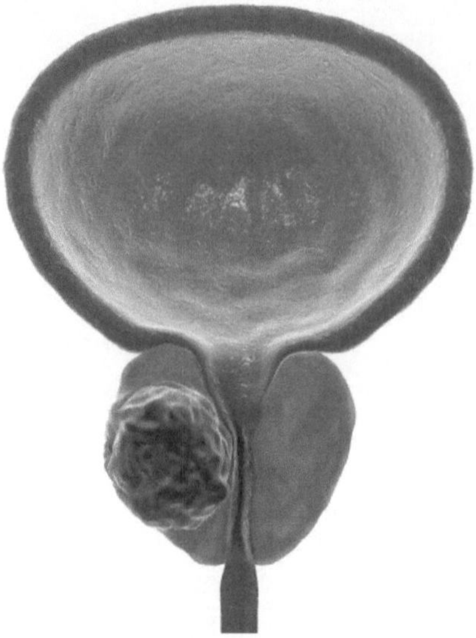

Figure 14.7 Prostate cancer

Source: Cancer Research UK, 2020a based on Brown *et al.*, 2018. Reproduced with permission from Cancer Research UK.

Colorectal/bowel cancer

Colorectal cancer and bowel cancer are interchangeable terms. They refer to cancer in the rectum, anus or large bowel, collectively known as the large intestine.

Common symptoms of bowel cancer include

- bleeding from the rectum and blood in the stools
- a change in normal bowel habits
- a feeling of needing to visit the toilet even after having been
- weight loss
- pain in the rectum or abdomen
- fatigue

Stomach cancer

Stomach cancer, also called gastric cancer, is situated within the stomach, or stomach walls.

Common symptoms of stomach cancer include

- swallowing difficulties
- weight loss
- persistent indigestion
- feeling full after eating only a small amount
- nausea or vomiting

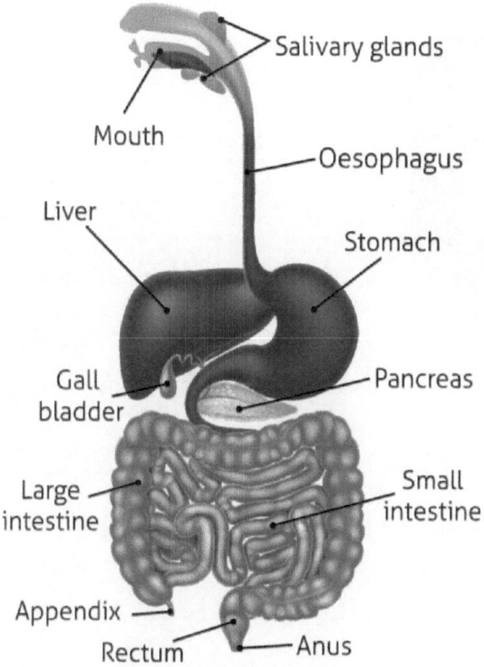

Figure 14.8 The digestive system
Source: Cancer Research UK, 2020a, based on Brown *et al.*, 2018. Reproduced with permission.

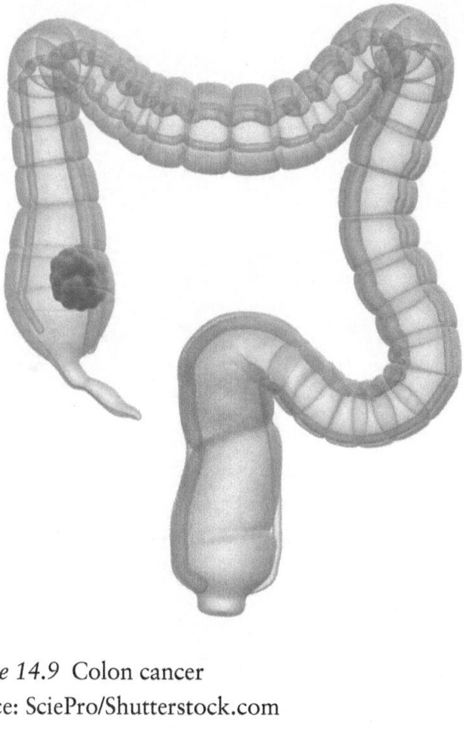

Figure 14.9 Colon cancer
Source: SciePro/Shutterstock.com

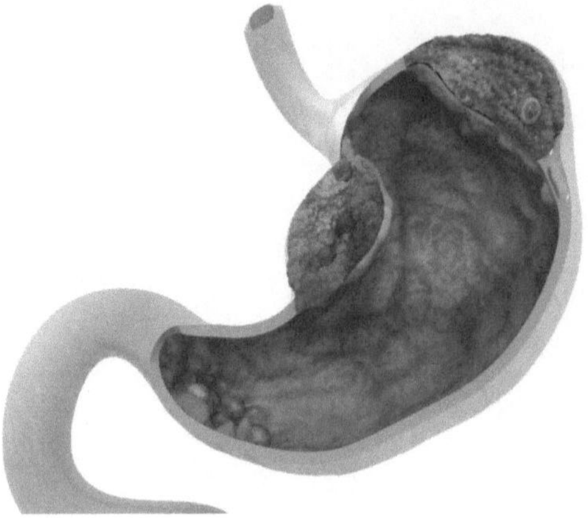

Figure 14.10 Stomach cancer
Source: crystal light/Shutterstock.com

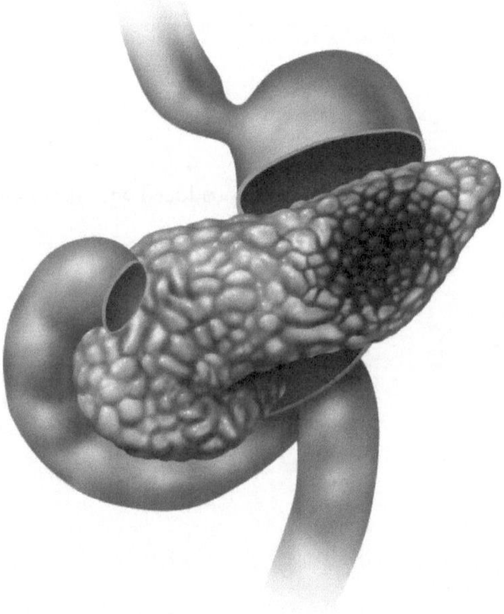

Figure 14.11 Pancreatic cancer
Source: Lightspring/Shutterstock.com

Pancreatic cancer

The pancreas is a gland that produces enzymes to support digestion and insulin, which helps to regulate blood sugar.

Common symptoms of pancreatic cancer include

- pain in the mid abdomen, close to the stomach, or the back
- weight loss

- jaundice, which is a yellowing of the skin and whites of the eyes, along with dark urine

Female reproductive cancers

Within the female reproductive system cervical, ovarian, uterine, vaginal and vulval cancers can develop.

Like many other cancers, cervical cancer may be present without a woman being aware of any symptoms. If they are present, they include

- unusual vaginal bleeding or discharge
- pain during sex

Common symptoms of ovarian cancer include

- bloating, feeling 'full' of wind, an increased tummy
- frequent urination

Common symptoms of uterine cancer include

- abnormal or unusually heavy bleeding, especially post menopause
- vaginal discharge

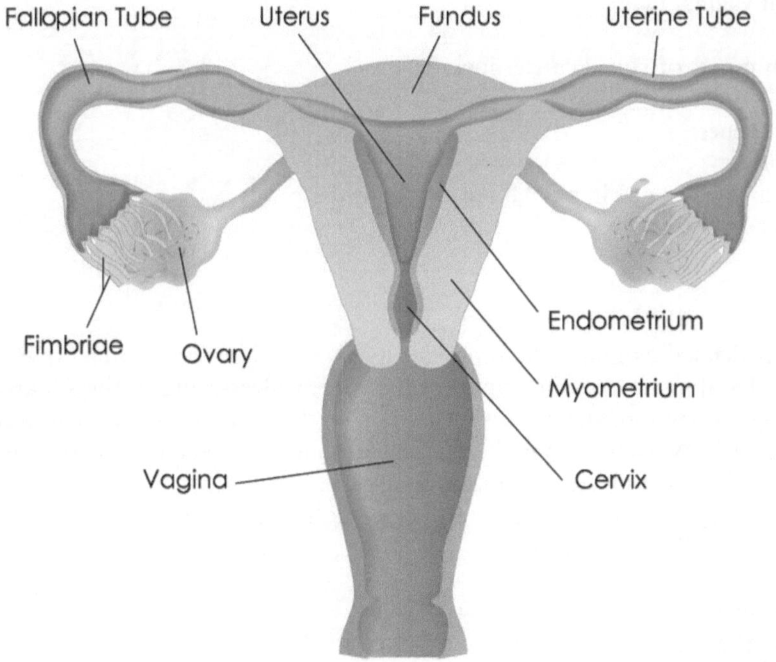

Figure 14.12 The female reproductive system
Source: snapgalleria/Shutterstock.com

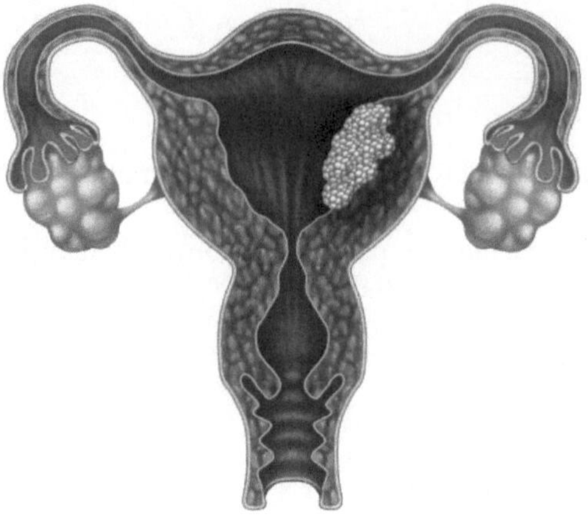

Figure 14.13 Uterine cancer in the endometrium
Source: Lightspring/Shutterstock.com

Common symptoms of vaginal cancer include

- bleeding after sex or between periods
- vaginal discharge
- pain during sex
- lump in the vagina
- persistent vaginal itch

Common symptoms of vulval cancer include

- pain or soreness
- persistent itch
- thickened patches which may be red, white or dark
- a lump or an open sore

Skin cancer

Skin cancer is defined as non-melanoma and melanoma. Non-melanoma comprises cancer in the basal skin cells, sometimes called rodent ulcers, and in the squamous skin cells. These rarely spread, whereas melanoma, in the melanocyte cells, can spread if not treated early. Melanocytes make the pigment melanin which gives the skin its colour. A cluster of melanocyte cells make up a mole.

A melanoma begins with a change in a freckle, mole or patch of skin. Examination comprises the 'ABCDE' approach.

A – symmetrical
Melanomas are uneven in shape and asymmetrical
B – border
The edges of a melanoma are irregular, blurred or jagged
C – colour

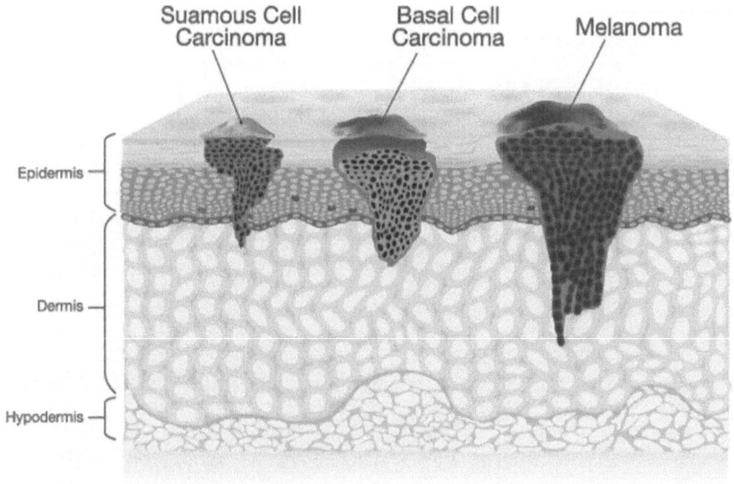

Figure 14.14 Skin cancer
Source: Solar22/Shutterstock.com

Melanomas are often an uneven colour with more than one shade
D – diameter
Most melanomas are more than 6 mm wide
E – evolving
Melanomas may change in shape, size or colour. They may bleed, itch or become crusty

Secondary sites

Any site in the body may be the recipient of floating cancer cells, which travel from the primary tumour in the blood or lymph, settle, and develop into secondary tumours. The most common places for secondary cancer to develop are the lungs, liver, lymph nodes, bones and brain (Cancer Research UK, 2017d).

Malignant primary tumours can begin anywhere in the body. Cells may break off and travel through the body to start a secondary tumour.

The burden of cancer

Cancer data are presented as incidence, risk, prevalence, survival and mortality. In the UK, data are collected by each of the four nations at different times. Cancer Research UK waits for all these to be published before being able to calculate the figures for the whole of the UK.

Incidence

Incidence means the number of people, or the number per 100,000 people, who are diagnosed with a type of cancer each year (Cancer Research UK, 2020a). In 2018,

Table 14.3 World and UK incidence of common cancers

Site/type	*World 2018*	*UK 2017*	*UK 2017*	
	Percentage of all cancers		*Percentage of male cancers (n = 187,000)*	*Percentage of female cancers (n = 179,000)*
Breast	12%	15%		30%
Lung	12%	13%	13%	13%
Colorectal/bowel	10%	11%	13%	10%
Prostate	7%	13%	26%	
Stomach	5%	2%		
Liver	5%	2%		
Uterus		3%		5%
Cervix uteri	3%			
Ovary		2%		4%
Cervix		<1%		2%
Skin (melanoma)		4%	4%	4%
Other sites	46%	34%	44%	31%

Sources: GCO (2019); Cancer Research UK (2020a).

there were 18,078,957 new cases of cancer across the world, with most (48.4%) occurring in Asia followed by 23.4% in Europe, 13.2% in North America, 7.8% in Latin America and the Caribbean, 5.8% in Africa and 1.4% in Oceania (GCO, 2019).

Box 14.1 Not me

First comes, the fear. You dread the worst
Trembling … It cannot be …
I'll be all right. No need to fuss
It won't happen to me.
Next comes the shock …

(Source: Catherine Brown in Hendry, undated p.60)

In the UK, Cancer Research UK (2020a) reports about 367,000 new cases every year, about 1,000 every day, about one every two minutes. In 2017, 179,000 of women and 187,000 of men were diagnosed with cancer. In the UK, more than half of all newly diagnosed cancers are situated in the breast, lung, bowel or prostate.

Projected future incidence of cancer

The incidence of people with cancer across the world is expected to increase by 45%, comparing 2008 to 2030, and 80% of this is expected to occur in low-income countries (WHO, 2020a). In the UK, Smittenaar and colleagues (2016) describe how the increase will affect more males than females. In the year 2035, 270,261 males are expected to be diagnosed with cancer. Cancerous tumours in the prostate will remain the most common (29%), followed by lung (12%) and bowel (11%). In the same year, 243,690 females are expected to be diagnosed with cancer. Tumours in the breast (29%), lung (12%) and bowel (10%) will remain the most common.

Thinking point:

Which health-related behaviours and exposures are increasing in low-income countries and might explain the anticipated 80% rise in cancers?

Incidence of cancer across socio-economic groups

Across the UK, like many chronic diseases, there is more cancer among people who live in poorer socio-economic circumstances than those who live in more affluent socio-economic circumstances. For example, in Scotland, the incidence of cancer among those who live in the most deprived areas is 28% higher than among those who live in the least deprived areas (PHS, 2020) (Figure 14.15).

Thinking point:

Consider what health-related behaviours and exposures may help to explain the different incidence of cancer across different socio-economic groups.

Incidence of cancer and ethnicity

Collecting data about cancer and ethnicity is complex; for example, Fazil (2018) explains that ethnic categorisations have been modified over time, and those who are White are assumed to be of British origin and English-speaking, thus other White

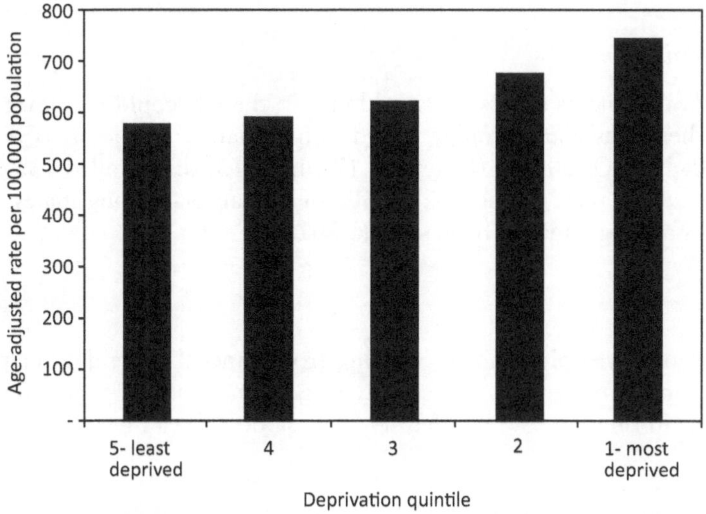

Figure 14.15 Age-adjusted cancer incidence rates for all cancers* by deprivation quintile, Scotland 2014 to 2018 (*excludes non-melanoma skin cancer)

Source: Public Health Scotland, 2020 p.9. Reproduced under the terms of the Open Government Licence v.3.0

people are invisible. Overall, there is less cancer in ethnic minority groups than the White population. It is more common among

- White and Black males than Asian males
- White females than in Black or Asian females

(Cancer Research UK, 2020a)

However, the incidence of cancer is rising among ethnic minority groups and the incidence of some specific cancers is already higher than in the White population. Compared to the comparable White population, UK studies show

- people from Black ethnic groups have a higher incidence of multiple myeloma
- Black Caribbean and Black African men have a higher incidence of prostate cancer
- Asian people have a higher incidence of liver cancer
- Asian women have a higher incidence of mouth cancer, and cervical cancer in the over 65s
- South Asian women have a higher incidence of breast cancer
- Bangladeshi women have a higher incidence of oesophageal cancer

(Fazil, 2018)

Some ethnic groups in the UK population are relatively young, and as they age, so their incidence of cancer will rise.

Incidence of cancer by age

The incidence of cancer in the UK rises with age, particularly from the mid to late 50s (Cancer Research UK, 2020a) (Figure 14.16).

Incidence of preventable cancers

Approximately 40% of cancers across the world and in the UK could be prevented each year because their causes are strongly linked to modifiable risk factors (Cancer Research UK, 2020a; WHO, 2020b) (Figure 14.17). In 2015, this totalled 135,507 diagnoses of preventable cancer in the UK: 38.6% of all cancers among males and 36.8% of all cancers among females (Brown *et al.*, 2018).

Risk

Risk means the risk of developing cancer or dying from cancer. These data help to identify who, at a population level, is more likely to get cancer. Risk figures may be presented 'at a point in time' or 'over a lifetime'. The same risk can be presented in two ways.

- The life-time risk for a man to develop lung cancer is 1 in 14. Out of every 14 men, one will get cancer during his lifetime and 13 will not
- The life-time risk for a man to develop lung cancer is 7%. (Divide 100% by 14 men to give 7% per man)

(Cancer Research UK, 2017e)

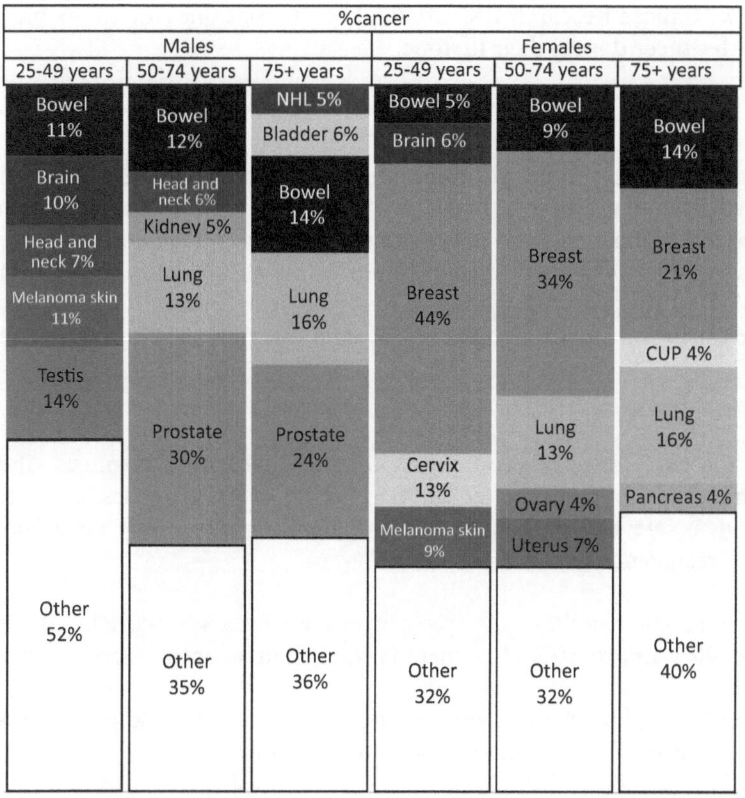

Figure 14.16 Site of incidence of cancers by age, UK 2015 to 2017 (NHL – Non Hodgkins Lymphoma; CUP – cancer of unknown primary origin).

Source: adapted from Cancer Research UK, 2020a

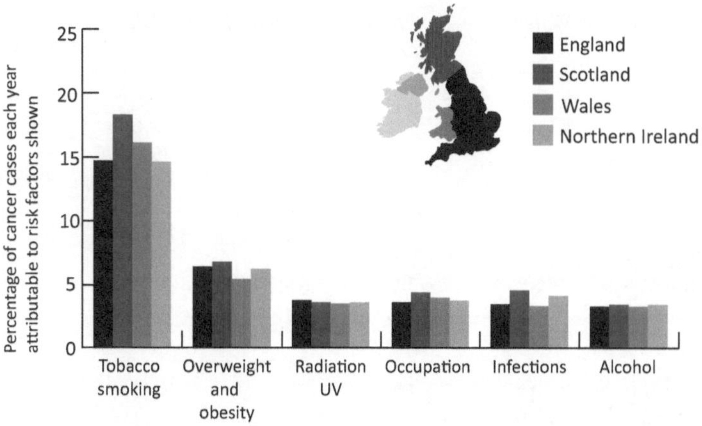

Figure 14.17 Percentage of UK cancer cases which may have been prevented in 2015, by risk factor

Source: Cancer Research UK, 2020a based on Brown *et al*, 2018

Life-time risk builds as we age, so older people have a greater risk than younger people. In the UK, Cancer Research UK (2020a) reports that one in two people will be diagnosed with cancer during their lifetime.

Prevalence

Prevalence means the number of people in the population who have had a cancer diagnosis. Some may have had a diagnosis in the past and are now cancer-free, others may have had a more recent diagnosis and are currently living with it. In 2018, the prevalence of cancer over a five-year period across the world was 43,841,302 cases. Most were in Asia (39.7%) followed by Europe (27.7%), North America (18.5%), Latin America and the Caribbean (7.6%), Africa (4.4%) and Oceania (2.1%) (GCO, 2019).

Survival

Survival means the percentage of people who are still alive, after diagnosis, after a certain time. Often, this is recorded after one year (Table 14.4), five years or 10 years. Disease-free survival refers to the number of people who are not only alive but are also well with no recurrence of cancer. In the UK

- the number of people who have survived cancer for 10 years or more has doubled over the last 40 years to 50%, but there is significant variation across different cancer types
- survival from breast, bowel and prostate cancers is highest in middle age, but survival of other cancers is best in those under 40 years old

Table 14.4 Age-standardised rate of survival after cancer diagnosis after one year in England, Wales and Northern Ireland, 2012 to 2016

Site	*Males*			*Females*		
	England	*Wales*	*Northern Ireland*	*England*	*Wales*	*Northern Ireland*
Prostate	96.5%	97%	97.0%			
Skin melanoma	97.4%	97%	97.3%	98.6%	97.6%	99.2%
Breast				95.8%	96.0%	96.0%
Uterus				90.0%		89.3%
Rectum	83.7%	82.3%	85.9%	82.4%	82.5%	83.1%
Cervix				81.1%	82.2%	84.9%
Colorectal	79.6%	78.3%	83.1%	77.3%	76.4%	79.3%
Bladder	78.4%	77.8%	75.7%	65.7%	67.3%	63.9%
Kidney	78.6%	77.6%	81.0%	78.4%	77.8%	85.4%
Colon	77.1%	75.7%	81.5%	75.3%	73.6%	77.5%
Ovary				71.1%		69.3%
Leukaemia	72.4%	74.4%	70.7%	70.6%	71.4%	73.3%
Stomach	47.3%	44.1%	46.2%	47.0%	45.1%	46.2%
Lung	36.3%	33.2%	35.4%	43.2%	41.1%	39.6%
Pancreas	23.7%	27.2%	26.5%	25.3%	30.5%	24.9%

Sources: PHW (2019); Cancer Research UK (2020a); NICR (2020).

- between 1971 and 2010/11, the UK saw notable improvements in the survival of cancer in prostate, malignant melanoma, non-Hodgkin lymphoma, leukaemia, bowel cancer and female breast cancer
- between 1971 and 2010/11, the UK has seen very little improvement in the survival of cancer in the brain, oesophagus and lung, and no change in pancreatic cancer

(Cancer Research UK, 2020a)

In the UK, people living in more deprived areas experience a shorter survival period. For example, Public Health Wales (2019) compared people who had been diagnosed with lung cancer in the most deprived areas of Wales with those who lived in the least deprived areas. They found a 5.6% difference, with those in the least deprived areas being less likely to survive five years after diagnosis.

Mortality

Mortality means the number of people, diagnosed with cancer, who have died. This may be within one year, or within a greater time interval. The Global Cancer Observatory (2019) shows 9,555,027 people died of cancer across the world in 2018. Most deaths were in Asia (57.3%) followed by Europe (20.3%). The most common cancers were in the lung (18.4%), bowel (9.2%), liver (8.2%), stomach (8.2%), breast (6.6%), oesophagus (5.3%), pancreas (4.5%) and prostate (3.8%).

In the UK, Cancer Research UK (2020a) reports about 165,000 people die of cancer every year, about 450 people per day, one person every four minutes. This makes up about a quarter of all UK deaths. In 2017, 77,700 women and 88,900 men died from cancer, with 53% of total deaths being among people 75 years and over. A further breakdown of the data is shown in Table 14.5.

Death from cancer is higher among those in lower socio-economic circumstances compared to the rest of the population. For example, this means about 19,000 deaths per year in England would not have occurred if there were no socio-economic differences. The greatest proportion of these related to lung cancer (Cancer Research UK, 2020a).

In the UK a person is diagnosed with cancer every two minutes, and another dies from cancer every four minutes. Rates of cancer are expected to rise. Lung, breast and bowel cancer are the most common cancers in the UK.

Causes of cancer

Like atherosclerosis and cardiovascular disease, obesity and type 2 diabetes, cancer is often described as a chronic low-grade inflammatory disease. Acute inflammation occurs when we sustain an injury. Blood vessels dilate, blood flow increases and white blood cells cluster around the wound to alert cytokines, activate the immune system and support healing. If the body exhibits persistent inflammation at a low level and 'doesn't switch off', it causes damage and disease. Low-grade inflammation may be triggered by internal and external threats, and these include age, excess body fat, a diet rich in saturated fat, trans fat and sugar, tobacco smoking and stress (Pahwa *et al.*, 2020). The causes of cancer can be divided into the non-modifiable risk factors that we can't change, and the modifiable ones that we can. Many may initially prompt low-grade inflammation which, in turn, may encourage cancer.

Table 14.5 Percentage of UK cancer deaths by sex and site of cancer, UK and Scotland

Site of cancer	*Males*		*Females*	
	Percentage male cancer deaths		*Percentage female cancer deaths*	
	UK 2017	*Scotland 2018*	*UK 2017*	*Scotland 2018*
Lung	21.2%	23.9%	21.0%	25.4%
Breast			14.6%	12.6%
Colorectal/bowel	10.3%	11.3%	9.7%	10.2%
Prostate	13.5%	11.1%		
Pancreas	5.4%	5.1%	6.0%	5.0%
Oesophagus	6.2%	7.0%	3.1%	3.7%
Site of primary tumour unknown	4.8%		6.3%	
Ovary			5.3%	4.9%
Liver	3.9%	4.6%		2.5%
Bladder	4.3%	3.7%		
Head and neck	3.3%	4.0%		
Brain/central nervous system	3.4%		3.0%	2.5%
Uterus			3.1%	2.4%
Non-Hodgkin lymphoma			2.9%	2.5%
Kidney		2.9%		
Other sites around the body	24.3%	23.0%	25.7%	28.2%

Sources: Cancer Research UK (2020a); National Statistics (2019).

Non-modifiable risk factors for cancer

The common non-modifiable risk factors for cancer are age, inherited genes and, rarely, the Epstein Barr virus.

Age

Cancer can start at any age, but most cancer starts after middle age because we accumulate damage to cells from normal wear and tear, and we also accumulate gene mutations through exposure to carcinogens.

Inherited genes

Inherited mutated genes are relatively rare but, because they are within the sperm or egg, they are carried into the next generation.

- Tumour-suppressor genes are protective because they monitor cell division, make repairs to DNA and control when a cell dies. If these genes are not working well, cells start to grow uncontrollably and form a tumour
- DNA-repair genes can be both acquired and inherited. These genes repair mutated strings of DNA within the genes of cells. Like tumour-suppressor genes, if they are not working well, fewer mutations in cells are repaired and the risk of developing a tumour increases

Inherited mutated genes are associated with cancers in a range of sites including ovaries, pancreas, prostate, skin, uterus, colon, stomach, bones, testicles and brain. Mutated *BRCA1* and *BRCA2* genes are both tumour-suppressor and mutated DNA-repair genes. Men who inherit mutated *BRCA* genes have a higher risk of cancer than those who don't, particularly prostate cancer and breast cancer (Ibrahim *et al.*, 2018). Women who inherit both, or one, of these mutated genes are at high risk of developing ovarian or breast tumours. About 2% of breast cancers are related to these two genes (Cancer Research UK, 2020a).

Epstein Barr virus (EPV)

Epstein Barr (EPV) is a common type of herpes virus, usually acquired in childhood and spread through saliva. Many people never get cancer, but a few develop lymphomas and nasopharyngeal cancers.

Additional non-modifiable factors

For some cancers, in specific locations, research points to some other non-modifiable risk factors. For example

- breast cancer seems to occur more in women who had an early menarche, before aged 12, and late menopause, after 55 years. It is higher among White women, and among women who are slightly taller than average
- testicular cancer is more likely in men with undescended testicles, men who have an inguinal (groin) hernia, men who are taller than average, men who have fertility problems
- prostate cancer is more common in men with Black-African heritage and high levels of growth hormone IGF-1

Modifiable risk factors for cancer

Some modifiable risk factors increase the risks of cancer developing across many sites; some relate to specific sites.

Carcinogens

The International Agency for Research on Cancer (2020) evaluates international evidence to determine how certain we can be that something causes cancer. Carcinogens are classified into three groups.

Group 1: carcinogenic to humans – the evidence is conclusive. For example

- alcohol
- asbestos
- betel quid with tobacco
- coal emissions
- *Helicobacter pylori* infection
- oestrogen therapy, postmenopausal
- processed meat

Table 14.6 Sites of cancer and examples of group 1 carcinogens

Site of cancer	*Examples of carcinogens*
Bladder	Arsenic, X-rays, gamma rays, painting, tobacco smoking
Bone	X-rays, gamma rays, plutonium, radium-226
Brain/central nervous system	X-rays, gamma rays
Breast	Alcohol, X-rays, gamma rays, oestrogen-progestogen contraceptives
Cervix/uterus	Human papilloma virus type 16, tobacco smoking
Colon and rectum	Alcohol, smoking tobacco, X-rays, gamma rays
Kidney	Tobacco smoking, X-rays, gamma rays
Larynx	Alcohol, smoking tobacco, asbestos
Leukaemia and lymphoma	*Helicobacter pylori*, hepatitis C, HIV type 1, rubber production, tobacco smoking, X-rays, gamma rays
Liver and bile duct	Alcohol, hepatitis B and C, oestrogen-progestogen contraceptives
Lung	Aluminium production, asbestos, coal emissions, tobacco smoke, X-rays, gamma rays, soot, silica dust
Oesophagus	Alcohol, tobacco, X-rays, gamma rays
Oral cavity	Alcohol, tobacco
Ovary	Asbestos, smoking tobacco
Pancreas	Tobacco
Penis	Human papilloma virus type 16
Skin (melanoma)	Solar radiation, tanning devices, arsenic, X-rays, gamma rays
Stomach	*Helicobacter pylori*, smoking tobacco, X-rays, gamma rays
Multiple or unspecified sites	X-rays, gamma rays

Source: Adapted from Cogliano *et al.* (2011 pp.1835–1836).

Group 2A: probably carcinogenic to humans – the evidence is compelling, but not conclusive. For example

- anabolic steroids
- exposures associated with hair dressing
- frying emissions at high temperature
- lead compounds, inorganic
- nitrites
- red meat

Group 2B: possibly carcinogenic to humans – the evidence is limited and not conclusive. For example

- aloe vera, whole leaf extract
- exposures associated with fire fighting
- exposures associated with printing
- magnetic fields at low frequency
- petrol
- radiofrequency, electromagnetic fields

Group 3: not classifiable as to its carcinogenicity in humans – the evidence is inadequate in humans and inadequate/limited in experimental animals. For example

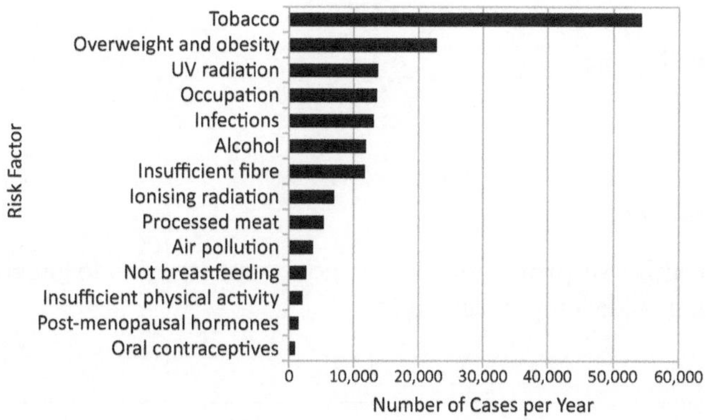

Figure 14.18 Estimated number of UK cases of cancer that could have been prevented by modifiable risk factors, 2015

Source: Cancer Research UK, 2020a, based on Brown *et al.*, 2018

Table 14.7 Percentage and number of UK cancer cases by modifiable risk factor and sex, 2015

	England		*Scotland*		*Wales*		*Northern Ireland*	
	Males	*Females*	*Males*	*Females*	*Males*	*Females*	*Males*	*Females*
Smoking tobacco	17.3%	12.1%	21.1%	15.6%	18.6%	13.4%	17.8%	11.3%
Cases	*26,375*	*17,738*	*3,204*	*2,532*	*1,832*	*1,241*	*830*	*519*
Overweight/ obesity	5.2%	7.5%	6.0%	7.6%	4.6%	6.4%	5.3%	7.0%
Cases	*7,960*	*11,036*	*909*	*1,244*	*450*	*590*	*248*	*324*
Occupation	4.9%	2.4%	5.8%	2.8%	5.3%	2.6%	5.0%	2.5%
Cases	*7,458*	*3,528*	*875*	*462*	*364*	*241*	*174*	*114*
Ultraviolet radiation	3.9%	3.8%	3.9%	3.5%	3.7%	3.4%	3.8%	3.4%
Cases	*5,899*	*5,541*	*587*	*570*	*364*	*311*	*174*	*157*
Insufficient dietary fibre	3.1%	3.3%	3.5%	3.5%	3.3%	3.4%	3.7%	3.5%
Cases	*4,713*	*4,917*	*529*	*564*	*322*	*316*	*171*	*161*
Alcohol	3.0%	3.5%	3.8%	3.3%	3.2%	3.3%	3.5%	3.5%
Cases	*4,634*	*5,202*	*572*	*538*	*319*	*301*	*164*	*163*
Processed meat	2.0%	0.9%	2.3%	0.9%	2.1%	0.8%	2.4%	1.0%
Cases	*3,096*	*1,330*	*346*	*145*	*204*	*73*	*112*	*46*
Air pollution	1.1%	1.0%	1.0%	0.9%	0.8%	0.8%	0.8%	0.7%
Cases	*1,636*	*1,442*	*146*	*142*	*82*	*74*	*38*	*32*
Inactivity	0.5%	0.5%	0.6%	0.5%	0.5%	0.5%	0.6%	0.5%
Cases	*794*	*801*	*85*	*86*	*51*	*49*	*27*	*25*
Oral contraceptives		0.5%		0.5%		0.3%		0.7%
Cases		*667*		*79*		*32*		*30*

Source: Adapted from Brown *et al.* (2018 p.1132).

- drinking coffee
- coal dust
- chlorinated drinking water
- electric fields, static
- fluorescent lighting

Primary prevention of cancer

Individuals, employers, healthcare professionals and governments can do much to prevent cancer from starting to develop in the body.

Box 14.2 Eleven ways to prevent cancer

- No tobacco
- Healthy weight and shape
- Radiation protection
- Healthy employment
- Protection from infection
- Limit alcohol
- Healthy eating
- Physical activity
- Prevent adverse childhood experiences (ACEs)
- Clean air
- Hormonal intelligence

No tobacco

Tobacco is the greatest cause of avoidable cancer in the world. Many of the chemicals in tobacco and tobacco smoke are carcinogenic.

- Smoking tobacco is strongly associated with cancer in the lung, larynx, oesophagus, mouth, throat, kidney, bladder, pancreas, stomach and cervix
- Second-hand smoke, also called environmental smoke, causes lung cancer in non-smokers though passive smoking
- Smokeless tobacco, such as snuff or chewing tobacco, causes oral, oesophageal and pancreatic cancer

(WHO, 2020b)

We can avoid cancer by

- avoiding the use of smoking and smokeless tobacco, including heated tobacco products
- encouraging smoke-free environments
- adopting e-cigarettes, with no nicotine, as a much safer alternative to tobacco

Healthy weight and shape

Being overweight or obese is the second largest cause of avoidable cancer in the UK. There are three main pathways:

- as the number of fat cells rise, so will their production of insulin and growth factors. These cause cells to divide more frequently and increase the chances of cell mutation
- an increase in fat cells encourages low-grade inflammation, which encourages cells to divide more frequently, thus increasing the chances of cell mutation
- after menopause, fat cells make oestrogen, which encourages cells in the uterus and breasts to divide more frequently, increasing the chances of mutation

(Cancer Research, 2018a)

Independent of weight, there is some evidence that risks of cancer increase with larger waist circumferences (Lee *et al.*, 2018).

We can avoid cancer by

- reducing overweight, maintaining healthy weight relative to height
- reducing abdominal fat, avoiding a large waist measurement
- encouraging environments which offer healthy eating options, activity and reduced sedentariness

Radiation protection

Exposure to all types of ionising radiation increases the risks of cancer. They include X-rays and gamma rays. The radiation comprises protons, electrons or neutrons produced by unstable atoms. Ionising radiation is emitted in the natural world from certain minerals, such as radon gas in the ground, or from outer space. Radon gas, a natural radioactive gas in the soil and rocks, is linked to 4% of lung cancer cases in the UK. Cancer is more likely to develop where it is particularly prevalent, and if it accumulates indoors, it can cause cancer (Cancer Research UK, 2019). Ionising radiation can also be produced by activities associated with industry, medical imaging, nuclear medicine or radiotherapy.

Ultraviolet (UV) radiation, from the sun (solar radiation) or sunbeds, causes skin cancer. The radiation damages the skin cells and the mutated cells replicate. Sunburn means the skin may feel tender or itchy, and fair skin may turn pink or red – a tan is a sign of damage. If someone gets sunburnt once every two years, it triples their risk of developing skin melanoma (Cancer Research UK, 2019).

We can avoid cancer by

- ensuring workplaces abide by the Ionising Radiation Safety Regulations
- checking the website UKradon for places with high radon levels
- protecting the skin and eyes from the sun, using clothes, sunglasses, shade or sunscreen of at least SPF15 and a four or five star rating
- accepting and positively promoting natural skin tones
- using tanning lotion in place of tanning sun beds
- developing environments with shade

Table 14.8 Estimated number of annual cancer deaths related to an occupational carcinogen, Great Britain 2013 to 2017

Carcinogen	*Bladder*	*Breast*	*Lung*	*Mesothelioma*	*Oesophagus*
Asbestos			2400	2400	
Silica			800		
Diesel-engine exhausts			600		
Mineral oils	200		400		
Shift work		500			
Painting-related chemicals			200		
Environmental tobacco smoke			300		
TCDD			200		
Radon			200		
Welders			200		
All*	300	500	5300	2400	200

Note: *Includes incidences of cancer that are less than 100 and not shown

Source: Adapted from HSE (2019 p.4).

Healthy employment

Every year, about 17,600 new diagnoses of cancer in Great Britain are probably related to someone's occupation (HSE, 2019). The construction industry, which includes builders, plumbers, carpenters, electricians, painters and decorators, roofers, road workers and paviours, accounts for 40% of these. These are mostly caused by the carcinogens asbestos, mineral oils, solar radiation, silica, painting and TCDD (2,3,7,8-tetracholordibenzodioxin) (Table 14.8). Other vulnerable occupations with a high incidence of cancer include

- shift workers, mostly due to night shifts
- metal workers, mostly due to mineral oils
- personal and household services, mostly due to asbestos
- land transport, mostly due to diesel-engine exhaust fumes and asbestos
- mining, mostly due to asbestos
- printing/publishing, mostly due to mineral oils

(HSE, 2019)

Mesothelioma is a carcinoma which usually starts in the double outer linings of the lungs, the pleura. Typically, it spreads to lung tissue and the diaphragm. Peritoneal mesothelioma is found in the surface linings of other organs in the abdomen. It is quite a rare cancer which is strongly linked to asbestos, an insulation material banned in 1999 in the UK. Table 14.9 compares the psychological impact of mesothelioma with lung cancer.

Box 14.3 Safety versus profit

"It has not been in the interests of politicians, employers, and even some civil society groups like cancer charities to research, recognize, and compensate workers for occupationally caused and related cancers and even less to develop effective cancer prevention programs in the workplace ... some ... governments within the UK have protected many employers who create hazardous work. The human, social and economic costs of occupational cancers are therefore picked up by society as a whole ... by the NHS, the victims, their families and communities ... There are even cases in which chemical and pharmaceutical companies produce or use carcinogens and so expose workers; then they sell carcinogens to the public, and finally, they produce cancer-treatment drugs ... This cycle of production and profit is frequently condoned by government, whose interests can be close to such manufacturers. Science has often been manipulated, funding skewed, decision makers influenced, and critics attacked by industries to allow companies to continue to make, use, and sell carcinogens when the science indicates they should not ... industries create doubt about the science that identifies their products as risks and hazards."

"The role of trade unions ... has generally been tardy and ambiguous ... placing wages and conditions above health and safety ... [They have] restricted or stopped cancer investigations and cancer campaigns among vulnerable membership groups, especially those exposed to asbestos ... Some have been captured by the lifestyle approach of charities and the NHS ... the Trades Union Congress (TUC), appear to have accepted the 'Doubt is their Product' arguments ... but neglected cancer prevention until very recently ..."

"Government statistics usually significantly underestimate or downplay occupational cancers; industrial injury schemes rarely recognize them, and insurers under-record them. With the exception of asbestos-related cancers, civil law claims are also few in number ..."

(Source: Watterson, 2013 p.141, 142)

We can avoid cancer by

- referring concerns about employees' cancer risks to an occupational health service, UK Health and Safety Executive or a health and safety representative of a trade union
- increasing awareness and education about occupational health risks
- questioning whether the responsibility for a cancer risk rests with the individual employee or the employer

Protection from infection

Some infections increase the risk of developing cancer.

- *Helicobacter pylori* is a type of bacteria that infects the stomach lining, often acquired through contaminated food or water in childhood. It rarely causes problems, but it can cause stomach ulcers from which cancer may develop. It is also associated with non-Hodgkin lymphoma, bowel cancer and oesophageal cancer.
- Hepatitis B (HBV) and hepatitis C (HBC) viruses are carried in body fluids, including blood. If the body is unable to fight the viruses, they can cause non-Hodgkin lymphoma and liver cancer.

Table 14.9 Comparison of psychological experiences between people with mesothelioma versus lung cancer

Themes	*Feelings in both*	*Mesothelioma*	*Lung cancer*
		Feelings expressed more frequently by people with mesothelioma	*Feelings expressed more frequently by people with lung cancer*
Uncertainty	Feelings of being 'out of control', worries about progression of the disease		Concerns about side-effects and outcomes of treatment
Normality	Strong need for a normal, purposeful life, fulfilling social/family roles		
Hope	Hope and hopelessness	Hopelessness due to disease being incurable and lack of effective treatment	Hope due to availability of treatment, hope is a way to manage the situation and gain a sense of control
Blame/stigma		Anger, betrayal, blaming former employers who exposed them to asbestos. Some have conflicting loyalty, recognising the benefit of employment	Feelings of stigma because of the association between lung cancer and smoking, but put their own smoking behaviour down to 'fashion' rather than blaming anyone
Family	Fear of becoming a burden to family, causing upset		
Impact of symptoms	Intensity of symptoms, impact on independence and social roles, markers of disease and impending death		
Diagnosis	Delays caused distress, late commencement of treatment	Delayed claims for compensation from employers, possibly too late. Messages of hopelessness from healthcare professionals	
Distress caused by healthcare staff and system	Poor communication	Fragmented, uncoordinated, unsupportive care	Impersonal, poor communication skills and attitudes. Patients' psychological concerns disregarded and 'their time was not respected'
Financial/legal		Distress caused by forms, meeting solicitors, evidence for compensation claims	
Death/dying	Fear of how they might die, e.g. suffocating, and a need to ensure their affairs were 'in order'		

Source: Ball *et al.* (2016).

- Human immunodeficiency virus (HIV) is mostly spread through contact with an infected person's fluids such as blood, semen and breast milk. It lowers immunity, making people less able to fight viruses that cause cancer, including rare viruses such as Kaposi's sarcoma herpes virus.
- There are hundreds of types of human papillomavirus (HPV), but only 13 cause cancer. HPV spreads by skin-to-skin contact. Genital and oral HPV can cause cancer in the cervix, vagina, vulva and penis, and anal and some mouth and tongue cancers.

(Cancer Research UK, 2019)

We can avoid cancer by

- discussing concerns about *Helicobacter pylori* with a doctor, who might carry out a test and prescribe antibiotics
- using barrier methods during sex and avoiding sharing razors, needles or other objects which may carry body fluids containing HBV, HCV or HIV
- taking antiretroviral treatment to reduce HIV transmission. For example, the World Health Organization (2009) recommends HIV-positive mothers breast feed their babies alongside taking antiretroviral treatment.
- accessing the HPV vaccine or using barrier methods during sex if not vaccinated

Limit alcohol

There is convincing evidence that alcohol increases the risk of seven cancers in the mouth, pharynx, oesophagus, larynx, breast, bowel and liver (WCRF/AICR, 2018). Alcohol in combination with tobacco use is particularly harmful. Alcohol converts to acetaldehyde in the mouth, oesophagus, stomach and then mostly in the liver. Acetaldehyde damages the DNA in genes of cells, then the mutation is replicated. Alcohol also causes liver cirrhosis, which, in turn, increases the risk of malignancy (Cancer Research UK, 2018b).

We can avoid cancer by

- limiting or avoiding alcohol
- reducing the availability and accessibility of alcohol

Healthy eating

Diets which are high in processed foods, and high in fat and sugar, are associated with cancer not only because they encourage weight gain, but because the diet is likely to contain a greater proportion of foods which are strongly associated with cancer risks (Table 14.10), such as processed meat.

- Where storage facilities are poor, in hot, damp climates, food can become contaminated with fungi/moulds and toxins, including aflatoxins
- Processed meat includes bacon, corned beef, ham, luncheon meats, pancetta, patés, pepperoni, salami and sausages. The meat has been salted, cured, fermented, or smoked to preserve and improve flavour

Table 14.10 Food which increases the risks of developing cancer

	Exposure	*Site of cancer*
Convincing strong evidence	Aflatoxins	Liver
	Processed meat	Colorectal/bowel
Probable strong evidence	Red meat	Colorectal/bowel
	Foods preserved by salting	Stomach
	Cantonese-style salted fish	Nasopharynx

Source: WCRF/AICR (2018).

Table 14.11 Food which protects against developing cancer

	Exposure	*Site of cancer*
Probable strong evidence	Wholegrains	Colorectal/bowel
	Foods containing dietary fibre	Colorectal/bowel
	Non-starchy fruit and vegetables	Aerodigestive cancers
	Dairy products	Colorectal/bowel

Source: WCRF/AICR (2018).

- Red meat includes beef, lamb/mutton, pork, veal and venison
- Salting is a method of preserving food, especially where refrigeration is unavailable. Cancer is increased among those whose diets contain a substantial amount of salted meat, fish, vegetables and fruit
- Cantonese-style salted fish undergoes a high degree of fermentation during the drying process

(WCRF/AICR, 2018)

Some foods protect against cancer (Table 14.11).

- Wholegrains contain compounds which have anti-carcinogenic properties. Some are antioxidants and some may bind with carcinogens, which limits their contact with the intestine wall
- Dietary fibre encourages regular evacuation and helps to prevent harmful chemicals from building up in the bowel. It also combines with bowel bacteria to make butyrate, which helps the bowel to stay healthy
- Non-starchy fruit and vegetables contain 'anti-cancer' ingredients such as dietary fibre, carotenoids, vitamins C and E, flavonoids, phenols and plant sterols
- Dairy products are high in calcium and lactic acid-producing bacteria which both protect against cancer

(WCRF/AICR, 2018)

We can avoid cancer by

- decreasing intakes of foods which increase the risks of cancer
- increasing intakes of foods which protect against developing cancer

- environmental, social and financial incentives to eat healthy food

Physical activity

Sedentary behaviour encourages weight gain, affects the body's hormones and causes the normal peristaltic movements through the gastrointestinal system to slow down. Kerr and colleagues (2017) report on several large studies that show that sedentary behaviour, such as sitting for work or watching television, is associated with an increased risk of developing colorectal/bowel cancer, endometrial and breast cancer. It is also associated with increased death from all cancers.

Being active reduces the levels of oestrogen and insulin, both of which encourage cells to divide. Lowering the hormones may help to prevent cancer. Being active encourages motility of the bowel and reduces inflammation. Physical activity is thought to prevent 15% of colon cancers (Oruc and Kaplan, 2019).

We can avoid cancer by

- being less sedentary and more active
- standing/walking/cycling-friendly environments

Prevent adverse childhood experiences

Adverse childhood experiences (ACEs), which include child maltreatment, household illness, violence or imprisonment and parental separation/divorce, are associated with an increased risk of developing cancer in adulthood (Holman *et al.*, 2016; Hughes *et al.*, 2017). Ports and colleagues (2018) examined all the known risk factors for cancer and found evidence for ACEs being associated with adult obesity and greater use of tobacco and alcohol. These may explain the link between ACEs and cancer, but as there are gaps in research these findings are tentative at present.

We can avoid cancer by

- preventing/safeguarding children from serious adverse experiences
- raising awareness that adverse childhood experiences are associated with adult disease, including cancer

Clean air

Across the world, air pollution has been associated with cancer in the bladder and leukaemia, but it is most associated with lung cancer, causing 29% of all deaths from lung cancer (Samet, 2013; WHO, 2020c). In the UK, air pollution is on average lower than in many other countries, and it causes approximately 10% of lung cancer cases (Cancer Research UK, 2019). Tiny particles called PM10 and PM2.5 cause lung cancer.

We can avoid cancer by

- using UK Air to monitor air pollution levels in the UK
- avoiding using polluting transport, encouraging walking and cycling
- supporting clean air zones; action to improve air quality in certain UK geographical areas

Hormonal intelligence

Hormone replacement therapy (HRT) comprises pills, patches, gels or implants. It is usually prescribed during or after menopause when a woman's ovaries have stopped producing oestrogen and progesterone, and often because she is experiencing uncomfortable symptoms such as hot flushes, vaginal dryness and mood swings.

- Any type of HRT increases the risk of developing breast cancer, but the risk is higher if HRT is taken for more than five years and if the HRT contains a combination of both oestrogen and progesterone
- Oestrogen-only and combined HRT increases the risk of ovarian cancer, but once HRT is stopped, the risk reduces
- Oestrogen-only HRT increases the risk of uterus cancer

(Cancer Research UK, 2019)

The contraceptive pill is a form of birth control.

- Women taking the combined contraceptive pill have a slightly increased risk of breast cancer and, over time, cervical cancer. These risks fall once it is stopped being taken. The longer the combined pill is taken, the greater protection against uterus and ovarian cancers
- The mini-pill, containing progestogen, is associated with a slightly increased risk of breast cancer

(Cancer Research UK, 2019)

Transgender women, undergoing hormone treatment, increase their risk of getting breast cancer compared to cisgender men, but the risk is lower than in cisgender women (de Blok *et al.*, 2019). More research is needed. There is some evidence that hormones, such as growth factor (IGF-1), may increase the risk of prostate cancer in men (Cancer Research UK, 2020b)

We can avoid cancer by

- making fully informed choices about taking hormones and alternatives

Forty percent of cancers may be prevented if we address the modifiable risk factors: the known carcinogens.

Secondary prevention of cancer

Secondary prevention comprises the ways in which we pick up the very early signs of cancer in healthy people and, hopefully, stop its advance.

Genetic screening

Genetic screening is testing for mutated genes which are known to increase risks of cancers such as those in the breast, bowel, ovary, uterus and prostate. People are referred for testing via their general practitioner. It normally comprises a blood test. Generally, a 'strong family history' of cancer means two close family members who have had the same type of cancer. Before having a test, a genetic counsellor helps people to work through the pros and cons of the decision. Someone who knows they are carrying a mutated gene may be advised to alter their health-related behaviours, be offered more regular screening and/or be supported with choices about talking with relatives and having children.

Body checking screening

Cancer Research UK (2018c) recommends people should

- be aware of what is normal for their bodies, and alert to anything that is not, e.g. a persistent cough or unusual changes in the skin
- occasionally check breasts and testicles, but this should not be done regularly or in a set way

UK national screening programmes

Invitations to attend the UK National Health Service screening programmes are sent to all those registered with a general practitioner.

- Breast cancer screening is offered to all women aged 50 to 70 in the UK. It comprises a mammogram, an X-ray of the breasts
- Cervical cancer screening is offered to women aged 25 to 64 in the UK. It comprises a 'smear test', where a small brush scrapes a sample of cells from the cervix and these are examined for the HPV virus
- Bowel cancer screening is offered to men and women aged 60 to 74 in Wales, Northern Ireland and England, and to those aged 50 to 74 in Scotland. This utilises a posted kit. A sample of faeces is tested for blood. Some people may have a sigmoidoscopy, where a tube containing a camera is inserted into the large bowel
- Those with a high family risk of developing cancer may be recommended to attend for more or different tests

(Cancer Research UK, 2018d)

Screening allows us to pick up cancer at an early stage.

Tertiary prevention

Tertiary prevention comprises treatments which aim to eradicate, reduce or slow down the growth of the malignant tumour(s) and to prolong the quantity and quality of life. These include

- surgery to remove the tumour(s)
- chemotherapy, taking drugs to kill the cancer cells, but these also kill other cells in the body, which is why it can cause whole-body symptoms such as nausea or hair loss
- immunotherapy, taking drugs to enhance the body's immune system to fight the cancer
- hormone therapy, taking drugs to alter hormones and slow down or stop the development of cancer

- radiotherapy, using radiation to kill cancer cells and, like sunburn, it can damage skin and tissues
- stem cell or bone marrow transplants are used for cancers in the blood or lymph. They are also used to help the body to recover after chemotherapy or radiotherapy
- targeted cancer drugs have very specific functions
- gene therapy uses genes to treat cancer, it involves inserting genes into cancer cells

(Cancer Research UK, 2017f)

Box 14.4 Chemotherapy

I did not imagine being bald
at forty four. I didn't have a plan.
Perhaps a scar or two from growing old,
hot flushes. I'd sit fluttering a fan.

But I am bald, and hardly ever walk
by day, I'm the invalid of these rooms,
stirring soups, awake in the half dark,
not answering the phone when it rings.

I never thought that life could get this small,
that I would care so much about a cup,
the taste of tea, the texture of a shawl,
and whether or not I should get up.

I'm not unhappy. I have learnt to drift
and sip. The smallest things are gifts.

(Source: Julia Darling, in Darling, 2003 p.50)

Complementary therapies such as acupuncture, herbal medicine, yoga, aromatherapy and massage therapy can help with the symptoms of cancer and those related to medical treatment, but they will not cure cancer. Palliative treatment and care aim to reduce the side effects of treatment, may extend life and, importantly, seek to improve people's quality of life while living with terminal cancer.

Summary

This chapter has

- described the development of cancer and how it can spread in the body
- outlined the extent and impact of cancer in the UK
- described the non-modifiable and modifiable risk factors for cancer
- examined several well-known carcinogens and discussed how cancer can be prevented in the general population
- outlined how we detect cancer early, and try to eradicate or limit its damage

Further reading

Fung, J. (2020) *The cancer code*. New York: Harper Weave

International Agency for Research on Cancer/World Health Organization (2019) IARC handbooks of cancer prevention. Available at: https://handbooks.iarc.fr/publications/index.php

Useful websites

Cancer Research UK www.cancerresearchuk.org

Health and Safety Executive www.hse.gov.uk

UK Air https://uk-air.defra.gov.uk

UKradon www.ukradon.org

References

Ball, H., Moore, S., and Leary, A. (2016) 'A systematic literature review comparing the psychological care needs of patients with mesothelioma and advanced lung cancer', *European Journal of Oncology Nursing*, 25, pp.62–67

Brown, K.F., Rumgay, H., Dunlop, C., Ryan, M., Quartly, F., Cox, A., Deas, A., Deas, A., Elliss-Brookes, L., Gavin, A., Hounsome, L., Huws, D., Ormiston-Smith, N., Shelton, J., White, C., and Parkin D.M. (2018) 'The fraction of cancer attributable to modifiable risk factors in England, Wales, Scotland, Northern Ireland, and the United Kingdom in 2015', *British Journal of Cancer*, 118(8), pp.1130–1141

Cancer Research UK (2017a) Cancer cells. Available at: www.cancerresearchuk.org/about-cancer/what-is-cancer/how-cancer-starts/cancer-cells (Accessed 19th May 2020)

Cancer Research UK (2017b) Types of cancer. Available at: www.cancerresearchuk.org/what-is-cancer/how-cancer-starts/types-of-cancer (Accessed 20th May 2020)

Cancer Research UK (2017c) Stages of cancer. Available at: www.cancerresearchuk.org/about-cancer/what-is-cancer/stages-of-cancer (Accessed 20th May 2020)

Cancer Research UK (2017d) Where cancer can spread. Available at: www.cancerresearchuk.org/what-is-cancer/how-cancer-can-spread/where-cancer-can-spread (Accessed 24th May 2020)

Cancer Research UK (2017e) Understanding cancer statistics – incidence, survival, mortality. Available at: www.cancerresearchuk.org/about-cancer/what-is-cancer/understanding-cancer-statistics-incidence-survival-mortality (Accessed 21st May 2020)

Cancer Research UK (2017f) Treatment for cancer. Available at: https://about-cancer.cancerresearchuk.org/about-cancer/cancer-in-general/treatment (Accessed 9th June 2020)

Cancer Research UK (2018a) Does obesity cause cancer? Available at: www.cancerresearchuk.org/about-cancer/causes-of-cancer/obesity-weight-and-cancer/does-obesity-cause-cancer (Accessed 27th May 2020)

Cancer Research UK (2018b) Does alcohol cause cancer? Available at: www.cancerresearchuk.org/about-cancer/causes-of-cancer/alcohol-and-cancer/does-alcohol-cause-cancer (Accessed 27th May 2020)

Cancer Research UK (2018c) How do I check for cancer? Available at: www.cancerresearchuk.org/about-cancer/cancer-symptoms/how-do-i-check-for-cancer (Accessed 9th June 2020)

Cancer Research UK (2018d) What is screening? Available at: https://bit.ly/36Ef282 (Accessed 9th June 2020)

Cancer Research UK (2019) Causes of cancer and reducing your risk. Available at: www.cancerresearchuk.org/about-cancer/causes-of-cancer (Accessed 27th May 2020)

Cancer Research UK (2020a) Cancer statistics for the UK. Available at: www.cancerresearchuk.org/health-professional/cancer-statistics-for-the-uk#heading-Zero (Accessed 21st May 2020)

Cancer Research UK (2020b) Prostate cancer. Risks and causes. Available at: www.cancerresearchuk.org/about-cancer/prostate-cancer/risks-causes (Accessed 28th May 2020)

Cogliano, V.J., Baan, R., Straif, K., Grosse, Y., Lauby-Secretan, B., Ghissassi, F., Bouvard, V., Benbrahim-Tallaa, L., Guha, N., Freeman, C., Galichet, L., and Wild, C.P. (2011) 'Preventable exposures associated with human cancers', *Journal of the National Cancer Institute*, 103(24), pp.1827–1839

Darling, J. (2003) *Sudden collapses in public places*. Todmorden: Arc

De Blok, C.J.M., Wiepjes, C.M., Nota, N.M., van Engelen, K., Adank, M.A., Dreijerink, K.M.A., Barbé, E., Konings, I.R.H.M., and den Heijer, M. (2019) 'Breast cancer risk in transgender people receiving hormone treatment: nationwide cohort study in the Netherlands', *BMJ*, 365 doi.org/10.1136/bmj.l1652

Fazil, Q. (2018) Better health briefing 47. Cancer and black and minority ethnic communities. Race Equality Foundation. Available at: http://raceequalityfoundation.org.uk/wp-content/uploads/2018/07/REF-Better-Health-471-1.pdf (Accessed 23rd May 2020)

Global Cancer Observatory (2019) All cancers. Available at: https://gco.iarc.fr/today/data/factsheets/cancers/39-All-cancers-fact-sheet.pdf (Accessed 21st May 2020)

Health and Safety Executive (2019) Occupational cancer statistics in Great Britain, 2019. Available at: www.hse.gov.uk/statistics/causdis/cancer.pdf (Accessed 27th May 2020)

Hendry, D. (ed) (undated) *Words from the wards*. The Scottish Arts Council/Dumfries and Galloway NHS Trust

Holman, D.M., Ports, K.A., Buchanan, N.D., Hawkins, N.A., Merrick, M.T., Metzler, M., and Trivers, K.F. (2016) 'The association between adverse childhood experiences and risk of cancer in adulthood: a systematic review of the literature', *Pediatrics*, 138(Suppl 1), S81–S91 doi:10.1542/peds.2015-4268L

Hughes, K., Bellis, M.A., Hardcastle, K.A., Sethi, D., Butchart, A., Mikton, C., Jones, L., and Dunne, M.P. (2017) 'The effect of multiple childhood experiences on health: a systematic review and meta-analysis', *Lancet Public Health*, 2, e356–366 doi:10.1016/S2468-2667(17)30118-4

Ibrahim, M., Yadav, S., Ogunleye, F., and Zakalik, D. (2018) 'Male *BRCA* mutation carriers: clinical characteristics and cancer spectrum', *BMC Cancer*, (18)179 doi:10.1186/s12885-018-4098-y

International Agency for Research on Cancer (2018) Red meat and processed meat. Volume 114. Available at: https://monographs.iarc.fr/wp-content/uploads/2018/06/mono114.pdf (Accessed 27th May 2020)

International Agency for Research on Cancer (2020) IARC monographs on the identification of carcinogenic hazards to humans. Available at: https://monographs.iarc.fr/list-of-classifications (Accessed 24th May 2020)

Kerr, J., Anderson, C., and Lippman, S.M. (2017) 'Physical activity, sedentary behaviour, diet, and cancer: an update and emerging new evidence', *The Lancet Oncology*, 18(8) e457–471 doi:10.1016/S1470-2045(17)30411–4

Lee, K.R., Seo, M.H., Han, K.D., Jung, J., and Hwang, C. (2018) 'Waist circumference and risk of 23 site-specific cancers: a population-based cohort study of Korean adults', *British Journal of Cancer*, 119(Suppl 2), pp.1018–1027

National Statistics (2019) Cancer mortality in Scotland. Annual update to 2018. Available at: www.isdscotland.org/Health-Topics/Cancer/Publications/2019-10-29/2019-10-29-Cancer-Mortality-Report.pdf (Accessed 21st May 2020)

Northern Ireland Cancer Registry (2020) 2018 Cancer incidence, survival, mortality and prevalence data. Available at: www.qub.ac.uk/research-centres/nicr/CancerInformation/official-statistics/ (Accessed 21st May 2020)

Oruc, A., and Kaplan, M.A. (2019) 'Effect of exercise on colorectal cancer prevention and treatment', *World Journal of Gastrointestinal Oncology*, 11(5), pp.348–366

Pahwa, R., Goyal, A., Bansai, P., and Jialal, I. (2020) 'Chronic inflammation', in StatPearls. Treasure Island (FL). Available at: www.ncbi.nlm.nih.gov/books/NBK493173/ (Accessed 2nd September 2020)

Ports, K.A., Holman, D.M., Guinn, A.S., Pampati, S., Dyer, K.E., Merrick, M.T., Buchanan Lunsford, N., and Metzler, M. (2018) 'Adverse childhood experiences and the presence of cancer risk factors in adulthood: a scoping review of the literature from 2005 to 2015', *Journal of Pediatric Nursing*, 44(2019), pp.81–96

Public Health Scotland (2020) Cancer incidence in Scotland (to December 2018). Available at: https://beta.isdscotland.org/find-publications-and-data/conditions-and-diseases/cancer/cancer-incidence-in-scotland/ (Accessed 21st May 2020)

Public Health Wales (2019) Cancer survival in Wales, 1995–2016. Available at: www.wcisu.wales.nhs.uk/sitesplus/documents/1111/2016%20data%20survival%20commentary_FINAL.pdf (Accessed 21st May 2020)

Samet, J.M. (2013) 'Chapter 13. Combined effect of air pollution with other agents', in Straif, K., Cohen, A., and Samet, J. (eds) *Air pollution and cancer*. Lyon: International Agency for Research on Cancer/World Health Organization

Smittenaar, C.R., Petersen, K.A., Stewart, K., and Moitt, N. (2016) 'Cancer incidence and mortality projections in the UK until 2015', *British Journal of Cancer*, 115(9), pp.1147–1155

Watterson, A. (2013) 'Competing interests at play? The struggle for occupational cancer prevention in the UK', in Nichols, T., and Walters, D. (eds) *Safety or profit? International studies in governance, change and the work environment*. New York: Baywood Publishing

World Cancer Research Fund/American Institute for Cancer Research (2018) *Diet, nutrition, physical activity and cancer: a global perspective*. London: World Cancer Research Fund International

World Health Organization (2009) 'Breast is always best, even for HIV-positive mothers', *Bulletin of the World Health Organization*, 88(1), pp.1–80

World Health Organization (2020a) Cancer. Key statistics. Available at: www.who.int/cancer/resources/keyfacts/en/ (Accessed 25th May 2020)

World Health Organization (2020b) Cancer prevention. Available at: www.who.int/cancer/prevention/en/ (Accessed 24th May 2020)

World Health Organization (2020c) Tobacco free initiative. Available at: www.who.int/tobacco/quitting/benefits/en/ (Accessed 28th May 2020)

15 Diabetes

Sally Robinson

Key points

- Introduction
- The rise of diabetes
- Blood glucose regulation
- Diabetes
- Long-term complications of diabetes/high blood glucose
- Types and causes of diabetes
- Primary prevention of diabetes
- Secondary prevention of diabetes
- Tertiary prevention of diabetes
- Summary

Introduction

Diabetes is rising at a rapid rate across the world and in the UK. This chapter explains blood glucose regulation, the acute symptoms of having too much or too little glucose in the blood and the long-term health complications that can be caused by diabetes. It describes three most common types of diabetes, type 1, type 2 and gestational, along with their causes. Although some diabetes cannot be prevented, most cases of type 2 diabetes can. As type 2 makes up 90% of all UK diabetes, the primary prevention of type 2 is a public health priority. It concludes with an outline of the secondary and tertiary prevention of diabetes.

The rise of diabetes

Across the world, 463 million people are living with diabetes and this figure is expected to rise to 700 million by 2045. Diabetes causes about 4.2 million deaths per year and 46.2% of deaths due to diabetes occur before the age of 60 years (Karuranga *et al.*, 2019). In February 2020, the charity Diabetes UK reported 3.9 million people in the UK were living with a diagnosis of diabetes. As many people have diabetes but have not been diagnosed, they estimate the true figure to be 4.8 million, a figure which will rise to about 5.3 million by 2025 (Diabetes UK, 2020a). The charity reports that more than 500 people die prematurely every week because of diabetes.

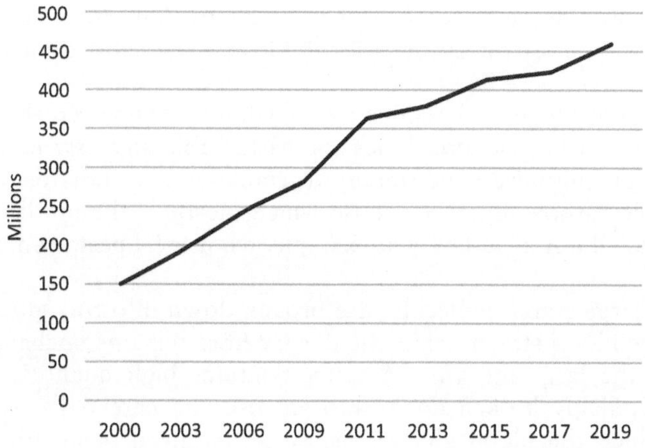

Figure 15.1 World prevalence of diabetes in 20- to 79-year-olds
Source: adapted from Karuranga *et al.*, 2019 p.6

Table 15.1 Prevalence of diabetes in the UK, 2018 to 2019

	Number of people diagnosed with diabetes
UK	3,919,505
England	3,319,266
Scotland	301,523
Wales	198,883
Northern Ireland	99,833

Source: Adapted from Diabetes UK (2020a).

Diabetes costs the National Health Service across England and Wales £1.5 million per hour; £25,000 per minute (Diabetes UK, 2019a).

Blood glucose regulation

Diabetes means that there is a problem with blood glucose regulation.

Blood glucose

The digestion of food means that large molecules are broken down into smaller molecules with the help of mechanical movements, gastric juices and enzymes. Protein, fat and carbohydrate molecules are broken down until they are small enough, just one molecule, to travel from the small intestine across the blood vessel wall into the bloodstream. Although they can all influence the level of glucose in the blood, the ones that have the greatest effect are the digestible carbohydrates (Russell *et al.*, 2016). The digestible carbohydrates include starch and sugars, such as fructose, sucrose and lactose. About 10 to 15 minutes after eating starches or sugars, the glucose in the blood will rise. The blood stream takes the glucose to the cells of the liver, muscles and tissues where it enters and provides fuel/energy for their functions. Any glucose that is not used is stored as glycogen, mostly in the muscles and liver. Eventually, some may be stored as body fat.

Foods and drinks which are high in digestible carbohydrates include cereals and cereal products such as breakfast cereal, bread, rice and pasta; table sugar, sweets and preserves; alcohol; fruit and fruit juices; and starchy vegetables such as potatoes and carrots. The non-digestible carbohydrates are those which mostly make up dietary fibre which is neither digested nor absorbed. For example, wholemeal pasta contains starch and dietary fibre.

During digestion, the large starch molecules are broken down into tiny glucose molecules which enter the blood stream while the dietary fibre remains unchanged and continues down to the large intestine. A toffee contains high quantities of sugar, and all of this is quickly broken down into glucose and enters the blood stream. The speed at which the blood glucose rises after eating depends on the glycaemic index and how much it rises depends on the glycaemic load, which are discussed in Chapter 7. A bag of toffees has a higher glycaemic load than a portion of wholemeal pasta.

The amount of glucose in the blood can be checked by a finger-prick of blood transferred to a small card strip which is inserted into a glucose meter. The meter displays

Table 15.2 The amount of digestible carbohydrates in some foods and drinks

100 grams of food	*Carbohydrate (grams)*	*100 millilitres of drink*	*Carbohydrate (grams)*
Cheese, cheddar	0.1	Spirits, 40% volume	trace
Chicken slices	2	Wine, red	0.2
Cauliflower, boiled	3.5	Wine, sparkling, white	5.1
Carrots, boiled	6	Lager, alcohol-free	1.5
Potatoes, mashed with butter	15.9	Lager, extra-strong	2.4
Chips, fine cut from takeaways	39.7	Beer, bitter	2.2
Pasta, wholewheat, boiled	27.g	Fruit juice, no added sugar	0.9
Pasta, white, boiled	31.5	Fruit juice	10.3
Rice, wholegrain, boiled	29.2	Cola	10.9
Rice, white, boiled	31.1	Tea, black, water and semi-skimmed milk	0.7
Porridge, made with whole milk	13.3	Coffee, instant, water and semi-skimmed milk	0.7
Shredded Wheat with semi-skimmed milk	35	Milk, soya, sweetened	2.4
Flapjacks	55.7	Milk, semi-skimmed	4.7
Fruit cake, homemade	61.5	Milk, skimmed	4.8
Flour, white, plain	80.9	Drinking chocolate, made with semi-skimmed milk	10.9
Sugar, Demerara	104.5	Horlicks, made with semi-skimmed milk	13.5
Sugar, white	105	Milkshake, thick, takeaway	15.3

Source: PHE/FSA (2015).

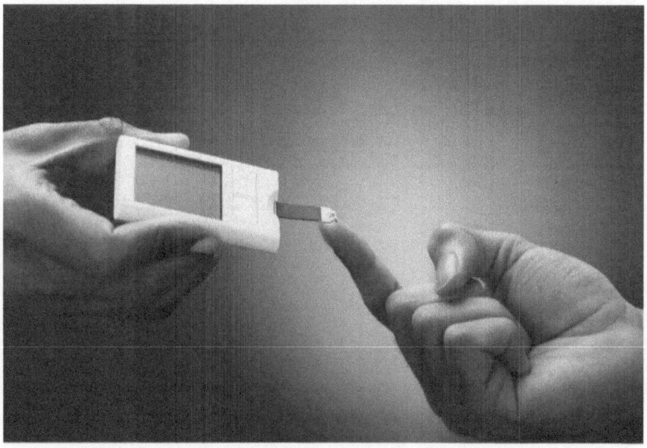

Figure 15.2 Blood glucose testing with a blood glucose meter
Source: Andrey_Popov/Shutterstock.com

the result on the screen. Alternatively, there are continuous glucose-monitoring systems which involve the long-term insertion of a sensor into the body. It picks up the glucose levels in the interstitial fluid in and around the body's cells. In healthcare settings a HbA1c blood test may be taken; the result indicates the average blood glucose level over time.

In the context of diabetes, we are concerned with the total amount of digestible carbohydrate that is eaten.

The pancreas

The pancreas is a gland in the abdomen. About 90% of its function is to produce digestive enzymes which travel into the small intestine and help to digest proteins, carbohydrates and fats into smaller molecules. The remaining 10% is concerned with producing pancreatic hormones, including insulin and glucagon, which work in opposite ways to keep blood glucose levels within an optimum range ready to respond to the body's needs. This is called blood glucose regulation (Figure 15.3).

Glucagon helps to prevent blood glucose from dropping too low, for example between meals. It does this by encouraging the liver to break down glycogen and release some glucose into the blood. If necessary, such as in starvation, it can also convert amino acid molecules to become glucose.

Insulin helps to keep the blood glucose level down and prevent it from becoming too high. When we eat, and the blood glucose rises, the pancreas is prompted to release the correct amount of insulin into the blood stream. Diabetes UK (2020b) describes insulin as like a door key which travels to a cell, opens a lock, and lets the glucose enter. In this way, the level of blood glucose falls, and the muscles, liver and tissues gain the fuel they need to do their work. Insulin will also stimulate the liver to store glucose in the form of glycogen, so the amount left in the blood is not too high.

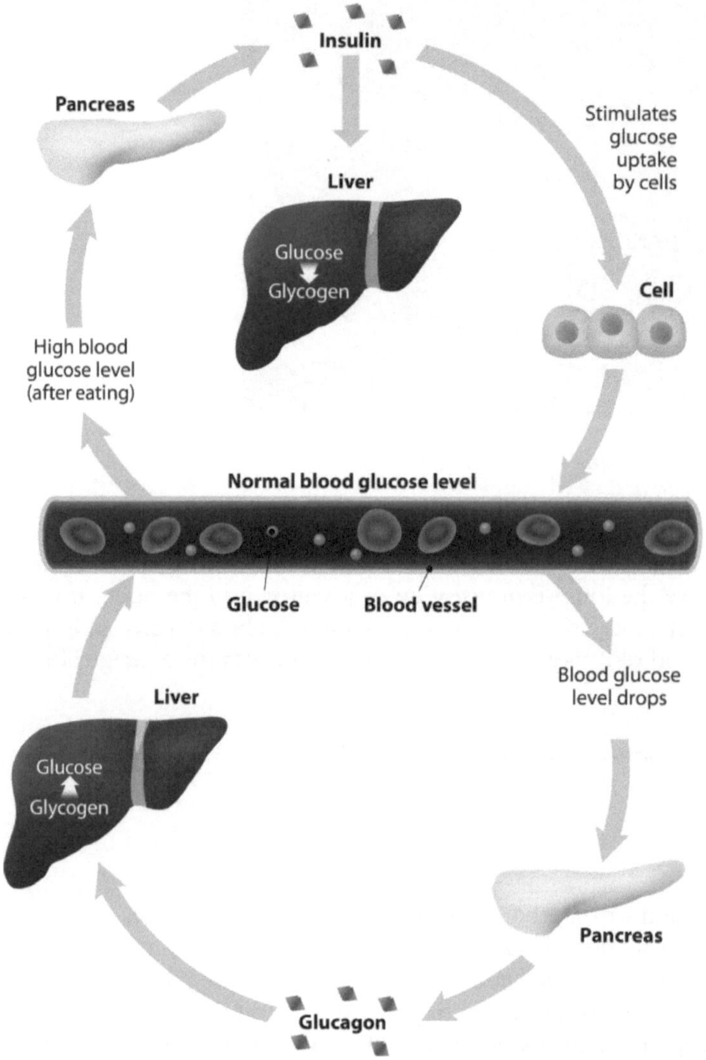

Figure 15.3 Glucose regulation
Source: Designua/Shutterstock.com

Diabetes

Diabetes mellitus is a condition where the blood glucose level is too high because the glucose is unable to enter the cells. This happens because the body does not produce enough 'door key' insulin and/or cannot effectively use the insulin that it does produce.

Box 15.1 Diabetes mellitus

Diabetes is the Greek word for 'siphon': to draw liquid from one place to another. It refers to frequent urination. Mellitus is a Latin word for sweet-tasting or honey-like. It refers to glucose in the urine. Diabetes mellitus is a different condition to the rarer diabetes insipidus, which also causes frequent urination. The symptoms of diabetes mellitus were first recorded in 1550 BC by the Egyptians.

Blood glucose regulation in diabetes

There are different types of diabetes, but they share common symptoms caused by the level of blood glucose being too high. In order to regulate their blood glucose, people may be prescribed insulin, administered by an injection/insulin pen or via an insulin pump. The aim is to balance the quantity of insulin administered to the quantity of digestible carbohydrates they are about to consume. Physical activity may also need to be considered. In this way glucose regulation can be achieved. Some people take tablets, which work in various ways, to help with glucose regulation.

Symptoms of diabetes

People with diabetes are most likely to complain of

- extreme thirst
- frequent urination
- thrush or genital itching
- slow-healing wounds
- blurred vision

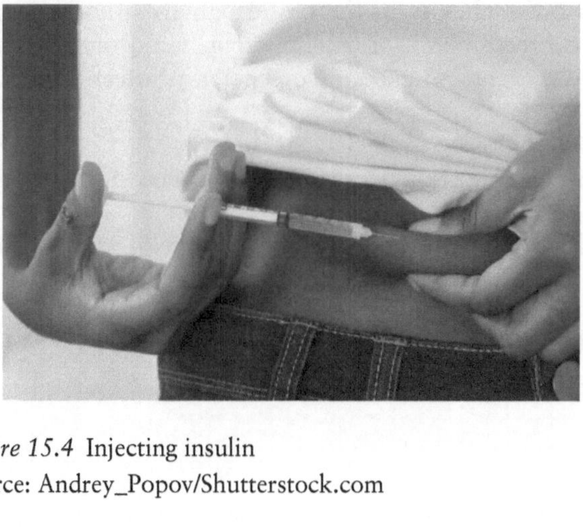

Figure 15.4 Injecting insulin
Source: Andrey_Popov/Shutterstock.com

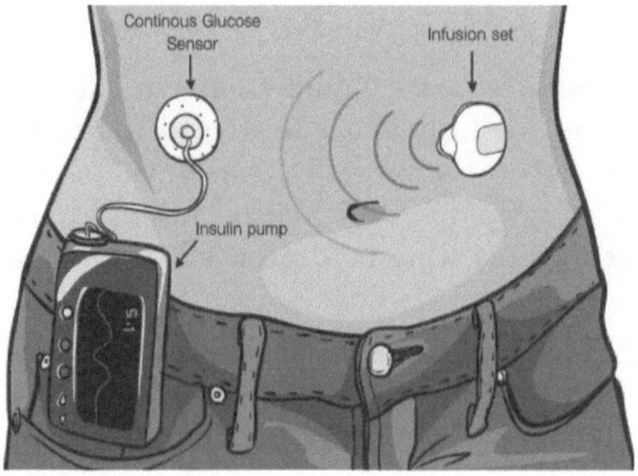

Figure 15.5 An insulin pump
Source: corbac40/Shutterstock.com

- tiredness
- hunger
- weight loss

These symptoms relate to having too much glucose in the blood, hyperglycaemia.

Hyperglycaemia

Too much glucose in the blood causes

- extreme thirst and frequent urination because the body is trying to flush out the excess glucose by filtering it through the kidneys. The filtering needs plenty of water, so the body encourages thirst
- thrush or genital itching because glucose in the urine provides a breeding ground for fungal or bacterial infection
- slow-healing wounds because the glucose in the blood damages blood vessels, which reduces blood flow and the amount of healing oxygen and nutrients that can reach the wound. Also, the glucose encourages bacterial infection around the wound
- blurred vision because glucose builds up in the lens of the eye
- tiredness because the cells are lacking the glucose/energy that they need
- hunger because the cells are needing glucose
- over time, the body breaks down its own stores of fat as a source of energy, which leads to weight loss

The person should check their blood sugar level. They may need to administer insulin. Drinking water will help to prevent dehydration.

Diabetic ketoacidosis

Prolonged and very high blood glucose is a medical emergency called diabetic ketoacidosis. Due to lack of insulin, the cells are starved of glucose, so the body breaks down its own fat, which releases acidic ketone bodies. These cause an unusual fruity breath odour. Other symptoms include dehydration, thirst, laboured breathing, rapid heartbeat, confusion, nausea, vomiting, loss of consciousness and coma.

Hyperosmolar hyperglycaemic state

A hyperosmolar hyperglycaemic state is a medical emergency which only occurs in people with type 2 diabetes. It means people have very high blood glucose levels, but this is not due to lack of insulin. It usually progresses over a few weeks despite the usual diabetes medication being taken. It is often the result of illness and dehydration. The symptoms include frequent urination, thirst, nausea and dry skin; it can progress to drowsiness, disorientation and loss of consciousness.

Hypoglycaemia

If there is too much insulin circulating in the blood, the blood glucose can fall too low. For example, hypoglycaemia can happen if an individual injects their normal dose of insulin and then a meal is unexpectedly missed or changed. People will experience

- difficulty with concentrating, drowsiness, dizziness, headache and confusion because glucose is not entering the brain cells
- shaking and weakness because glucose is not entering the peripheral nerves and muscles
- rapid heart rate because the lack of glucose to the central nervous system activates a range of changes to counter the threat and improve the heart's output and blood pressure

When possible, the person should check their blood sugar level. If they are conscious and able to swallow, they should be given carbohydrate, such as a solution of sugar in water, fruit juice or some glucose tablets which dissolve in the mouth.

Severe hypoglycaemia

Very low blood glucose is a medical emergency as it can lead to convulsions and unconsciousness.

Illness and blood glucose regulation

Any illness can interfere with blood glucose regulation. People with diabetes are vulnerable to experiencing serious swings. For example, the body may break down glycogen to raise the glucose in the blood to help fight the illness. This hyperglycaemia may become life-threatening diabetic ketoacidosis or a hyperosmolar hyperglycaemic state.

Other conditions

It is worth noting that both hyperglycaemia and hypoglycaemia can occur in people without diabetes; medical advice should be sought.

Long-term complications of diabetes/high blood glucose

Regulating the level of glucose in the blood stream is important because, over time, excess glucose damages blood vessels, tissues and nerves. This can affect the whole body and lead to serious complications which cause premature death.

Compared to people without diabetes in the UK, those with diabetes are

- nearly 2.5 times more likely to have a heart attack
- more than 2.5 times more likely to experience heart failure
- more than twice as likely to have a stroke
- 20 times more likely to have an amputation
- more likely to develop preventable sight loss
- five times more likely to need kidney dialysis or a kidney transplant
- twice as likely to suffer from depression and be depressed for longer

(Diabetes UK, 2019b)

Cardiovascular disease

A high quantity of glucose in the blood reduces the rate of blood flow, increases the risk of fatty plaques (atheroma) developing inside the blood vessels and irritates the inner lining of the vessel walls. The blood vessels become narrow and hardened. Together these cause poor blood circulation, high blood pressure and high blood cholesterol, which affects the whole body from the peripheries to the major organs, including the heart. Heart failure means the heart muscle is unable to pump the blood as efficiently as it once did. If a blood vessel in the heart becomes blocked, the oxygen to some of the heart muscle is cut off, causing it to die. This is a heart attack (myocardial infarction). A blocked blood vessel in the brain will cause brain tissue to die. This is a stroke (cerebrovascular accident). In the UK, diabetes causes 530 heart attacks and 680 strokes every week (Diabetes UK, 2020c).

Peripheral arterial disease

Peripheral arterial disease is an aspect of cardiovascular disease that often develops with high blood glucose. The blood stream is unable to take enough oxygen and nutrients to the periphery of the body to feed the tissues. Early signs in the hands and feet include feeling cold or numb, having dry skin and lighter skins may appear pale blue. Deteriorated tissue reveals itself as a sore, wound or ulcer that does not heal. The high glucose in the blood also provides an attractive environment for infection. The tissue damage can be hard to treat even with combinations of antibiotics and careful wound care – sometimes with types of maggots which remove bacteria. With no treatment, or in those severe cases which do not respond well to treatment, the tissue dies, a condition called ischaemia, and gangrene sets in.

Diabetic foot disease

Peripheral arterial disease means that any small abrasion or cut in the toes or foot may become a bigger wound as it fails to heal and may become infected. Any unusual signs in the feet, including being cold, numb, swollen or aching, require immediate

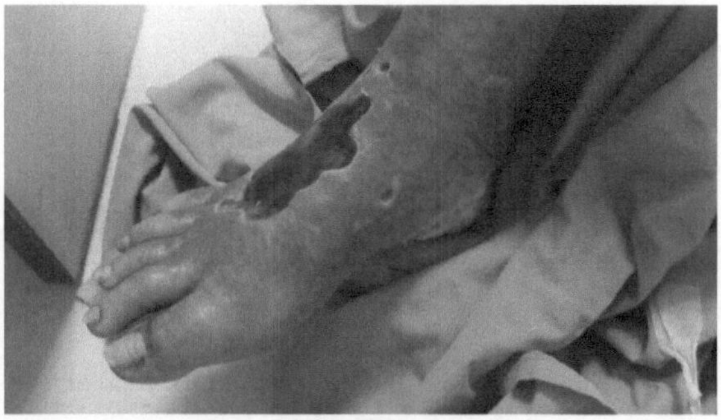

Figure 15.6 Diabetic foot ulcer with gangrene
Source: Casa nayafana/Shutterstock.com

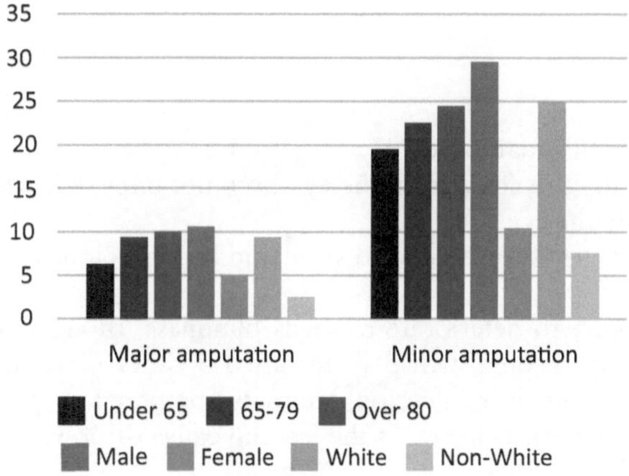

Figure 15.7 Major and minor diabetic lower-limb amputation rates 2015/16 to 2017/18 by age and sex per 10,000 population-years, England
Source: adapted from Public Heath England, 2019 p.3

medical attention. Surgery, in some cases amputation, is recommended to prevent gangrene spreading throughout the body and causing death. A person with diabetes is 20 times more likely to need an amputation compared to other people (Diabetes UK, 2020c). For example, in Scotland 1,401 people with diabetes had a major lower limb amputation in 2018, which represented 0.5% of all people with diabetes (Scottish diabetes data group, 2019). In England 2015/16 to 2017/18, there were 7,545 similar amputations, which can be standardised to 8.2 per 10,000 population-years (Figure 15.7).

Diabetic eye disease

The blood vessels of the eye are tiny and can be easily damaged by high blood glucose and high blood pressure. In response, blood vessels may grow abnormally. The eyes may develop

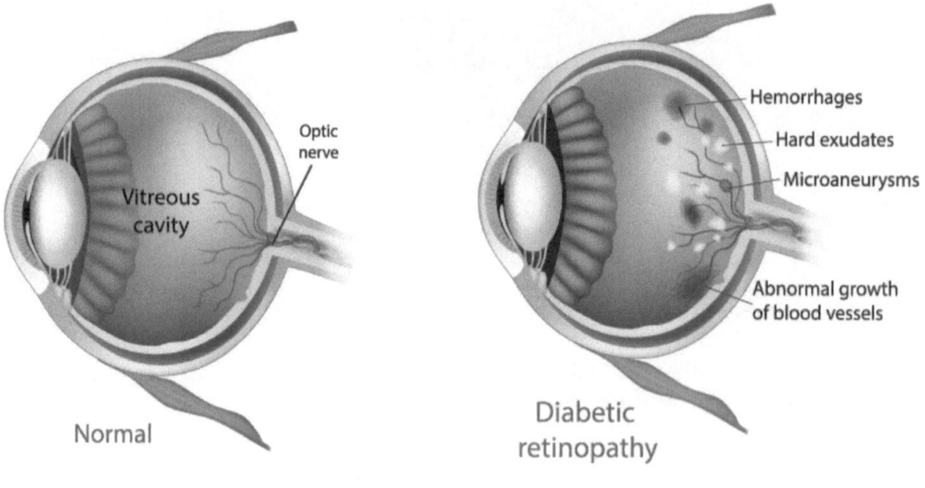

Figure 15.8 Diabetic retinopathy
Source: Sakurra/Shutterstock.com

- diabetic retinopathy – the retina is damaged
- glaucoma – the normal draining of fluid from the eye becomes impeded, which leads to raised pressure inside the eye
- cataract – the glucose encourages the eye's lens to swell and become cloudy

All three conditions cause vision to deteriorate towards blindness, though there are eye treatments which can help. People with diabetes are 1.5 times more likely to develop glaucoma and twice as likely to develop cataracts compared to people without diabetes (Diabetes UK, 2020c). Diabetes is the leading cause of preventable sight loss in the UK (Diabetes UK, 2019b).

Diabetic kidney disease

The role of the two kidneys are to filter the blood. They filter approximately one litre of blood every minute, which is about a fifth of all the blood circulating in the body. Blood enters the kidneys, via the renal arteries, to be filtered inside the kidney (Figure 15.9). The kidney sorts out what needs to be conserved, such as water and other useful substances including protein molecules, from what can be disposed of, the waste. The useful substances are diverted to the blood in the renal vein, which transports them out of the kidney to other parts of the body. The waste is released as urine down the ureters, out of the kidneys, and into the bladder.

Cystitis is a type of urinary tract infection which means inflammation of the bladder. It may develop because the body tries to get rid of the excess glucose in the urine. The symptoms include painful urination, frequent urination and pain in the lower abdomen. Drinking plenty of water and cranberry juice may be enough for symptoms to subside but taking antibiotics may be necessary.

The combination of high blood glucose and high blood pressure can damage the main renal artery as well as the tiny blood vessels inside the kidneys, which interferes with the filtration process. Useful substances, such as water and protein, are not fully

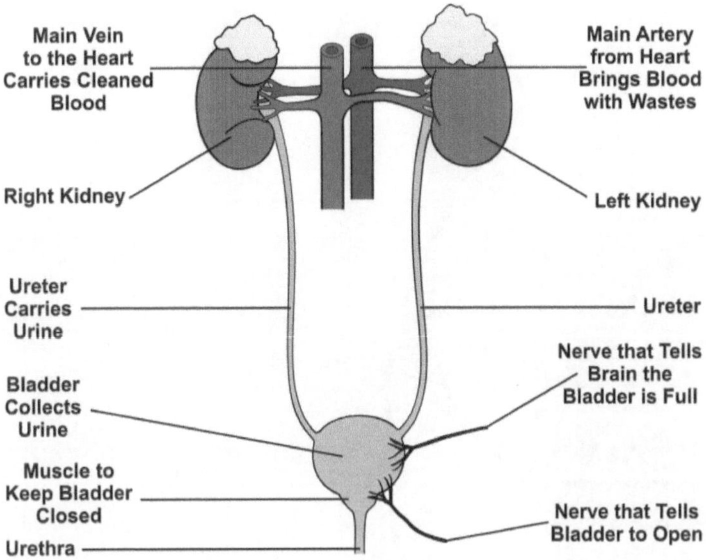

Figure 15.9 The renal system
Source: udaix/Shutterstock.com

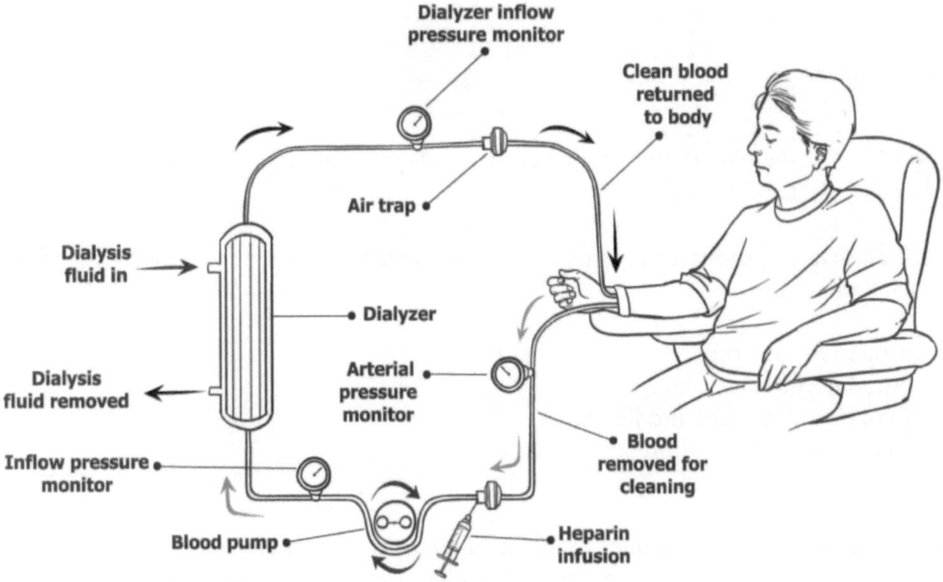

Figure 15.10 Haemodialysis: filtering the blood via a dialysis machine
Source: corbac 40/Shutterstock.com

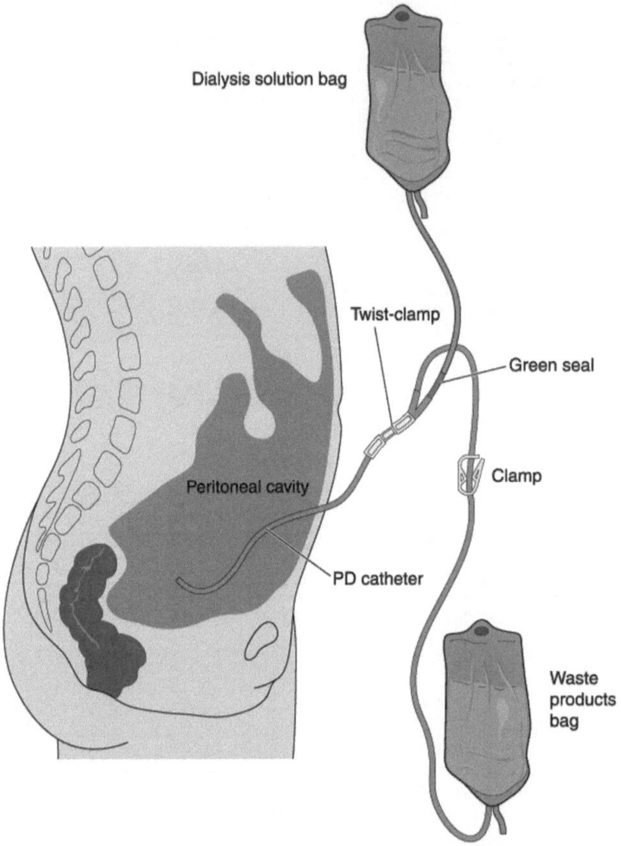

Figure 15.11 Peritoneal dialysis: filtering the blood via the lining of the abdomen
Source: Blamb/Shutterstock.com

saved and waste products may not be properly excreted, so we feel unwell. Signs of kidney damage are

- protein in the urine
- blood in the urine
- swollen ankles, feet and hands
- feeling tired, short of breath and nauseous

(Diabetes UK, 2020c)

The filtration parts of the kidney are called nephrons, and kidney damage due to diabetes is called diabetic nephropathy. The kidneys become less able to function and artificial filtering of the blood, dialysis (Figures 15.10 and 15.11), may be required or a kidney transplant. In the UK, diabetes is the leading cause of kidney failure, and about a fifth of people who start dialysis have diabetes (Kidney Research UK, 2020).

Diabetic gum disease

The tiny blood vessels in gums can become damaged by high glucose levels in the blood. The gums receive poor levels of oxygen and nutrients, making them vulnerable

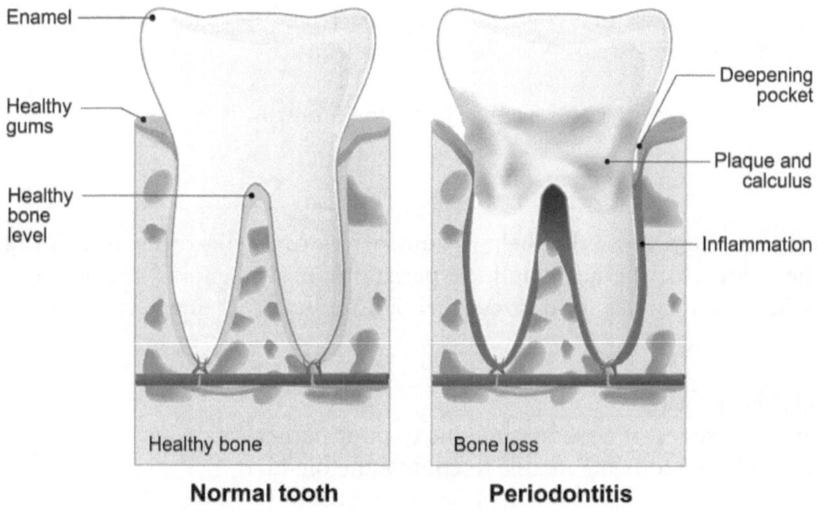

Figure 15.12 Periodontitis
Source: Designua/Shutterstock.com

to the bacteria that make up dental plaque. Also, a high level of glucose in the blood encourages excess glucose in the saliva. Sugary saliva attracts and feeds the plaque bacteria. Plaque bacteria produce acid which damages gums and can lead to

- gingivitis – red, swollen and bleeding gums
- xerostomia – a dry mouth
- tooth decay and tooth loss
- oral thrush
- sore mouth and abscesses
- periodontitis – damage to the soft tissues and bones that support the teeth (Figure 15.12)

(Diabetes UK, 2020c)

Severe periodontitis can upset the body's immune system and, in turn, affect the body's blood glucose regulation (Midwood and Hodge, 2018).

Diabetic nerve problems

Diabetic neuropathy refers to the damage to nerves caused by raised blood glucose travelling through the small blood vessels that supply the nerves. The nerves do not receive the nutrients that they need and become damaged. Diabetes UK (2020c) describe the three types of nerves that are affected.

Sensory nerves are those that allow people to feel pain, touch and temperature as well as other sensations from bones, muscles and skin. If these nerves are damaged, a person may experience

- numbness, tingling
- an absence of pain or shooting/burning pains
- an inability to detect changes in temperature
- loss of coordination as the position of joints becomes unclear

Loss of sensation increases the risk of people with diabetes damaging their feet.

Motor nerves are those that control movement. When these are damaged, muscles are used less and become weak. Muscle weakness leads to

- falls or difficulties with tasks such as fastening a button
- muscle wasting
- muscle twitches and cramps

Autonomic nerves are those that help to control key functions of the body's organs such as the beating of the heart and the peristaltic movements of the gastrointestinal system, which carries food down through the body. Damage to these nerves includes

- irregular heart beats
- bloating, diarrhoea or constipation due to poor peristalsis
- incontinence due to being unable to control the bladder
- impotence due to being unable to sustain an erection
- problems with sweating such as intolerance to heat or reduced ability to sweat

Diabetic reproductive problems

The high glucose in the blood damages the blood vessels and nerves in the reproductive organs. After the blood is filtered by the kidneys, the glucose travels in the urine from the kidneys to the bladder. Both these processes cause urinary and reproductive-related health concerns (Diabetes UK, 2020c).

- Erectile dysfunction

Men may find it difficult to get or keep an erection. This may be caused by nerve damage and/or poor blood flow. Men with diabetes are three times more likely to have erectile dysfunction compared to men without diabetes (Diabetes UK, 2020c). It is noteworthy that erectile dysfunction can be caused by age, drugs and alcohol as well. Treatment may include tablets and/or counselling.

- Vaginal dryness

The blood vessels in the vagina may be damaged by high blood glucose and cause vaginal dryness. The lack of lubrication can make having sex painful. If nerves are damaged by the blood glucose, the woman may experience less sensation. Treatments include lubricants, tablets and/or counselling.

- Thrush

Sugary urine encourages the bacteria which encourage the yeast infection thrush to thrive. Both diabetic men and women are vulnerable to thrush, but it is more common in women. Symptoms in women include

- genital itching
- white discharge
- painful sex
- stinging on urination

and in men

- genital itching
- white discharge
- white patches on the head of the penis

(Diabetes UK, 2020c)

Treatment is available as tablets and creams.

Thinking point:

Imagine you have been diagnosed with diabetes and are now aware of the acute symptoms and the long-term complications that can happen to your body if you do not manage your blood glucose levels well. How would you feel and what would be your practical concerns?

Psychological concerns

Managing diabetes is associated with a range of emotional difficulties connected to the diagnosis, the distress of managing the condition, fear and the development of mental disorders. These can be summarised as

- emotional/crisis reactions – shock, denial, anger, guilt, anxiety
- diabetes distress – overwhelmed about self-managing diabetes, frustrated, difficulties with communication, distress about dietary needs within the family
- phobia reactions – fear, e.g. insulin, injections, needles, hypoglycaemia, long-term complications, obsessive behaviour
- mental health disorders – depression, anxiety, delirium, eating disorders, schizophrenia

(Kalra *et al.*, 2018)

Box 15.2 Case study: Sally

"Sally Morris had Type 1 diabetes that was very difficult to control, meaning that her [blood glucose] levels would swing from high to low without warning – something she found hard to cope with. Her husband, Gary, was used to this situation and didn't take the things Sally said to heart, such as her shouting that he should leave her alone when she was trying to help reverse her hypoglycaemia with sweet tea. Gary would assure Sally that her moods were not her fault. One day Gary's parents came to stay, and Sally had a bad hypo followed by prolonged hyperglycaemia because her liver had released stored glucose – Sally was battling to reduce it. Gary's parents didn't understand the situation and had never seen Sally act in this 'snappy and sarcastic' way before. Sally later overheard her mother-in-law describing her as hostile. This upset Sally greatly and she was overwhelmed with a sense that people just didn't understand. She decided to apologise, although she strongly felt she shouldn't have to. When she said sorry, she expected her parents-in-law to understand that it was her [blood glucose] levels but instead they said, "We don't know why you had to act like that". Sally was angry at the injustice for a long while afterwards and felt isolated by the experience."

(Source: Wilson, 2019 p.45)

There is a bi-directional relationship between diabetes and the mental disorders depression and anxiety (Kolb and Martin, 2017; Kalra *et al.*, 2018):

> Individuals with depression, but no diabetes, are at higher risk for developing diabetes at follow-up. Conversely, individuals with no depression, but receiving diabetes treatment, are at higher risk of developing depression at follow-up.
>
> (Lin *et al.*, 2010 p.264)

Lin and colleagues' (2010) study of 3,922 adults with type 2 diabetes over five years showed that major depression increased the risk of cardiovascular complications by 25% and peripheral vascular complications by 36%. Grigsby and colleagues (2002) examined 18 research studies which included a total of 2,584 people with diabetes. They concluded that 14% of those with diabetes had generalised anxiety disorder and 40% had raised anxiety symptoms.

Diabetes-related conditions

Diabetes UK (2020b) lists several other physical conditions that are associated with diabetes for varying reasons. These include coeliac disease, thyroid disease, mastopathy, muscular conditions such as frozen shoulder and carpel tunnel syndrome, haemochromatosis and pancreatitis.

> *The immediate symptom of poor blood glucose regulation is hyperglycaemia. Over time, hyperglycaemia can damage blood vessels, tissues and nerves throughout the body, causing serious health complications.*

Types and causes of diabetes

There are several types of diabetes. The main ones are type 1, type 2 and gestational diabetes. Although the main symptoms and longer-term complications are the same because they share a problem with blood glucose regulation, the causes of each type differ and some are preventable, and some are not.

Type 1 diabetes

Type 1 diabetes means that a person does not produce any insulin, or only minute amounts, so the glucose remains in the blood and cannot enter the cells. This happens because the body's immune system destroys the cells in the pancreas which produce insulin. The cause of this autoimmune disorder is not completely understood, but researchers believe that it may be triggered by a virus, vaccines or low levels of vitamin D in the blood and/or is encouraged by certain genes (Diabetes UK, 2019c). Researchers are learning that within type 1 diabetes there are sub-types (Leete *et al.*, 2020). Type 1 diabetes is often diagnosed in childhood, but it is also diagnosed in adulthood, as was the case with the UK prime minister Theresa May. It is treated by injecting insulin.

Type 1 diabetes is characterised by the onset of hyperglycaemia, high blood glucose, because of the lack of insulin.

Type 2 diabetes

Type 2 diabetes means that the body produces insulin but either it does not produce enough due to a problem with the pancreas or, using the 'door key' metaphor, it is unable to unlock the door of the cells and let the glucose enter. The glucose remains in the blood stream and rises. The cells do not receive the fuel that they need to work. The pancreas produces more insulin as it tries to rectify the problem and the cycle continues. Over time, the strain on the pancreas causes it to tire, its ability to produce insulin falls and the blood glucose level rises higher.

Type 2 diabetes is characterised by a combination of hyperglycaemia, hyperinsulinemia and insulin resistance.

Insulin resistance

Insulin resistance means that the body's cells are less responsive to insulin than 'normal', which leads to high levels of blood glucose, hyperglycaemia. It is also called having reduced insulin sensitivity. It can lead to high blood pressure and high blood cholesterol (Patel and Abate, 2013). The most common cause of insulin resistance is too much body fat.

Hyperglycaemia

Hyperglycaemia means a high blood glucose level.

Hyperinsulinemia

In response to a high blood glucose level, the pancreas produces more insulin. Hyperinsulinemia means an abnormally high level of insulin in the blood. It is often caused by insulin resistance, but not always. Symptoms of hyperinsulinemia may include

- weight gain
- intense hunger
- cravings for sugar
- feeling frequently hungry
- difficulty concentrating
- fatigue
- poor concentration

Type 2 diabetes is often treated in one or more ways: tablets which may stimulate the pancreas to produce insulin, insulin injections, weight loss, healthy diet and physical activity. Unlike type 1 diabetes, type 2 diabetes is largely preventable and sometimes reversible.

Causes of type 2 diabetes

Table 15.3 shows that prediabetes and metabolic syndrome are precursors to type 2 diabetes, though not everyone who develops type 2 diabetes has these conditions. Both conditions suggest that the pancreas is working very hard and the insulin is having difficulty entering the cells. The risks of developing prediabetes, metabolic syndrome and type 2 diabetes are increased by chronic low-grade inflammation (Furman *et al.*, 2019). All three precursors are encouraged directly or indirectly by the modifiable risk factors: excess body fat/abdominal fat, poor diet, physical inactivity, sedentary behaviour, smoking and alcohol.

Genetics, ethnicity and age have a part to play, and these explain why some people exposed to similar environments and health-related behaviours may be more vulnerable to developing type 2 diabetes than others. Type 2 diabetes is a disorder that develops due to a complex interaction between multiple genes, health-related behaviours and environmental factors.

Prediabetes

The terms 'prediabetes', 'non-diabetic hyperglycaemia', 'intermediate hyperglycaemia', 'borderline diabetes', 'impaired fasting glucose', 'impaired glucose tolerance' and 'impaired glucose regulation' are all used to describe a problem with glucose regulation. The blood glucose is higher than normal, but not high enough to warrant

Table 15.3 Risk factors for type 2 diabetes

Common precursors to type 2 diabetes	*Non-modifiable risk factors*	*Modifiable risk factors*		
	These increase risks of developing precursors and/or type 2 diabetes			
		Health-related behaviours	*Environmental factors*	*Adverse childhood experiences*
Prediabetes	Genetics	Excess body/ abdominal fat	Obesogenic environment	Emotional abuse Physical abuse
Metabolic syndrome	Ethnicity	Poor diet	Traffic	Sexual abuse Emotional neglect Physical neglect
Oxidative stress/ low-grade inflammation	Age	Physical inactivity	Noise pollution	Domestic violence Alcohol or drug misuse in household
		Sedentary behaviour	Air pollution	Mental health problem in household
		Smoking tobacco Alcohol	Persistent organic pollutants	Parental separation/ divorce Imprisonment of household member

a diagnosis of diabetes. It may progress to type 2 diabetes and should be treated as a warning (Karuranga *et al.*, 2019; Diabetes UK, 2020d).

Metabolic syndrome

Metabolic syndrome is a collection of risk factors that increase a person's risk of developing type 2 diabetes and cardiovascular disease. They include large waist circumference/abdominal obesity, high blood cholesterol, high blood pressure and insulin resistance/poor glucose regulation. At least three of these factors need to be present for a diagnosis of metabolic syndrome. Grundy (2006) explains that metabolic syndrome starts with abdominal obesity. As someone ages, both the obesity and the metabolic factors worsen.

> Many persons with metabolic syndrome eventually develop type 2 diabetes. As the syndrome advances, risk for cardiovascular disease and its complications increase. Once diabetes develops, diabetic complications other than cardiovascular disease often develop. The metabolic syndrome encompasses each stage in the development of risk factors and type 2 diabetes.
>
> (Grundy, 2006 p.1094)

Oxidative stress and low-grade inflammation

Low-grade inflammation, caused by oxidative stress, is associated with an increased risk of developing type 2 diabetes. The body produces free radicals as part of its normal metabolism, but also absorbs them from sources such as X-rays and pollution in the environment. These atoms are unstable because they have one or more unpaired electrons, negative charges. They seek out and snatch electrons from other atoms so that they can make their own pair and become balanced. The snatching process is called oxidative stress and it causes chronic low-grade inflammation in the body. Low-grade inflammation is

> ... a prolonged pathological condition recognised by tissue destruction and fibrosis, culminating in cell damage due to [free radical] over production from inflammatory cells.
>
> (Oguntibeju, 2019 p.52)

Oxidative stress and chronic low-grade inflammation are encouraged by

- obesity/excess body fat
- physical inactivity/sedentary behaviour
- chronic infections
- poor diet
- chronic stress
- loneliness/isolation
- disturbed sleep, blue light
- pollutants, hazardous waste and other industrial chemicals
- tobacco smoke

- drugs/chemicals, e.g. personal care, prescription/non-prescription, household products
- imbalance within the microbiome, the microbiota in the intestine

(Furman *et al.*, 2019; Bishehsari *et al.*, 2017)

More low-grade inflammation has been found in people with type 2 diabetes than those without. Oguntibeju (2019) explains that hyperglycaemia, high blood glucose, encourages oxidative stress, but the reasons why are unclear. For example, it may be that oxidative stress damages the insulin-producing cells in the pancreas. The process of oxidative stress and the processes that lead to and maintain chronic low-grade inflammation can amplify each other. Also, type 2 diabetes is thought to cause oxidative stress. Low-grade inflammation

- appears to be present in the muscle, tissues and the insulin-producing pancreatic cells in people who are obese with type 2 diabetes
- is associated with insulin resistance and some of the long-term complications of diabetes such as nerve damage (diabetic neuropathy) and kidney damage (diabetic nephropathy)
- is associated with greater physical inactivity and abdominal body fat

(Oguntibeju, 2019; Burini *et al.*, 2020)

Genetics

A person is 40% more likely to develop type 2 diabetes if one parent has the condition; the risk rises to 70% if both parents have it (Ali, 2013). Many of the genes which have been found to be associated with type 2 diabetes contribute to the functioning of the insulin-producing cells in the pancreas, and some are linked to fat metabolism and atheroma, the fatty plaque that clogs the arteries in cardiovascular disease. These findings are of relevance to understanding metabolic syndrome as well as type 2 diabetes (Ali, 2013).

People's genes may encourage their risk of developing type 2 diabetes because genes influence the way that people adapt to their environment. As an environment becomes obesogenic, that is one that promotes high-calorie eating and a sedentary lifestyle, so people's genes such as those which affect appetite, taste and food preferences play a part in how we respond and whether we gain weight. Greater weight is strongly associated with type 2 diabetes.

Another way that the environment may influence genes and the development of type 2 diabetes is through epigenetics. Epigenetics refers to the way that genes express themselves in response to the environment. The human body contains the DNA that makes up its inherited genes. The shape and function of a skin cell and a liver cell differ because of the combination of genes inside the cell that are turned on (expressed) or turned off (repressed). This process of gene expression/repression is influenced by the environment within the cells and outside of the cells. One example, which relates to type 2 diabetes, is the effect of the uterine environment on the cells of the foetus.

David Barker examined the relationship between low-birth-weight babies and later adult disease. He argued that in times of adversity such as during periods of starvation, the developing foetus in the woman's uterus adapts its metabolism in ways that encourage a 'thrifty phenotype', a body that retains as much nutritional energy/glucose as possible. The foetus 'programmes' itself in anticipation that the environment after birth, and throughout life, will remain one with little food. However, the low-birth-weight baby may find itself growing up in the 'obesogenic land of plenty' and the 'thrifty phenotype' body is 'mismatched' (Calkins and Devaskar, 2011). The baby has a pre-existing susceptibility to develop obesity, insulin resistance and then type 2 diabetes, high blood pressure, high blood cholesterol and coronary heart disease (Edwards, 2017). Barker's work is collectively called the Foetal Origins of Adult Disease. More recently the mechanism has been described as epigenetic; the repression and expression of genes in the developing foetus programmes itself to be more vulnerable to developing type 2 diabetes and related conditions later in life.

Ethnicity

People of Asian, sub-Saharan African and Caribbean descent develop prediabetes more frequently than Caucasians (Yip *et al.*, 2017; Diabetes UK, 2019e, Fazli *et al.*, 2019). The relationship between people's ethnicity and metabolic syndrome is less clear (Krishnadath *et al.*, 2016). For example:

> Despite more than 80% of the world's population being of non-European descent, the overwhelming majority of research on [metabolic syndrome], from prevalence to treatment, is in predominantly European-derived populations.
>
> (Lear and Gaevic, 2020 p.8)

Type 2 diabetes is more common among people of Afro-Caribbean or South Asian ethnicities compared to European. In the UK, although people of South Asian origin make up 4% of the population, they are six times more likely to have type 2 diabetes compared to the rest. This makes them three times more likely to develop cardiovascular disease (Diabetes UK, 2019e). The evidence suggests, compared to people of European origin, they

- inherit six genes which make them susceptible to type 2 diabetes
- have a propensity for storing excess fat around the abdomen
- may have muscles which do not break down fat as well as Europeans, and this may be linked to insulin resistance

(Diabetes UK, 2019e)

There is urgent need for more research with people of South Asian origin to better understand the factors which contribute to the higher rates of type 2 diabetes. An in-depth report (Khunti *et al.*, 2009) recommended that research needs to

- enable greater participation in research by those of South Asian ethnicity
- study large cohorts of South Asians born in the UK over time to identify risks
- understand health-related behaviour such as diet, physical activity and smoking within the South Asian culture
- understand how best to deliver culturally sensitive healthcare, including screening for diabetes and its complications during pregnancy

(Khunti *et al.*, 2009)

Age

Ageing is an important risk factor for type 2 diabetes, as most cases of prediabetes and type 2 diabetes are diagnosed in people over 40 years old (Diabetes UK, 2019d; Karuranga *et al.*, 2019). With age, the body's cells develop greater insulin resistance associated with body fat, muscle wasting and inactivity; there is a deterioration in the functioning of the insulin-producing cells of the pancreas and the body has accumulated more chronic low-grade inflammation (Kirkman *et al.*, 2012; Furman *et al.*, 2019).

Excess body/abdominal fat

Excess body fat is the main modifiable risk factor for type 2 diabetes. As a population's weight relative to their height, their body mass index (BMI), increases so does type 2 diabetes and those who have been obese for some time are the most likely to develop the condition (PHE, 2014). However, BMI does not consider sex, the distribution of fat or ageing and the loss of muscle mass. Recent studies suggest that the percentage of body fat is a stronger predictor of prediabetes and type 2 diabetes than BMI (Jo and Mainous, 2018).

Body fat comprises visceral fat around the organs and subcutaneous fat under the skin. Visceral fat is more strongly associated with cardiovascular disease than sub-cutaneous fat. Insulin resistance is different. Both visceral and sub-cutaneous fat contribute to insulin resistance because subcutaneous fat under the skin of the abdomen, but not elsewhere, takes on some properties of visceral fat, which encourages insulin resistance (Patel and Abate, 2013; Kojta *et al.*, 2020). Diabetes UK (2019e) suggests that a waist size more than 31.5 inches/80 cm for women and more than 37 inches/94 cm for men increases the risk of developing type 2 diabetes. People who are 'apple'-shaped are more at risk than those who are 'pear'-shaped.

Up to a fifth of people with type 2 diabetes are not particularly overweight or obese; they do not have a high BMI but they have a metabolism that behaves like that

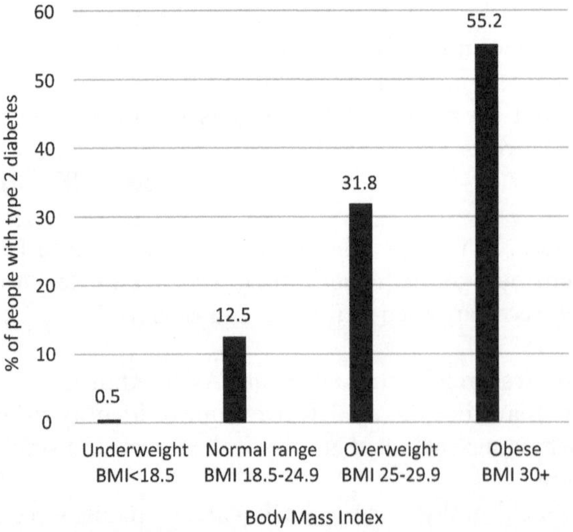

Figure 15.13 Percentage of adults with type 2 diabetes by BMI, Scotland, 2018 (*n* = 48,994)
Source: Scottish diabetes group, 2019

of an obese person. Overall, they may be lean but have abdominal fat or other areas of fatty tissue; older people may have a high proportion of body fat relative to decreasing muscle mass and they may have a marked deterioration in the insulin-producing cells of the pancreas (Oloagun *et al.*, 2020; Patel and Abate, 2013). Together these may explain their type 2 diabetes.

Poor diet

As excess body fat is associated with type 2 diabetes, diets which are high in calories are implicated. Diets which are high in refined grains such as flour and sugar are associated with increased oxidative stress, excess weight and type 2 diabetes (Kolb and Martin, 2017; Tan *et al.*, 2018). Diets which include the regular consumption of sugary drinks are associated with an increased risk of developing type 2 diabetes (Drouin-Chartier *et al.*, 2019; Imamura *et al.*, 2016) by as much as 20 to 30% (Kolb and Martin, 2017).

Physical inactivity/sedentariness

Lower levels of physical activity, such as doing no more than casual walking, and sedentary behaviours, such as sitting to watch television, are both associated with a greater risk of developing type 2 diabetes because they are associated with increased body fat and more insulin resistance (Joseph *et al.*, 2016; Bowden Davies *et al.*, 2018).

Smoking tobacco

Tobacco smoking, either actively or passively, increases the risk of developing type 2 diabetes by between 30% and 40% because the nicotine encourages insulin resistance, and other tobacco chemicals encourage low-grade inflammation (Zhang *et al.*, 2011; CDC, 2019). Even among former smokers, the risk of type 2 diabetes remains higher compared to people who have never smoked (Spijkerman *et al.*, 2014).

Alcohol

Heavy drinking can encourage type 2 diabetes because alcohol

- is highly calorific and adds to excess body fat
- encourages insulin resistance
- can cause chronic inflammation of the pancreas, pancreatitis, which effects its insulin production

(Drinkaware, 2020)

Environment

The more developed/industrialised the country, the more we see obesogenic environments and type 2 diabetes. As there is more overweight and obesity in areas of deprivation compared to more affluent areas, we see type 2 diabetes following the same gradient. For example, type 2 diabetes is 60% more common in the most deprived areas of England compared to the most affluent (PHE, 2018).

Studies have shown that people living with higher levels of traffic, noise and air pollution are at greater risk of developing type 2 diabetes, even when their age, sex, BMI and health-related behaviour are accounted for (Kolb and Martin, 2017). Air pollution, particularly particulate matter PM2.5, is strongly associated with all types of diabetes (Bowe *et al.*, 2018).

> The global toll of diabetes attributable to $PM_{2.5}$ is significant. Reduction in exposure will yield substantial health benefits.
>
> (Bowe *et al.*, 2018 p.e301)

Persistent organic pollutants, which are industrial chemicals, are also associated with type 2 diabetes. Even though some have been banned, many are found in water and soil and enter the food chain via animal fats in meat, fish and dairy products (Mambiya *et al.*, 2019).

Adverse childhood experiences

Adverse childhood experiences (ACEs), such as abuse, parental mental health problems, substance misuse in the household, neglect and domestic violence, are associated with the development of type 2 diabetes in adulthood (Hughes *et al.*, 2017). The more adverse experiences a child suffers, the greater the risk of developing type 2 diabetes (Deschênes *et al.*, 2018). ACEs cause children to suffer toxic stress, which triggers chronic low-grade inflammation, and ACEs are associated with adult obesity, and the use of tobacco and alcohol (Ports *et al.*, 2019). These may explain the pathway to type 2 diabetes, but more research is needed.

Comparisons of type 1 and type 2 diabetes

The key differences between type 1 and type 2 diabetes are shown in Table 15.4 and Figure 15.14.

COVID-19

An analysis of those who died with COVID-19 coronavirus in England, between March and May 2020, showed that 26% had diabetes (Barron *et al.*, 2020). This reflects similar findings from the United States of America (Stokes *et al.*, 2020). About 90% of people with diabetes have type 2 and the majority of those with type 2 diabetes are over 60 years old. Overweight and obesity are strongly associated with type 2 diabetes, and older and obese people are more vulnerable to the effects of the virus. Once age, sex and ethnicity are accounted for, the data suggest that compared to people with no diabetes, people with type 1 diabetes were 3.5 times and people with type 2 diabetes were twice as likely to die from COVID-19 in early 2020 (Diabetes UK, 2020f).

Gestational diabetes

Gestational diabetes means

> Women with elevated blood glucose concentrations during pregnancy.
>
> (Karuranga *et al.*, 2019 p.159)

Table 15.4 Comparison of type 1 and type 2 diabetes

Type 1 diabetes	*Type 2 diabetes*
Is not preventable	Is largely preventable
Approximately 8% of people diagnosed with diabetes in the UK	Approximately 90% of people diagnosed with diabetes in the UK, about 3.9 million people
More common in young people	More common in middle-aged and older people
The body destroys the pancreatic cells that produce insulin	The body cannot make enough insulin, or the insulin cannot enter the cells
Causes are not well understood	Causes are quite well understood, and it is largely preventable. Obesity counts for 80% to 85% of someone's risk
Symptoms associated with hyperglycaemia appear quite quickly	Symptoms associated with hyperglycaemia, insulin resistance and hyperinsulinemia appear slowly and are easier to miss. Six out of 10 people diagnosed with type 2 diabetes have no symptoms
Managed by injecting insulin to control the blood glucose	Managed in a number of ways, including tablets, insulin, activity, diet and weight loss
There is no cure	There is no cure, but it can be put into remission

Source: Adapted from Diabetes UK (2019c; 2020a; 2020e).

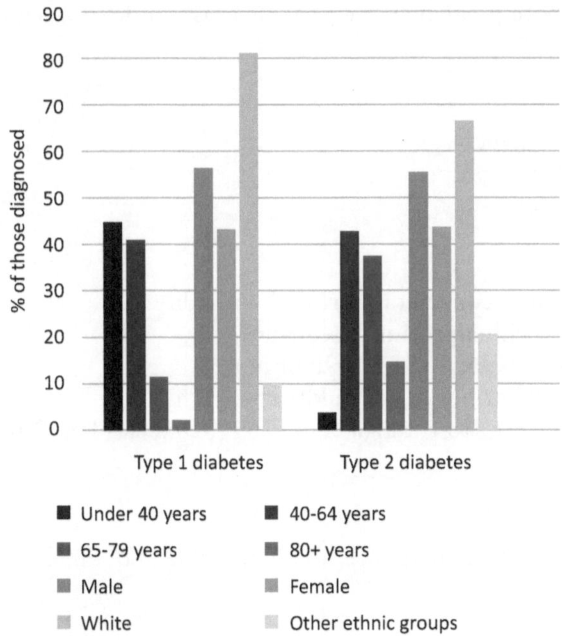

Figure 15.14 Type 1 and type 2 diabetes in England by age, sex and ethnicity, 2018 to 2019
Source: PHE, 2020

During pregnancy the mother's blood glucose transfers across the placenta to the foetus. This stimulates the foetus to produce insulin. Insulin is important for foetal growth and development. During pregnancy, due to hormonal changes, the mother normally develops some insulin resistance. If it becomes pronounced, the mother's blood glucose level will rise. This is maternal hyperglycaemia.

Maternal hyperglycaemia may occur for the first time in pregnancy and end after the birth. It can also occur in women who have diabetes before, during and after pregnancy. It is a concern because continuous high blood glucose levels are associated with

- a high-birth-weight baby, which can be painful for the mother and stressful for the baby
- birth injuries, e.g. shoulder dystocia, where a shoulder(s) get stuck inside the mother during birth, slowing down the birth and sometimes causing fractures and nerve damage to the baby
- increased risk of preeclampsia, where the mother's blood pressure is so high that organs such her liver and kidneys can be damaged
- caesarean sections, a surgical birth due to concerns about the health of the mother and/or baby
- a baby being born with low blood glucose or other complications that may necessitate intensive care or increase the possibility of death
- an increased risk of the mother developing type 2 diabetes in later life
- an increased risk of the baby developing into a child with some insulin resistance and becoming overweight or obese

(Karuranga *et al.*, 2019)

Women who are not diabetic before pregnancy are at greater risk of developing gestational diabetes if they

- are at an older age
- gain excess weight during pregnancy
- have a family history of diabetes
- have polycystic ovary syndrome
- are a regular smoker
- have had a still birth
- have given birth to a baby with a congenital (birth) abnormality
- have had gestational diabetes with a previous pregnancy
- have given birth to a very large baby (4.5 kg/10 lb or more)
- have South Asian, Black, Afro-Caribbean or Middle Eastern heritage

(Karuranga *et al.*, 2019; Diabetes UK, 2020g)

Thinking point:

> Which risk factors for gestational diabetes are non-modifiable and which could be modified?

In England and Wales, more women with type 2 diabetes are becoming pregnant than those with type 1, and they often come from areas of social deprivation. The data show:

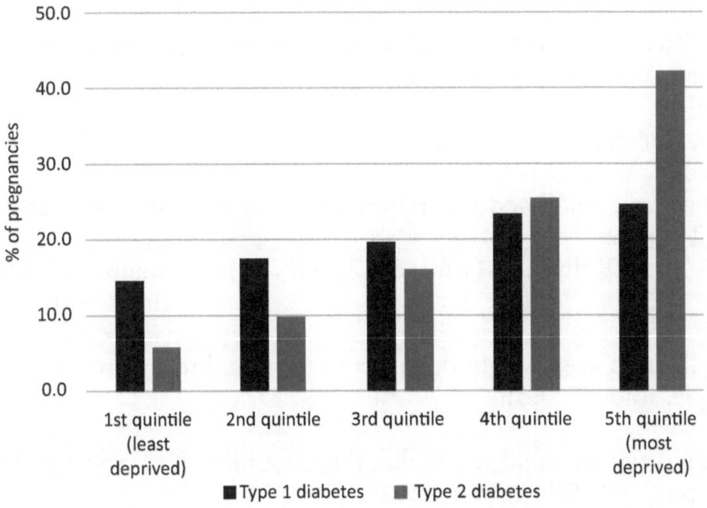

Figure 15.15 Percentage of pregnancies with gestational diabetes in areas of low to high deprivation in England and Wales, 2018

Source: NHS Digital, 2019 p.23. Reproduced under the terms of the Open Government Licence v3.0

> Neonatal death, still birth, congenital anomaly, large and small for dates babies and neonatal unit admission all remain very high by comparison with non-diabetic pregnancies and so are of considerable concern.
>
> (NHS Digital, 2019 p.4)

There are three common types of diabetes: type 1, type 2 and gestational. Most type 2 and some gestational diabetes can be avoided by healthy behaviours and a healthy environment.

Primary prevention of diabetes

The primary prevention of diabetes means focusing on the modifiable risk factors. Currently, type 1 diabetes cannot be prevented. The priorities for preventing type 2 diabetes and gestational diabetes (with no previous history) are to reduce or avoid

- high body fat, including abdominal fat
- obesogenic environments
- built-up environments with high air, noise and traffic pollution
- smoking tobacco
- high alcohol consumption
- regular consumption of sugary drinks
- inactive and sedentary behaviour
- adverse childhood experiences

and to encourage

- healthy, plant-based diets, such as a Mediterranean-style diet which contains plenty of fruit, vegetables and wholegrains
- physical activity
- increased green, walkable environments with low traffic, air and noise pollution
- good mental health
- awareness that adverse childhood experiences are associated with adult disease, including type 2 diabetes

(Kolb and Martin, 2017; PHE, 2018; Dendup *et al.*, 2018; Ashton *et al.*, 2016)

Healthy behaviours help to keep weight down, but they also directly prevent type 2 diabetes. For example, studies indicate

- the higher the intake of fruit and vegetables, the more the risk of type 2 diabetes is reduced, by up to 50% (Zheng *et al.*, 2020)
- eating wholegrains two or more times per week reduces the risk of type 2 diabetes by up to 29% (Hu *et al.*, 2020)
- high physical activity may reduce type 2 diabetes by about 30%. The muscle work reduces insulin resistance. Substituting 30 minutes of sedentary time for vigorous physical activity can improve insulin sensitivity by up to 15% (Kolb and Martin, 2017)
- both regular physical activity and weight loss, where needed, protect against low-grade inflammation (Burini *et al.*, 2020)

Secondary prevention of diabetes

Pregnant women are routinely screened for gestational diabetes by an oral glucose tolerance test (OGTT). This comprises fasting for eight to 10 hours, drinking glucose and having a blood test two hours later to check the level of blood glucose.

Once someone is diagnosed with any type of diabetes, the aim is to prevent the long-term complications caused by high blood glucose. The healthcare priorities are to educate, encourage an individual to self-manage their blood glucose regulation and to check for early signs of harm within the body. It is estimated that

> Over two thirds of people don't fully understand their diabetes.
>
> (Diabetes UK, 2019c p.50)

In the UK, the National Health Service offers 15 essential diabetes checks and services.

- Blood glucose tests
- Blood pressure checks
- Blood cholesterol checks
- Eye screening
- Leg and foot checks
- Kidney tests
- Dietary advice
- Emotional and psychological support

- Courses providing education about managing diabetes
- Care from diabetes specialists such as diabetic nurses and doctors
- Free flu injections
- Diabetes care whilst in hospital
- Support with sexual concerns
- Smoking-cessation services
- Specialist care if planning a pregnancy

(Diabetes UK, 2020h)

Across the UK,

> Fewer than one in five people with type 1 diabetes [and] ... two in five people with type 2 diabetes are meeting the recommended treatment targets that will reduce their risk of complications.
>
> (Diabetes UK, 2019c p.50, 51)

Healthcare professionals need to be aware that adults who suffered ACEs in childhood may have reduced self-control and difficulties with social interactions and are vulnerable to depression, anxiety and self-harm (Ashton *et al.*, 2016). They will need greater support with the management of diabetes, and asking about childhood stress needs to be incorporated into care.

In type 2 diabetes, regulation of blood glucose can be helped by medication, but it is also helped by weight loss, which may occur alongside changes in health-related behaviour such as diet and physical activity. A change in weight and health-related behaviours may encourage the reduction of insulin resistance (increase insulin sensitivity) to a degree that the blood glucose level falls below the threshold for a diabetes diagnosis. This is diabetes going into remission and it may be possible to stop medication.

Tertiary prevention of diabetes

Tertiary prevention concerns treating the diabetes-related symptoms and long-term complications to avoid physical, and potentially life-threatening, deterioration. For example, treatments often focus on cardiovascular, including peripheral vascular, diseases and their consequences, and may include medication for high blood pressure, renal dialysis, treating ischaemic wounds and amputation. Psychological support is a priority and ongoing.

People with diabetes often die from similar conditions to the rest of the population, though heart failure and certain cancers are over-represented and they may die earlier. End-of-life care includes

- minimising the effects of treatments on glucose regulation
- avoiding hyperglycaemia or hypoglycaemia
- care to avoid the skin breaking down into pressure sores and care of the feet
- supporting the individual's self-management of their diabetes for as long as possible

(ABCD/Trend UK/Diabetes Frail, 2018)

Summary

This chapter has

- explained why the rise of diabetes is a public health priority
- described blood glucose regulation, hyperglycaemia and hypoglycaemia
- explained the long-term health complications of hyperglycaemia
- clarified the most common types of diabetes and their causes
- detailed the non-modifiable and modifiable risk factors for type 2 diabetes
- described the primary, secondary and tertiary prevention of diabetes

Further reading

Wilson, V. (2019) *How to live well with diabetes. A comprehensive guide to taking control of your life with diabetes.* London: Robinson

Useful websites

Diabetes UK. Available at: www.diabetes.org.uk
International Diabetes Federation *IDF Diabetes Atlas.* Available at: www.diabetesatlas.org/en

References

Ali, O. (2013) 'Genetics of type 2 diabetes', *World Journal of Diabetes*, 4(4), pp.114–123

Ashton, K., Bellis, M.A., Davies, A.R., Hardcastle, K., and Hughes, K. (2016) *Adverse childhood experiences and their association with chronic disease and health service use in the Welsh adult population.* Cardiff: Public Health Wales NHS Trust

Association of British Clinical Diabetologists/Trend UK/Diabetes Frail (2018) End of life diabetes care. Clinical care recommendations. 3rd edn. Diabetes UK. Available at: www.diabetes.org.uk/resources-s3/2018-03/EoL_Guidance_2018_Final.pdf (Accessed 21st July 2020)

Barron, E., Bakhai, C., Kar, P., Weaver, A., Bradley, D., Ismail, H., Knighton, P., Khunti, K., Sattar, N., Wareham, N., Young, B., and Valabhji, J. (2020) 'Type 1 and type 2 diabetes and COVID-19 related mortality in England: a whole population study', pre-publication copy. Available at: www.england.nhs.uk/wp-content/uploads/2020/05/valabhji-COVID-19-and-Diabetes-Paper-1.pdf (Accessed 14th July 2020)

Bishehsari, F., Magno, E., Swanson, G., Desai, V., Voigt, R.M., Forsyth, C.B., and Keshavarzian, M.D. (2017) 'Alcohol and gut-derived inflammation', *Alcohol Research*, 38(2), pp.163–171

Bowden Davies, K.A., Sprung, V.S., Norman, J.A., Thompson, A., Mitchell, K.L., Halford, J.C.G., Harrold, J.A., Wilding, J.P.H., Kemp, G.J., and Cutherbertson, D.J. (2018) 'Short-term decreased physical activity with increased sedentary behaviour causes metabolic derangements and altered body composition: effects in individuals with and without a first-degree relative with type 2 diabetes', *Diabetologia*, 61(6), pp.1282–1294

Bowe, B., Xie, Y., Li, T., Yan, Y., Xian, H., and Al-Aly, Z. (2018) 'The 2016 global and national burden of diabetes mellitus attributable to $PM_{2.5}$ air pollution', *Lancet Planet Health*, 2(7), e301–312 doi:10.1016/S2542-5196(18)30140–2

Burini, R.C., Anderson, E., Durstine, J.L., and Carson, J.A. (2020) 'Inflammation, physical activity, and chronic disease: an evolutionary perspective', *Sports Medicine and Health Science*, 2(1) doi:10.1016/j.smhs.2020.03.004

Calkins, K., and Devaskar, S.U. (2011) 'Fetal origins of adult disease', *Current Problems in Pediatric and Adolescent Health Care*', 41(6), pp.158–176

Centers for Disease Control and Prevention (2019) Smoking and diabetes. Available at: www.cdc.gov/diabetes/library/features/smoking-and-diabetes.html (Accessed 20th July 2020)

Dendup, T., Feng, X., Clingan, S., and Astell-Burt, T. (2018) 'Environmental risk factors for developing type 2 diabetes mellitus: a systematic review', *International Journal of Environmental Research and Public Health*, 15(1) doi:10.3390/ijerph15010078

Deschênes. S.S., Graham, E., Kivimäki, M., and Schmitz, N. (2018) 'Adverse childhood experiences and the risk of diabetes: examining the roles of depressive symptoms and cardiometabolic dysregulations in the Whitehall II cohort study', *Diabetes Care*, 41(10), pp.2120–2126

Diabetes UK (2019a) Cost of diabetes. Available at: www.diabetes.co.uk/cost-of-diabetes.html (Accessed 22nd July 2020)

Diabetes UK (2019b) Us, diabetes and lots of facts and stats. Available at: www.diabetes.org.uk/resources-s3/2019-02/1362B_Facts%20and%20stats%20Update%20Jan%202019_LOW%20RES_EXTERNAL.pdf (Accessed 15th July 2020)

Diabetes UK (2019c) Type 1 diabetes. Available at: www.diabetes.co.uk/type1-diabetes.html (Accessed 8th July 2020)

Diabetes UK (2019d) Type 2 diabetes. Available at: www.diabetes.co.uk/type2-diabetes.html (Accessed 15th July 2020)

Diabetes UK (2019e) Diabetes in South Asians. Available at: www.diabetes.co.uk/south-asian/ (Accessed 16th July 2020)

Diabetes UK (2020a) Diabetes prevalence 2019. www.diabetes.org.uk/professionals/position-statements-reports/statistics/diabetes-prevalence-2019 (Accessed 15th July 2020)

Diabetes UK (2020b) Diabetes: the basics. Available at: www.diabetes.org.uk/diabetes-the-basics (Accessed 2nd July 2020)

Diabetes UK (2020c) Complication of diabetes. Available at: www.diabetes.org.uk/guide-to-diabetes/complications (Accessed 13th July 2020)

Diabetes UK (2020d) Prediabetes. Available at: www.diabetes.org.uk/preventing-type-2-diabetes/prediabetes (Accessed 10th July 2020)

Diabetes UK (2020e) Differences between type 1 and type 2 diabetes. Available at: www.diabetes.org.uk/diabetes-the-basics/differences-between-type-1-and-type-2-diabetes (Accessed 9th July 2020)

Diabetes UK (2020f) Updates: coronavirus and diabetes. Available at: www.diabetes.org.uk/about_us/news/coronavirus#deaths (Accessed 14th July 2020)

Diabetes UK (2020g) What is gestational diabetes? Available at: www.diabetes.org.uk/diabetes-the-basics/gestational-diabetes (Accessed 13th July 2020)

Diabetes UK (2020h) Your 15 diabetes healthcare essentials. Available at: www.diabetes.org.uk/guide-to-diabetes/managing-your-diabetes/15-healthcare-essentials/what-are-the-15-healthcare-essentials (Accessed 21st July 2020)

Drinkaware (2020) Alcohol and diabetes. Available at: www.drinkaware.co.uk/facts/health-effects-of-alcohol/alcohol-related-diseases/alcohol-and-diabetes (Accessed 20th July 2020)

Drouin-Chartier, J., Zheng, Y., Li, Y., Malik, V., Pan, A., Bhupathiraju, S.N., Tobias, D.K., Manson, J.E., Willett, W.C., and Hu, F.B. (2019) 'Changes in consumption of sugary beverages and artificially sweetened beverages and subsequent risk of type 2 diabetes: results from three large prospective U.S. cohorts of women and men', *Diabetes Care*, 42(12), pp.2181–2189

Edwards, M. (2017) 'The Barker hypothesis', in Preedy,V., and Patel, V. (eds) Handbook of famine, starvation and nutrient deprivation. Springer. Available at: https://link.springer.com/referenceworkentry/10.1007%2F978-3-319-40007-5_71-1 (Accessed 18th July 2020)

Fazli, G.S,. Moineddin, R., Bierman, A.S., and Booth, G.L. (2019) 'Ethnic differences in prediabetes incidence among immigrants to Canada: a population-based cohort study', *BMC Medicine*, 17(100) doi.10.1186/s12916-019-1337-2

Furman, D., Campisi, J., Verdin, E., Carrera-Bastos, P., Targ, S., Franceschi, C., Ferrucci, L., Gilroy, D.W., Fasano, A., Miller, G.W., Miller, A.H., Mantovani, A, Weyand, C.M., Barzilae, N., Goronzy, J.J., Rando, T.A., Effros, R.B., Lucia, A., Kleinstreuer, N., and Slavich, G.M. (2019) 'Chronic inflammation in the etiology of disease across the life span', *Nature Medicine*, 25(12), pp.1822–1832

Grigsby, A.B., Anderson, R.J., Freedland, K.E., Clouse, R.E., and Lustman, P.J. (2002) 'Prevalence of anxiety in adults with diabetes: a systematic review', *Journal of Psychosomatic Research*, 53(6), pp.1053–1060

Grundy, S.M. (2006) 'Metabolic syndrome: connecting and reconciling cardiovascular and diabetes worlds', *Journal of the American College of Cardiology*, 47(6), pp.1094–1100

Hu, Y., Ding, M., Sampson, L. Willett, W.C., Mason, J.E., Want, M., Rosner, B., Hu, F.B., and Sun, S. (2020) 'Intake of whole grain foods and risk of type 2 diabetes: results from three prospective cohort studies', *BMJ*, 370 doi:10.1136/bmj.m2206

Imamura, F., O'Connor, L.,Ye, Z., Mursu, J., Hayashino, Y., Bhupathiraju, S.N., and Forouhi, N.G. (2016) 'Consumption of sugar sweetened beverages, artificially sweetened beverages, and fruit juice and incidence of type 2 diabetes: systematic review, meta-analysis, and estimation of population attributable fraction', *British Journal of Sports Medicine*, 50(8), pp.496–504

Jo, A., and Mainous III A.G. (2018) 'Informational value of percent body fat with body mass index for the risk of abnormal blood glucose: a nationally representative cross-sectional study', *BMJ Open*, 8(4) doi:10.1136/bmjopen-2017–019200

Joseph, J.J., Echouffo-Tcheugui, J.B., Golden, S.H., Chen, H., Jenny, N.S., Carnethon, M.R., Jacobs, D., Burke, G.L., Vaidya, D., Ouyang, P., and Gertoni, A.G. (2016) 'Physical activity, sedentary behaviours and the incidence of type 2 diabetes mellitus: the multi-ethnic study of atherosclerosis (MESA) ', *BMJ Open Diabetes Research and Care*, 4(·1) doi:10.136/bmjdrc-2015-000185

Kalra, S., Jena, B.N., and Yeravdekar, R. (2018) 'Emotional and psychological needs of people with diabetes', *Indian Journal of Endocrinology and Metabolism*, 22(5), pp.696–704

Karuranga, S., Malanda, B., Saeedi, P., and Salpea, P. (eds) (2019) *IDF Diabetes atlas.* 9th edn. Brussels: International Diabetes Federation

Khunti, K., Kumar, S., and Brodie, J. (eds) (2009) *Diabetes UK and South Asian Health Foundation recommendations on diabetes research priorities for British South Asians*. South Asian Foundation/Diabetes UK

Kidney Research UK (2020) Diabetes. Available at: https://kidneyresearchuk.org/conditions-symptoms/diabetes/ (Accessed 13th July 2020)

Kirkman, M.S., Briscoe, V.J., Clark, N., Florez, H., Haas, L.B., Halter, J.B., Huang, E.S., Korytkowski, M.T., Munshi, M.N., Odegard, P.S., Pratley, R.E., and Swift, C.S. (2012) 'Diabetes in older adults', *Diabetes Care*, 35(12), pp.2650–2664

Kojta, I., Chacińska, M., and Błachnio-Zabielska, A. (2020) 'Obesity, bioactive lipids, and adipose tissue inflammation in insulin resistance', *Nutrients*, 12(5) doi.10.3390/nu12051305

Kolb, H., and Martin, S. (2017) 'Environmental/lifestyle factors in the pathogenesis and prevention of type 2 diabetes', *BMC Medicine*, 15(131) doi:10.1186/s12916-017-0901-x

Krishnadath, I.S.K., Toelsie, J.R., Hofman, A., and Jaddoe, V.W.V. (2016) 'Ethnic disparities in the prevalence of metabolic syndrome and its risk factors in the Suriname Health Study: a cross-sectional population study', *BMJ Open*, 6(12) doi:10.1136/bmjopen-2016–013183

Lear, S.A., and Gasevic, D. (2020) 'Ethnicity and metabolic syndrome: implications for assessment, management and prevention', *Nutrients*, 12(1) doi:10.3390/nu12010015

Leete, P., Oram, R.A., McDonald, T.J., Shields, B.M., Ziller, C., TIGI study team, Hattersley, A.T., Richardson, S.J., and Morgan, N.G. (2020) 'Studies of insulin and proinsulin in pancreas and serum support the existence of aetiopathological endotypes of type 1 diabetes associated with age at diagnosis', *Diabetologia*, 63(6), pp.1258–1267

Lin, E.H.B., Rutter, C.M., Katon, W., Heckbert, S.R., Chiechanowski, P., Oliver, M.M., Ludman, E., Young, B.A., Williams, L.H., McCulloch, D.K., and Von Korff, M. (2010) 'Depression and advanced complications of diabetes', *Diabetes Care*, 33(2), pp.264–269

Mambiya, M., Shang, M., Wang, Y., Li, Q., Liu, S., Yang, L., Zhang, Q., Zhang, K., Liu M., Fangfang, N., Zeng, F., and Liu, W. (2019) 'The play of genes and non-genetic factors on type 2 diabetes', *Frontiers in Public Health*, 7(349) doi:10.3389/fpubh.2019.00349

Midwood, I., and Hodge, P. (2018) 'Diabetes and gum disease: does oral health matter?', *Journal of Diabetes Nursing*, 22(3), pp.17–25

NHS Digital (2019) National pregnancy in diabetes (NPID) audit report 2018. England, Wales and the Isle of Man. Available at: https://files.digital.nhs.uk/CF/4791D9/National%20 Pregnancy%20in%20Diabetes%20Audit%20Report%202018.pdf (Accessed 21st July 2020)

Oguntibeju, O.O. (2019) 'Type 2 diabetes mellitus, oxidative stress and inflammation: examining the links', *International Journal of Physiology, Pathophysiology and Pharmacology*, 11(3), pp.45–63

Olaogun, I., Farag, M., and Hamid, P. (2020) 'The pathophysiology of type 2 diabetes mellitus in non-obese individuals. An overview of the current understanding', *Cureus*, 12(4) doi.10.7759/cureus.7614

Patel, P., and Abate, N. (2013) 'Body fat distribution and insulin resistance', *Nutrients*, 5(6) doi.10.3390/nu5062019

Ports, K.A., Holman, D.M., Guinn, A.S., Pampati, S., Dyer, K.E., Merrick, M.T., Buchanan Lunsford, N., and Metzler, M. (2018) 'Adverse childhood experiences and the presence of cancer risk factors in adulthood: a scoping review of the literature from 2005 to 2015', *Journal of Pediatric Nursing*, 44(2019), pp.81–96

Public Health England (2014) Adult obesity and type 2 diabetes. Available at: https://assets.publishing.service.gov.uk/government/uploads/system/uploads/attachment_data/file/338934/Adult_obesity_and_type_2_diabetes_.pdf (Accessed 18th July 2020)

Public Health England (2018) Health matters: preventing type 2 diabetes. Available at: www.gov.uk/government/publications/health-matters-preventing-type-2-diabetes/health-matters-preventing-type-2-diabetes (Accessed 20th July 2020)

Public Health England (2019) Diabetes foot care profile April 2019. Available at: https://app.box.com/s/pmdl91gf2d6pscttb9avqwan6mcbs296/file/432108631907 (Accessed 14th July 2020

Public Health England (2020) Public health profiles 2020. Available at: https://fingertips.phe.org.uk (Accessed 15th July 2020)

Public Health England/Food Standards Agency (2015) *McCance and Widdowson's the composition of foods*, 7th edn. London: Royal Society of Chemistry

Russell, W.R., Baka, A., Björck, I., Delzenne, N., Gao, D., Griffiths, H.R., Hadjilucas, E., Juvonen, K., Lahtinen, S., Lansink, M., van Loon, L., Mykkänen, H., Őstman, E., Riccardi, G., Vinoy, S., and Weickert, M.O. (2016) 'Impact of diet composition on blood glucose regulation', *Food Science and Nutrition*, 56(4), pp.541–590

Scottish diabetes data group (2019) Scottish diabetes survey 2018. Available at: www.diabetesinscotland.org.uk/wp-content/uploads/2019/12/Scottish-Diabetes-Survey-2018.pdf (Accessed 27th July 2020)

Spijkerman, M.W., van der A., D.L., Nilsson, P.M., *et al.* (2014) 'Smoking and long-term risk of type 2 diabetes: the EIPC-InterAct Study in European populations', *Diabetes Care*, 37(12), pp.3164–3171

Stokes, E.K., Zambrano, L.D., Anderson, K.N., Marder, E.P., Raz, K.M., Suad El Burai, F., Tie, Y., and Fullerton, K.E. (2020) 'Coronavirus disease 2019 case surveillance – United States, January 22-May 30, 2020', *Morbidity and Mortality Weekly Report*, 69(24), pp.759–765

Tan, B.L., Norhaizan, M.E., and Liew, W. (2018) 'Nutrients and oxidative stress: friend or foe?', *Oxidative Medicine and Cellular Longevity*, 2018(6) doi:10.1155/2018/9719584

Whincup, P.H., Kaye, S.J., Owen, C.G., *et al.* (2008) 'Birth weight and risk of type 2 diabetes: a systematic review', *Journal of the American Medical Association*, 300(24), pp.2886–2897

Wilson, V. (2019) *How to live well with diabetes. A comprehensive guide to taking control of your life with diabetes*. London: Robinson

Yip, W.C.Y., Sequeira, I.R., Plank, L.D., and Poppitt, S.D. (2017) 'Prevalence of pre-diabetes across ethnicities: a review of impaired fasting glucose (IFG) and impaired glucose tolerance (IGT) for classification of dysglycaemia', *Nutrients*, 9(11) doi:10.3390/nu9111273

Zhang, L., Curhan, G.C., Hu, F.B., and Forman, J.P. (2011) 'Association between passive and active smoking and incident type 2 diabetes in women', *Diabetes Care*, 34(4), pp.892–897

Zheng, J., Sharp, S.J., and Imamura, F., *et al.* (2020) 'Association of plasma biomarkers of fruit and vegetable intake with incident type 2 diabetes: EPIC-InterAct case-cohort study in eight European countries', *BMJ*, 370 doi:10.10.1136/bmj.m2194

16 Dementia

Pat Chung and Trish (Patricia) Vella-Burrows

Key points

- Introduction
- Defining dementia
- Common types of dementia
- Rising rates of dementia
- The impact of dementia
- Risk factors for dementia
- Primary prevention of dementia
- Secondary prevention of dementia
- Tertiary prevention of dementia
- Summary

Introduction

This chapter will explain why dementia is a public health priority for the world, with a focus on the UK. It will define dementia and describe four common types. It will present data to show the anticipated significant rise in the number of people living with dementia over the next few decades. The challenges of dementia for countries, families, carers and individuals are examined through a discussion about the costs of care, the impact on the wider economy and the personal impacts for individuals and those around them. The chapter describes the non-modifiable and modifiable risk factors for developing dementia. It concludes with an overview of the primary, secondary and tertiary prevention of dementia.

Defining dementia

Dementia is not a disease, but a cluster of symptoms that can include memory loss, psychiatric and psychological changes, disturbances in language and impairments in daily living (Burns and Illiffe, 2009). The World Health Organization defines dementia as a syndrome which is usually chronic or progressive in nature. There is a

> ... deterioration in cognitive function ... beyond what might be expected from normal ageing. It affects memory, thinking, orientation, comprehension, calculation, learning capacity, language, and judgement. Consciousness is not affected.

> The impairment in cognitive function is commonly accompanied … by deterioration in emotional control, social behaviour, or motivation.
>
> (WHO, 2019a)

Dementia is caused by a variety of injuries or diseases that either directly or indirectly affect the brain, such as Alzheimer's disease. It comprises signs and symptoms that range from mild, such as when forgetfulness starts to affect a person's functioning, to the most severe, when the person becomes dependent on others to assist with most aspects of their daily living.

Mild cognitive impairment

Mild cognitive impairment means that an individual has problems with thinking or memory, but this alone does not lead to a diagnosis of dementia (NICE 2019). Between 5% and 20% of people aged over 65 in the UK have mild cognitive impairment. Of those, about half are likely to develop dementia (NICE, 2019; Alzheimer's Society, 2020a).

Common types of dementia

There are about 200 types of dementia (Foley and Swanwick, 2014). Each is characterised according to the area and type of damage to the brain (WHO 2019a; NICE, 2019). Dementia that is diagnosed under the age of 65 is called 'early-onset' or 'young-onset' dementia. Here we describe Alzheimer's disease, vascular dementia, dementia with Lewy bodies and frontotemporal dementia.

It is important to note that dementia is more complex than this medical model suggests. During the 1990s, post-mortem research with people who had been diagnosed with dementia showed that damage to brain tissue does not always correlate with the person's behaviour or expression of cognition (Snowdon, 1997). Some people with moderate to severe brain tissue damage were higher functioning than expected and vice versa. The science of dementia is by no means the complete story, and today emphasis is placed on looking for social, psychological and other personal factors which provide a more holistic understanding of each individual person's experience of dementia (Vella-Burrows, 2015).

Alzheimer's disease

Alzheimer's disease was named after the clinician Alois Alzheimer in 1906. It is the most common cause of dementia, accounting for 60% to 70% of all cases across the world and 50% to 75% of cases in the UK (WHO, 2019a; NICE, 2019). It is caused by

- a build-up of amyloid plaques. These are types of proteins that clump together between the nerve cells in the brain
- an increase in neurofibrillary tangles, twisted fibres, in the brain
- a reduction of neurotransmitters, the chemicals that transmit messages between the brain cells

Together, these cause brain cells to die (Alzheimer's Society, 2020a; RCP, 2019).

Key features include

- memory loss, which is usually gradual and sometimes insidious
- difficulty in recalling recent events and learning new information
- progressive changes in personality and behaviour

(NICE 2019)

Whilst Alzheimer's disease often affects older people, around 5% of cases in the UK and world-wide are under 65. Some people living with Alzheimer's disease also experience symptoms and signs of vascular dementia or dementia with Lewy bodies. In these cases, a diagnosis of mixed dementia is given (ARUK, 2018a; NICE, 2019).

Vascular dementia

Vascular dementia makes up about 20% of all cases of dementia in the UK (NICE, 2019). It is caused when the blood fails to deliver enough oxygen to the brain cells, which then die (BHF, 2019; NICE, 2019). This can be due to a stroke or other damage to blood vessels.

Key features will vary according the location of damage in the brain. They include

- confusion
- difficulty in attention and speech
- memory loss
- gait/mobility problems
- changes in personality

(NICE, 2019)

Dementia with Lewy bodies

Dementia with Lewy bodies is the third most common type of dementia, accounting for 10% to 15% of all people living with dementia in the UK (ARUK, 2019). It is caused by

- abnormal deposits of protein inside the nerve cells in the brain. These are called Lewy bodies after Frederick Lewy who discovered them in 1912
- disruption to brain chemicals
- the loss of connections between nerve cells

Together, these cause brain cells to die (McKeith *et al.*, 2017; Alzheimer's Society, 2020a).

Key features will depend on the location of the Lewy bodies and include

- visual hallucinations
- fluctuating levels of cognitive impairment
- problems with movement, sometimes like the tremors or slow movements associated with Parkinson's disease

- rapid eye movement (REM) sleep behaviour disorder, which means someone may act out vivid dreams with sound and bodily movements

(Kane *et al.*, 2018; McKeith *et al.*, 2017; Outeiro *et al.*, 2019)

Frontotemporal dementia

Frontotemporal dementia, formerly called Pick's disease, occurs in around 2% of all dementia cases in the UK (NICE, 2019). About one-third have some family history of dementia (Alzheimer's Society, 2020a). It is a significant cause of dementia in people aged under 65 and is the third most common cause of young-onset dementia. It is caused by an accumulation of tau proteins, called Pick bodies, in the brain which cause the gradual deterioration of the brain's frontal and/or temporal lobes (NICE 2019).

Key features include

- changes in personality and behaviour, such as poor judgement and foresight
- problems with understanding, speaking and writing
- problems with walking, balance and coordination
- problems with vision and mood
- muscle weakness and wasting

(Alzheimer's Society, 2020a; Alzheimer's Association, 2020)

There are about 200 types of dementia with different underlying causes and consequences for the lives of individuals.

Rising rates of dementia

About 50 million people are living with dementia across the world, and this figure is expected to reach 150 million by 2050, because about 10 million people are diagnosed each year (WHO, 2019a). Of these, almost 60% are expected to live in low- and middle-income countries (Prince *et al.*, 2014) (Figure 16.1).

In Europe, rates of dementia are expected to almost double by 2050 compared to 2019 (Alzheimer Europe, 2019) (Figure 16.4). This is because the prevalence of dementia rises with age, and life expectancy across Europe is increasing (Figure 16.2). More women are affected than men, so the anticipated increase is expected to fall disproportionately on women (Figure 16.3).

In the UK, there are around 885,000 people living with dementia. The number is expected to rise to 1.6 million people by 2040, and over two million by 2050 (Prince *et al.*, 2014; Wittenberg *et al.*, 2019) (Tables 16.1 and 16.2). The prevalence across age and sex mirrors the European data, across the four nations of the UK (Alzheimer Europe, 2019).

A person's dementia can be described as mild, moderate or severe. By 2040, researchers anticipate a 55% rise in mild dementia, a 33% rise in moderate dementia and a 109% rise in severe dementia in the UK (Wittenberg *et al.*, 2019). Northern Ireland is expected to see the greatest rise because it is anticipated that they will see a 58% increase in the number of over-65-year-olds by 2040. By contrast, the numbers of over-65s are expected to rise by 47% in England, 41% in Scotland and 33% in Wales (Wittenberg *et al.*, 2019) (Figure 16.5).

Across the world, the rates of dementia are expected to rise as people live longer, and this will affect relatively poorer countries the most.

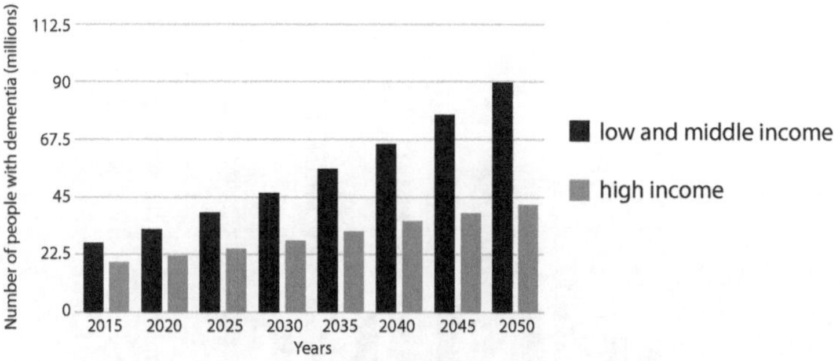

Figure 16.1 Projected rise in people with dementia according to country income, 2015 to 2050
Source: Prince *et al*, 2015

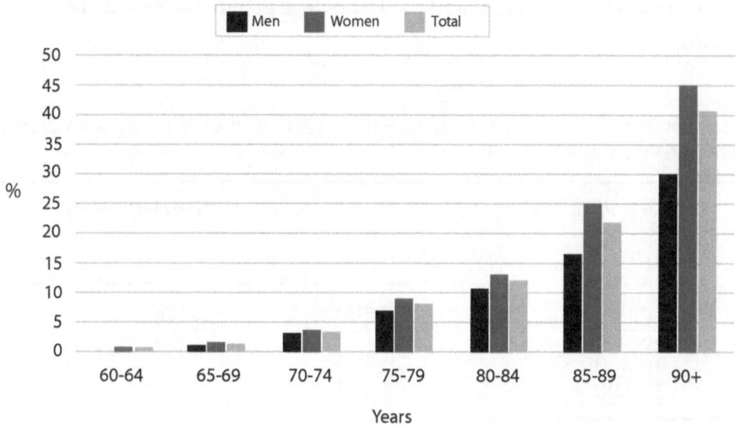

Figure 16.2 Prevalence of dementia in EU countries (including UK) by age and sex, 2019
Source: Alzheimer Europe, 2019

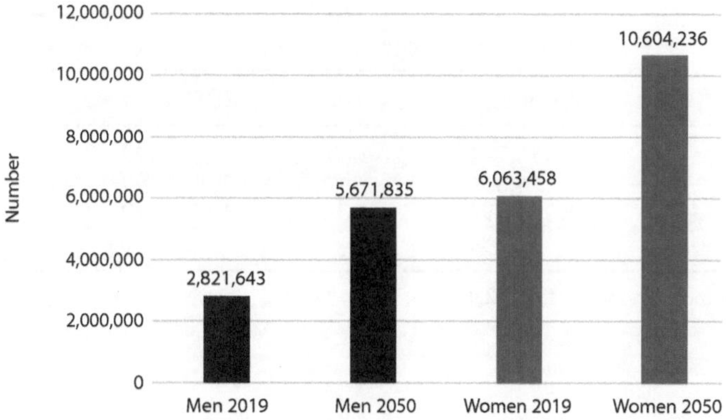

Figure 16.3 Predicted rise in numbers of men and women with dementia in EU countries (including UK), 2019 to 2050
Source: Alzheimer Europe, 2019

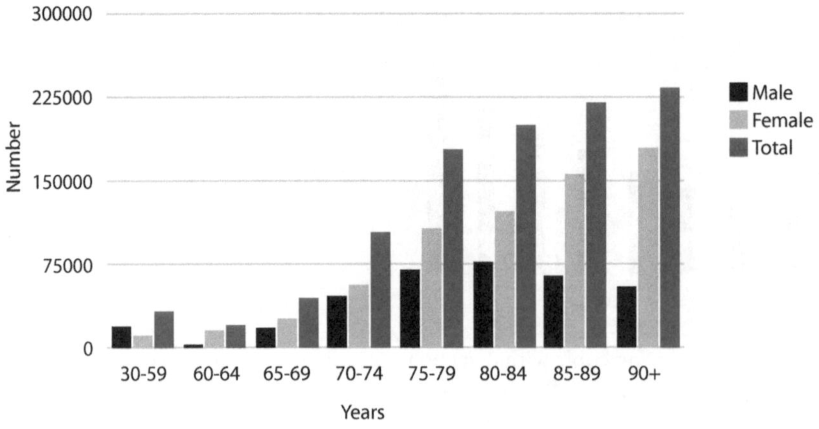

Figure 16.4 Number of people with dementia in the UK by age group and sex, 2018
Source: Alzheimer Europe, 2019

Table 16.1 Projected rise in the number of people aged 65 years and over living with dementia in the UK, 2019 to 2040

UK nation	*Number of people*		*Percentage rise*
	2019	*2040*	
England	748,000	1,352,400	81%
Scotland	66,200	115,100	74%
Wales	46,800	79,700	70%
Northern Ireland	22,100	42,800	95%

Source: Adapted from Wittenberg *et al.* (2019 p.4).

Table 16.2 Projected rise in the number of people living with dementia in the UK by sex, 2018 to 2050

	Number of people	
	2018	*2050*
Men	356,741	743,399
Women	674,656	1,233,999
Total	1,031,396	1,977,399
Percentage of UK population	1.56%	2.67%

Source: Adapted from Alzheimer Europe (2019 p.12,15).

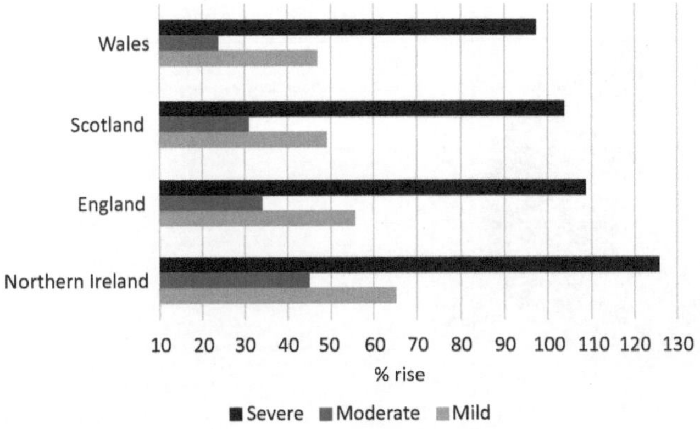

Figure 16.5 Projected percentage rise in older people living with mild, moderate and severe dementia in the UK, 2019 to 2040

Source: Wittenberg *et al*, 2019

Thinking point:

> As the number of people living with dementia rises, what challenges does this present for countries?

The impact of dementia

The impacts of dementia to countries, families and individuals are financial, social and personal. They include the cost of care, wider economic impacts, changes to people's social experiences and relationships as well as profound personal changes.

The financial cost of caring for people with dementia

The costs of caring for people with dementia are considerable and expected to rise. Dementia cost the UK £34.7 billion in 2019 (Wittenberg *et al.*, 2019). This was double the £15.8 billion spent on heart disease, and four times the £7.6 billion spent on cancer (Hilhorst and Lockey, 2019; PHE, 2019). By 2040, dementia is predicted to cost £94.1 billion, equating to a 172% rise from 2019 (Wittenberg *et al.*, 2019).

In the UK, how dementia is defined influences how the person's needs are defined and met.

- Dementia defined in the medical language of diagnosis, clinical tests, treatment and medication leads to a person's needs being defined as healthcare needs
- Dementia defined in terms of a person's need for help with dressing or shopping will lead to their needs being defined as social care needs
- Dementia defined in terms of a person's needs that can be, or are, met by family and friends are defined as unpaid/informal care needs

The type of care individuals need determines whether the costs of care will be paid by the state's healthcare or social care budget, or from neither. The consequences

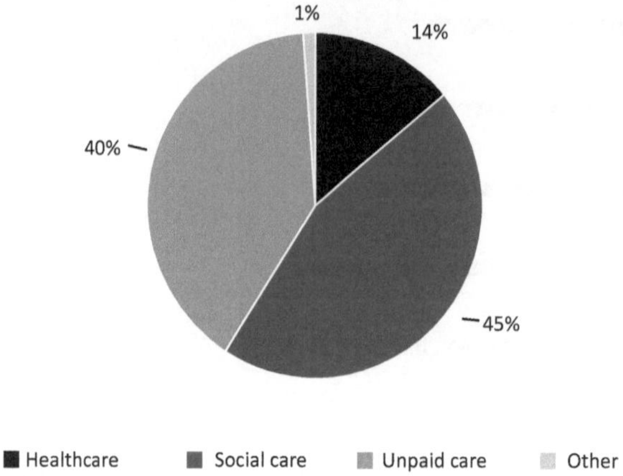

Figure 16.6 Proportionate costs of healthcare, social care and unpaid care for dementia in the UK, 2019

of such a complex system alongside the changing care needs of a person living with dementia, and the varying ability of individuals and families to be able to meet needs and access funding, has been the subject of much controversy over many decades (Balsinha *et al.*, 2019).

Healthcare costs

Healthcare costs are met by the National Health Service in the four nations of the UK. These include paying for diagnostic investigations, appointments, medication, hospital care and services such as physiotherapy, eye and hearing tests and foot care. In some areas, healthcare includes dementia-specialist Admiral Nurses (Dementia UK, 2020). The predicted rise in healthcare costs includes the higher needs of those with late-stage dementia requiring continuing care, although nursing home fees are not normally met by the healthcare budget.

Table 16.3 Predicted rise in UK dementia healthcare costs, 2019 to 2040

UK nation	*£ million*		*Percentage rise*
	2019	*2040*	
England	£4,100	£10,600	156%
Scotland	£370	£900	146%
Wales	£260	£630	143%
Northern Ireland	£120	£330	174%
UK total	£4,900	£12,500	155%

Source: Adapted from Wittenberg *et al.* (2019 p.7).

Social care costs

Social care is defined as:

> [Support for people] who are older or living with disability or physical or mental illness [to] live independently and stay well and safe.
>
> (Bottery *et al.*, 2019a)

Social care carried out in people's homes, called domiciliary care, aims to keep people living in their familiar community for as long as possible and to help them stay active and socially engaged. It may involve:

> ... routine household tasks within or outside the home, personal care of the client and other associated domestic services necessary to maintain an individual in an acceptable level of health, hygiene, dignity, safety and ease in their home.
>
> (DH, 2019 p.8)

Social care can also include short-term, temporary respite care or long-term care in a residential or nursing care home (Bottery *et al.*, 2019a). In the UK, the cost of social care is paid for by both local authorities and individuals. Those with higher assets/wealth, including their home, receive less from the local authority and need to pay proportionately more for services. In Scotland, individuals may receive more support from their local authority for personal care, compared to the rest of the UK (Alzheimer's Society, 2020b). In 2018, it was estimated that over 70% of older people residing in UK care homes had some form of dementia (Hutchings *et al.*, 2018). Nursing homes, unlike residential homes, provide nursing care in addition to personal care and are more likely to care for people with moderate to severe dementia (Prince *et al.*, 2014).

In 2018, in England, the average weekly cost of domiciliary care for an older person was £591, compared to the average care home cost of £933 (Bottery *et al.*, 2019b). However, for people living with dementia, the unit costs of domiciliary care rise as their condition progresses, and the cost of looking after someone in the later stages of dementia in their own home can match or exceed the cost of caring for a person in a nursing care home (Prince *et al.*, 2014).

Table 16.4 Predicted rise in UK dementia social care costs, 2019 to 2040

UK nation	*£ million*		*Percentage rise*
	2019	*2040*	
England	£13,500	£39,200	191%
Scotland	£1,100	£3,030	183%
Wales	£770	£2,130	176%
Northern Ireland	£340	£1,050	212%
UK total	£15,700	£12,500	190%

Source: Adapted from Wittenberg *et al.* (2019 p.7).

Unpaid care costs

Unpaid care, or informal care, is a

> ... private arrangement whereby someone cares for a family member, friend, or neighbour.
>
> (POST, 2018, p.1)

The carers of people living with dementia are a 'silent army' (Alzheimer's Society, 2018). In just one year, these carers provide the equivalent of 150,000 years, 1,340,000,000 hours, of care (Prince *et al.*, 2014). This army of over 700,000 people save the UK economy £13.9 billion a year, around one-third of the total annual cost of dementia care (Alzheimer's Society, 2018).

The costs of care to individuals and families

For people living with dementia and their families, financing care is complex, confusing and worrying. Typically, individuals spend up to £100,000 on their dementia care, which is about 40% more than the cost of social care for people without dementia (Hutchings *et al.*, 2018). The Alzheimer's Society reports that they often hear from people

> ... who have spent everything they have on care and have even sold their home. Others who need significant support have felt forced not to access care because of the expense. This puts their health, and sometimes the health of those around them, at risk.
>
> (Hutchings *et al.*, 2018 p.17)

The struggle to pay for care is also impacted by carers needing to reduce their employment income to be able to care (NHS Digital, 2017). In the UK, people with reduced incomes as a result of dementia may be entitled to some financial state benefits in the form of help with housing costs, personal support or local tax reductions (Gov. UK, 2020).

Table 16.5 Predicted rise in UK unpaid care contributions, 2019 to 2040

UK nation	*£ million*		*Percentage rise*
	2019	*2040*	
England	£11,700	£30,100	157%
Scotland	£1,100	£2,800	150%
Wales	£740	£1,770	141%
Northern Ireland	£350	£960	178%
UK total	£13,900	£35,700	156%

Source: Adapted from Wittenberg *et al.* (2019 p.7).

The wider economic impact of dementia

A large study into the impact of dementia on English businesses concluded that £4.2 billion of revenue was lost due to the syndrome, and this figure would rise to £5 billion by 2040. Financial losses related to

- the reducing skills of people with dementia
- the premature retirement of people with dementia
- presenteeism of carers; they are present at work, but less productive due to exhaustion, stress or other health problems
- carers reducing working hours to spend more time caring
- carers withdrawing from the workforce completely

(CEBR, 2019)

An additional impact on the wider economy relates to households that include a person living with dementia and the occupants as consumers. In England, in 2019, this group of the population spent £16.7 billion on recreational and cultural activities, household fuel/power, and food and non-alcoholic beverages. This figure is expected to nearly double to £33.9 billion by 2040 (CEBR, 2019). Although spending may be limited due to a reduction in income, 80% of carers of people with dementia report 'shopping' as a favourite activity (Bould and Hill, 2018). It remains to be seen whether commercial economic gains offset the rising costs of dementia over future decades, and the consequences for household expenditure.

The impact of dementia on carers

The impact of living with someone with dementia for families and friends who become their carers presents many challenges. In 2016/17 research in England found

- 68% of carers did not have as much social contact as they would like
- 63% had no or too little support
- 48% had long-standing illnesses
- 47% said they could not look after themselves well enough
- 36% spent more than 100 hours per week in their caring role
- 30% had been in their caring role for between 5 and 10 years
- 22% had been in their role for over 10 years
- 18% worried about their personal safety

(NHS Digital, 2017)

During the process of diagnosis, carers report feeling let down by healthcare professionals, feeling unheard and distressed by the burdensome bureaucratic dementia care system (Cruse Bereavement Care, 2019). As the relationship with the cared-for changes, carers report a sense of loss:

> You lose the support of your partner because they can't support you anymore.
> (Cruse Bereavement Care, 2019 p.14)

Some carers express a loss of identity:

> I can't be the wife, I've got to be the carer. I am different people, so I don't know who I am half the time when he is asking me questions.
>
> (Skingley *et al.*, 2020 p.8)

Carers often feel alone in making efforts to keep their cared-for engaged in a meaningful relationship and activities. Here, a wife encourages her husband to dance and sing with limited success:

> He stands up and I put my arms around him, I know he is not very steady but he remembers what he has to do more or less and I do a lot of singing you know, to cheer myself up and I will say come on, you know this.
>
> (Chung, 2013 p.11)

Carers' physical health is hampered by broken sleep, having to 'eat on the go' and having few opportunities for being outside and exercising (Carers UK, 2019; Cruse Bereavement Care, 2019). Their exhaustion is compounded by the weight of responsibility and a dichotomy of emotions:

> [Caring is] frustrating and draining … and can lead to you losing your temper and then feeling guilty afterwards.
>
> (Cruse Bereavement Care, 2019 p.18)

While many carers appreciate their ability to support the cared-for when most needed, this can create tensions for them; for example,

> I have to be rude sometimes during social occasions to put my husband and his wellbeing first.
>
> (Cruse Bereavement Care, 2019 p.18)

Many carers report feeling lonely, being socially isolated and losing their independence (Carers UK, 2019). One UK survey found 57% of carers reported losing touch with family and friends due to their caring responsibilities (Carers UK, 2019). This may be because of poor understanding on the part of others, or it may be because the carer wishes to protect others from stress.

> They've [other family members] got their own problems. They're so busy with their working lives … I don't want to burden them with it.
>
> (ARUK, 2015 p.25)

The personal impact of dementia

Every person with dementia is unique and is influenced by their own subjective experiences. The late Professor Tom Kitwood suggested that a person's experience and expression of their dementia are the result of five interrelated factors, their

- neurological impairment
- personality
- biography
- health
- social-psychological environment

(Kitwood, 1993)

People with dementia often express confusion and uncertainty. They have concerns about a lack of support and feelings of being stigmatised.

> When I was diagnosed with dementia it felt like falling off a cliff into a dark hole, I struggled to find information and access services ... viewed by medical professionals as a hopeless case, not a person with a disability needing support and services to live as well as possible.
>
> (Alzheimer Europe, 2018 p.16)

Some are frustrated due to a lack of public understanding about dementia.

> They don't always believe me, they say you don't look like you've got it and I say, 'What should I look like then?'
>
> (Dementia Action Alliance, 2017 p.11)

Many report experiencing depression, guilt, fear, anxiety and a loss of self-worth. In turn, this leads to isolation.

> ... I went into absolute depression and guilt, lost ... my confidence and ... self-worth ... I felt ... I'd put my family in this position.
>
> (Alzheimer's Society, 2017, p.5)

> My biggest fear is not being able to help my family in future.
>
> (Quinn, 2020)

> You can't socialise because ... people sometimes don't understand.
>
> (Alzheimer's Society, 2017 p.5)

They face challenges to adapt their daily life and worry about the cost of their care.

> Everything has to be structured and routine.
>
> (Alzheimer's Society, 2017 p.5)

> My writing used to be small, but now it is diabolical.
>
> (Dementia Action Alliance, 2017 p.8)

> ... the cost is enormous I would fear.
>
> (Alzheimer's Society, 2017 p.19)

Despite the challenges faced by people with dementia, many become advocates for change, providing a voice in literature, research and policy (e.g. Swaffer, 2016; Oliver, 2019). They challenge the stereotypes and myths of dementia and want the public and professionals to see them as *a person (with dementia)* who has self-agency, a desire to be part of the community and wants to continue to use their remaining abilities, just like everyone else.

> I am still the same person that I was yesterday.
>
> (Dementia Action Alliance, 2017 p.7)

> [you have to] just get on with life as it hits you ... You have to be resilient and you take life as it treats you ... we have to look at ourselves with a sense of humour.
>
> (Chung, 2019 p.719)

> What is important to me is being part of a community – meeting other people.
>
> (Dementia Action Alliance, 2017 p.7)

Dementia and mortality

Dementia is the leading cause of death in the UK (ONS, 2019). It accounts for 12.8% of all deaths in England and Wales; 15.1% of deaths in males over 80 and 23.6% of deaths in females over 80. This reflects the fact that dementia tends to occur in older age, recent improvements in the diagnosis of dementia and better reporting of dementia on death certificates. Dementia actively damages the brain and, as the brain is the 'control centre' for the whole body, the body can no longer function properly, and a person becomes susceptible to infections. Once body systems begin to shut down, death becomes inevitable.

> *Dementia has a significant impact on the economy and individuals. The burden of dementia is largely borne by people living with the condition, their families and carers.*

Risk factors for dementia

There is no single approach to preventing all types of dementia, but here are the main non-modifiable and modifiable risk factors that seem to be important.

Non-modifiable risk factors

The non-modifiable risk factors for dementia relate to age, sex, genetics/family history and ethnicity.

Age and sex

- The risk of developing dementia doubles every five years after the age of 65
- Age-related dementia is associated with an increase in the prevalence of other common age-related diseases
- Women are more likely than men to develop dementia throughout their lifetimes

(Jorm and Jolley, 1998; Corrada *et al.*, 2010; ARUK, 2018c; Alzheimer Europe, 2019)

Genes and family history

- Genetic links have been found in some people with early-onset Alzheimer's disease, behavioural variant frontotemporal dementia and a rare form of vascular dementia, called cerebral autosomal dominant arteriopathy with subcortical infarcts and leukoencephalopathy
- Certain genetic factors increase the risk of Parkinson's disease, which precipitates dementia in around 50% of cases
- Many people with Down's syndrome have protein deposits in the brain characteristic of Alzheimer's disease. About 30% develop the condition by age 50 and 50% by age 60

(Hanagasi *et al.*, 2017; ARUK, 2018a; BPS, 2015; NICE 2019)

Ethnicity

- In the UK, the risk of dementia is higher among black ethnic groups (African, Caribbean, or other black background) than in white ethnic groups (British or other white background)
- The risk of dementia is lower in UK Asian ethnic groups (Indian, Pakistani, Bangladeshi, Chinese, or other Asian) than white ethnic groups
- Current data may include some underdiagnoses among some ethnic groups, and more research is needed to understand the reasons for the differences

(Pham *et al.*, 2018; Rocca, 2017)

Modifiable risk factors for dementia

People may be able to decrease their chances of developing dementia by reducing the risks associated with cardiovascular disease and type 2 diabetes, social isolation and loneliness, intellectual inactivity and enduring depressive disorders (Table 16.6).

Cardiovascular disease and type 2 diabetes

The modifiable risk factors for both cardiovascular disease and type 2 diabetes are linked. For example, both are strongly associated with excess weight and the causes of weight gain such as inactivity and a high-calorie diet. Both conditions damage blood vessels and impede the healthy flow of blood, which can lead to high blood pressure, atherosclerosis (fatty cholesterol plaques which narrow vessels) or thromboses (clots). Both conditions affect the blood circulation through the brain, reducing its functioning and increasing risks of dementia (Justin *et al.*, 2013; Vijayan and Reddy, 2016). In addition, tobacco smoking, a poor-quality diet, inactivity and heavy drinking directly damage blood vessels, the quality of the blood and its circulation. Excess alcohol also causes nerve damage. These health-related behaviours are discussed in more detail in other chapters of this book. They all contribute to a stroke (clot or haemorrhage in the brain) and may contribute to developing dementia.

Social isolation and loneliness

Social isolation and feelings of loneliness are both directly associated with an increased risk of developing dementia (Kuiper *et al.*, 2015; Sutin *et al.*, 2018). Social isolation increases the risk of developing cardiovascular disease, including high blood pressure, and can lead to depressive behaviours (Xia and Li, 2018). Even individuals who have relatively frequent interactions with others, but who feel lonely, have an increased risk of developing dementia (Rafnsson *et al.*, 2017). There are three ways in which loneliness is thought to affect people's conscious mental processes, their cognition, and increase their risks of dementia.

- People who are lonely are more likely to smoke tobacco and be inactive
- Loneliness is associated high blood pressure, obesity and type 2 diabetes
- Loneliness is associated with disruptions in the physical workings of the body, including chronic low-grade inflammation, which is linked to increased risk of dementia
- Loneliness includes negative emotions, which are a risk factor for general poor health and dementia

(Sutin *et al.*, 2018)

Intellectual inactivity

The hypothesis that dementia may be prevented by mental activities has emerged from the concept of cognitive reserve. Stern (2009) explains there are individual differences in how people respond to similar brain damage. Some people's cognition, their memory, thinking and learning, hardly change, while others experience cognitive impairments. Cognitive reserve means

> The brain actively copes with brain damage using pre-existing cognitive processes or by enlisting compensatory processes.
>
> (Stern, 2009 p.2)

The more cognitive reserve one has, the better one can tolerate and cope with equal brain damage compared with someone with lower cognitive reserve, who will show signs of impairment sooner. The thinking is that intellectual and other activities may induce neuroplasticity in the brain. This is a 'rewiring process' where nerve cells grow new connections with one another. Neuroplasticity is the way that the brain constantly adapts to events, including recovering from physical or psychological traumas; it is how it learns and lays down memories. Christie and colleagues (2017) explain that research studies have suggested that lower levels of education and occupational attainment are associated with lower levels of cognitive reserve and then earlier signs of dementia.

Enduring depressive disorders

There is a strong relationship between people suffering from enduring depressive disorders and poor health-related behaviours such as tobacco smoking, low levels of physical activity, heavy alcohol consumption, high-calorie/high-fat diets and metabolic syndrome: all significant risk factors for cardiovascular disease (Cabello *et al.*, 2017; Bonnet *et al.*, 2005). In addition, low social engagement and lowered cognitive activity increase the risks of developing dementia.

Table 16.6 Risk factors and mediating conditions that increase risks of dementia

Risk factor	*Resulting conditions lead to increased risk of dementia*
Physical inactivity	Cardiovascular disease Overweight/obesity Type 2 diabetes
Unhealthy diet (e.g. high calorie, high saturated fat, salt and sugar)	Cardiovascular disease Overweight/obesity Type 2 diabetes
Smoking tobacco	Cardiovascular disease Oxidative stress leading to brain cell damage
Hazardous and harmful intakes of alcohol	Cardiovascular disease Damage to nervous system including brain cells Vitamin B1 deficiency leading to Korsakoff's syndrome, a type of dementia
Social isolation and loneliness	Cardiovascular disease Low mood, depression Smoking Obesity
Intellectual inactivity	Cognitive decline
Enduring depressive disorders	Health-related behaviours that are strongly linked to cardiovascular disease Low social engagement Low cognitive engagement

Other modifiable risk factors

The risks of dementia are also increased by long-term exposure to air pollution; hearing impairment, which is thought to limit cognitive stimulation; less childhood education, which may be associated with lower cognitive reserve; and traumatic brain injury through sports such as boxing or riding, and traffic accidents (Peters *et al.*, 2019; Grande *et al.*, 2020; Livingston *et al.*, 2020).

> *Although age is the strongest risk factor for cognitive decline, risks from health-related behaviours can be modified.*

Thinking point:

> To what extent do you think the general public are aware that we can reduce our risks of developing dementia?

Primary prevention of dementia

The primary prevention of dementia means addressing the modifiable risk factors in earlier life to prevent cognitive decline. As many of the modifiable risk factors overlap with other major diseases, such as cardiovascular disease, preventing dementia can easily be integrated with other preventive programmes. The strength of the evidence for preventing cognitive decline is stronger for some interventions than others.

Table 16.7 Primary prevention of cognitive decline and/or dementia

Risk factor	*Recommended action to reduce cognitive decline*	*Strength of the recommendation that it prevents cognitive decline in adults with normal cognition* (percentage reduction in population prevalence if risk factor is eliminated**)*	*Benefits of recommended action to health and prevention of cognitive decline*
Physical inactivity	Encourage activity	Strong (2%)	Activity improves mobility, balance, mood and cognitive ability. It also decreases risk of falls. Reduces risks of cardiovascular disease. All decrease chances of cognitive decline.
Unhealthy diet (e.g. high calorie, high saturated fat, salt and sugar)	Encourage Mediterranean-style diet	Unsure. Different choices may be appropriate for some individuals.	Reduces risks of cardiovascular disease. Encourages lower weight, lower blood glucose and lower insulin resistance which will decrease risk of type 2 diabetes. Both decrease chances of cognitive decline.
Overweight and obesity	Weight management towards a 'normal range' body mass index	Unsure. Different choices may be appropriate for some individuals. (1%)	Reduces risks of cardiovascular disease and type 2 diabetes. Both decrease chances of cognitive decline.
Hypertension (high blood pressure)	Management towards a 'healthy range' blood pressure	Unsure. Different choices may be appropriate for some individuals. (2%)	Decreases pressure and damage to blood vessels and therefore chances of cognitive decline.
Smoking tobacco	Smoking cessation and protect others from smoke	Strong (5%)	Reduces risk of cardiovascular disease which decreases chances of cognitive decline.
Diabetes	Management towards a 'healthy range' blood glucose level	Unsure. Different choices may be appropriate for some individuals. (1%)	Reduces damage to blood vessels and risks of cardiovascular disease, which decreases chances of cognitive decline
Hazardous or harmful intakes of alcohol	Reduce or cease hazardous or harmful drinking	Unsure. Different choices may be appropriate for some individuals. (1%)	Reduces risks of cardiovascular disease and damage to nerve/ brain cells. Both decrease chances of cognitive decline.

Table 16.7 Cont.

Risk factor	*Recommended action to reduce cognitive decline*	*Strength of the recommendation that it prevents cognitive decline in adults with normal cognition* (percentage reduction in population prevalence if risk factor is eliminated**)*	*Benefits of recommended action to health and prevention of cognitive decline*
Intellectual inactivity	Cognitive interventions	Unsure. Different choices may be appropriate for some individuals.	Mental activities add to cognitive reserve which may prevent or delay cognitive decline.
Hearing impairment	Hearing checks/ hearing aids	(8%)	Helps to maintain cognitive stimulation.
Less childhood education	Prioritise childhood education for all	(7%)	Increases cognitive ability/reserve.
Traumatic brain injury	Road, military and sports safety measures	(3%)	Protects the brain from injury.
Air pollution	Reduce exposure to air pollution	(2%)	Reduces damage to blood vessels.
Social isolation and loneliness	Social activity	Insufficient evidence (4%)	Social participation and social inclusion are strongly connected with general health and wellbeing and may help to provide mental stimulation.
Enduring depressive disorders	Use of antidepressants and psychological interventions	Insufficient evidence (4%)	People with better mental health are more likely to be motivated towards healthy behaviours such as activity, healthy eating.

Sources: Peters *et al.* (2019); *WHO (2019b); **Livingstone *et al.* (2020); BHF, 2019.

Secondary prevention of dementia

The secondary prevention of dementia concerns screening, early diagnosis and interventions at the earliest stages of cognitive decline before symptoms cause disability (Savica and Peterson, 2011). Misconceptions and negative attitudes towards dementia can act as barriers to people seeking early diagnosis and care (ADI, 2019). In the UK, a person suspected of having dementia is commonly referred to a specialist memory clinic by their general practitioner. Here, the healthcare professional asks about the individual's health/medical history, reviews any current medicines, asks the individual to complete a cognitive test, takes blood tests and may suggest that they have a brain scan.

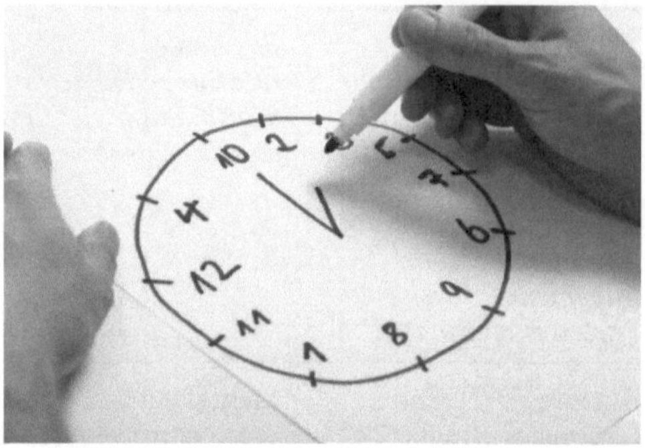

Figure 16.7 A screening test for dementia
Source: Andrey_Popov/Shutterstock.com

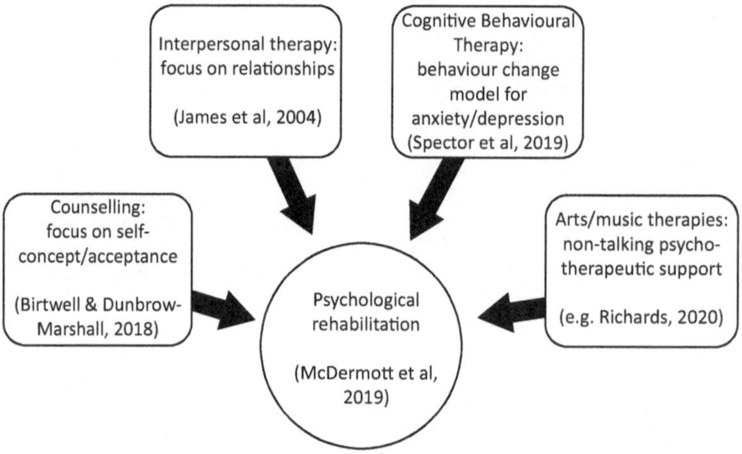

Figure 16.8 Psychological therapies to help people to adjust to their diagnosis of dementia

Once dementia is diagnosed, the individual is referred to the healthcare professionals who can best meet their needs. These include psychiatrists, geriatricians, psychologists, occupational therapists and dementia-specialist nurses (RCP, 2019). Many will be prescribed medicines to help with the cognitive symptoms, such as difficulties with learning and memory, alongside medicines to help with any additional medical needs (NICE, 2019). Some may benefit from psychological therapies to help them to come to terms with their diagnosis.

Social prescribing

In the UK, many people living with dementia benefit from social prescribing. Social prescribing is partly funded by the government, who recognise it makes an important contribution to maximising and prolonging people's functioning and wellbeing, as well as the wellbeing of their carers (NICE, 2018; Alzheimer's Society, 2020c).

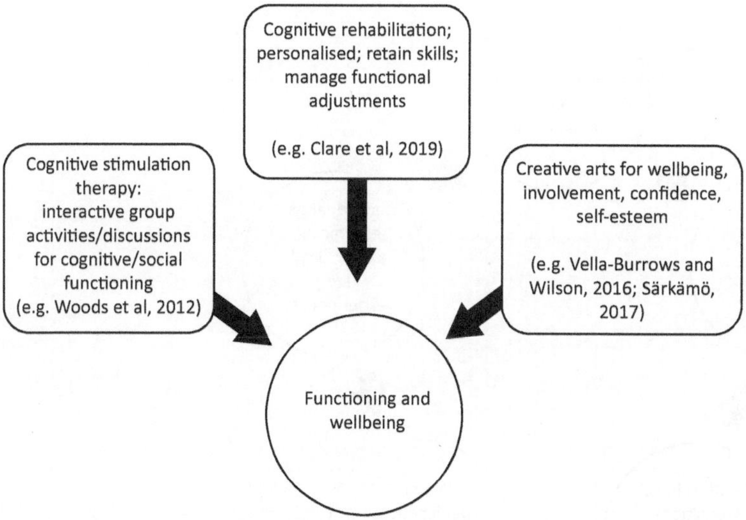

Figure 16.9 Interventions to maximise functioning and wellbeing for people with dementia

Healthcare professionals can make a referral and, normally, a social prescribing link worker directs the individual to appropriate social activities, such as art, music or dance, in the local community (Baker and Irving, 2015). The prime aim is to maintain the individual's quality of life, and in so doing, reduce the personal, social and economic burden to individuals, carers, households and to the wider society.

Person-centred care

In the UK, the aim is to provide every person diagnosed with dementia with personalised, meaningful care throughout the course of their condition. Person-centred care (Figure 16.10) means prioritising

- the human value of the person living with dementia, their carers and families
- the individuality of the person living with dementia
- the person's perspective
- relationships and interactions for the person living with dementia
- support for carers

(NICE, 2018)

Tertiary prevention of dementia

Tertiary prevention

> ... focuses on reducing [the] negative impact of an existing disease through restoring function and reducing complications.
>
> (Alzheimer's Society, 2020d)

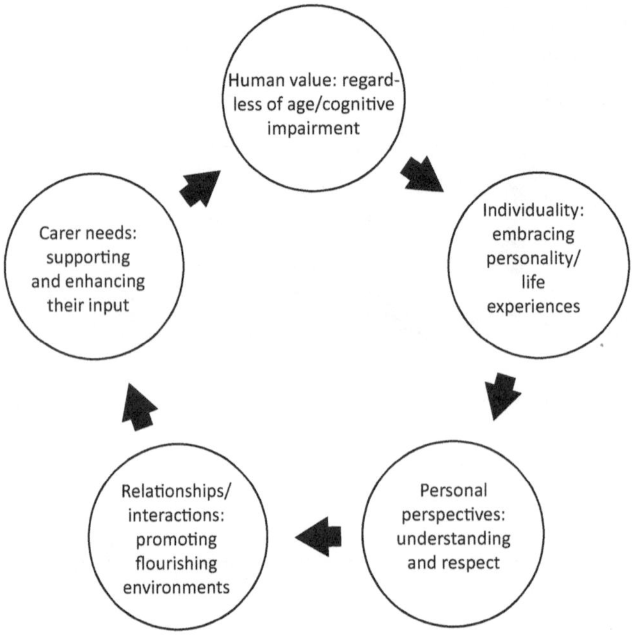

Figure 16.10 Principles of person-centred care for people living with dementia and carers
Source: NICE, 2018

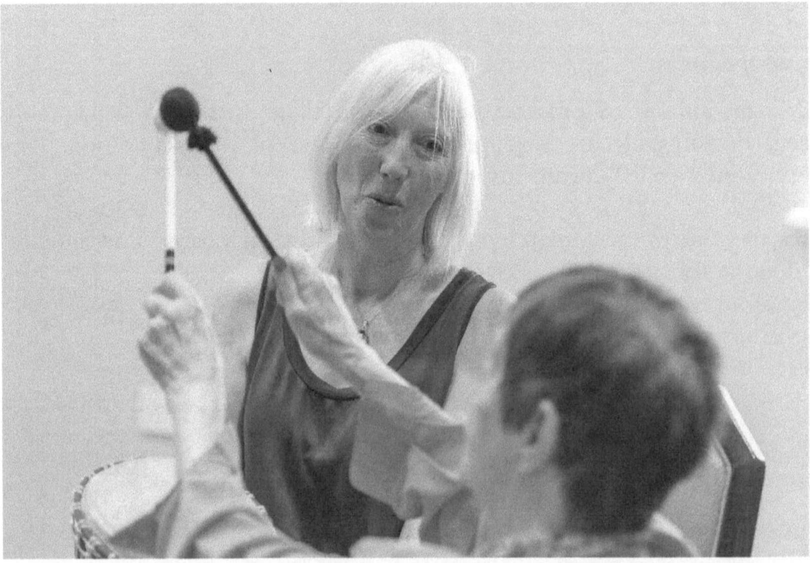

Figure 16.11 Therapeutic music activities can enhance involvement, self-confidence and self-esteem
Source: Reproduced with permission from Alan Langley

A whole range of complex and individual factors influence the progression of dementia. Medicines may do little or nothing to halt the changes in cognition, but individuals are sometimes prescribed medicines to help with symptoms such as depression or agitation (Knapp *et al.*, 2017). Attention turns to providing holistic, meaningful and personalised psychosocial interventions that support a good quality of life, personal growth and fulfilment, regardless of someone's cognitive abilities (Joplin, 2017; NCCMH, 2018; NICE, 2018). These include

- information on living well with dementia, e.g. daily living, staying well, finance, legal advice, sources of support
- education, e.g. dementia awareness, training for carers
- supportive communities, e.g. understanding and stigma-free groups
- support for carers, e.g. respite care, peer support for carers
- cognitive support groups, e.g. cafés and clubs that host groups for social activities
- individualised therapeutic activities, e.g. group singing, walking, gardening, outings to heritage sites

Box 16.1 A dementia-friendly community

A dementia-friendly community is a place, such as a village, town or city, where people living with dementia are understood, respected and supported. It is a place where everyone, from those in local shops and local government, to churches and book shops, understands dementia and helps to create an environment where people with the syndrome feel included, active, engaged and valued.

The City of York was one of the first multidisciplinary, intergenerational dementia-friendly communities. It has put in place several initiatives, including:

- GCSE drama students at the Joseph Rowntree Foundation School devised a theatre piece to raise awareness about people living with dementia among young people
- the Energise Leisure Centre provided games such as Jiminy Wicket (croquet-based) for people living with dementia to try out new fitness routines
- training about dementia was provided for British Transport Police, which helped people living with dementia and their families to feel more confident when travelling by rail

Today, there are 137 dementia-friendly communities across England and Wales. A champion group leads the work and provides guidance for all sectors, including business, finance, technology, housing and utilities, sport and leisure, tourism, retail, health and social care, those in rural areas and faith communities. For example, faith groups can help people living with dementia who are isolated by encouraging volunteers to provide support, ensuring people have phone numbers for food deliveries and providing specific dementia telephone help-lines. Heritage organisations can distribute printed reminiscence packs.

(Source: Alzheimer's Society, 2020e; Joseph Rowntree Foundation, 2012).

Individual interventions need to sit within a deep social acceptance of people living with dementia, the 'social model of disability', which means

- listening to personal experiences
- focusing on people's abilities not their losses
- working towards dementia-friendly communities that draw on people's strengths and capabilities
- providing timely, accessible and person-centred support services, such as post-diagnosis services and advice web sites
- developing housing, transport, technology and care services to enable people to live well with dementia
- ensuring that both the social and built environment enables people living with dementia to thrive
- addressing discrimination/marginalisation
- respecting human rights and rights to equal citizenship

(Joplin 2017)

The primary, secondary and tertiary prevention of dementia is about preventing and delaying cognitive decline, maximising people's quality of life, supporting carers, full social inclusion and decreasing the strain on national economies.

Summary

This chapter has

- defined dementia as a cluster of symptoms caused by a variety of injuries or diseases that affect the brain
- described four of the more common types of dementia
- discussed the rising rates of dementia across the world, including the UK
- explained the economic, social and personal impacts of dementia for countries, families, carers and individuals
- discussed the non-modifiable and modifiable risk factors for developing dementia
- described the primary, secondary and tertiary prevention of dementia

Further reading

Brooker, D. (ed), and Kitwood, T.M. (2019) *Dementia reconsidered, revisited. The person still comes first.* 2nd edn. London: Open University Press

Oliver, K. (2019) *Dear Alzheimer's. A diary of living with dementia.* London: Jessica Kingsley

World Health Organization (2017) *Global action plan on the public health response to dementia 2017–2025.* Geneva: World Health Organization

Useful websites

Age UK Available at: www.ageuk.org.uk
Arts 4 Dementia Available at: https://arts4dementia.org.uk
Alzheimer's Society Available at: www.alzheimers.org.uk
Alzheimer Europe Available at: www.alzheimer-europe.org

References

Alzheimer's Association (2020) Frontotemporal dementia. Available at: www.alz.org/alzheimers-dementia/what-is-dementia/types-of-dementia/frontotemporal-dementia (Accessed 7th March 2020)

Alzheimer Europe (2018) *Dementia in Europe year book 2018. Comparison of national dementia strategies in Europe*. Luxembourg: Alzheimer Europe

Alzheimer Europe (2019) *Dementia in Europe year book 2019. Estimating the prevalence of dementia in Europe*. Luxembourg: Alzheimer Europe

Alzheimer's Disease International (2019) World Alzheimer report 2019. Attitudes to dementia. Available at: www.alz.co.uk/research/WorldAlzheimerReport2019.pdf (Accessed 21st March 2020)

Alzheimer's Research UK (2015) Dementia in the family. The impact on carers. Available at www.alzheimersresearchuk.org/wp-content/uploads/2019/09/Dementia-in-the-Family-The-impact-on-carers1.pdf. (Accessed 12th May 2020)

Alzheimer's Research UK (2018a) Types of dementia. Available at: www.alzheimersresearchuk.org/about-dementia/types-of-dementia/ (Accessed 21st March 2020)

Alzheimer's Research UK (2018b) Dementia attitudes monitor. Wave 1 2018. Available at: www.dementiastatistics.org/wp-content/uploads/2019/02/Dementia-Attitudes-Monitor-Wave-1-Report.pdf (Accessed 21st March 2020)

Alzheimer's Research UK (2018c) Prevalence by age in the UK. Available at: www.dementiastatistics.org/statistics/prevalence-by-age-in-the-uk/ (Accessed 21st March 2020)

Alzheimer's Research UK (2019) Dementia with Lewy bodies. Available at: www.alzheimersresearchuk.org/about-dementia/types-of-dementia/dementia-with-lewy-bodies/about/ (Accessed 21st March 2020)

Alzheimer's Society (2017) Turning up the volume: unheard voices of people with dementia. Available at: www.alzheimers.org.uk/sites/default/files/migrate/downloads/turning_up_the_volume_unheard_voices_of_people_with_dementia.pdf (Accessed 15th June 2020)

Alzheimer's Society (2018) Carers for people with dementia struggling in silence. Available at: www.alzheimers.org.uk/news/2018-06-22/carers-people-dementia-struggling-silence (Accessed 20th February 2020)

Alzheimer's Society (2020a) Types of dementia. Available at: www.alzheimers.org.uk/about-dementia/types-dementia (Accessed 21st March 2020)

Alzheimer's Society (2020b) How much does dementia care cost? Available at: www.alzheimers.org.uk/blog/how-much-does-dementia-care-cost (Accessed 4th March 2020)

Alzheimer's Society (2020c) Personalised care, social prescribing, assessment and improvement. Available at: www.alzheimers.org.uk/dementia-professionals/dementia-experience-toolkit/need-measure-experience//personalised-care-social-prescribing (Accessed 5th May 2020)

Alzheimer Society (2020d) Alzheimer's Society's view on public health, prevention and dementia. Available at: www.alzheimers.org.uk/about-us/policy-and-influencing/what-we-think/public-health-prevention-dementia (Accessed 1st January, 2020)

Alzheimer's Society (2020e) Making your community more dementia friendly. Available at: www.alzheimers.org.uk/get-involved/dementia-friendly-communities/making-your-community-more-dementia-friendly (Accessed 16th June 2020)

Baker, K., and Irving, A. (2015) 'Co-producing approaches to the management of dementia through social prescribing', *Social Policy and Administration*, 50(3), pp.379–397

Balsinha, C., Gonçalves-Pereira, M., Iliffe, S., Freitas, J.A., and Grave, J. (2019) 'Health-care delivery for older people with dementia in primary care', in de Mendonça Lima, C., and Ivbijaro, G. (eds) *Primary care mental health in older people*. New York: Springer International, pp.311–329

Birtwell, K., and Dubrow-Marshall, L. (2018) 'Psychological support for people with dementia: a preliminary study', *Counselling and Psychotherapy Research*, 18(1), pp.79–88

Bonnet, F., Irving, K., Terra, J.L., Nonym, P., Berthezene, F., and Moulin, P. (2005) 'Depressive symptoms are associated with unhealthy lifestyles in hypertensive patients with metabolic syndrome', *Journal of Hypertension*, 23(3), pp.611–617

Bottery, S., Ward. D., and Fenney, D. (2019a) Key facts and figures about adult social care. The Kings Fund. Available at www.kingsfund.org.uk/audio-video/key-facts-figures-adult-social-care (Accessed 5th May 2020)

Bottery, S., Ward, D., and Fenney, D. (2019b) Social care 360. The Kings Fund. Available at: www.kingsfund.org.uk/publications/social-care-360 (Accessed 5th May 2020)

Bould, E. and Hill, H. (2018) The dementia friendly retail guide. Available at: www.alzheimers.org.uk/sites/default/files/2019-07/AS_NEW_DF_Retail_Guide_Available_09_07_19.pdf. (Accessed 15th March 2020)

British Heart Foundation (2019) Vascular dementia. Available at: www.bhf.org.uk/informationsupport/conditions/vascular-dementia (Accessed 21st March 2020)

British Psychological Society (2015) Dementia and people with intellectual disabilities. Guidance on the assessment, diagnosis, interventions and support of people with intellectual disabilities who develop dementia. Available at: www.bps.org.uk/sites/www.bps.org.uk/files/Member%20Networks/Faculties/Intellectual%20Disabilities/Dementia%20and%20People%20with%20Learning%20Disabilities%20%282015%29.pdf (Accessed 5th May 2020)

Burns, A., and Iliffe, S. (2009) 'Dementia', *British Medical Journal*, 338 doi:10.1136/bmj.b75

Cabello, M., Miret, M., Caballero, F.F., Chatterji, S., Naidoo, N., Kowal, P., D'Este, C., and Ayuso-Mateos, J. (2017) 'The role of unhealthy lifestyles in the incidence and persistence of depression: a longitudinal general population study in four emerging countries', *Global Health*, 13(18) doi:10/1186/s12992-017-0237-5

Carers UK (2019) State of caring. A snapshot of unpaid care in the UK. Available at: www.carersuk.org/images/News__campaigns/CUK_State_of_Caring_2019_Report.pdf (Accessed 12th May 2020)

Centre for Economics and Business Research (2019) The economic cost of dementia to English businesses-2019 update. A report for Alzheimer's society. Available at: www.alzheimers.org.uk/sites/default/files/2019-09/The%20economic%20cost%20of%20dementia%20to%20English%20businesses%20-%20edited.pdf (Accessed 7th January 2020)

Christie, G.J., Hamilton, T., Manor, B.D., Farb, N.A.S., Farzan, F., Sixsmith, A., Temprado, J., and Moreno, S. (2017) 'Do lifestyle activities protect against cognitive decline in ageing? A review', *Frontiers in Aging Neuroscience*, 9(381) doi:10.3389/fnagi.2017.00381

Chung, P. (2013) 'Professionals partnering with family carers in home-based activity for those with dementia', *World Federation of Occupational Therapists Bulletin*, 67(1), pp.9–16

Chung, P. (2019) 'Experiences of older people with dementia: homecare enablement to support transitions in daily life at home', *British Journal of Occupational Therapy*, 82(12), pp.716–725

Clare, L., Kudlicka, A., Oyebode, J., Jones, R., Bayer, A., Leroi, I., Kopelman, M., James, I.A., Culverwell, A., Pool, J., Brand, A., Henderson, C., Hoare, Z., Knapp, M., Morgan-Trimmer, S., Burns, A., Corbett, A., Whitaker, R., and Woods, B. (2019) 'Goal-oriented cognitive rehabilitation for early-stage Alzheimer's and related dementias: the GREAT RCT', *Health Technology Assessment*, 23(10), pp.1–242

Corrada, M.M., Brookmeyer, R., Paganini-Hill, A., Berlau, D., and Kawas, C.H. (2010) 'Dementia incidence continues to increase with age in the oldest old: the 90+ study', *Annals of Neurology*, 67(1), pp.114–121

Cruse Bereavement Care (2019) Carers' stories: loss along the journey. Supporting people living with dementia. A guide for carers written by carers. Available at: www.cruse.org.uk/sites/default/files/default_images/pdf/Documents-and-fact-sheets/Cruse_Carers_Stories_Booklet_AW_DIGITAL%20FINAL.pdf (Accessed 7th May 2020)

Dementia Action Alliance (2017) Review of the dementia statements. Companion paper. Available at: www.dementiaaction.org.uk/assets/0003/3965/Companion_document_August_2017_branded_final.pdf (Accessed 16th June 2020)

Dementia UK (2020) What is an admiral nurse and how can they help? Available at: www.dementiauk.org/get-support/admiral-nursing/ (Accessed 5th May 2020)

Department of Health (2019) Domiciliary care services for adults in Northern Ireland in 2019. Available at: www.health-ni.gov.uk/articles/domiciliary-care (Accessed 2nd January 2020)

Foley, T., and Swanwick, G. (2014) Dementia: diagnosis and management in general practice. Irish College of General Practitioners Quality in Practice Committee. Available at: http://dementia.ie/images/uploads/site-images/ICGP_QIP_Dementia.pdf (Accessed 5th May 2020)

Gov.UK (2020) Carers and disability benefits. Available at: www.gov.uk/browse/benefits/disability (Accessed 4th February 2020)

Grande, G,, Ljungman, P.L.S., Eneroth, K., Bellander, T., and Rizzuto, D. (2020) 'Association between cardiovascular disease and long-term exposure to air pollution with the risk of dementia', *JAMA Neurology*, 77 doi10.1001/jamaneurol.2019.4914

Hanagasi, H., Tufekcioglu, Z., and Emre, M. (2017) 'Dementia in Parkinson's disease', *Journal of Neurological Sciences*, 374, pp.26–31

Hilhorst, S., and Lockey, A. (2019) Cancer costs. Demos/Pfizer UK Ltd. Available at: https://demos.co.uk/wp-content/uploads/2020/01/Cancer-Costs-FINAL-Jan-2020.pdf (Accessed 10th February 2020)

Hutchings, R., Carter, D., and Bennett, K. (2018) Dementia – the true cost. Fixing the care crisis. Alzheimer's Society. Available at: www.alzheimers.org.uk/sites/default/files/2018-05/Dementia%20the%20true%20cost%20-%20Alzheimers%20Society%20report.pdf (Accessed 4th January 2020)

James, I., Postma, K., and Mackenzie, L. (2004) 'Using an IPT conceptualisation to treat a depressed person with dementia', *Behavioural and Cognitive Psychotherapy*, 31(4), pp.451–456

Joplin, K. (2017) Promising approaches to living well with dementia. Age UK. Available at: https://bit.ly/36CTaKs (Accessed 1st December 2019)

Jorm, A.F., and Jolley, D. (1998) 'The incidence of dementia: a meta-analysis', *Neurology*, 51(3), 728–733

Joseph Rowntree Foundation (2012) Creating a dementia-friendly York. Available at: www.jrf.org.uk/report/creating-dementia-friendly-york (Accessed 10th May 2020)

Justin, B.N., Turek, M., and Hakim, A.M. (2013) 'Heart disease as a risk factor for dementia', *Clinical Epidemiology*, 5(1), pp.135–145

Kane, J.P.M., Surendranathan, A., Bentley, A., Barker, S.A.H., Taylor, J., Thomas, A.J., Allan, L.M., McNally, R.J., James, P.W., McKeith, I.G., Burn, D.J., and O'Brien, J.T. (2018) 'Clinical prevalence of Lewy body dementia', *Alzheimer's Research and Therapy*, 10(19) doi:10.1186/s13195-018-0350-6

Kitwood, T. (1993) 'Person and process in dementia', *International Journal of Geriatric Psychiatry*, 8(7), pp.541–545

Knapp, M., Park, A., and Burns, A. (2017) Medications for treating people with dementia: summary of evidence on cost-effectiveness. PSSRU, London School of Economics and Political Science. Available at: www.england.nhs.uk/wp-content/uploads/2018/01/dg-medications-for-treating-people-with-dementia.pdf (Accessed 20th March 2020)

Kuiper, J.S., Zuidersma, M., Oude Voshaar, R.C., Zuidema, S.U., van den Heuvel, E.R., Stolk, R.P., and Smidt, N. (2015) 'Social relationships and risk of dementia: a systematic review and meta-analysis of longitudinal cohort studies', *Ageing Research Reviews*, 22, pp.39–57

LaingBuisson (2019) *Care of older people UK market report*. 30th edn. London: LaingBuisson

Livingston, G., Huntley, J., Sommerlad, A., *et al.* (2020) 'Dementia prevention, intervention, and care: 2020 report of the Lancet Commission', *The Lancet*, 396(10248), pp.413–446
McDermott, O., Charlesworth, G., Hogervorst, E., Stoner, C., Moniz-Cook, E., Spector, A., Csipke, E., and Orrell, M. (2019) 'Psychosocial interventions for people with dementia: a synthesis of systematic reviews', *Aging and Mental Health*, 23(4), pp. 393–403
McKeith, I.G., Boeve, B.F., Dickson, D.W., *et al.*, (2017) 'Diagnosis and management of dementia with Lewy bodies: fourth consensus report of the DLB consortium', *Neurology*, 89(1), pp.88–100
National Collaborating Centre for Mental Health (2018) *The dementia care pathway. Full implementation guidance.* London: National Collaborating Centre for Mental Health
National Institute for Health and Care Excellence (2018) Dementia: assessment, management and support for people living with dementia and their carers. *Guideline [NG97]*. Available at: www.nice.org.uk/guidance/ng97/resources/dementia-assessment-management-and-support-for-people-living-with-dementia-and-their-carers-pdf-1837760199109 (Accessed 21st March 2020)
National Institute for Health and Care Excellence (2019) Dementia. Background information. Available at: https://cks.nice.org.uk/dementia#!background (Accessed 16th June 2020)
NHS Digital (2017) Personal social services survey of adult carers in England (SACE) 2016–17. Available at: https://files.digital.nhs.uk/publication/a/o/sace_report_2016-17.pdf (Accessed 23rd March 2020)
Office for National Statistics (2019) Deaths registered in England and Wales: 2018. Available at: www.ons.gov.uk/peoplepopulationandcommunity/birthsdeathsandmarriages/deaths/bulletins/deathsregistrationsummarytables/2018 (Accessed 16th June 2020)
Oliver, K. (2019) *Dear Alzheimer's: a diary of living with dementia.* London: Jessica Kingsley
Outeiro, T.F., Koss, D.J., Erskine, D., Walker, L., Kurzawa-Akanbi, M., Burn, D., Donaghy, P., Morris, C., Taylor, J., Thomas, A., Attems, J., and McKeith, I. (2019) 'Dementia with Lewy bodies: an update and outlook', *Molecular Neurodegeneration*, 14(5) doi:10.1186/s13024-019-0306-8
Parliamentary Office of Science and Technology (2018) Unpaid care. Available at: https://post.parliament.uk/research-briefings/post-pn-0582/ (Accessed 16th June 2020)
Peters, R., Booth, A., Rockwood, K., Peters, J., D'Este, C., and Anstey, K.J.(2019) 'Combining modifiable risk factors and risk of dementia: a systematic review and meta-analysis', *BMJ Open*, 9 doi: 10.1136/bmjopen-2018–022846
Peters, R., Ee, N., Peters, J., Booth, A., Mudway, I., and Anstey, K.J. (2019) 'Air pollution and dementia: a systematic review', *Journal of Alzheimer's Disease*, 70(s1), S145-S163 doi:10.3233/JAD-180631
Pham, T.M., Petersen, I., Walters, K., Raine, R., Manthorpe, J., Mukadam, N., and Cooper, C. (2018) 'Trends in dementia diagnosis rates in UK ethnic groups: analysis of UK primary care data', *Clinical Epidemiology*, 10, pp.949–960
Prince, M., Knapp, M., Guerchet, M., McCrone, P., Prina, M., Comas-Herrera, A., Wittenberg, R., Adelaja, B., Hu, B., King, D., Rehill, A., and Salimkumar, D. (2014) *Dementia UK. Second edition -overview. Alzheimer's Society.* Available at: http://eprints.lse.ac.uk/59437/1/Dementia_UK_Second_edition_-_Overview.pdf (Accessed 5th May 2020)
Prince, M., Wimo, A., Guerchet, M., Ali, G., Wu, Y., and Prina, M. (2015) World Alzheimer report 2015. The global impact of dementia. Alzheimer's disease international. Available at: www.alz.co.uk/research/WorldAlzheimerReport2015.pdf (Accessed 5th May 2020)
Public Health England (2019) Dementia: comorbidities in patients – data briefing. Available at: www.gov.uk/government/publications/dementia-comorbidities-in-patients/dementia-comorbidities-in-patients-data-briefing (Accessed 3rd March 2020)

Quinn, C. (2020) 'The best of today: accepting who I am', *Dementia Together Magazine*, December 2019 /January 2020. Available at: www.alzheimers.org.uk/dementia-together-magazine-dec-19jan-20/best-today-accepting-who-i-am (Accessed 15th June 2020)

Rafnsson, S.B., Orrell, M., d'Orsi, E., Hogervorst, E., and Steptoe, A. (2017) 'Loneliness, social integration, and incident dementia over 6 years: prospective findings from the English longitudinal study of ageing', *The Journals of Gerontology, Series B: Psychological Sciences and Social Sciences*, 75(1), pp.114–124

Richards, C. (ed) (2020) *Living well with dementia through music.* London: Jessica Kingsley

Rocca, W. (2017) 'Time, sex, gender, history, and dementia', *Alzheimer's Disease and Associated Disorders*, 31(1), pp.76–79

Royal College of Psychiatrists (2019) Memory problems and dementia. Available at: www.rcpsych.ac.uk/mental-health/problems-disorders/memory-problems-and-dementia (Accessed 2nd April 2020)

Särkämö, T. (2017) 'Music for the ageing brain: cognitive, emotional, social and neural benefits of musical leisure activities in stroke and dementia', *Dementia*, 17(6) doi.10.1177/1471301217729237

Savica, R., and Petersen, R. (2011) 'Prevention of dementia', *Psychiatric Clinics of North America*, 34(1), pp.127–145

Skingley, A., Billam, D., Clarke, D., Hodges, R., Jobson, I., Jobson, R., Moore, J., Vella-Burrows, T., Vickers, P., Walker, J., and West, H. (2020) 'Carers create: carer perspectives of a creative programme for people with dementia and their carers on the relationship within the (carer and cared-for) dyad', *Dementia*, June doi.10.1177/1471 301220933121

Snowdon, D. (1997) 'Aging and Alzheimer's disease: lessons from the Nun Study', *The Gerontologist*, 37(2), pp.150–156

Spector, A., Charlesworth, G., King, M., Sadek, S., Marston, L., Rehill, A., Hoe, J., Qazi, A., Knapp, M., and Orrell, M. (2019) 'Cognitive behavioural therapy (CBT) for anxiety in dementia: a pilot randomised controlled trial', *British Journal of Psychiatry*, 206(6), pp.509–516

Stern, Y. (2009) 'Cognitive reserve', *Neuropsychologia*, 47(10), pp.2015–2018

Sutin, A.R., Stephan, Y., Luchetti, M., and Teracciano, A. (2018) 'Loneliness and risk of dementia', *Journals of Gerontology: Series B: Psychological Sciences and Social Sciences*, doi:1093/geronb/gby112

Swaffer, K. (2016) *What the hell happened to my brain? Living beyond dementia.* London: Jessica Kingsley

Vella-Burrows, T. (2015) 'Prescription for music', in Franklin Gould, V. (ed) *Music reawakening. Musicianship and access for dementia. The way forward.* Arts 4 Dementia, pp.17–23. Available at: https://arts4dementia.org.uk/wp-content/uploads/2017/09/Music_Reawakening.pdf (Accessed 5th May 2020)

Vella-Burrows, T., and Wilson, L. (2016) *Remember to dance. Evaluating the impact of dance activities for people in different stages of dementia.* Canterbury: Canterbury Christ Church University

Vijayan, M., and Reddy, P.H. (2016) 'Stroke and vascular dementia and Alzheimer's disease – molecular links', *Journal of Alzheimer's Disease*, 54(2), pp.427–443

Wittenberg, R., Hu, B., Barraza-Araiza, L., and Rehill, A. (2019) *Projections of older people living with dementia and costs of dementia care in the United Kingdom, 2019–2040. CPEC working paper 5.* London School of Economics and Political Science. Available at: lse.ac.uk/cpec/assets/documents/Working-paper-5-Wittenberg-et-al-dementia.pdf (Accessed 19th December 2019)

Woods, B., Aguirre, E., Spector, A., and Orrell, M. (2012) 'Cognitive stimulation to improve cognitive functioning in people with dementia', *Cochrane Database of Systematic Reviews*, 2 doi:10.1002/14651858.CD005562.pub2

World Health Organization (2019a) *Dementia*. Available at: www.who.int/news-room/fact-sheets/detail/dementia (Accessed 21st March 2020)

World Health Organisation (2019b) *Risk reduction of cognitive decline and dementia: WHO guidelines*. Geneva: World Health Organisation

Xia, N. and Li, H. (2018) 'Loneliness, social isolation, and cardiovascular health', *Antioxidants and Redox Signalling*, 28(9), pp.837–851

Index

Note: Page numbers in *italics* indicate figures and in **bold** indicate tables on the corresponding pages.